T0195151

The Health Care Professional's Guide to Cultural Competence

SECOND EDITION

The Health Care Professional's Guide to Cultural Competence

Edited by

RANI H. SRIVASTAVA, RN, MScN, PhD, FCAN

Dean, School of Nursing, Thompson Rivers University
Adjunct Professor, School of Nursing, Dalhousie University
Adjunct Professor, Faculty of Health, York University

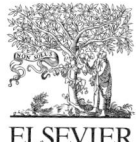

ELSEVIER

Managing Director, Global Content Partners: Kevonne Holloway
Senior Content Strategist (Acquisitions, Canada): Roberta A. Spinosa-Millman
Director, Content Development Manager: Laurie Gower
Content Development Specialist: Lenore Gray-Spence
Senior Copyeditor: Jerri Hurlbutt
Publishing Services Manager: Shereen Jameel
Senior Project Manager: Nadhiya Sekar
Design Direction: Margaret Reid

Printed in India

Last digit is the print number: 9 8 7 6 5 4 3 2 1

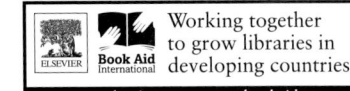
Working together to grow libraries in developing countries

www.elsevier.com • www.bookaid.org

Discovering the Difference

We go looking for culture and cultural meanings
Only to find issues of equity and power
Our hidden expressions and lack of compliance
Are really a reflection of limitations
Imposed on us by a system, a society
That says it values difference and diversity
But what it really wants is conformity
The issue is racism, the challenge discrimination
The patterns are lost in processes of racialization
Being an "other" is to be inferior
Why can't it be equal or even superior
I do what I do because of who I am
But also what you have made me to be
"Different" can be strong or it can be weak
The answer, the choice is ours to seek
It's only when we embrace the difference
And deal with forces that impose conformity
That we will discover cultures
And the true value of diversity

Rani Srivastava (2006)

CONTENTS

ABOUT THE AUTHOR

RANI HAJELA SRIVASTAVA, RN, MScN, PhD, FCAN

Dr. Rani Srivastava is currently the Dean of Nursing at Thompson Rivers University in Kamloops, British Columbia. She is a nurse leader with a track record for leading change through building relationships and translating vision into concrete strategies across stakeholder jurisdictions. She is recognized for her leadership in cultural competence, bridging academia and practice environments, and creating practice-based research roles. Her career has included senior leadership positions in professional practice and quality improvement.

Dr. Srivastava is passionate about patient- and family-centred care for culturally diverse and marginalized populations. In addition to being the author and editor for *The Health Care Professional's Guide to Cultural Competence* (first published in 2007), she has written several book chapters and articles on topics of cultural identity, religion, ethics, and family-centred care.

She regularly serves as a consultant, speaker, and workshop facilitator and has worked with hospitals, universities, and regulatory and professional associations in nursing to develop guidelines for developing and integrating culture into care. In 2017, for her leadership on cultural competence, diversity, and equity, Dr. Srivastava was named by the Canadian Nurses Association as one of the 150 nurses in Canada who are strong public advocates and leaders in advancing patient-centred care. In 2021, Dr. Srivastava was inducted into the Canadian Academy of Nursing. Becoming a Fellow of the Canadian Academy of Nursing (FCAN) represents the highest honour for Canada's most accomplished nursing leaders.

On a personal level, Dr. Srivastava identifies as a first-generation immigrant, racialized woman, and South Asian parent navigating the complexities of tradition, cultural evolution, discrimination, and growth opportunities. Her personal life and professional experiences have been the inspiration, catalyst, and motivator for her work on cultural competence, diversity, equity, and antiracism.

Dr. Srivastava received a Bachelor of Nursing with Honours from Dalhousie University; earned a Master of Science in Nursing; and a PhD from the University of Toronto. She also holds adjunct appointments at York University in Toronto, Ontario, and Dalhousie University in Halifax, Nova Scotia.

BRANKA AGIC, MD, PhD, is the Director of Knowledge Exchange and an Independent Scientist at the Centre for Addiction and Mental Health (CAMH). She is also an Assistant Professor in the Clinical Public Health Division and the Associate Director of the Master of Science in Community Health (MScHS) in the Addiction and Mental Health Program at the Dalla Lana School of Public Health, University of Toronto. Dr. Agic holds a PhD in Health and Behavioural Sciences and a Master of Health Science (MHSc) degree from the University of Toronto, along with a Medical Degree from the University of Sarajevo, Bosnia and Herzegovina. Dr. Agic has worked on key provincial and national initiatives focusing on immigrant and refugee populations, including the United Nations High Commissioner for Refugees (UNHCR) Global Strategy Beyond Detention – National Action Plan Canada; Immigration, Refugees and Citizenship Canada (IRCC)-funded Refugee Mental Health Project; Health Equity Impact Assessment (HEIA) Immigrant Populations Supplement; and many others. Her primary research resides in the area of mental health and substance use among immigrants, refugees, and ethnocultural and racialized groups, including factors affecting access, quality, and outcomes of care.

MICHELLE ANDERSON, BSc, MD, is a psychiatry resident at the University of Calgary and a graduate of the University of Alberta Doctor of Medicine program. She also holds a BSc in Biological Sciences and Psychology from the University of Alberta. Dr. Anderson has presented research on LGBTQ2 education both nationally and internationally and has participated in revising the LGBTQ2 curriculum at the University of Alberta's MD program.

R. LISA (MONA) BOURQUE BEARSKIN, RN, PhD, a tenured Associate Professor at Thompson Rivers University, is an inaugural Canadian Institutes of Health Research (CIHR) Chair holder in Indigenous Health Research for Nursing in British Columbia, and a Fellow of the Canadian Academy of Nursing (FCAN) and the American Academy of Nursing (FAAN). Her research contributes to supporting community knowledge as a generative process to advancing Indigenous health in nursing. Globally, Dr. Bourque Bearskin is recognized for her relational and rights- and strengths-based approach and as a leader in reconciling parallel pathways of traditional Indigenous health care in the context of community wellness. A former president of the Canadian Indigenous Nursing Association (CINA), she led organizational changes that focused on creating collaborative partnerships and mentorship of Indigenous nurses implementing cultural safety and security as key educational outcomes for improving nursing practice. She is a proud nehiyaw iskwew, a sur-thriver of the residential school and Sixties Scoop era, who maintains a solid connection to her community and cultural and ancestral roots.

JULIA CHRONOPOULOS, BSc, MD, CCFP, FCFP, is a family physician working at MacEwan University Health Centre in Edmonton, Alberta. There, she is the clinical lead for the Rainbow Health Centre, providing inclusive health care services for folks in the queer community and transition support for gender-diverse individuals. Dr. Chronopoulos is an Associate Clinical Professor at the University of Alberta, focusing on educating medical learners and professionals about providing inclusive medical care to sexually and gender-diverse people. It is her mission to see a world in which every door is the right door for all people seeking safe and supportive medical care.

LAURIE CLUNE, RN, BA, BScN, MEd, PhD, is an Associate Professor at the University of Regina, Faculty of Nursing. She has completed a post-doctoral fellowship at the Institute for Work and Health in Toronto. Dr. Clune came to Saskatchewan in 2013 to set up a Master of Nursing Nurse Practitioner Program in collaboration with University of Regina and Saskatchewan Polytechnique. Prior to moving west, Dr. Clune was a faculty member at Toronto Metropolitan University's Daphne Cockwell School of Nursing and an active member of the Registered Nurses Association of Ontario. Before moving to academia, Dr. Clune worked in a variety of tertiary and rural practice settings including pediatrics, neonatal, women's health, pain and regional anaesthesia management, women's health, palliative care, and community nursing. In these settings, she held the roles of staff nurse, patient care coordinator, nurse manager, clinical consultant, and clinical nurse specialist.

SALMA DEBS-IVALL, RN, BScN, MScN, is founder and president of Debs-Ivall Consulting, a management consulting firm in Ontario. She draws on her experiences as a nurse and leader in health care during a career that spans four decades. She also works as a diversity and inclusion consultant and had been involved on a panel of experts with the development of the Registered Nurses Association of Ontario's Healthy Workplace Environment Best Practice Guideline titled "Embracing Cultural Diversity: Developing Cultural Competence." Most recently, she facilitated the articulation of the Canadian Nurses Association's declarations regarding anti-Black and anti-Indigenous racism.

MELBA SHEILA D'SOUZA, RN, CMSN, PhD, MPhilN, MScN, BScN, is an Assistant Professor at Thompson Rivers University and a practising nurse at Abbotsford Regional Hospital and Cancer Centre. She is an ethnocultural, racialized person born, nurtured, raised, and having lived in the Kingdom of Bahrain, Sultanate of Oman, Thailand, and East India. She is committed to improving her professional practices in Canada. This land is a gathering place for nations of the Indigenous people whose histories, languages, and cultures continue to positively influence her journey to make sustainable efforts in advocacy and health care. Dr. D'Souza has been engaged in co-developing self-management and health promotion through patient engagement in care and with an equity-oriented lens. She has focused her initiatives of applying self-determination and meaningful experiences in nurturing, caring, and healing for patients and caregivers. She has harnessed vital partnerships and collaborations for promoting justice and sovereignty using an intersectionality and critical cultural analysis. Dr. D'Souza has maintained strong connections and fostered optimal professional relationships for co-creating a foundation in comprehensive cancer care.

ROBERT Jr. (R. J.) EDRALIN, RN, BScN, MN, is a clinical nurse specialist for the Medical Assistance in Dying (MAiD) program at the University Health Network in Toronto. As one of the first advanced practice nurses in Canada to pioneer a dedicated MAiD role, R. J. has acquired specialized knowledge in relevant legislation, process coordination, and interprofessional collaboration within this progressive field in end-of-life care. He has contributed to the advancement of nursing practice, interprofessional education, and operational service delivery of MAiD across several clinical settings in a large academic health organization, while sustaining safe, compassionate, and ethical care for culturally diverse patient populations. R. J. has held previous roles as a clinical coordinator, project manager, and emergency nurse. R. J. received his BScN and MScN from Toronto Metropolitan University, where he worked as a contract lecturer in their undergraduate and post-diploma nursing program.

NIKITA GUPTA, RN, BScN, is currently working toward her graduate education in nursing at Queen's University in Kingston, Ontario. Her clinical background entails working under step-down critical care and cardiac settings. She is involved in teaching in the undergraduate program. This is her first publication, and she hopes to dive further into research after her graduate studies.

BARBARA-ANN HAMILTON-HINCH, BSc, BEd, MA, PhD, is from the historical African Nova Scotian communities of Beechville and Cherry Brook. Dr. Hamilton-Hinch is an Associate Professor with the Faculty of Health in the School of Health and Human Performance and the Assistant Vice-Provost, Equity and Inclusion, at Dalhousie University, Halifax, Nova Scotia. Her work examines the impact of structural, systemic, and institutional racism on diverse populations, particularly people of African descent. Her research examines the "opportunity gap" for African Nova Scotians in the public school system and addresses supporting the reintegration of individuals and their families involved in the justice system; creating a sense of belonging for students of African descent in medicine and dentistry and with the Faculty of Health; and optimizing services for communities that have been marginalized. Dr. Hamilton-Hinch has published in areas of education and higher education, recreation and leisure, mental health, public health, racism and health, and nutrition. At Dalhousie University, Dr. Hamilton-Hinch is the co-team lead for the Health of People of African Descent Research Cluster with Healthy Populations Institute; one of the founders of Imhotep Legacy Academy (ILA, a program that is developed to increase the number of students of African descent in science, technology, engineering, and math); and co-chair of Promoting Leadership in Health for African Nova Scotians (PLANS, a program to increase the number of African Nova Scotian students in health). Dr. Hamilton-Hinch has been a lifelong advocate, researcher, trainer, and teacher for equity and inclusion to ensure health and well-being for individuals and groups who have been marginalized.

PHILLIP HAU, Registered Psychologist, BA, MC, is a clinical psychologist in private practice in Edmonton, Alberta. He works with patients from all walks of life, with specialization in trauma work and LGBTQ2 patients. He holds a BA from the University of Alberta, with a double major in psychology and sociology, and an MC from Athabasca University, majoring in counselling psychology. His academic research has focused on topics related to promoting the emotional and mental health of post-secondary students through fostering resiliency, connectedness among peers, and multicultural impacts. He has presented his research at regional, provincial, and national as well as international conferences. His longstanding interests include identity development, post-traumatic growth, mental health, minority stress, and resiliency development.

EMMA HILLIER, BASc, is a medical student at the University of Alberta in Edmonton. Previously she completed a Bachelor's degree at McGill University in Psychology and International Development. Beyond health care she dedicates her time to research and volunteer experience that focuses on Indigenous, low-socioeconomic status, and LGBTQ2 communities. She has been involved with the Edmonton Men's Health Collective and the Indigenous Medical and Dental Students Association, among others, and is currently a council member on the Nîsohkamâkewin Council with the Edmonton Police Service. She approaches all her work with an intersectional lens and seeks to determine how health care can be best administered in a culturally safe and respectful manner.

SONYA L. JAKUBEC, RN, PhD, is a professor with the Faculty of Health and Community Studies at Mount Royal University, Calgary, Alberta. Her area of practice and research is community mental health across the lifespan, with a focus on social interventions and health promotion. Her clinical practice has involved rural and northern community mental health in Canada and West Africa, teaching and training for preservice and inservice, refugee care, crisis, and emergency mental health, as well as teaching and research. Dr. Jakubec has a 30-year background in community mental health nursing, with practice, leadership, and research in rural and remote and global health contexts. Her research concentrates on health promotion across the lifespan, including palliative and grief care, with a particular interest in health and environment connections. Dr. Jakubec has researched and published in the areas of community mental health services; older persons and community health; mental health and sexual assault/intimate partner violence in rural communities; and community recreation (including outdoor nature interventions and community gardening) and social inclusion in mental health promotion.

KARIMA KARMALI, RN, BScN, MBA, has over 25 years of leadership experience in nursing and health care and is currently the Director of the Centre for Innovation & Excellence in Child- and Family-Centred Care at The Hospital for Sick Children (SickKids®) in Toronto. In this role, she provides strategic and operational leadership in the design and delivery of pediatric health care that is patient and family centred. She champions and leads strategic initiatives aimed at improving patient experience and health equity. Karima has published and speaks regularly at national and international conferences on these topics. She is a strong proponent of volunteerism and gives of her time both locally and internationally. She is the Vice-President of the Board of Ronald McDonald House Charities Canada and recently completed a 4-year term as the Vice-President of the Aga Khan Council for Canada. Karima obtained her BScN from McGill University and MBA from Queens University.

ANDREA KENNEDY, RN, PhD, is a nurse, an educator, and a researcher dedicated to Indigenous health and education equity. She holds a deep respect for her diverse relations, including Italian, Celtic, and Métis ancestry and traditionally adopted Tsuut'ina and hānai Hawaiian families. Dr. Kennedy teaches undergraduate nursing at Mount Royal University with a decolonizing approach that honours the wisdom of Elders as valued knowledge holders. Dr. Kennedy is engaged in scholarly work on advancing reconciliation and equity in higher education and health care through social innovation, mentorship, and relational learning with communities.

JULIE LEISING, BSCH, MD, is completing her psychiatry residency at the University of British Columbia at the time of this publication, after earning her MD at the University of Toronto. In her research and practice, Dr. Leising is interested in critically examining systemic barriers to culturally competent care and advocating for change at both the individual and systemic levels. Her research has been published in the *Journal of Clinical Psychopharmacology*.

PAIGE LESLIE, RM, BHSc, is a graduate from the McMaster Midwifery Education program and currently works as a Registered Midwife in southern Ontario. She has extensive experience working with vulnerable populations and providing culturally competent care. She has a keen interest in fostering success for Black, Indigenous, and People of Colour (BIPOC) midwifery students and at the time of press was working with the Clinical Skills for Midwifery Practice course at McMaster University in addition to being in clinical practice.

STEPHEN G. LINCOLN, MA, CPhil, is currently a Patient Engagement Facilitator with the Patient and Family Experience Team at the Centre for Addiction and Mental Health (CAMH). He has also previously served as the Client Relations Officer and Coordinator of Risk Management. He is a trained sociologist and criminologist with an extensive background in teaching and social research at the University of California, San Diego (UCSD), as well as numerous other nongovernmental and governmental institutions in the United States and Canada. His research and publications have included work on such diverse phenomena as sexuality and sexual health; mental health and mental illness; stigma and discrimination; law enforcement; and substance use and misuse. His interests include more precise efforts to understand the situational motivations behind crime, delinquency, and deviance with a particular focus on the emotional and other experiential aspects of these behaviours. He is the recipient of the Paul J. Saltman Distinguished Teaching Award (UCSD), the Faculty Excellence in Teaching Award (UCSD), and Congressional Teaching Citations from both the United States Senate and House of Representatives.

NANCY MacVICAR, RN, MScN, is a consultant at the Nova Scotia Department of Health and Wellness. She has over 15 years of experience working in diverse areas of public health in both Ontario and Nova Scotia, such as the COVID-19 response, health protection, health promotion, and healthy development. Her thesis from the University of Ottawa (2006) was "Exploring the Role and Turnover among Heart Health Coordinators in the Ontario Heart Health Program: A Qualitative Study." Nancy's clinical background includes working with children and their families, as well as teaching mental health at the University of New Brunswick.

ALEXANDRA MARSHALL, BEd, has been teaching for over 14 years in a wide range of contexts. She has an education degree from the University of Alberta and a passion for advocacy. She is the rural education coordinator at the Institute for Sexual Minority Studies and Services (ISMSS) at the University of Alberta.

JANET MAWHINNEY, BA, MA, is currently the Director of Community Engagement at the Centre for Addiction and Mental Health (CAMH). She has held leadership roles in equity and human rights at the CAMH and completed a 10-year partnership on equity capacity building with the Factor-Inwentash Faculty of Social Work, University of Toronto. Her work includes consulting with numerous social service and health care organizations on education and equity change strategies.

CATHARINE (KATIE) McCANN, BSc, MD, is a resident physician in obstetrics and gynaecology at the University of British Columbia. She holds a BSc from McGill University and an MD from the University of Toronto. She will be pursing further fellowship training in maternal fetal medicine at the University of Manitoba at the completion of her residency.

ANN POTTINGER, RN, MN, has extensive experience in providing nursing care, in both hospital and community settings, to diverse patients and families who have experienced mental illnesses and addictions. She has focused on care approaches that honour the values and preferences of diverse individuals and groups. Ann has held clinical and leadership positions at the Centre for Addiction and Mental Health (CAMH), including Staff Nurse, Advanced Practice Nurse, Director of Quality, Patient Safety, and Risk, and Clinical Director. As an educator, Ann has co-designed mental health, cultural competence, and health equity curricula that she has delivered to interprofessional health care providers. Ann is currently an Assistant Professor in the School of Nursing, Faculty of Health, York University, where she is a course director for the undergraduate mental health nursing course and the coordinator for the International Educated Nurse (IEN) Post-Registered Nurse Program.

MONAKSHI SAWHNEY, NP(Adult), PhD, has worked in hospital-based pain services since 1995 at a variety of hospitals in Toronto, and in Kingston, Ontario. Her research interest is in pain management following surgery. Dr. Sawhney currently works as an Associate Professor at the School of Nursing at Queen's University and has a clinical practice in the chronic pain clinic at Hotel Dieu Hospital in Kingston.

ORIANA SHAW, HBSc, is in the Doctor of Medicine (MD) program at the University of Alberta (anticipated completion in 2022) in a stream that includes additional training in social justice and community service. In 2017, she completed BSc(Hons) at the University of Toronto with a specialization in neuroscience and minors in psychology and physiology. She has held several positions related to education and science communication and had volunteer roles working with a variety of populations, including people who have experienced sexual abuse and other forms of trauma, people with disabilities, and Indigenous youth. She has conducted research at the University of Toronto and University of Alberta, with studies ranging from cellular research to clinical trials and focus groups. She has co-authored several publications and presented work at local and international conferences.

LINDA PURUSHUTTAM, RPN, BSc, earned her degree from the University of Toronto. Linda's interests are in health equity, clinical research, patient-centred care, and pharmacological and complementary therapies. She has held various roles in health care and industry. She was the Manager of Clinical Research in the Radiation Medicine Program at the Princess Margaret Hospital; Clinical Manager at the Toronto Institute of Pharmaceutical Technology (TIPT); and Manager of Clinical Operations at Alpha Medical Research and Pharma Medica Research Inc. Linda also worked for the Centre for Addiction and Mental Health (CAMH) as a Project Manager and Manager of Operations and Special Projects in the Professional Practice Office. Linda is an instructor in the Personal Support Worker program at the Toronto Institute of Pharmaceutical Technology and is pursuing her BScN degree.

KAREN SAPPLETON, MSED, MSW, RSW, is the Senior Manager for Child & Family-Centred Care, Health Equity, & Interpreter Services in the Centre for Innovation and Excellence in Child & Family-Centred Care at the Hospital for Sick Children (SickKids®) in Toronto, Ontario. Prior to joining SickKids, Karen was an educator in New York City, specializing in learning disabilities and special education for students from kindergarten to grade 12. She has held multiple roles in the hospital in her 16 years at SickKids, including clinical social worker, clinical research project manager, interprofessional education specialist, and transition specialist. Currently, Karen is the Manager of the Office of the Patient and Family Experience, the Family Centre, Interpreter Services Department, Toronto District School Board (TDSB) schooling program, and the partnership with Ronald McDonald House Family Room. She is also the staff co-chair of the hospital Family Centred Care Advisory Council. These programs aim to provide equitable access, enhance communication, elevate patient and family engagement, and ensure delivery of services that promote positive, inclusive experiences for this very diverse patients and families. Karen has spent over 30 years of her life learning, unlearning, and teaching others about antibias, antiracist, and anti-oppressive practices. Karen is a member of the Ontario Council on Community Interpreting Advisory Board, and she has been actively engaged in promoting the profession of medical interpreters as an integral member of the health care team.

Heather Bensler, RN, MSN
Instructor, Faculty of Nursing
Director of Indigenous Initiatives
University of Calgary
Calgary, Alberta

Laura Bulmer, RN, BScN, MEd
Professor, Sally Horsfall Eaton School of Nursing
George Brown College
Toronto, Ontario

Elizabeth Burgess-Pinto, BScN, RN, MH, PhD, IBCLC
Assistant Professor, Faculty of Nursing
MacEwan University
Edmonton, Alberta

Steve Cairns, BScN, BEd, MEd, PhD (c)
Assistant Professor, RPN to BScN Blended
    Learning Program, School of Nursing
Nipissing University
North Bay, Ontario

Lisa Doucet, RN, BTHM, MN
Adjunct Assistant Professor, School of Nursing
Dalhousie University
Yarmouth, Nova Scotia

Lisa-Marie Forcier, RN, BSc, BScN (Hons), MN
Professor, Bridging to University Nursing
    Program
School of Community and Health Studies
Centennial College
Toronto, Ontario

Caroline Foster-Boucher, BScN, RN, MN
Assistant Professor, Faculty of Nursing
MacEwan University
Edmonton, Alberta

Bonnie Fournier, RN, BScN, MSc, PhD
Adjunct Professor, School of Nursing
Thompson Rivers University
Kamloops, British Columbia

Crystal Garvey, RN, BScN, MScN, PhD (c)
Professor, Collaborative BScN Program
Durham College/Ontario Tech University
Oshawa, Ontario

Manon Lemonde, RN, PhD
Associate Professor, Faculty of Health Sciences
Ontario Tech University
Oshawa, Ontario

Eric MacMullin, RN, MSN
Professor, Bridging to University Nursing
    Program
School of Community and Health Studies
Centennial College
Toronto, Ontario

Elaine Mordoch, RN, BN, MN, PHD
Associate Professor, College of Nursing
Rady Faculty of Health Sciences
University of Manitoba
Winnipeg, Manitoba

Cindy Kuster Orban, RN, BScN, MN
Instructor, Faculty of Nursing
University of Regina
Regina, Saskatchewan

Em M. Pijl-Zieber, BScN, MEd, PhD, RN
Assistant Professor, Faculty of Health Sciences
University of Lethbridge
Lethbridge, Alberta

Bukola Salami, RN, MN, PhD
Associate Professor, Faculty of Nursing
University of Alberta
Edmonton, Alberta

Gisèle Thibodeau, BScN, RN
Faculty, Practical Nursing Program, School of
    Health and Human Services
Nova Scotia Community College
Yarmouth, Nova Scotia

Barbara Thompson, RN, BScN, MScN
Professor of Nursing, Health Programs
Sault College
Sault Ste. Marie, Ontario

Jacqueline Williamson, RN, BScN, MEd, PhD
Professor, Practical Nursing Program
School of Health and Community Services
Durham College
Oshawa, Ontario

PREFACE

It is hard to believe that 15 years have passed since the first edition. The response from students, faculty, and community organizations has been humbling, heartwarming, and beyond my wildest expectations! I am grateful to many individuals who have adopted, applauded, adapted, debated, and challenged my thinking over the past 15 years—I have learned much from all these conversations and feedback. This new Second Edition is a reflection of that learning and is offered with my gratitude.

While much has changed in the last 15 years, much remains the same. This Second Edition offers expanded content in depth and in breadth. The words of the poem *Discovering the Difference* still ring true. Over the years the lines *"I do what I do because of who I am, But also what you have made me to be"* have become more prominent in understanding culture and cultural competence. While the previous edition clearly recognized the impact of dynamics of difference, this edition explicitly describes culture as patterns and culture as power. There is greater discussion of privilege, colonialism, intersectionality, equity, and the impact of social determinants including racism and marginalization on health across the chapters. As well, there are new chapters on Indigenous health, gender and sexual diversity, and community health.

This edition reflects significant diversity in contributing authors with respect to geography, cultural identity, professional discipline, and perspectives as students, educators, clinicians, and policy leaders (please see contributor biographies). The diverse voices and experiences are evident in the varied writing styles across the chapters. The diversity of voices is important and has greatly enriched the discourse. I am confident that readers will benefit from the diverse voices and the insights that come with the blending of personal and professional experiences. I am grateful to all the authors who have shared their time and expertise so generously, while navigating a global pandemic with unprecedented demands on health care providers and society.

The Second Edition is yet another a milestone in a journey that began nearly 40 years ago, when I first became a nurse. Full of enthusiasm and committed to providing the best possible care, I recognized that patients reflected a range of ethnocultural, religious, and social backgrounds and felt unprepared to provide care for all the different cultures I would encounter. Globalization and increasing diversity, along with evidence of health inequities, continue to make the need to integrate culture into care an urgent priority. A recognition of the importance of the influence of culture in safe and effective care was, and continues to be, the driving force behind this work.

The year 2020 has become a defining period in history with the outbreak of a global pandemic that further highlighted inequities in all aspects of society; social movements that highlight racism, discrimination, and inequities across a number of populations; and perhaps most importantly, a shift in societal response from denial and minimization toward recognition, acceptance, reconciliation, and a commitment to do better. Perhaps this will be the turning point in history when meaningful change and transformation occur and the goals of cultural safety, cultural competence, and health equity are no longer elusive.

This book is written mainly for students in the health disciplines and for health care providers who wish to develop a deeper understanding of cultural competence in clinical care. Health is defined broadly and includes many social services that aim to address inequities and foster well-being of individuals, families, and communities. It is also designed for educators who desire to integrate the issues of culture and diversity into their health care curricula.

The term *cultural competence* can mean different things to different people. A variety of theoretical perspectives underlie discussions about cultural diversity, and all of them need to be understood for their strengths as well as their limitations. This book presents an integrated approach to cultural competence, highlighting critiques as well as strengths of various approaches, while acknowledging that our understanding of equity pedagogy and cultural competence in health care continues to evolve. It is my sincere belief that the goal of equity and culturally appropriate care is what matters most. I humbly encourage the reader to go beyond terminology and focus on core concepts, inclusive processes, and integrative health care options that will drive care toward the desired outcomes. Language matters, and language is limiting.

Format and Style

The Health Care Professional's Guide to Cultural Competence is divided into three sections: the first looks at the fundamentals of clinical cultural competence, the second at cultural knowledge of processes and populations that is needed across clinical settings, and the third section looks at cultural competence in working with specific clinical populations. The three sections all reflect an application of both the fundamentals of clinical cultural competence and generic cultural knowledge. Where any overlap occurs in the chapters as a result, it is meant to illustrate how similar issues assume different guises among different populations. The style of this book reflects an attempt to integrate theory into practice—using learning tools labelled "Cultural Considerations in Care" and "Cultural Competence in Action." The purpose of these tools and exercises is to invite reflection. The end-of-chapter activities are a way of testing and consolidating learning. Developing cultural competence means developing new eyes, new ears, and new ways of thinking.[1] Readers are invited to use their new eyes, ears, and ways of thinking to challenge their own assumptions and to explore alternative meanings and opportunities within everyday occurrences. Exploring reasons behind responses will strengthen insight into various dimensions of our own cultural identity. Pay attention to the emotions that may be invoked. Learning happens by engagement. Challenge the ideas in the book with what you see and experience in practice.

Providing culturally responsive care to individual patients, families, and communities requires knowledgeable health care providers as well as responsive organizations that support this practice. This book, however, largely focuses on the individual level and the practitioner, reflecting a belief that individual health care providers are at the heart of health care. Knowledgeable, committed health care providers are providing, and will continue to provide, leadership for wider system-level change. Policymakers need to be influenced. Health care providers are encouraged to challenge and develop their own practices and be a catalyst for broader team and system-level change.

Organization

The three sections of this book break down as follows:

Section I, *Foundation Stones*, provides an overview of culture as a determinant of health; associated concepts and terminology; and approaches of cultural safety, cultural competence, and patient-centred care. Addressed are common myths, misconceptions, and evolving perspectives on multiculturalism, diversity and equity, and key events with respect to Indigenous experiences of colonization that shape contemporary discourse and practice. Varied perspectives on diversity are presented that provide a frame of understanding for what we are attempting to do, where we may get stuck, and how we can move forward. Also in this section is an introduction to the Culture Care Framework, an approach to integrating culture into health care. The framework

---

[1] My thanks to Felix Munger and Diversity Level II: Clinical Cultural Competence Education Team at the Centre for Addiction and Mental Health, Toronto, for this metaphor.

describes the elements of cultural sensitivity, cultural knowledge, and cultural resources along with a recognition of the dynamics of difference that are inherent across the elements. This section ends with a discussion on strategies to navigate difference at the individual, team, and organizational levels with implications for allyship and policy development.

Section II, *Universally Applicable Cultural Knowledge*, examines the foundational knowledge that is relevant across cultural groups and clinical populations. Cross-cultural communication, caring for diverse families, and fundamental understanding of what health and illness can mean across populations are all important to cultural competence. The section also includes chapters on Indigenous people, immigrants and refugees, and people from the sexual and gender minorities communities. While these can be regarded as distinct populations, health providers will work with patients and families from these groups across the entire health care system. There is also considerable diversity within each group, and thus recognizing the potential unique needs, challenges, and strengths of the individuals we care for is critical.

Section III, *Specific Cultural Considerations*, presents a discussion of cultural considerations in a few specific clinical populations. The chapters in this section are the work of individuals with expertise in and passion for specialized areas of practice, and each chapter reflects the individual authors' experiences as it highlights issues that are significant for the clinical population and associated care processes. The intent is to illustrate how basic understanding of culture and diversity needs to be combined with foundational cultural knowledge for examination of issues and approaches involving specific groups. Readers are invited to consider what this process could or would be like for the population(s) with whom they may be working.

Scope

Like any book, this one is limited in its scope. Culture is a broad term, and during the course of a professional career, we can expect to encounter many cultural groups—some that are readily visible and others that are invisible on the surface. Readers are invited to develop their understanding of culture and reflect on its application to cultures that are not addressed explicitly in this book. The principles are the same—the approaches may be different. Readers will approach this book with varying levels of familiarity and perspectives on culture and diversity. Developing a common ground for the dialogue means that, at times, information may seem too basic for some; the aim is not to insult any reader's intelligence, only to make explicit what may be obvious to some and difficult to see for others.

Assumptions and Bias of the Editor and the Contributors

There are different ways of knowing, and although all of the authors have drawn on literature that is theoretical or research based or represents expert opinion, we have also drawn on our own lived experiences as practitioners and as cultural beings. In my (the editor's) case, the experience is that of nurse in a multicultural society working in pediatric critical care, with adults with chronic illness, as an educator, administrator, and a health care executive. My perspective also reflects experiences of a bicultural youth developing my own identity in a Eurocentric multicultural society, an immigrant woman of colour, and a racialized immigrant parent. Many of the examples used in the text are from the authors' experiences and practice. Where specific cultural groups are referenced, the intention is neither to stereotype nor to limit the example to that group only; a specific cultural group is used as a reference point and an illustration for the issue. It is the issue that needs to be understood in the context of culture. Readers are invited to use the examples as triggers for discussions that raise their own individual and collective awareness—not about just what is there but also about how it could be shaped differently in a different context.

A Note on Terminology

Last, a note on terminology. Communication is not just about what is intended or said but also what is perceived or heard. Both the content and the words in the text are obviously reflective of the author's perspective. Language evolves over time and is contextual in its interpretation. The "correct" language changes and evolves. Over the years, the term *ethnocultural communities* has been replaced by *ethnoracial, racialized communities,* and, finally, by *marginalized, underserved,* and *equity priority* groups; *Aboriginal population* has been replaced by *Indigenous people* in some contexts. There are also inconsistencies in how the terms are understood. For example, "multicultural health" can be understood superficially with respect to beliefs and rituals, or as a more complex concept that encompasses individual- and system-level factors. Wherever possible, the terms have been defined (see Glossary); any readers who feel that there are glaring omissions or that terminology falls short are urged to forward their feedback.

The authors and contributors of the text recognize and acknowledge the diverse histories of the First peoples of the lands now referred to as Canada. It is recognized that individual communities identify themselves in various ways; within this text, the term *Indigenous* is used to refer to all First Nations, Inuit, and Métis people within Canada unless there are research findings that are presented uniquely to a population.

In the text, gender-neutral language is used to be respectful of and consistent with the values of equality recognized in the *Canadian Charter of Rights and Freedoms*. Using gender-neutral language is professionally responsible and mandated by the Canadian Federal Plan for Gender Equality. Knowledge and language concerning sex, gender, and identity are fluid and continually evolving. The language and terminology presented in this text endeavour to be inclusive of all peoples and reflect what is, to the best of our knowledge, current at the time of publication.

Evolve for The Health Care Professional's Guide to Cultural Competence

Located at https://evolve.elsevier.com/Srivastava/culturalcompetence/, the Evolve website for this textbook includes the following materials for instructors and students:

For Instructors

    PowerPoint Slides
    Image Library
    Answers to Case Studies

For Students

    Review Questions
    Case Studies for Clinical Reasoning and Clinical Judgement
    Answers to In-Text Review Questions
    Glossary
    Online Resources

ACKNOWLEDGEMENTS

Many people have contributed to this book and worked to make the second edition a reality. I have been humbled by notes of thanks and requests from students, peers, and colleagues to update the content so they can continue to use this as a tool and resource in their classrooms and clinical settings. I thank you for your encouragement and support—this edition is for you!!

The biggest debt of gratitude goes to my family—Rajiv, Ratika, Raman, and Reji—for their ongoing questions, encouragement, and loving critique (thank you, Raman beta) and believing in me when I am not so certain. You have been my support, my motivation, and my inspiration, without which this book would not have been possible. To my family and friends, thank you for always being there for the conversations, stories, and just listening to my thinking. I am grateful to my parents and am sorry that my father is not alive to see this milestone, yet his love and faith in me have been a constant companion for this work.

A very special gratitude is extended to Dr. Madeline Leininger, a mentor whom I was also privileged to call friend, for the foundation on which this work is built, and for her blessing and support for the first edition. Thank you to the many colleagues and students across the health disciplines, whose stories, comments, questions, ideas, and challenges shaped the ideas.

My deepest appreciation to all the staff at Elsevier Canada. I would especially like to thank Roberta Spinosa-Millman (Senior Content Strategist) for making the second edition a possibility and Lenore Gray-Spence (Content Development Specialist) for her constant support, suggestions, and stickhandling the logistics to make this a reality. Thanks also to Nadhiya Sekar (Senior Project Manager) and Jerri Hurlbutt (copyeditor).

The book would be incomplete without the valuable work of the contributors, and the same is true for the reviewers, whose thoughtful questions, suggestions, and words of encouragement were invaluable. I am grateful for your feedback and for your belief in the value of this work—thank you, merci, shukriya, dhanyavaad, gracias, meegwetch, kia-ora, and kukwstsétsemc.

Rani Srivastava
Kamloops, British Columbia

Foundation Stones

Rani H. Srivastava

Section Outline

1. Cultural Competence in Health Care: Overview of Issues
2. Myths, Misconceptions, and Evolving Perspectives
3. The Culture Care Framework
4. Navigating Difference

This opening section focuses on issues that help us understand and develop the set of behaviours, attitudes, and policies known as cultural competence. Each chapter builds on the previous one(s) to lay the foundation for understanding and navigating differences and cultural complexities in care.

Chapter 1 examines the need for cultural competence and the meaning of the term. The chapter begins with a brief discussion of the impact of culture on health along with the historical issues and demographics that make this a critical imperative. Culture as a determinant of health is examined through the concept of health equity and explicating the difference between equity and equality. We discuss the evolution of the concepts of cultural safety and cultural competence along with their limitations. The elusive concept of culture is defined and described in terms of patterns as well as power. Key concepts such as diversity, equity, racism, intersectionality, marginalization, and unconscious bias are also explored. We look at the various degrees of cultural competence (or lack of it), as well as the interdependence among the individual, organizational, and system levels of cultural competence. The chapter ends with a brief discussion on differentiating cultural safety and cultural competence from patient-centred care.

Chapter 2 examines the evolution of thought and knowledge concerning culture and diversity. The chapter begins with a discussion of some common myths and misconceptions about culture. We explore the developing social and academic perspectives on culture and diversity through a discussion of the evolution of multiculturalism in Canada, along with a parallel history of relevant legislation affecting the health and well-being of Indigenous people. These evolving perspectives allow for deeper understanding of the complexity and paradoxes associated with the intersection of cultural, racial, and social issues and their impact on health.

Chapter 3 presents the Culture Care Framework as a practical approach to understanding cultural issues and blending cultural knowledge into health care. The framework evolved from practice and experience and has been used in practice settings to make culture visible. The Culture Care Framework provides health care providers an approach to understanding and working with cultural complexities and influences on health and health care. Building on the foundational understanding of "culture" in earlier chapters, Chapter 3 provides an overview of the framework with respect to its three core elements of cultural sensitivity, cultural knowledge, and cultural resources. For too long, understanding cultural issues has generally meant learning about the "other" without examining our own impact on any cultural interaction. Cultural sensitivity focuses on respect, humility, awareness, and understanding. Self-awareness is not only about our own values, biases, and responses to difference, but also how we might be perceived by others. Cultural knowledge includes knowledge of other cultures and knowledge of legacies, structures, and systems that continue to perpetuate health inequities. Cultural resources need to be developed at the individual as well as the organizational level through critical appraisal of information and collaborative connections.

Chapter 4 completes the discussion of the Culture Care Framework and focuses on navigating difference at the individual, team, and organizational level. Understanding cultural issues is an initial step, but cultural competence requires application of that understanding. We explore barriers such as privilege and unconscious bias at the individual and organizational level and discuss strategies to make the unconscious visible and engage in allyship and advocacy. Navigating difference in practice builds on and integrates clinical, leadership, and practice skills and requires intentional leveraging of resources within the personal, professional, organizational, and social domains. The chapter ends with a discussion of key dimensions that require attention at the organizational level to achieve the goal of culturally congruent, equitable care for all.

CHAPTER 1

Cultural Competence in Health Care: Overview of Issues

Rani H. Srivastava

At the end of this chapter, the learner will be able to:

- Recognize the need for cultural competence in health care
- Describe the cultural diversity that exists in Canadian society
- Describe culture as a determinant of health
- Define the terms *culture, cultural competence, cultural safety, cultural imposition, diversity, ethnicity, ethnocentrism, health equity,* and *worldview*
- Identify the similarities and differences between cultural competence, cultural safety, and patient-centred care[1]
- Discuss the interdependence between the micro, meso, and macro levels of cultural competence

Biomedical	Cultural racism	Marginalization
BIPOC (Black, Indigenous, People of Colour)	Cultural safety	Microaggressions
	Culture	Minority
Cultural bias	Discrimination	Prejudice
Cultural blindness	Diversity	Race
Cultural competence	Ethnicity	Racism
Cultural competence continuum	Ethnocentrism	Stereotype
	Everyday racism	Structural racism
Cultural destructiveness	Health equity	Systemic racism
Cultural humility	Health inequality	Unconscious bias
Cultural imposition	Health inequity	Visible minorities
Cultural incapacity	Implicit bias	Western culture
Cultural pre-competence	Institutional racism	Worldview
Cultural proficiency	Intersectionality	

---

[1] We acknowledge that while some may have a preference, in this text *patient-centred care* is used interchangeably with *client-centred care.*

Canada is a settler nation and prides itself on being an ethnocultural mosaic nation that values and celebrates diversity. Every aspect of society, including health care, is culturally diverse. Culture, health, and illness are inextricably linked, and culture is recognized as a determinant of health (Government of Canada, 2020). However, our track record of caring for patients from a variety of cultures has been inconsistent at best, leading to poor quality of care and poor health outcomes for many individuals, groups, and communities. The need for cultural competence in health care has been articulated globally and across a variety of health disciplines, including nursing, medicine, social work, dietetics, and pharmacy (Alizadeh & Chavan, 2016; Azzopardi & McNeill, 2016; Cai, 2016; Danso, 2018; Jongen et al., 2018; Kurtz et al., 2018; McCabe et al., 2020; Okoro et al., 2015; Olaussen & Renzaho, 2016; Shepherd et al., 2019; Tehee et al., 2020; Watt et al., 2016; Yoshikawa et al., 2020).

Indigenous people are the original inhabitants of Canada. They had well-established social, political, economic, and cultural systems long before the European settlers arrived on this land. However, with White settlement and colonization, much of their traditions and culture was lost or altered in ways that had, and continue to have, significant negative consequences for individuals and communities in all aspects of life, including health and well-being (Allan & Smylie, 2015; National Collaborating Centre for Determinants of Health, 2017; Truth and Reconciliation Commission [TRC], 2015b).

The study of cultural issues has a long history in the field of anthropology. In the early 1970s, Madeleine Leininger, an anthropologist and nurse theorist, and Arthur Kleinman, a psychiatrist and medical anthropologist, identified the need to integrate aspects of anthropology into health care. Leininger (1991) proposed the Theory of Culture Care Diversity and Universality and launched the field of transcultural nursing. Leininger's theory is further discussed in Chapters 3 and 4.

Kleinman et al. (1978) highlighted the limitations of the **biomedical** model of traditional Western clinical practice (which is based on the biological and physiological sciences), making a case for applying social science to medical practice, and argued for the need to focus on the illness experience of the patient. Since then, much has been written about the need for recognizing and addressing the importance of cultural issues in health care across a variety of health disciplines. In recent years there has been an increasing call for recognition and reconciliation for the impact of colonization on the health and well-being of Indigenous people (TRC, 2015a). There has been a resurgence of seeking, acknowledging, and promoting Indigenous health through traditional teachings and ways of being.

The purpose of this chapter is to provide an overview of the issues related to the need for cultural competence in health care. The chapter begins with a brief discussion of the impact of culture on health and health care, as well as the historical and current issues and demographics that are making this a critical imperative. Culture as a determinant of health is examined through the concept of health equity and explicating the difference between equity and equality. The chapter explores key concepts that need to be understood along with terms such as *diversity, equity, racism, intersectionality, marginalization,* and *unconscious bias.* Terminology in this field is continuously evolving, with new terms and new interpretations emerging. We encourage the reader not to focus excessively on terminology, but rather to understand the essence of the concept while at the same time probing how it might be used differently over time and context. We explore the origin and approach of frameworks such as cultural safety and cultural competence, as well as their limitations and critiques. Cultural competence is discussed with respect to the micro, meso, and macro levels and as a continuum ranging from cultural destructiveness to cultural proficiency. The chapter ends with a brief discussion on differentiating cultural safety and cultural competence from person-centred care. Subsequent chapters present more in-depth discussions on many of the issues introduced in this chapter.

Impact of Culture on Health

Culture and health are inextricably linked. Culture influences health and illness behaviour, including how illness is perceived and experienced, what symptoms are reported, what remedies are sought, and who is consulted in the process. However, the health systems in Canada are largely built on a Western biomedical model of health beliefs and health care delivery (including who is regarded as a legitimate provider of health care services); hence, it is often challenging for health care providers to understand and accommodate all ethnocultural health beliefs and expectations.

The culture clash between the Canadian health care system—with its roots in **Western culture**[2]—and the individual patient's values and beliefs, along with a failure on the part of the health care provider to recognize diverse ways of expressing distress, can lead to miscommunication, misdiagnosis, and inappropriate care (National Collaborating Centre for Determinants of Health, 2017; Public Health Agency of Canada, 2018). For example, not recognizing that some Eastern cultures present psychological distress through physical symptoms can lead to an overtreatment of physical symptoms and a failure to recognize the root cause. At the same time, the way health and illness are viewed in different cultures can pose a challenge to the biomedical model and the Western health care system. In many cultures, illness and recovery are seen as signs from God, the universe, or some other power, and are often reflective of past good or bad deeds, and healing involves natural and spiritual connections as well as the use of plants and minerals. Consequently, health care organizations struggle to provide culturally appropriate care to diverse communities, while communities struggle with issues related to access and ability to receive culturally appropriate health care (Khanalou et al., 2017; Shepherd et al., 2019; Turpel-Lafond, 2020; Yoshikawa et al., 2020).

The health care system's initial approach to understanding culturally diverse communities was to focus on learning about the cultural stranger, the "other," whose ways were different from what was regarded as the mainstream norm. Cultural issues were perceived as a "problematic difference" (misconceptions and unusual beliefs or practices), often viewed as an impediment to a shared understanding and regarded as belonging exclusively to patients. Cultural concerns were then objectified, and health care providers could distance themselves from the need to address cultural issues. Addressing cultural diversity in the health care system was perceived as a nice thing to do, but nonessential. The unstated assumption was that the problem was with the patient, and the values, assumptions, and approaches inherent in the system and within the providers were not questioned or challenged. These assumptions are indicative of both ethnocentrism and cultural bias. **Ethnocentrism** refers to the belief that one's own cultural values, beliefs, and behaviours are the best, preferred, and most superior ones. **Cultural bias**, a closely related concept, refers to the view that the values and beliefs of a particular culture must guide the situation or decisions (Leininger, 1995). To some extent, we are all ethnocentric and biased toward our own culture. We prefer our own way of doing things, believing that to be the best way; however, problems arise when ethnocentrism and bias are so strong that we are unable to consider alternative viewpoints and these views are imposed on others. The latter is considered **cultural imposition**.

Over the years, there has been increasing recognition that the culture of the health care provider and the health care system matters as much as that of the patient. In 2003, a landmark report entitled *Unequal Treatment* was published by the Institute of Medicine (IOM) that identified differences in health outcomes, based on race and ethnicity, across geographic and clinical populations documented in the literature. The IOM report (2003) went on to identify three possible sets of factors that contributed to these differences: (1) patient preference (what people consider good care); (2) health care

---

[2]The term *Western culture* is used to describe values and social norms associated with European culture and Christian religion, where modern technologies, efficiency, and scientific approaches are emphasized and seen as progressive.

system structures, policies, and regulatory context (i.e., where and how care is provided); and (3) bias, prejudice, and stereotypes on the part of well-intentioned and competent health care providers. While the IOM report was US based, it had been extremely influential in amplifying a discourse across the United States, Canada, and internationally that had been previously based on anecdotal and less robust evidence. It became clear that when it comes to health quality and outcomes, culture matters, and the culture of the health care system and the health care provider matters as much as the culture of the patient and community it serves (Srivastava & Srivastava, 2019). Cultural differences must consider the personal and professional background of the health care provider, as well as the social context of practice (Yoshikawa et al., 2020). Cultural challenges arise from differences between the patient's and the health care provider's values, beliefs, and expectations regarding health, illness, and treatment. The cultural attitudes of the health care providers and health care system affect diagnosis, treatment, and organization of services, including the hours and types of services offered, all of which have a noticeable impact on access to and quality and effectiveness of health care services.

Cultural Considerations In Care

How Do You Treat a Cold?

If you get cold, what do you do?
a) Do nothing—it will get better on its own.
b) Eat hot chicken soup.
c) Drink ginger tea.
d) Get medications, vitamins, and supplements to shorten the duration.
e) Get fresh air and exercise.
    How did you arrive at your preferred method—was it something you experienced in your childhood? Has it changed over the years? What happens if your preferred options are not available to you when needed?

Although the need for culturally appropriate health care has long been recognized in Canada, this need has become increasingly urgent for multiple reasons, including:

- The changing demographics of the country, with respect to patients as well as the health care workforce, means that diversity is more visible and more frequently encountered.
- An increasing amount of literature documents persistent and, in many cases, widening gaps in health outcomes for various cultural groups (e.g., Ramraj et al., 2016; Veenstra & Patterson, 2016; Veenstra et al., 2020).
- The Truth and Reconciliation Commission (TRC) recommendations call for increased cultural competency education for all health professionals that reflects respect, understanding, and integration of Indigenous healing practices and abilities to effectively address human rights, cultural conflicts, and racism (TRC, 2015a).
- There is increasing recognition of anti-Black and anti-Indigenous racism, along with understanding of the impact of racism on health, and the social movement Black Lives Matter (BLM) has emerged in response to police brutality and racially motivated violence against Black people (Maynard, 2017; Potvin, 2020; Turpel-Lafond, 2020; Williams et al. 2019).

Thus the need to address culture in health care has shifted away from being a supplementary consideration to an urgent and necessary one.

Changing Demographics

Canadian society, by virtue of its First Peoples and immigration heritage, has been described as a kaleidoscope of cultures, languages, and nationalities. Canada is one of the most multicultural countries in the world, accepting 341 180 permanent residents in 2019 from many different countries (Immigration, Refugees and Citizenship Canada, 2020). At the start of this century, statistics indicated that nearly 20% of the population in Canada was foreign-born; in 2016, the percentage was similar, at 21.9% (Statistics Canada, 2017d). The 2016 census data identified over 250 groups with respect to ethnic ancestry (Statistics Canada, 2017b), clearly validating Canada's identity as a multicultural society.

Although immigration has always been a part of Canada's heritage, the immigration patterns have shifted in the past few decades. Before 1961, 90% of the immigrants to Canada came from Europe and only 3% were born in Asia. In 2016, these numbers changed dramatically, where less than 12% of recent immigrants came from Europe and nearly 62% came from Asia and the Middle East (Statistics Canada, 2017d). There is now a greater proportion of recent immigrants from Africa compared with newcomers from Europe (Statistics Canada, 2017d). In 2019, the top five source countries of immigrants were India, China, the Philippines, Nigeria, and Pakistan (Immigration, Refugees and Citizenship Canada, 2020). The shifting immigration and settlement patterns translate into considerable variation in diversity across the nation. In some areas, such as Regina, Saskatchewan, residents are largely descended from the first wave of European settlers, whereas in Richmond, British Columbia, **visible minorities**,[3] primarily Chinese, South Asians, and Filipinos, account for more than 75% of the total population (Statistics Canada, 2017c). The new arrivals also add to the growing differences between urban and rural Canada, as approximately 91% of immigrants settle in metropolitan areas (Statistics Canada, 2017d: Table 1). Tables 1.1 and 1.2 show the percentage and distribution of some visible-minority groups across Canada.

According to the 2016 census, Indigenous people (including First Nations, Métis, and Inuk [Inuit]) accounted for 4.9% of Canadians (Statistics Canada, 2017a). The population of approximately 1.7 million is increasing and is relatively young compared with the non-Indigenous population (Statistics Canada, 2017a). At least 70 Indigenous languages are spoken in Canada; however, the percentage of Indigenous people with knowledge of these languages has decreased since 2006 (Statistics Canada, 2017a, 2019a).

Canada's Black population is also increasing and doubled to almost 1.2 million in the 20 years prior to the 2016 census, now representing 3.5% of the total population of Canada (Statistics Canada, 2019b). Approximately 44% of this population was born in Canada, and about 9% have multigenerational status (Statistics Canada, 2019b). Since 2001, most of the Black population has originated from African countries (e.g., Nigeria, Ethiopia, and Somalia), whereas before 1991, a higher proportion of immigrants came from the Caribbean and Bermuda regions, although Jamaica and Haiti remained the top source countries in 2016 (Statistics Canada, 2019b).

In addition to race and ethnicity, diversity also exists based on gender identification, sexual orientation, disability, social class, religion, and many other variables. Cultural clashes and racialization are not limited to individuals from foreign lands; they can occur across a wide number of communities perceived as minorities. During the COVID-19 pandemic, there has been a reported exacerbation of the impact of inequities on minority populations (Statistics Canada, 2020).

Culture as a Determinant of Health

Culture is acknowledged as a key determinant of health (Public Health Agency of Canada, 2018). It can also mediate the impact of other social factors, such as perceptions of social status, ability to secure stable employment and housing, family roles and obligations, and historical legacies of discrimination, disadvantage, and trauma (Kirmayer & Jarvis, 2019). The Indigenous health

---

[3]*Visible minority* is a Statistics Canada term that refers to people who are not White, with the exclusion of Indigenous people (Statistics Canada [2017e]. *Visible minority* and *population group reference guide: Census population, 2016*. Statistics Canada Catalogue no. 98-500-X2016006.)

TABLE 1.1 ■ Percentage of Visible Minorities Relative to Total Population (2016)

Province/Territory	% Visible Minorities
Newfoundland, Labrador	2.3
Prince Edward Island	4.8
Nova Scotia	6.5
New Brunswick	3.4
Quebec	13
Ontario	29.3
Manitoba	17.5
Saskatchewan	10.8
Alberta	23.5
British Columbia	30.3
Yukon	8.5
Northwest Territories	9.6
Nunavut	2.5

Statistics Canada. (2016). *Immigration and ethnocultural diversity highlight tables: Visible minority, 2016 census data.* https://www12.statcan.gc.ca/census-recensement/2016/dp-pd/hlt-fst/imm/Table.cfm?Lang=E&T=41&Geo=00&SP=1&vismin=2&age=1&sex=1.

TABLE 1.2 ■ Visible Minority Groups Ranked as Percentage of Total Population (2016)

Visible Minority Group	Highest %	Second Highest %	Third Highest %
Chinese	11.2% – BC	5.7% – Ontario	4% – Alberta
South Asian	8.7% – Ontario	8% – BC	5.8% – Alberta
Filipino	6.4% – Manitoba	4.2% – Alberta	3.4% – Yukon
Black	4.7% – Ontario	4% – Quebec	3.3% – Alberta
Arab	2.7% – Quebec	1.6% – Ontario	1.4% – Alberta
Latin American	1.7% – Quebec	1.5% – Ontario	1.4% – Alberta

Statistics Canada. (2016). *Immigration and ethnocultural diversity highlight tables: Visible minority, 2016 census data.* https://www12.statcan.gc.ca/census-recensement/2016/dp-pd/hlt-fst/imm/Table.cfm?Lang=E&T=41&Geo=00&SP=1&vismin=2&age=1&sex=1.

perspective recognizes interconnections among the physical, social, environmental, and spiritual dimensions and notes the influence of culture on all aspects of health and well-being. Three levels of social determinants are recognized: (1) proximal determinants, which have a direct impact on health (e.g., health behaviours); (2) intermediate determinants, which are the origins of the proximal determinants (e.g., community infrastructure, kinship networks, ceremonies, and knowledge sharing); and (3) distal or structural determinants, which represent the political, economic, and social contexts, including colonialism, racism, Indigenous worldviews, and self-determination (Public Health Agency of Canada, 2018).

Language barriers pose a major threat to patient safety and quality of care (Alimezelli et al., 2015; Gil et al., 2016; Minnican & O'Toole, 2020; Yoshikawa et al., 2020). Canada is a bilingual country with two official languages, French and English. According to the 2016 statistics, 22.8% of the population reported French as their first official language. The majority of Francophones (approximately 85%) live in the province of Quebec, and the province of New Brunswick is the only officially bilingual province (Heritage, 2019). Despite being an official language, French language health care services are limited outside of these two provinces, and Francophone people, who are an official language minority, experience challenges to quality care and increased risk of adverse events due to linguistic and cultural barriers (de Moissac & Bowen, 2018).

The resettlement process for immigrants and refugees presents inherent challenges as these individuals experience difficulties in employment, housing, and access to social support. Individuals may also face health risks because of marginalization and lack of access to culturally appropriate diet, activity, and health care services. Disruptions in traditional lifestyles and discrimination can lead to greater social exclusion and increased risk for substance use; lack of culturally appropriate services can result in delayed help seeking; and concerns about symptoms being minimized or ignored may lead to a lack of follow through with prescribed treatments (McKenzie et al., 2016). It must be emphasized that although culture is regarded as a determinant of health, it should not be confused with being the *cause* of illness or health inequities; rather, the inequities are rooted in the social and structural factors that can and must be addressed. Culture is often a positive mediator that is "… significantly and positively associated with physical health, social and emotional wellbeing, and reduces risk-taking behaviours" (Bourke et al., 2018, p. 11), and challenges arise when culture is ignored.

Health Equity

Increasing recognition of issues such as health inequity has made the need for cultural competence more compelling. It is important to distinguish between health inequality and health inequity. **Health inequality** refers to differences in health status between different groups. These differences can be attributed to many factors, including biological factors, individual choices, and chance. However, there is clear evidence that differences can also be attributed to "the unequal distribution of the social and economic factors that influence health" such as income, education, employment, and social conditions that are largely beyond individual control and are recognized as unfair or unjust (Public Health Agency of Canada, 2018, p. 14). **Health inequity** refers to this subset of factors that are deemed to be "unfair or unjust." **Health equity** refers to the "absence of unfair and avoidable or remediable differences in health among population groups defined socially, economically, demographically or geographically" (Public Health Agency of Canada, 2018, p. 14). Health equity creates equal opportunities for good health for everyone by (1) decreasing the negative effect of the social determinants of health and (2) improving services to enhance access and reduce exclusion.

Health equity can occur when all health disparities have been addressed and removed (Fiscella & Sanders, 2016). Fournier and Karachiwalla (2020) identify how key determinants of health affect health and equity. For example, the lack of suitable housing and income can lead to unsafe exposure to environmental contaminants and increased stress. Experiences of racism and discrimination can result in lack of access to proper health services and feelings of exclusion and further marginalization. While it is recognized that elimination of disparities requires systemic solutions, such as expanded health insurance coverage, and multilevel strategies that engage patients, communities, health providers, and health organizations (Fiscella & Sanders, 2016), health care providers must also recognize the individual effects of inequity and understand how providers can make a difference through actions that promote engagement, empowerment, and advocacy. The Health Equity Impact Assessment tool (HEIA) is an excellent resource that can be used by health care planners and leaders to support decision making and be vigilant to recognizing unintended consequences of decisions regarding health services (Ontario Ministry of Health and Long-Term Care, 2019). Health care providers can promote health equity by recognizing cultural needs and strengths, understanding vulnerability, removing unnecessary barriers in care, and supporting informed choices.

In Canada, it is apparent that racialized individuals, Indigenous people, gender and sexual minority people, immigrants, and people living with disabilities experience health inequities (Public Health Agency of Canada, 2018). Racism and discrimination against Black Canadians have been linked to higher rates of diabetes and hypertension (Veenstra & Patterson, 2016). Poor socioeconomic conditions and the legacy of colonization have led to high rates of diabetes, cardiovascular disease, and tuberculosis (Greenwood et al., 2018; Public Health Agency of Canada, 2018; Ramraj et al., 2016). A recent study relating to COVID-19 infections in Canada indicates that visible minorities are disproportionately affected because of their lower socioeconomic status and greater risk of exposure to the virus (Subedi et al., 2020).

Over the past two decades it has been shown that immigrant populations are healthier on arrival than people born in Canada. Known as the "healthy immigrant effect," this advantage is largely attributed to the selection process associated with immigration. However, it is also clear that the healthy immigrant effect does not last, and immigrant health begins to deteriorate over a period of 10 years, particularly for immigrants from non-European countries. The reasons for deterioration of the healthy immigrant effect are not well understood but are thought to be related to acculturation, including potential changes in diet and lifestyle, as well as interaction of social factors such as under-employment, unemployment, racism, discrimination, and lack of culturally responsive health services (Fung & Guzder, 2018; McKenzie et al., 2016; Vang et al., 2017).

Exploring Cultural Concepts in Health Care

One of the greatest difficulties associated with developing cultural competence in health care has been a lack of clarity regarding the meaning of the terms *culture* and *cultural competence*, as well as related terms such as *diversity, minority, ethnicity,* and *race*. Some discussions about culture use the terms *culture, race,* and *ethnicity* interchangeably, while others argue for greater specificity and advocate using terms such as *ethnocultural* and *ethnoracial*. The terms *diversity* and *minority* also are being used with increasing frequency as alternative concepts that transcend culture, race, and ethnicity. In order to develop an understanding of a concept, we have to understand both the definition of the term and its contextual meaning. Cultural competence requires a basic understanding of core concepts such as culture, race, ethnicity, diversity, marginalization, and minority. Each of these concepts is examined briefly in the discussion that follows. The intent is to present the meaning of the terms so that readers can compare and challenge their own assumptions and interpretations and, at the same time, recognize when meanings are similar or different.

Cultural Competence In Action

What's Your Take on These Terms?

What comes to mind when you hear the following terms: *race, ethnicity, diversity,* and *culture*? Note the descriptors you think of as well as your feelings or emotions. What were some of the feelings: fear, confusion, frustration, anger, challenge, or excitement? Are there terms that you are more comfortable with or prefer? What are they? Are there any related terms that you prefer and, if so, what are they?

The first step toward developing cultural competence is to increase your own awareness of what the various terms mean and the emotions they generate. As you compare your answers with those of a colleague, note the similarities and differences in your perspectives. What life experiences might have shaped your perspectives?

RACE

The term **race** "refers to a group of people who share the same physical characteristics such as skin tone, hair texture and facial features" (Turpel-Lafond, 2020, p. 8). However, it is important to recognize that the physical attributes are often linked to social behaviour and status, largely based on assumptions and stereotypes. Thus in contemporary discourse, the concept of race is recognized as a "socially constructed way to categorize people and is used as the basis for discrimination by situating human beings within a hierarchy of social value" (Turpel-Lafond, 2020, p. 8). In the past, health care literature referenced the biological basis of race; this is being increasingly challenged and the language is now shifting to ancestry (Reich, 2018). Children of mixed-race couples can have varying degrees of skin pigmentation and shared physical characteristics, yet they share similarity in genetic makeup and social culture. Where race is used as an identifying variable, it is important to be cautious and explore the meaning and intention behind the term to determine its utility and appropriateness.

RACISM

The term *racism* has come to mean many different things. Essentially, racism occurs when preconceived, adverse judgement or opinion (prejudice) is formed on the basis of characteristics such as skin colour, facial features, or ethnicity. **Racism** can be defined as an organized social system in which the dominant group uses its power and privilege to devalue, disempower, and differentially allocate social resources and opportunities across racial or ethnic groups, leading to a lack of opportunities and resources to those deemed to be inferior and less deserving (Paradies et al., 2015; Williams et al., 2019).

Racism can take many forms. It is both an attitude and a behaviour resulting from that attitude. While individual-level racism can be seen in the actions and attitudes of individuals, **institutional racism** (also known as **systemic racism**) is less visible and manifests itself in organizational policies and practices, and **structural racism** refers to broader factors in society and the "discrimination through mutually reinforcing systems [such as] housing, education, employment … [and] health care" that lead to inequitable distribution of resources and outcomes (Bailey et al., 2017, p. 1453). Structural racism privileges "whiteness," is insidious, and persists even if there is no intent or individual(s) that explicitly express these views (Bailey et al., 2017; Hardeman et al., 2016; Williams et al., 2019).

Cultural racism manifests as implicit or unconscious bias (Williams et al., 2019) and forms the basis of both individual-level and institutional racism. **Cultural racism** asserts the inferiority of nondominant cultures through policies and practices or stereotypical negative representations of values, language, imagery, symbols, and worldviews. Through conscious and unconscious bias, discrimination is then normalized (Williams et al., 2019). Cultural racism can also lead to internalized racism or self-stereotyping, where "some members of stigmatized racial populations respond to the pervasive negative racial stereotypes in the culture by accepting them to be true" (Williams et al., 2019, p. 111). Members of minority groups may be encouraged to turn their backs on their own cultures and to become absorbed by the majority culture.

Unlike overt forms of racism that are easier to recognize, systemic racism is harder to address as it is reproduced largely through routine and taken-for-granted practices in everyday life. **Everyday racism**, a concept introduced by Essed (2000), highlights the everyday injustices that are reflected in unconscious assumptions (such as believing that groups are lazy, promiscuous, or lack ambition) and practices that systematically exclude individuals from particular events or opportunities. The persistent injustices can be difficult to pinpoint and are thus hard to address, but the persistent nature of such events can have a negative impact on mental and physical health (Bourabain & Verhaeghe, 2021). Acts of everyday racism are also described as **microaggressions**, Microaggressions which are everyday interactions that communicate a negative bias toward a marginalized group. While on the surface these interactions are usually not a "big deal" (hence the term "*micro*") and are therefore difficult to challenge without the person being labelled as being oversensitive, they are nonetheless demeaning and exclusionary (Hook et al., 2016). Microaggressions can also be described as "subtle acts of exclusion" (Jana & Baran, 2020) or casual racism (Australian Human Rights Commission, 2014). Microaggressions can be organized into three categories: microassaults, microinsults, and microinvalidations. *Microassaults* are intentional overt actions such as telling a racist joke and claiming it's only a joke. *Microinsults* are more subtle and refer to actions that are disparaging and insulting—comments such as "You speak good English" or "Your people must be so proud of your success as a xxx." *Microinvalidations* are actions that are exclusionary or dismissive; examples include questions such as "Where are you really from?" that imply a challenge to belonging, statements that imply a racialized person is being oversensitive to racist comment, or countering Black Lives Matter discussion with "all lives matter," thereby negating or dismissing the experiences of Black people (Ehie et al., 2021; Hopper, 2019).

Reviews of research into the effects of racism on identity, health, and well-being indicate that perceived racism jeopardizes the health of those who experience it. Racism is linked to poor mental and physical health (Paradies et al., 2015). Multiple exposures to racial discrimination can significantly affect mental health and have a long-lasting effect (Wallace et al., 2016). Microaggressions can have a cumulative impact on individuals and have been associated with decreased mental health outcomes, including suicide ideation, compromised therapeutic alliance with counsellors, and decreased intention to seek care (Hollingsworth et al., 2017; Hook et al., 2016). Racism is also recognized to be "inextricably intertwined" with colonization (Allan & Smylie, 2015, p. 5), and the health and well-being of Indigenous people continue to be greatly compromised due to negative racial assumptions and stereotypes (Leyland et al., 2016).

STEREOTYPE, PREJUDICE, AND DISCRIMINATION

Stereotype, prejudice, and discrimination are related terms that lead to exclusion and inequities. A **stereotype** is "a preconceived generalization of a group of people. This generalization ascribes the same characteristic(s) to all members of the group, regardless of their individual differences" (Canadian Race Relations Foundation, 2019). **Prejudice** is a belief, feeling, or attitude, usually negative and lacking in legitimacy, toward another person or persons (Canadian Race Relations Foundation, 2019). **Discrimination** refers to actions or behaviours, based on stereotypes and prejudices, that reflect unequal, unfair access and unequal, unfair treatment of people and that lead to inequitable outcomes (Canadian Race Relations Foundation, 2019). The relationship between the three concepts is depicted in Fig. 1.1.

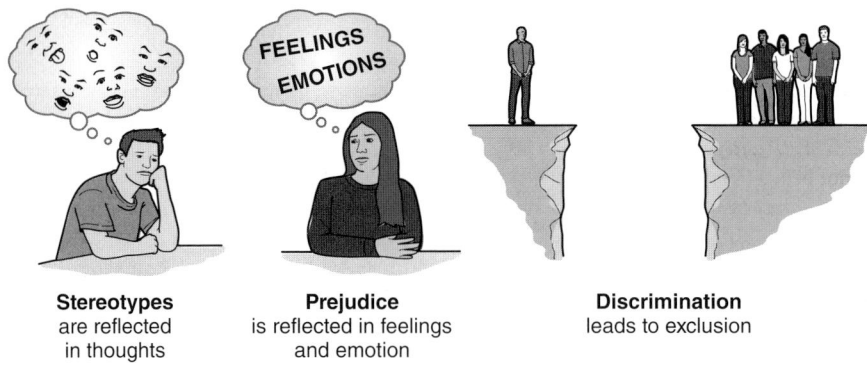

Stereotypes
are reflected
in thoughts

Prejudice
is reflected in feelings
and emotion

Discrimination
leads to exclusion

Fig. 1.1 Relationship Between Stereotype, Prejudice, and Discrimination.

MARGINALIZATION

To marginalize people is to confine them to an outer limit or edge (the margins), thus questioning their right to belong and be full participants. **Marginalization** is an exclusionary social process that refers to "the experience of persons outside the dominant group who face barriers to full and equal participating members of society. It also refers to the process of being 'left out' of or silenced in a social group" (Canadian Race Relations Foundation, 2019). Marginalization is often a result of unconscious bias. **Unconscious** or **implicit bias** "describes associations or attitudes that reflexively alter our perceptions, thereby affecting behavior, interactions, and decision making" (Marcelin et al., 2019, S62). In other words, the bias is not intentional; however, altered perceptions impact actions and decisions. Research from neuroscience has shown that implicit attitudes are formed through early development, and implicit bias "appears to be the result of being raised in a culture of subtle racism" (Stevens & Abernethy, 2018, p. 563). Even when there is a recognition of racial bias and explicit racism is controlled, unconscious and implicit bias can remain. A review of literature on implicit bias in health care across the United States found that most health care providers have "implicit biases against Black, Hispanic, American-Indian and dark-skinned individuals" (Maina et al., 2018, p. 224). There is no reason to believe that Canada is much different. In addition to race, unconscious bias also exists among other identity characteristics such as gender, sexual orientation, and religion.

Implicit bias leads to marginalization and subtle acts of exclusion; marginalization, in turn, leads to a continuation of social and structural inequities with harmful health effects (Browne et al., 2016). In Canada, references to marginalized groups include members of visible-minority communities, immigrants, refugees, Indigenous people, homeless people, sexual minorities, and persons with physical or mental disabilities. Marginalized groups also are referred to as "vulnerable populations" as they are more likely to be exposed to or unprotected from health-damaging environments and are less likely to receive appropriate care. Browne et al. (2016) note that when it comes to Indigenous people, "marginalization is entrenched in the history of relations between Indigenous people and the nation-state, resulting in a disproportionate burden of ill health and social suffering within Indigenous populations" (p. 14).

MINORITY

Within the health care context, **minority** group status is associated with marginalized status, meaning that such groups have limited access to opportunity, power, and resources, including health care services. Minority group status, then, is not simply referring to a population that is numerically small; rather, it can also refer to populations that are disadvantaged, underprivileged, discriminated against, exploited, or disempowered in the governing structures of the dominant society because of lack of access to power or ability to influence the outcome(s) (Canadian Race Relations Foundation, 2019). Even in instances where the actual number of individuals with minority group status reaches 50% or more of the population, such as the visible-minority population in large Canadian cities such as Toronto, they are still likely to experience systemic inequities within the dominant social systems. The term *racialized* is often preferred because a racialized community in a particular area may not be a numerical "minority"; it also recognizes that barriers faced by people are reflective of historical social prejudice and not individual or group inadequacies (McKenzie et al., 2016).

The term **BIPOC (Black, Indigenous, People of Colour)** also gained popularity in 2020. Seen as an umbrella term to refer to people who experience skin colour racism, the term is inadequate in the representation of other racialized groups (e.g., gender and sexual-minority people). Although the term aspires to be inclusive, the term *people of colour* is controversial, and grouping disparate groups under one umbrella makes the individual experiences invisible, further exacerbating the challenge of making racism visible.

ETHNICITY

Although some use the term *ethnicity* interchangeably with *race*, **ethnicity** is a broader term and refers to the "multiplicity of beliefs, behaviours and traditions held in common by a group of people bound by particular linguistic, historical, geographical, religious and/or racial homogeneity" (Canadian Race Relations Foundation, 2019). The characteristics can include ancestry, language, kinship, family rituals, food preferences, clothing, and particular celebrations.

INTERSECTIONALITY

Intersectionality is an approach or framework for understanding how multiple social identities such as race, gender, sexual orientation, and disability interact with each other and influence individual experience. It is important to understand that each identity may reflect different levels of power, privilege, and oppression (i.e., racism, sexism, heterosexism, classism) at the macro social structural level (Overstreet et al., 2020). The multiple social identities cannot be simply added to one another; rather, they interact with each other to create something new with respect to exclusion and disadvantage (Henry et al., 2017). For example, consider the social inequality between men and women; now also consider what additional disadvantages a woman who is Black, Indigenous, or Asian might face. Although there are only two variables—race and gender—the combination can drastically change one's experience of discrimination, power, and inclusion (see Wilson et al., 2016 for further discussion).

DIVERSITY

Diversity is a broad term related to culture. The term can simply refer to differences or variations across individuals and social groups. However, in a social context, diversity does not simply refer to difference but rather implies difference from the majority, which is assumed to be the norm. In this context, diverse groups and communities refer to a marginalized status within society, and diversity initiatives become almost synonymous with freedom from discrimination, protecting human rights, social justice, and health equity (Beagan, 2015). As a term, *diversity* gained popularity in the cultural discourse as an expansion to the multicultural discourse that narrowly aligned culture with ethnicity; thus diversity came to be regarded as a broader, post-multicultural term that recognizes intersectionality and the complexity of diversity in Canada (Fleras, 2019).

A broad view of diversity can be problematic. One challenge involved with associating all marginalized groups under the diversity umbrella is that the actual diversity within diverse groups can easily be overlooked. For example, the terms *visible minority* or *people of colour* collapse a broad, heterogeneous group of people who are not White into a single category, thus masking ethnic differences. While diverse communities may be similar in that they share a marginalized status, they continue to differ in terms of history, traditions, beliefs, and values. In other words, each community has its own culture, and it is equally important to understand the similarities as well as differences across the communities. The term *diversity* therefore cannot serve as a substitute for the term *culture*. In any reference to diverse groups, it is important to be explicit about the context and note which differences we are referring to and why and how these differences matter.

CULTURE

Culture is a difficult concept to define. It is complex, elusive, and at times paradoxical. Definitions of culture generally refer to values, norms, and traditions that are shared, to varying

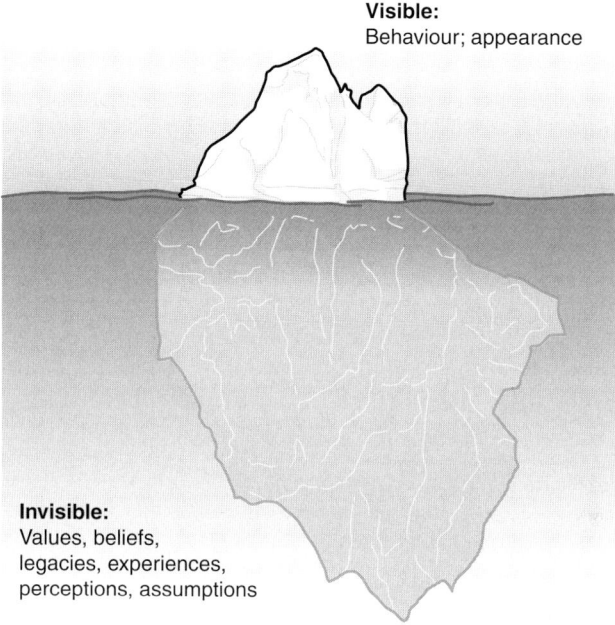

Visible:
Behaviour; appearance

Invisible:
Values, beliefs,
legacies, experiences,
perceptions, assumptions

Fig. 1.2   The Iceberg Analogy of Culture.

degrees, among a group of people and are used to guide behaviours in everyday life (Cai, 2016; Sharifi et al., 2019). While some definitions equate culture solely with ethnicity, race, religion, or country of origin, this is a narrow view that is problematic as it can reinforce a static view of culture and fails to recognize the diversity that exists within groups (Srivastava & Srivastava, 2019). It is important to recognize that culture is dynamic and includes broader social identities such as socioeconomic status, gender, sexual orientation, citizenship, and age (Blanchet Garneau & Pepin, 2015; Cai, 2016; Srivastava & Srivastava, 2019).

Culture is said to constitute several layers. The shallow first layer reflects behaviour and represents the explicit culture. It is what is seen and interpreted by others. The second layer, deeper and more implicit, is that of values, and the core of culture is formed by basic assumptions that often are hidden, even from those who belong to the cultural group. Two common analogies can be used to convey the complexities of culture (Figs. 1.2 and 1.3). Fig. 1.2 uses the visual of an iceberg to explain the concept of culture and highlights three key points: (1) the aspects of culture that we see, such as behaviours and appearance, are only a small portion of what actually exists; (2) what we see is influenced by what is not readily visible (i.e., values and beliefs drive behaviour); and (3) to understand culture we have to go deeper and seek out what is not readily visible. When cultural conflict or synergy occurs, it is due to the aspects of culture that are not readily visible.

Fig. 1.3 describes culture using the analogy of fish in water. The key points associated with this analogy are (1) the fish, as a cultural being, is immersed in water, yet the fish does not see the water (culture is often invisible to those who are in it); (2) water is necessary for the fish to survive—being a "fish out of water" leads to feeling uncomfortable and unsafe and ultimately can lead to death. Similarly, connection to culture and cultural identity is seen as a necessity for wellness and growth, while a loss of culture and cultural identity can lead to irreparable harm.

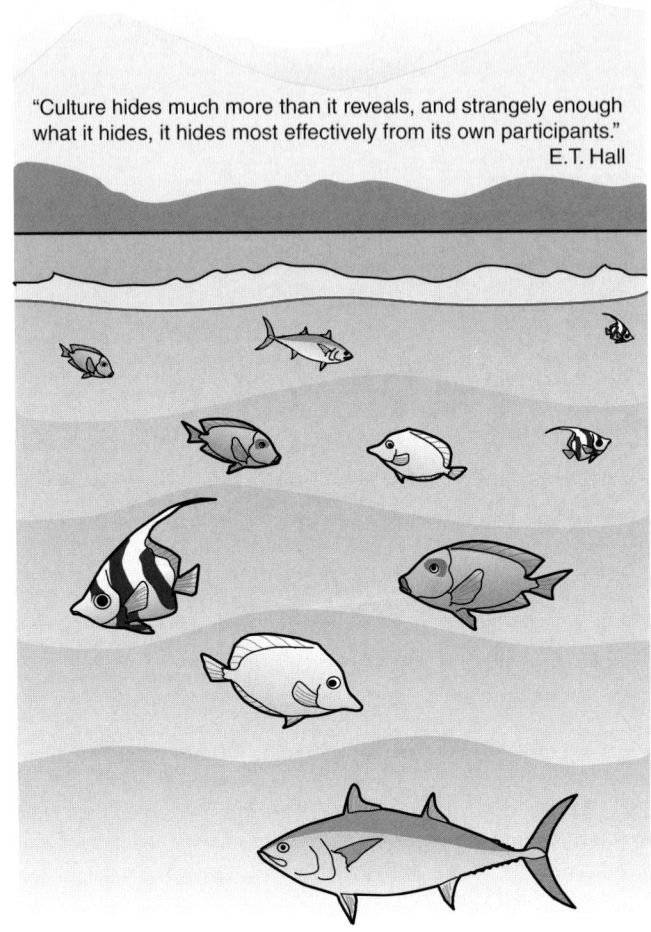

Fig. 1.3   Culture as Described Using the Analogy of Fish in Water.

Culture as Patterns

A simple description of culture is reflected by the letters *C.U.L.T.U.R.E.*

Description of Culture
Culture is …
Commonly
Understood
Learned
Traditions and
Unconscious
Rules of
Engagement

Culture is something that is commonly understood by those who share it—it is the common worldview, values, and beliefs that are clear to those who are a part of the cultural group, but foreign to others. A **worldview** is the "way in which an individual or group looks out on and understands their world about them as a value, stance, picture, or perspective about life or the world" (Leininger, 2002, p. 83). In other words, it is the way in which we perceive, interpret, and relate to the world around us.

Culture is learned from birth, through language acquisition and socialization. Individuals are not born with culture; they are born into a culture. Similarly, health care providers are socialized into professional cultures as they learn about and take on the norms, values, and expectations of the profession. Culture also is about traditions and rituals—what is done, when it is done (or not done), and how it is done. Different groups have different ways of doing things.

Culture is not only commonly understood, but it is unconscious and automatic. It reflects a norm based on values and assumptions about the world that are taken for granted and rarely examined or enacted consciously. Often, it is only when we are confronted with difference that traditions and rituals are recognizable for what they are and what they represent.

Lastly, cultural values determine the identity norms or rules of engagement with varying situations and events in our lives, including illness and health care. Cultural values influence perception of and reaction to people, events, and situations, including what is deemed acceptable and unacceptable behaviour.

The preceding description, like the iceberg analogy, points to the existence of explicit or implicit patterns of behaviour that influence thoughts and actions. However, it is critical to recognize that culture is a dynamic concept: cultural patterns exist but vary among individuals and can also change over time. Automatically assigning such patterns to behaviours or norms is stereotyping and harmful. This will be further discussed in Chapter 3.

Cultural Competence In Action

The Changing and Unchanging Nature of Values

Identify two values that your parents (or elders) taught you when you were growing up. Consider values like independence, co-operation, duty, desire, obedience, respect, honour, individuality, allegiance to family, and questioning or challenging the status quo.

From the above list, identify two values that you would like to teach your children (or your niece or nephew, or young people in general). Are the values the same as the ones that were taught to you? Are they different? Can you identify the reasons for any differences? Does the gender of the child or person influence your answer?

This exercise highlights the dynamic nature of culture. While some values and preferences may remain the same across generations, others may change over time, based on circumstances and life experiences.

Cultural Competence In Action

Values and Decision Making

Suppose you won a raffle for $1000. How would you spend your unexpected winnings?
a) Give it to family.
b) Go on a vacation.
c) Pay off debts or save it for future expenses.
d) Buy shoes or clothing.
e) Go out for dinner at a fancy restaurant.

Reflect on your answers: Do some of the options seem frivolous or ridiculous? Would you have made the same choices 5 years ago? What might be influencing your choices? Discuss your answers with colleagues who might have made a different choice. Identify one to two factors that led to determining what is "right." Note that the "right" answer is not always right for everyone at all times.

Culture as Power

It is important to note that culture is not just about patterns (worldviews or ways of being), it is also about power. Culture is a social construction, thus it "must be considered in historical, social, political, and economic contexts" (Garneau & Pepin, 2015, p. 10). In a diverse society, cultural differences lead to unequal power relations. How we navigate the world is shaped by our worldviews and by our experiences. Being part of the dominant culture can lead to safety and privilege, whereas minority group status can lead to experiences of discrimination and exclusion, which in turn influence actions and behaviours in different circumstances (Srivastava & Srivastava, 2019). Thus aspects of identity are also sites of "difference, oppression, marginalization, and privilege via systems and practices of power" (Overstreet et al., 2020, p. 780).

Cultural Competence and Cultural Safety

The concepts of cultural competence and cultural safety are both used as guidelines to ensure equitable patient-centred care in Canada and globally. Cultural safety originated in New Zealand within a "strictly Indigenous purpose and context" and "requires explicit, detailed recognition of the cultural identity of Indigenous people" (Yeung, 2016, p. 4). The main focus of **cultural safety** is on the impact of colonialism and power imbalances that disregard the ways of being and knowing (including health and illness beliefs) of Indigenous people and deny self-determination. Cultural safety has been considered an outcome of cultural competence (Sharifi et al., 2019) or as a distinct approach focusing on social and political power that emphasizes self-determination in the provider–patient relationship (Berg et al., 2019). Although the theoretical definition and origins of cultural safety are distinct from cultural competence, the two are similar in application (Yeung, 2016), with cultural safety being predominately applied to health care for Indigenous people. A key aspect of cultural safety is that it must be understood from the perspective of the person being served or cared for.

Cultural competence can be described as "a set of congruent behaviors, attitudes, and policies that come together in a system, agency, or among professionals and enable [them] to work effectively in cross-cultural situations" (Cross et al., 1989, p. 13). As a concept, cultural competence "exhibits adaptability to different ethno-cultural group interactions" (Yeung, 2016, p. 4) and recognizes the need for adapting assessment and treatment approaches to achieve equity in health quality and outcomes. Cultural competence is often described as a process or journey, not as a destination or an outcome.

Cultural competence requires an understanding of the concepts of culture and competence. As discussed earlier, "culture" refers to "integrated patterns of human behaviour" and "competence" implies having the requisite knowledge, skills, and judgement to function effectively (National Center for Cultural Competence, n.d.). Therefore, cultural competence should not be regarded as knowing everything about every culture or any culture; rather, competence implies the transformation of knowledge and understanding into effective health care responses or interventions. In this respect, cultural competence is like clinical competence and similarly requires ongoing, lifelong learning.

The complex, elusive, and ambiguous nature of culture and cultural competence has led to many critiques of the concept (Beagan, 2018; Blanchet Garneau et al., 2016; Danso, 2018). These critiques can be summarized as follows:

- Narrow, static definition of culture that focuses on race, ethnicity, and ignores other identities
- Focus on the individual and failure to recognize the structural or social determinants of health
- Focus on the "other" and centring the problem on the "other" while failing to recognize or scrutinize the dominant culture

- A simplistic, bicultural approach that portrays all health care providers as members of the dominant group and rendering "racialized and ethnic minority professionals as invisible" (Beagan, 2018, p. 123)
- Measuring cultural competence only in terms of provider comfort and confidence cannot be equated with working effectively

These critiques are valid but lack analytical rigour. They are valid to the extent that they should serve as caution for narrow definitions and simplistic interpretations of either culture or cultural competence. Danso (2018) argues that critiques of cultural competence are often based on invalid or contradictory assumptions: "Perhaps the problem with cultural competence is not the concept itself, but rather the myriad ways in which different researchers and practitioners in different places and times have (mis)conceptualized, (mis)understood, and (mis)interpreted the concept" (p. 9). The author further notes it is unrealistic to expect cultural competence to be an "omnibus or omnicompetent construct capable of addressing all culture-related or structural problems" (p. 9).

Alternatives to cultural competence include cultural humility, structural competency, and cultural competemility (a blend of cultural competence and cultural humility) (Campinha-Bacote, 2019). As a concept, **cultural humility** focuses on self-awareness, particularly in relation to issues of professional power and privilege. Cultural humility emphasizes the understanding of social structures and how they impact patients—and calls for advocacy toward systemic changes. By emphasizing self-critique and critical reflection, cultural humility points to the privilege that is associated with professional expertise and institutional structures (Beagan, 2015; Danso, 2018). Cultural humility is an important concept, but it is not a robust model or framework that offers significant advantage over cultural competence. (See Chapter 9 for further discussion of cultural humility.) Critical self-reflection, respecting difference, addressing power in provider–patient relationships, partnering with patients and families, and learning from patients are all fundamental tenets of professional practice across health disciplines, as well as foundational elements of anti-oppressive practice and hallmarks of patient-centred care (Danso, 2018). As a characteristic, humility is about being humble and unpretentious. In cultural competence terms, humility is about challenging one's own ethnocentrism and valuing the knowledge and wisdom that exist across diverse individuals and communities. While cultural competence may not be a perfect concept, it does offer a way forward to address the challenges of cultural differences and systemic and structural inequities. Tehee et al. (2020), following a comprehensive review and examination of cultural competence, recommend "scholars and practitioners to embrace the complexity of this construct and resist the urge to find a replacement construct with a neat definition but rather incorporate new knowledge and conceptualizations as they arise and celebrate the deeper and broader understanding that results from added concepts" (p. 20). Success will be dependent on robust understanding, thoughtful application, and critical evaluation.

The interconnections between culture, diversity, health equity, and cultural competence are presented in Table 1.3.

Levels of Cultural Competence

Research and scholarship in public and health care administration recognize three interconnected levels for analysis, goal and strategy development, and implementation of actions to achieve desired outcomes. The macro level refers to overall policy, priorities, and processes at the national level (e.g., coverage for health care and reimbursement); the meso level refers to the institution level where the priorities are enacted through structure and strategy; and the micro level reflects relationships and interactions between people and includes patient care approaches, options, and interventions (Sawatzky et al., 2021).

TABLE 1.3 ■ **Interconnections Between Culture, Diversity, Health Equity, and Cultural Competence**

Culture	Shared patterns and experiences that shape our ways of being and doing
Diversity	Includes the multiple ways of being and intersectional operations of power, privilege, and marginalization at the individual, institutional and systemic levels
Health Equity	Considers how diverse identities and social locations affect health status, with an emphasis on access and outcomes and provides a lens to bring diversity awareness and knowledge into (more equitable) health deliverables
Clinical Cultural Competence	Can be understood as a specific set of practices in care design and delivery, based on an awareness and knowledge of culture, diversity and power to support equitable health outcomes. In other words, cultural competence is a practice strategy to reach health equity goals informed by both culture and diversity

Adapted from Mawhinney, J. (2013). Diversity and equity competencies in clinical practice. In M. Herie & W. J. Skinner (Eds.), *Fundamentals of addiction: A practical guide for counsellors* (pp. 43–62). CAMH.

Within the health care literature, it is recognized that cultural competence is needed at the individual provider level (micro) and at the broader organizational and system level (macro) (McCalman et al., 2017; Srivastava & Srivastava, 2019; Tehee et al., 2020). The majority of literature on cultural competence is explicitly or implicitly aimed at the individual health care provider operating within the broader context of professional practice to understand the issues and apply them in practice.

An unrecognized level for cultural competence is that of team level (meso). This is important, particularly as health care is largely delivered via teams. Cultural competence at the team level means creating an environment that promotes healthy dialogue on differences by setting up mechanisms in the care process that allow for the exchange of diverse viewpoints and knowledge to develop innovative and transformative interventions (Srivastava, 2008). Team-level competence is seen as necessary to link the organization's espoused values to day-to-day care practice. Putting policy in place is often hampered by differing priorities of individual staff, particularly those in senior or more authoritative and leadership positions. For example, an individual's attempts at cultural assessment may not be valued or seen as legitimate if this is not part of the usual protocol or if the process will take too long and is thus considered impractical. Team-level cultural competence makes the group values explicit, establishes and/or clarifies group norms, and draws on the strength of the collective to support the group's culture.

Cultural Competence In Action

How to Advocate for a Patient

Helen is a relatively new registered nurse (RN) on a busy mental health unit of an urban hospital. She recognizes that Mr. Yuen has communication challenges due to limited English proficiency; however, despite this communication barrier, he is usually cooperative and nods a lot during conversations. His family visits regularly and no complaints have surfaced. In team rounds, it is evident that there is little information on how Mr. Yuen is feeling as no team member has had an opportunity to have a direct conversation with him. Helen is aware that the hospital has access to interpreter services and wants to use this service for Mr. Yuen. However, when she mentions this to the charge nurse, she is told it is not necessary—interpreters are expensive and not always reliable, and there is no immediate issue for which an interpreter is needed. How could Helen advocate for the team and Mr. Yuen's access to interpreter services? Is it necessary? Why or why not?

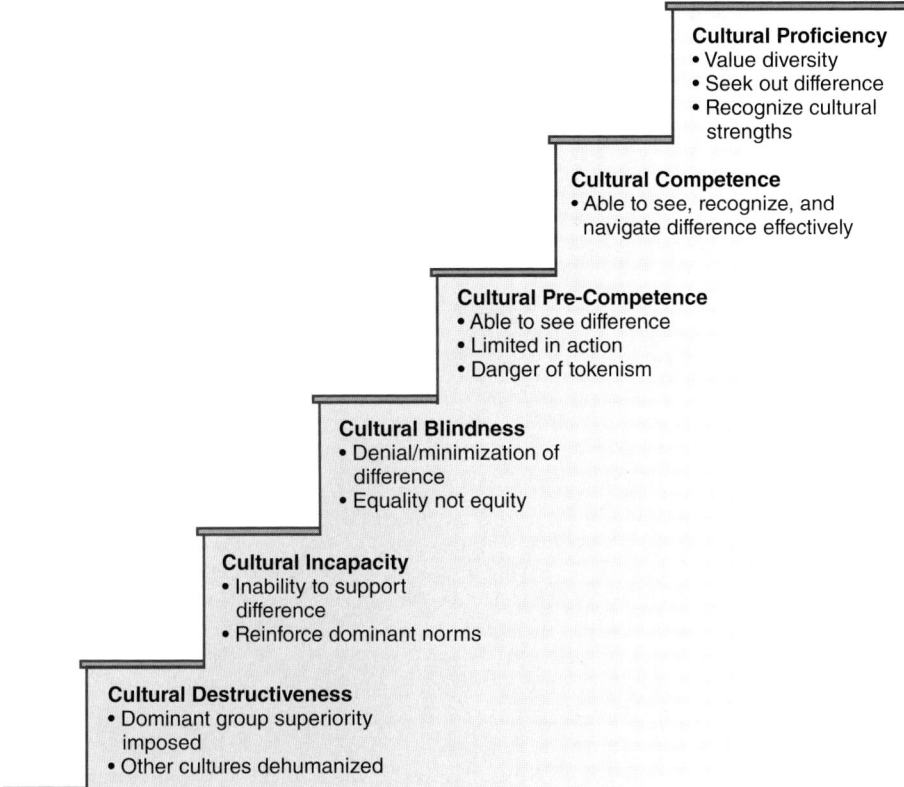

Cultural Proficiency
- Value diversity
- Seek out difference
- Recognize cultural
  strengths

Cultural Competence
- Able to see, recognize, and
  navigate difference effectively

Cultural Pre-Competence
- Able to see difference
- Limited in action
- Danger of tokenism

Cultural Blindness
- Denial/minimization of
  difference
- Equality not equity

Cultural Incapacity
- Inability to support
  difference
- Reinforce dominant norms

Cultural Destructiveness
- Dominant group superiority
  imposed
- Other cultures dehumanized

Fig. 1.4 Cultural Competence Continuum.

At the organizational level, cultural competence can be understood as "strategic effort made on a systems level to meet the needs of employees and patients of diverse backgrounds" (Kumra et al., 2020, p. 109). Although considerable literature exists on frameworks and guidelines regarding institutional or organizational diversity, there is a general lack of empirical research on organizational diversity, particularly from a Canadian context. Organizational interventions address systems issues in the following ways: (1) increase access—through language support, hours and location of service, removing complexity from referrals; and (2) build capacity—through strategies such as user engagement, workforce training, enhancing workforce diversity, outreach activities, and coordination with traditional healers. Although evidence that organizational strategies lead to positive outcomes for patients is limited, it is promising and continues to be an area for further examination and development (McCalman et al., 2017).

The Cultural Competence Continuum

Given that cultural competence is a process and an ongoing journey, it follows that cultural competence can be described on a continuum. Unlike other approaches that advocate cultural competence as a method for further enhancing the quality and effectiveness of care, the **cultural competence continuum** (Fig. 1.4), developed by Cross et al. (1989), clearly highlights that a lack of competence can be harmful and destructive. In other words, cultural competence is a necessary ingredient for effective care and cannot simply be equated with icing on the cake. Although the continuum is presented in a linear fashion, it should not be interpreted as a series of predetermined, rigid phases; rather, it presents possible ways to respond to cultural differences, and individuals can be at different stages with different groups (Goode, 2004).

At the extreme end of the continuum, **cultural destructiveness** refers to attitudes, practices, and organizational policies that focus on the superiority of one culture to the extent that other cultures are dehumanized and destroyed. Historical examples of cultural destructiveness can be found with respect to Indigenous people in Canada and the forced removal of Indigenous children from their families for placement in residential schools or non-Indigenous foster families. The explicit goal of this policy was to eradicate Indigenous culture and language (Allan & Smylie, 2015).

Cultural incapacity refers to the inability of health care providers and institutions to help patients from different cultures. The dominant patient group serves as the norm for all care, and systemic biases lead to paternalism or exclusionary approaches of diverse communities. The subtle and not-so-subtle messages are that members of communities that are different are not welcomed, valued, or able to fit into the systems of care. The expectation is that minority culture(s) will adapt to, accept, and even be grateful for the care provided. Cultural incapacity is characterized by ignorance, stereotypes, and unrealistic fears based on race (Goode, 2004). Individuals and agencies behave as "agents of oppression" by enforcing and supporting racist policies and structures (Cross, 1988, p. 2). The lack of language interpretation services may be one example of cultural incapacity.

Cultural blindness occurs when cultural differences are minimized or denied in a desire to be unbiased and treat everyone identically. Cultural blindness disregards longstanding systemic biases and fails to recognize the need for equitable practices. This is discussed further in Chapter 2 (see The Myth of Sameness). At the **cultural pre-competence** stage there is an awareness or recognition of needs based on culture; however, the ability to take appropriate action is limited. Organizations and individuals exhibit a genuine desire for learning and commitment toward inclusive policy and initiatives; however, there is a danger of a false sense of accomplishment or tokenism. Isolated initiatives do not lead to foundational change in practice or within an organization. There is also a danger of demoralization at this stage when providers encounter challenges during activities or initiatives. If such challenges are viewed as failures, there might be a reluctance to make any further effort and then the continuum is compromised (Goode, 2004).

The cultural competence stage is characterized by a recognition of, and respect for, difference and an ongoing effort toward self-assessment, enhancing awareness, and strengthening knowledge and skills in order "to provide safe and quality health care to patients with different cultural backgrounds" (Cai, 2016, p. 269). The final stage of the cultural competence continuum is described as **cultural proficiency**. Practitioners and organizations in this stage value diversity and seek out the positive role that culture can play in health and health care (Goode, 2004). Rather than just providing unbiased care, culturally proficient health care providers and agencies look for cultural strengths and opportunities to create new knowledge and innovative practices. They recognize and challenge health inequities across different populations and groups. Cultural diversity is embraced and can lead to transformative change that includes changes in the structural elements involving power and oppression. Examples of transformative interventions include programs that involve cultural communities in the design and delivery of health care, with a plan for sustainability driven by the cultural groups.

It is evident from the earlier discussion that cultural competence is a journey in which a disregard for or lack of cultural competence can be harmful or destructive; acceptance of status quo perpetuates inequities; and cultural proficiency, integration, and innovation tap into the strength of cultures to identify approaches and solutions whose benefit extends beyond the cultures from which they originated. Table 1.4 provides a brief self-assessment tool that can be used by individuals as a beginning exploration of their awareness, knowledge, and skills with respect to developing cultural competence.

TABLE 1.4 ■ Cultural Competence Self Assessment

Intercultural competence is an ongoing learning process. There are no right or wrong answers. As you complete this assessment, think about WHY you are choosing the particular rating. Note opportunities for change.

SCALE: 1 = Very well 2 = Well 3 = Fairly well 4 = Not at all

1. I can identify the cultures to which I belong and the significance of that membership.	1	2	3	4
2. I can recognize when the impact of my attitudes, beliefs, and values may be interfering with providing the best service/care to patients.	1	2	3	4
3. I can identify my emotional reactions, stereotypes, and preconceived notions of individuals and groups that are different from myself.	1	2	3	4
4. I am aware of my social status and privilege in relation to my colleagues and patients.	1	2	3	4
5. I am aware of the specific cultural knowledge of the diverse populations with whom I work, including worldviews, healing traditions, strengths, and health beliefs.	1	2	3	4
6. I can explain the concepts of culture, health equity, inclusion, and social determinants of health.	1	2	3	4
7. I recognize the effects and the implications of racism, sexism, and heterosexism in society and on the care I provide.	1	2	3	4
8. I can identify privileges and marginalization in society due to intersections of race, ethnicity, socio-economic status, sex and gender, sexual orientation, language, and physical abilities.	1	2	3	4
9. I know where to seek credible health information about the cultures with whom I work.	1	2	3	4
10. I can advocate on behalf of people who feel they were discriminated against.	1	2	3	4
11. I recognize that our health care services and approaches reflect particular cultural perspectives.	1	2	3	4
12. I understand and respect that age, gender, and family roles may vary among cultures and need to be considered in interactions.	1	2	3	4
13. I recognize how the meaning and value of medical treatment and health education may vary among cultures.	1	2	3	4

Adapted from Nova Scotia Health Authority. (2016). Diversity lens toolkit, based on Alberta Health Services (2009). *Enhancing cultural competency: A resource kit for health care professionals* (pp. 124–136).

Differentiating Cultural Competence From Person-Centred Care

A question that health care providers often ask is how clinical cultural competence is different from "patient-centred" or "person-centred" care. In a review, Håkansson Eklund et al. (2019) identified nine themes present in person-centred as well as in patient-centred care: (1) empathy; (2) respect; (3) engagement; (4) relationship; (5) communication; (6) shared decision-making; (7) holistic focus; (8) individualized focus; and (9) coordinated care. Clarke et al. (2017) conducted a critical interpretive review of patient-centred care literature and explicated six elements of the patient–health provider relationship: (1) engaging the patient as a whole person; (2) recognizing and responding to emotions; (3) fostering a therapeutic alliance; (4) promoting an exchange of information; (5) shared decision making; and (6) enabling continuity of care. In theory, there is significant overlap between patient-centred care and cultural competence; however, as noted by Mathers and Bansal (2016), patient-centred care can be difficult at the best of times, and it is particularly challenging with "someone from a culture very different from one's own" (p. 2). The person- and patient-centred approaches describe the person in terms of bio-psycho-social factors with some reference to the person's preferences or context; however, in the reviews cited earlier there was no explicit reference to culture (of the patient or provider) or issues of power, privilege, access, or equity. Patient- and person-centredness is a great start to culturally appropriate or responsive care; however, without the explicit and intentional attention to culture it can be argued that clinically competent, caring health care providers unknowingly provide care that is culturally ineffective or unsafe. The literature on health inequities would support such an argument. Actions related to the themes and principles that underlie patient- and person-centred care are greatly influenced by legacies of colonization and discrimination along with differences in ways of being and doing. Adding a cultural competence lens to patient- and person-centred care is essential to realize the promise of quality health care for all.

Summary

This chapter presents an overview of key terms and issues associated with cultural competence and why it is essential to incorporate cultural competence in health care. Canadian society is becoming increasingly diverse. There is increased recognition that historical and social factors have led to unequal access in health care and poorer health outcomes for many minority groups. Based on changing perspectives, culture is now fully recognized as an important determinant of health. The growing evidence and increased recognition of the impact of colonization and loss of culture for Indigenous people have prompted a renewed commitment to reconciliation, social justice, and equitable health outcomes for all cultural communities.

Provision of quality care in a culturally diverse context requires an understanding of culture, social justice, racism, and many other related concepts that impact the goal of health equity and quality care. Culture is a broad, ambiguous concept that is associated with *patterns* or ways of being, as well as *power* or ways in which individuals and groups experience inclusion, exclusion, privilege, and marginalization.

Frameworks such as patient- and person-centred care, cultural safety, and cultural competence are all focused on the delivery of high-quality patient care and have many similarities with respect to meaningful engagement with those we care for and serve. However, patient- and person-centred care approaches often ignore culture and its impact on health. Although cultural safety and cultural competence have differing origins with respect to populations and groups they were developed for, these frameworks are similar in the following ways: (1) recognizing the need for humility and inclusivity; (2) understanding the unique history, traditions, and beliefs of individuals and groups; (3) considering the impact of the social determinants on health; and (4) communicating in respectful, culturally appropriate ways.

The cultural competence continuum highlights that a lack of respect for diversity and culture is actually harmful to individuals and groups, whereas the ability to integrate cultural strengths can lead to innovation and positive transformation for individuals and the services provided by a team or agency. Culture and cultural competence exist at the level of the individual (micro), team (meso), and organization or institution (macro). It is important to understand the interplay across these levels. Cultural competence involves more than accepting diversity; it requires challenging systemic barriers and changing the existing structures and practices that perpetuate intolerance, oppression, and inequity.

Questions for Review and Discussion

1. Outline the differences between cultural competence and person-centred care. Describe why adding a cultural competence lens to person-centred care is important.
2. Briefly describe the key aspects of culture that are evident through the iceberg analogy.

3. What are the key aspects of culture that can be described by the analogy of culture as a fish in water?
4. Outline the difference between health equity and health equality.
5. List three reasons why cultural competence and cultural safety are essential to quality care.

Group Experiential/Reflection Activity

This experiential activity can be completed in small groups or individually as a reflection activity.

Microaggressions are everyday interactions that communicate a negative bias toward a marginalized group. They are part of everyday injustices that are reflected in unconscious assumptions (such as believing that groups are lazy, promiscuous, or lack ambition) and practices that systematically exclude individuals from particular events or opportunities.

In small working groups, watch one of the following video clips:

https://www.youtube.com/watch?v=ZahtlxW2CIQ

https://www.youtube.com/watch?v=ICrPkfwbMAc

Discuss your thoughts and feelings. Can you give examples of everyday racism that you have observed in your daily life?

Have you witnessed examples of microaggressions directed at another person?

Have you experienced microaggressions personally? What was your response?

List examples of microaggressions experienced or personally observed by members of your group.

Reflect on ways that you and your group members could increase awareness of these unconscious assumptions.

 http://evolve.elsevier.com/Srivastava/culturalcompetence/.

References

Alimezelli, H. T., Leis, A., Denis, W., et al. (2015). Lost in policy translation: Canadian minority Francophones and health disparities. *Canadian Public Policy*, *41*, 44–52.

Alizadeh, S., & Chavan, M. (2016). Cultural competence dimensions and outcomes: A systematic review of the literature. *Health & Social Care in the Community*, *24*(6), e117–e130.

Allan, B., & Smylie, J. (2015). *First Peoples, second class treatment: The role of racism in the health and well-being of Indigenous people in Canada.* Wellesley Institute.

Australian Human Rights Commission. (2014). *What is casual racism?* https://humanrights.gov.au/about/news/what-casual-racism

Azzopardi, C., & McNeill, T. (2016). From cultural competence to cultural consciousness: Transitioning to a critical approach to working across differences in social work. *Journal of Ethnic & Cultural Diversity in Social Work*, *25*(4), 282–299.

Bailey, Z. D., Krieger, N., Agénor, M., et al. (2017). Structural racism and health inequities in the USA: Evidence and interventions. *Lancet*, *389*(10077), 1453–1463.

Beagan, B. L. (2015). Approaches to culture and diversity: A critical synthesis of occupational therapy literature. *Canadian Journal of Occupational Therapy*, *82*(5), 272–282.

Beagan, B. L. (2018). A critique of cultural competence: assumptions, limitations, and alternatives. In C. Frisby & W. O'Donohue (Eds.), *Cultural competence in applied psychology*. Springer. https://doi.org/10.1007/978-3-319-78997-2_6.

Berg, K., McLane, P., Eshkakogan, N., et al. (2019). Perspectives on Indigenous cultural competency and safety in Canadian hospital emergency departments: A scoping review. *International Emergency Nursing*, *43*, 133–140.

Blanchet Garneau, A., Browne, A. J., & Varcoe, C. (2016). *Integrating social justice in health care curriculum: Drawing on antiracist approaches toward a critical antidiscriminatory pedagogy for nursing.* Sydney, Australia: 2nd International Critical Perspectives in Nursing and Healthcare Conference.

Blanchet Garneau, A., & Pepin, J. (2015). Cultural competence: A constructivist definition. *Journal of Transcultural Nursing*, *26*(1), 9–15.

Bourabain, D., & Verhaeghe, P. -P. (2021). The conceptualization of everyday racism in research on the mental and physical health of ethnic and racial groups: A systematic review. *Journal of Racial and Ethnic Health Disparities*, *8*, 648–660. https://doi.org/10.1007/s40615-020-00824-5.

Bourke, S., Wright, A., Guthrie, J., et al. (2018). Evidence review of Indigenous culture for health and wellbeing. *The International Journal of Health, Wellness, and Society*, *8*(4), 11–27.

Browne, A. J., Varcoe, C., Lavoie, J., et al. (2016). Enhancing health care equity with Indigenous populations: Evidence-based strategies from an ethnographic study. *BMC Health Services Research*, *16*(1), 544.

Cai, D. -Y. (2016). A concept analysis of cultural competence. *International Journal of Nursing Sciences*, *3*(3), 268–273.

Campinha-Bacote, J. (2019). Cultural competemility: A paradigm shift in the cultural competence versus cultural humility debate, Part I. *Online Journal of Issues in Nursing*, *24*(1). https://doi.org/10.3912/OJIN.Vol24No01PPT20.

Canadian Heritage. (2019). *Some facts on the Canadian Francapohonie*. https://www.canada.ca/en/canadian-heritage/services/official-languages-bilingualism/publications/facts-canadian-francophonie.html

Canadian Race Relations Foundation. (2019). *CRRF glossary of terms*. https://www.crrf-fcrr.ca/en/resources/glossary-a-terms-en-gb-1

Clarke, S., Ells, C., Thombs, B. D., et al. (2017). Defining elements of patient-centered care for therapeutic relationships: A literature review of common themes. *European Journal for Person Centered Healthcare*, *5*(3), 362–372.

Cross, T. (1988). Cultural competence continuum. *Focal Point: The Bulletin of the Research and Training Center, Regional Research Institute for Human Services, Portland State University*, *3*(1), 1–4.

Cross, T. L., Bazron, B. J., Dennis, K. W., et al. (1989). *Towards a culturally competent system of care: A monograph on effective services for minority children who are severely emotionally disturbed*. Georgetown University Child Development Center.

Danso, R. (2018). Cultural competence and cultural humility: A critical reflection on key cultural diversity concepts. *Journal of Social Work*, *18*(4), 410–430.

De Moissac, D., & Bowen, S. (2018). Impact of language barriers on quality of care for official language minority Francophones in Canada. *Journal of Patient Experience*, *6*(1), 24–32. https://doi.org/10.1177/2374373518769008.

Ehie, O., Muse, I., Hill, L., et al. (2021). Professionalism: Microaggression in the health setting. *Current Opinion in Anaesthesiology*, *34*(2), 131–136. https://doi.org/10.1097/ACO.0000000000000966.

Essed, P. (2000). *Towards a methodology to identify converging forms of everyday discrimination*. https://www.un.org/womenwatch/daw/csw/essed45.htm

Fleras, A. (2019). 50 years of Canadian multiculturalism: Accounting for its durability, theorizing the crisis, anticipating the future. *Canadian Ethnic Studies*, *51*(2), 19–59.

Fiscella, K., & Sanders, M. R. (2016). Racial and ethnic disparities in the quality of health care. *Annual Review of Public Health*, *37*, 375–394.

Fournier, B., & Karachiwalla, F. (2020). *Shah's public hand preventive health care in Canada* (6th ed.). Elsevier.

Fung, K., & Guzder, J. (2018). Canadian immigrant mental health. In D. Moussaoui, D. Bhugra, & A. Ventriglio (Eds.), *Mental health and illness in migration. Mental health and illness worldwide*. Springer.

Garneau, A. B., & Pepin, J. (2015). Cultural competence: A constructivist definition. *Journal of Transcultural Nursing*, *26*(1), 9–15.

Gil, S., Hooke, M., & Niess, D. (2016). The limited English proficiency patient family advocate role: Fostering respectful and effective care across language and culture in pediatric oncology setting. *Journal of Pediatric Oncology Nursing*, *33*(3), 190–198.

Goode, T. D. (2004). *Cultural competence continuum*. National Center for Cultural Competence. https://nccc.georgetown.edu/

Government of Canada. (2020). *Social determinants of health and health inequalities*. https://www.canada.ca/en/public-health/services/health-promotion/population-health/what-determines-health.html

Greenwood, M., de Leeuw, S., & Lindsay, N. (2018). Challenges in health equity for Indigenous people in Canada. *The Lancet*, *391*, 1645–1648.

Håkansson Eklund, J., Holmström, I. K., Kumlin, T., et al. (2019). "Same Kulin or different?" A review of reviews of person-centered and patient-centered care. *Patient Education and Counseling*, *102*(1), 3–11.

Hardeman, R. R., Medina, E. M., & Kozhimannil, K. B. (2016). Structural racism and supporting Black lives—the role of health professionals. *New England Journal of Medicine*, *375*(22), 2113–2115.

Henry, F., Dua, E., Kobayashi, A., et al. (2017). Race, racialization and Indigeneity in Canadian universities. *Race Ethnicity and Education*, *20*(3), 300–314.

Hollingsworth, D. W., Cole, A. B., O'Keefe, V. M., et al. (2017). Experiencing racial microaggressions influences suicide ideation through perceived burdensomeness in African Americans. *Journal of Counseling Psychology*, *64*(1), 104–111.

Hook, J. N., Farrell, J. E., Davis, D. E., et al. (2016). Cultural humility and racial microaggressions in counseling. *Journal of Counseling Psychology*, *63*(3), 269–277.

Hopper, E. (2019). *What is a microaggression? Everyday insults with harmful effects.* https://www.thoughtco.com/microaggression-definition-examples-4171853

Immigration, Refugees and Citizenship Canada. (2020). *2020 Annual Report to Parliament on immigration.* Immigration, Refugees and Citizenship Canada Catalogue No. Ci1E-PDF. https://www.canada.ca/en/immigration-refugees-citizenship/corporate/publications-manuals/annual-report-parliament-immigration-2020.html

Institute of Medicine. (2003). *Unequal treatment: Confronting racial and ethnic disparities in health care.* The National Academies Press.

Jana, T., & Baran, M. (2020). *Subtle acts of exclusion: How to understand, identify, and stop microaggressions.* Berrett-Koehler.

Jongen, C., McCalman, J., & Bainbridge, R. (2018). Health workforce cultural competency interventions: A systematic scoping review. *BMC Health Services Research*, *18*, 232.

Khanlou, N., Haque, N., Skinner, A., et al. (2017). Scoping review on maternal health among immigrant and refugee women in Canada: Prenatal, intrapartum, and postnatal care. *Journal of Pregnancy*, *2017*, 8783294. https://doi.org/10.1155/2017/8783294.

Kirmayer, L. J., & Jarvis, G. E. (2019). Culturally responsive services as a path to equity in mental health care. *HealthcarePapers*, *18*(2), 11–23.

Kleinman, A., Eisenberg, L., & Good, B. (1978). Culture, illness, and care: Clinical lessons from anthropologic and cross cultural research. *Annals of Internal Medicine*, *88*, 251–258.

Kumra, T., Hsu, Y. J., Cheng, T. L., et al. (2020). The association between organizational cultural competence and teamwork climate in a network of primary care practices. *Health Care Management Review*, *45*(2), 106–116.

Kurtz, D., Janke, R., Vinek, J., et al. (2018). Health sciences cultural safety education in Australia, Canada, New Zealand, and the United States: A literature review. *International Journal of Medical Education*, *9*, 271–285. https://doi.org/10.5116/ijme.5bc7.21e2.

Leininger, M. (1991). The theory of culture care diversity and universality. In M. Leininger (Ed.), *Culture care diversity and universality: A theory of nursing* (pp. 5–72). National League for Nursing.

Leininger, M. (1995). Transcultural nursing perspectives: Basic concepts, principles, and culture care incidents. In M. Leininger & M. R. McFarland (Eds.), *Transcultural nursing: Concepts, theories, research and practice* (2nd ed., pp. 57–92). McGraw Hill.

Leininger, M. (2002). Theory of culture care and the ethnonursing research method. In M. Leininger & M. R. McFarland (Eds.), *Transcultural nursing: concepts, theories, research and practice* (3rd ed., pp. 71–98). McGraw Hill.

Leyland, A., Smylie, J., Cole, M., et al. (2016). *Health and health care implications of systemic racism on Indigenous peoples in Canada: Indigenous health working group [Fact sheet].* The College of Family Physicians of Canada.

Maina, I. W., Belton, T. D., Ginzberg, S., et al. (2018). A decade of studying implicit racial/ethnic bias in healthcare providers using the implicit association test. *Social Science & Medicine*, *199*, 219–229.

Marcelin, J. R., Siraj, D. S., Victor, R., et al. (2019). The impact of unconscious bias in healthcare: How to recognize and mitigate it. *The Journal of Infectious Diseases*, *220*(2), S62–S73.

Mathers, N., & Bansal, A. (2016). Patient-centered care in a multicultural world. *Family Medicine and Community Health*, *4*(4), 1–3.

Maynard, R. (2017). *Policing Black lives: State violence in Canada from slavery to the present.* Fernwood.

McCabe, C. F., O'Brien-Combs, A., & Anderson, O. S. (2020). Cultural competency training and evaluation methods across dietetics education: A narrative review. *Journal of the Academy of Nutrition and Dietetics*, *120*(7), 1198–1209.

McCalman, J., Jongen, C., & Bainbridge, R. (2017). Organisational systems' approaches to improving cultural competence in healthcare: A systematic scoping review of the literature. *International Journal for Equity in Health*, *16*, 78.

McKenzie, K., Agic, B., Tuck, A., et al. (2016). *The case for diversity: Building the case to improve mental health services for immigrant, refugee, ethno-cultural and racialized populations*. Mental Health Commission of Canada.

Minnican, C., & O'Toole, G. (2020). Exploring the incidence of culturally responsive communication in Australian healthcare: The first rapid review on this concept. *BMC Health Services Research*, *20*, 20. https://doi.org/10.1186/s12913-019-4859-6.

National Center of Cultural Competence (n.d.). *Definition of terms*. Georgetown University Center for Child and Human Development. https://nccc.georgetown.edu/culturalbroker/8_Definitions/index.html

National Collaborating Centre for Determinants of Health. (2017). *Let's talk: Racism and health equity*. National Collaborating Centre for Determinants of Health, St. Francis Xavier University. https://nccdh.ca/images/uploads/comments/Lets_Talk_Racism_and_health_equity_EN_web.pdf

Okoro, O., Odedina, F., & Smith, W. T. (2015). Determining the sufficiency of cultural competence instruction in pharmacy school curriculum. *American Journal of Pharmaceutical Education*, *79*(4), 50.

Olaussen, S. J., & Renzaho, Andre M. N. (2016). Establishing components of cultural competence healthcare models to better cater for the needs of migrants with disability: A systematic review. *Australian Journal of Primary Health*, *22*, 100–112. https://doi.org/10.1071/PY14114.

Ontario Ministry of Health and Long-Term Care. (2019). *Health equity impact assessment*. http://www.health.gov.on.ca/en/pro/programs/heia/

Overstreet, N. M., Rosenthal, L., & Case, K. A. (2020). Intersectionality as a radical framework for transforming our disciplines, social issues, and the world. *Journal of Social Issues*, *76*, 779–795. https://doi.org/10.1111/josi.12414.

Paradies, Y., Ben, J., Denson, N., et al. (2015). Racism as a determinant of health: A systematic review and meta-analysis. *PLoS ONE*, *10*(9), e0138511.

Potvin, L. (2020). Black lives matter in Canada too! *Canadian Journal of Public Health*, *111*, 633–635.

Public Health Agency of Canada. (2018). *Key health inequities in Canada: A national portrait*. Pan-Canadian Health Inequities Reporting Initiative. https://www.canada.ca/content/dam/phac-aspc/documents/services/publications/science-research/key-health-inequalities-canada-national-portrait-executive-summary/hir-full-report-eng.pdf

Ramraj, C., Shahidi, F. V., Darity, W., et al. (2016). Equally inequitable? A cross-national comparative study of racial health inequalities in the United States and Canada. *Social Science & Medicine*, *161*, 19–26.

Reich, D. (March 23, 2018). How genetics is changing our understanding of 'race'. *The New York Times*. https://www.nytimes.com/2018/03/23/opinion/sunday/genetics-race.html

Sawatzky, R., Kwon, J., Barclay, R., et al. (2021). Implications of response shift for micro-, meso-, and macro-level healthcare decision-making using results of patient-reported outcome measures. *Quality of Life Research*. https://doi.org/10.1007/s11136-021-02766-9.

Sharifi, N., Adib-Haijbaghery, M., & Najafi, M. (2019). Cultural competence in nursing: A concept analysis. *International Journal of Nursing Studies*, *99*, 1–8.

Shepherd, S. M., Willis-Esqueda, C., Newton, D., et al. (2019). The challenge of cultural competence in the workplace: perspectives of healthcare providers. *BMC Health Services Research*, *19*, 135.

Srivastava, R. (2008). *Influence of organizational factors on clinical cultural competence*. Institute of Medical Sciences, University of Toronto. Unpublished doctoral dissertation.

Srivastava, R., & Srivastava, R. (2019). Impact of cultural identity on mental health in post-secondary students. *International Journal of Mental Health and Addiction*, *17*, 520–530.

Statistics Canada. (2017a). *Indigenous people in Canada: Key results from the 2016 census*. Statistics Canada Catalogue no. 11-001-X.

Statistics Canada. (2017b). *Ethnic and cultural origins of Canadians: Portrait of a rich heritage*. Statistics Canada Catalogue no. 98–200-X2016016.

Statistics Canada. (2017c). *Focus on Geography Series, 2016 census*. Statistics Canada Catalogue no. 98–404-X2016001. Data products, 2016 Census.

Statistics Canada. (2017d). *Immigration and ethnocultural diversity: Key results from the 2016 census.* Statistics Canada Catalogue no. 11-001-X.

Statistics Canada. (2017e). *Visible minority and population group reference guide: Census of population, 2016.* Statistics Canada Catalogue no. 98–500-X2016006.

Statistics Canada. (2019a). *2016 Census Indigenous community portrait – Canada.* Statistics Canada Catalogue no. 41260001.

Statistics Canada. (2019b). *Diversity of the Black population in Canada: An overview.* Statistics Canada Catalogue no. 89–657-X2019002.

Statistics Canada. (2020). *Experiences of discrimination during the COVID-19 pandemic.* Statistics Canada Catalogue no. 11-001-X.

Stevens, F. L., & Abernethy, A. D. (2018). Neuroscience and racism: The power of groups for overcoming implicit bias. *International Journal of Group Psychotherapy*, *68*, 561–584.

Subedi, R., Greenberg, L., & Turcotte, M. (2020). *COVID-19 mortality rates in Canada's ethno-cultural neighbourhoods.* Statistics Canada Catalogue no. 45280001.

Tehee, M., Isaacs, D., & Domenech Rodríguez, M. M. (2020). The elusive construct of cultural competence. In L. Benuto, F. Gonzalez, & J. Singer (Eds.), *Handbook of cultural factors in behavioral health* (pp. 11–24). Springer.

Truth and Reconciliation Commission of Canada. (2015a). *Truth and Reconciliation Commission of Canada: Calls to action.* Author.

Truth and Reconciliation Commission of Canada. (2015b). *Truth and Reconciliation Commission of Canada: Honouring the truth, reconciling for the future.* Author.

Turpel-Lafond, M. E. (2020). *In plain sight: Addressing Indigenous-specific racism and discrimination in B.C. health care.* Government of British Columbia. https://engage.gov.bc.ca/app/uploads/sites/613/2020/11/In-Plain-Sight-Full-Report.pdf

Vang, Z. M., Sigouin, J., Flenon, A., et al. (2017). Are immigrants healthier than native-born Canadians? A systematic review of the healthy immigrant effect in Canada. *Ethnicity & Health*, *22*(3), 209–241.

Veenstra, G., & Patterson, A. C. (2016). Black-White health inequalities in Canada. *Journal of Immigrant and Minority Health*, *18*(1), 51–57.

Veenstra, G., Vas, M., & Sutherland, D. K. (2020). Asian-White health inequalities in Canada: Intersections with immigration. *Journal of Immigrant and Minority Health*, *19*, 300–306.

Wallace, S., Nazroo, J., & Bécares, L. (2016). Cumulative effect of racial discrimination on the mental health of ethnic minorities in the United Kingdom. *American Journal of Public Health*, *106*(7), e1–e7. https://doi.org/10.2105/AJPH.2016.303121.

Watt, K., Abbott, P., & Reath, J. (2016). Developing cultural competence in general practitioners: An integrative review of the literature. *BMC Family Practice*, *17*, 158.

Williams, D. R., Lawrence, J. A., & Davis, B. A. (2019). Racism and health: Evidence and needed research. *Annual Review of Public Health*, *40*, 105–125.

Wilson, C., Flicker, S., Restoule, J.-P., et al. (2016). Narratives of resistance: (Re) telling the story of the HIV/AIDS movement – because the lives and legacies of Black, Indigenous, and People of Colour communities depend on it. *Health Tomorrow*, *4.*

Yeung, S. (2016). Conceptualizing cultural safety: Definitions and applications of safety in health care for Indigenous mothers in Canada. *Journal for Social Thought*, *1*, 1–13.

Yoshikawa, K., Brady, B., Perry, M. A., et al. (2020). Sociocultural factors influencing physiotherapy management in culturally and linguistically diverse people with persistent pain: A scoping review. *Physiotherapy*, *107*, 292–305.

CHAPTER 2

Myths, Misconceptions, and Evolving Perspectives

Rani H. Srivastava

LEARNING OBJECTIVES

At the end of this chapter, the learner will be able to:
- Identify the common myths and misconceptions associated with culture
- Discuss the evolution of multiculturalism policy in Canada
- Describe key events with respect to Indigenous rights that influence contemporary discourse and practice
- Discuss major perspectives on culture and diversity and their influence on integrating culture into health care
- Recognize the paradoxical dilemmas associated with cultural competence

KEY TERMS

Anti-racism/anti-oppression	Equity deserving groups	Inclusivity
Assimilation	Ethnic matching	Multiculturalism
Cultural literacy	Ethno-specific agencies	Perspectives
Cultural mosaic	Explanatory model of	Settlers
Cultural safety	illness	Stereotypes
Equity	Generalizations	

The purpose of this chapter is to provide an overview of the evolution of thought and knowledge concerning culture and diversity. Over the years, there have been different perspectives on how best to understand and apply cultural competence in health care practices. **Perspectives** can be thought of as conceptual landscapes or sets of ideas that form the overall picture on a given topic. To understand our current thinking about culture and diversity, it is important to understand the evolving social and academic perspectives on the subject.

This chapter begins with a discussion of some common myths and misconceptions about culture. This is followed by an exploration of multiculturalism and how it has evolved over time. One way to examine the evolving social context of diversity is to look at government policies. For Canada, this means an examination of multiculturalism—as it evolved in legislation and as it is experienced by Canadians. In this chapter, the legislative context is discussed separately from the conceptual perspectives in health care for ease of understanding, but in reality, the two are interrelated. The discourse on culture in health care has changed over time. How we understand and view culture has been debated from varying, and often conflicting, perspectives. These include the cultural literacy approach, relational approach, anti-racism/anti-oppression approach, and finally an integrative social justice approach. These evolving perspectives have allowed for a deeper and broader understanding of the complexity and paradoxes associated with the intersection of cultural and social issues and how they impact health and well-being.

Misconceptions and Myths[1]

Despite decades of discourse on concepts of culture and diversity, there continue to be myths and misconceptions that need to be identified and challenged to fully understand the issues related to culture and approaches to health care.

MYTH #1: THE MYTH OF EQUALITY

This myth refers to the view that fairness means equal treatment for all. It is characteristic of what is often described as a *meritocratist* perspective, which values hard work, self-reliance, and individualism. A meritocratist perspective cites success stories in which individuals of all ethnic, racial, and gender backgrounds have achieved goals and outcomes based on their hard work and merit. The argument is that all are equal and if some can succeed, so can all. However, this view lacks awareness of and sensitivity to systemic barriers and institutional racism. Further, it places the responsibility for success solely on the individual without acknowledging systemic inequities, and may lead to unconscious bias and prejudice against individuals and groups who are unable to achieve the desired outcomes.

It is widely recognized that while all people may be created equal, they are not created the same. Therefore, equality must be differentiated from and, in most instances replaced by, the concept of equity. **Equity** refers to equality with respect to opportunity, access, and outcome based on individual needs. Achieving equity often requires differential treatment of individuals to achieve the same results (see Fig. 2.1).

In the *equality* paradigm (Fig. 2.1), the resource (in this case the block to stand on) is shared equally among three individuals. If the goal was to assist people to see over the fence, success was only achieved for one of the three individuals and two-thirds of the resource was wasted. The tallest person did not need the block, the person of medium height benefitted from the support, and the shortest person remained unable to achieve access to see the ball game. In the *equity* paradigm, the resource is distributed according to need, where one person gets nothing and another gets twice as much; as a result, the goal of access to the ball game is achieved for all. Lastly, in the *justice* paradigm, the barrier itself is examined and changed to promote access. In these examples the difference in access is attributed to height. However, if one considers the difference based on social or cultural identity, it is important to recognize that the reason people do not have equal access is not due to their limitation or shortcoming but rather because the ground they are standing on is not level. As shown in Fig. 2.2, the tallest person begins with considerable advantage and the shortest is starting from a place of considerable disadvantage created by society; they are not starting on the same level. It is important to recognize that many populations experience significant barriers to equal participation in society based on factors such as age, ethnicity, disability, economic status, gender, nationality, race, sexual orientation, and transgender status. Such populations, who experience disadvantage that is socially created, are referred to as *marginalized populations* or, more recently, **equity deserving groups**.[2]

---

[1]Many of the myths presented here were initially identified by Dr. Ralph Masi (Masi, R. [1996]. Inclusion: How can a health system respond to diversity. In A. S. Zieberth [Ed.], *Pinched: A management guide to the Canadian health care archipelago* [pp.147–157]. Pinched Press).

[2]The term *equity deserving* was suggested by Professor Wisdom Tettey, Vice President and Principal of University of Toronto Scarborough in his 2019 Installation Address. See https://utsc.utoronto.ca/news-events/inspiring-inclusive-excellence-professor-wisdom-tetteys-installation-address.

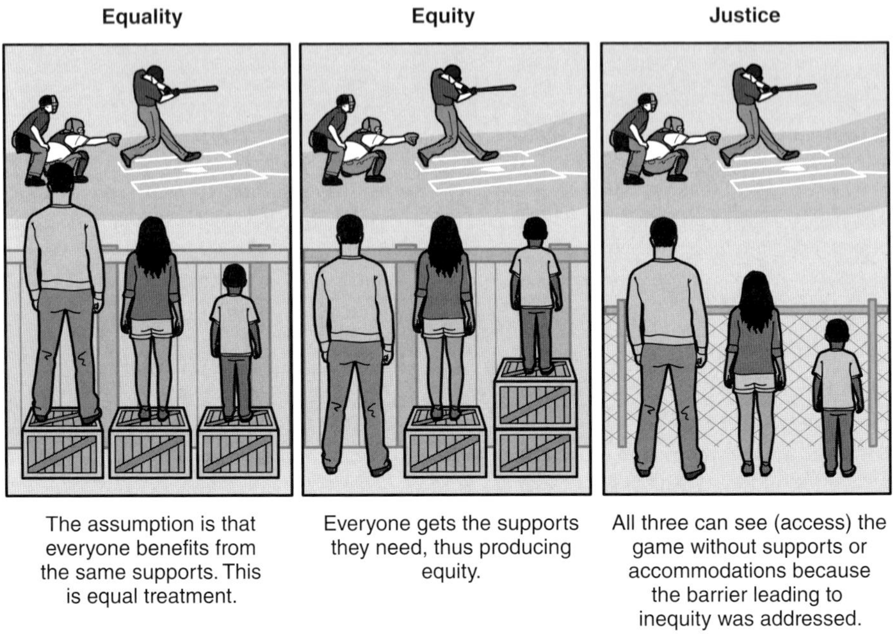

Equality   **Equity**   **Justice**

The assumption is that everyone benefits from the same supports. This is equal treatment.

Everyone gets the supports they need, thus producing equity.

All three can see (access) the game without supports or accommodations because the barrier leading to inequity was addressed.

Fig. 2.1 Equality, Equity, and Justice. Adapted from Craig Froehle's original concept. https://www.storybased-strategy.org/ the4thbox.

MYTH # 2: THE MYTH OF REVERSE RACISM

The myth of *reverse racism* grew out of a response by some toward affirmative action or targeted equity initiatives and suggests that reverse racism is experienced when an individual from a privileged group, such as a White male, is passed over for an opportunity (job, entrance to a competitive program, etc.) because preference is given to an individual from a historically under-represented group or equity deserving group (e.g., woman, person of colour or Indigenous heritage). This is inaccurate for two reasons: (1) reverse racism assumes that the world is a level playing field for all, and (2) it ignores the fundamental question of power and privilege (Alberta Civil Liberties Association, n.d.). While it is true that a person from the dominant group may experience discrimination as an individual, to say that those with years of privilege are experiencing racism implies that "injustice of not getting a particular job or not getting into a particular school is somehow morally equivalent to the over 350 years of enslavement" (Suiter, 2016, p. 18). Policies aimed at equity-oriented hiring are attempts at corrective action to social injustices and are not racism. Calls of reverse racism often occur in circumstances where White people may be a numerical minority, or people feel that as they did not personally or intentionally oppress anyone, they are not part of the system of racism. It can also be seen as avoidance of having to acknowledge one's privilege or the existence of systemic barriers for marginalized populations.

MYTH #3: THE MYTH OF SAMENESS

This myth suggests that patients receive the best care from health care providers of their own background. An attempt to match patients and health care providers of the same ethnic background is sometimes referred to as **ethnic matching**. Based on the premise that cultural

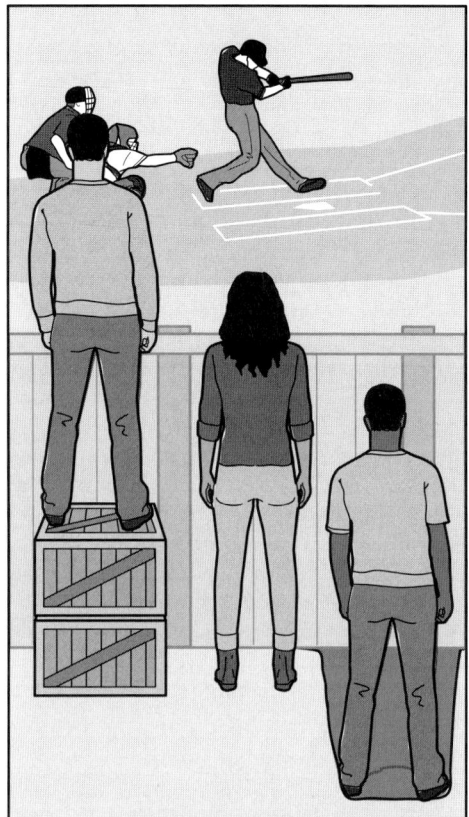

All three people are the same height.
The access, or lack of it, to the game is
based on the level of the ground they are on.
Thus advantage or disadvantage is in the
environment (structural), not in the person.

Fig. 2.2 Privilege, Equity, and Reality.

differences between patient and health care provider can lead to miscommunication, misdiagnosis, and inappropriate care, ethnic matching attempts to minimize difference by having a provider of the same ethnicity. Khambhaita, Willis, and Pathak (2017) refer to this in terms of having *insider* knowledge and understanding; however, the premise is limited and does not account for the dynamic and intersectional nature of cultural identity. Kirmayer and Jarvis (2019) note that assumption of ethnic matching can lead to further stereotyping and "unwarranted assumptions of similarity and mutual understanding or even de facto segregation in the healthcare system" (p. 16). Although the empirical evidence on ethnic matching is inconclusive and often contradictory, there is some support for racial matching as a "viable practice for enhancing the psychotherapeutic experience" (Steinfeldt et al., 2020, p. 2). The authors note that the racial identity takes into account experiences within a broader sociopolitical and cultural environment where "power is differentiated by race" (Steinfeldt et al., 2020, p. 2).

The assumption that someone who shares the patient's ethnicity will provide more effective health care is subject to challenge. The visible similarity may only be skin deep; individuals may not share language, culture, religion, or other aspects of identity that are important. Furthermore, since the capacity to deal with a specific culture depends on individuals, it is transient—as people leave, the ability to provide culturally appropriate health care is drastically reduced, leading to ongoing challenges in continuity and sustainability of care. It is, however, important to recognize the positive impact a diverse workforce can have in addressing health inequities. Increasing workforce diversity is a frequently cited approach for health services to become more culturally safe and responsive; however, a diverse workforce is one of multiple strategies and is often accompanied by health care provider training (Federation of Ethnic Communities' Councils of Australia [FECCA], 2019; McCalman et al., 2017; Truth and Reconciliation Commission [TRC], 2015).

Similarly, developing partnerships with **ethno-specific agencies** (agencies serving specific cultural groups) is a key aspect of organizational cultural supports. Ethno-specific agencies often have limited resources and provide targeted services (Mukhtar et al., 2016). A model of exclusive or over-reliance on such services is also not realistic or feasible, given the diverse needs of the population being served (Radermacher et al., 2009). Furthermore, it is important not to make assumptions about sameness in individuals' needs and preferences (Radermacher, 2009). There is, however, clear evidence that having access to culturally based services can be very positive, particularly when the services are designed and developed intentionally and in partnership with the specific population they serve (Churchill et al., 2020; Khanlou et al., 2017). All health care providers, regardless of their personal background, need to develop the necessary competence to provide quality care to a diverse, multicultural society and do so in collaboration with patients, families, and culturally specific organizations. Ultimately, it is the quality of respect and connection that will lead to experiences of cultural safety.

Cultural Considerations In Care

Similarity Is Not Always Similar

Julie, a nursing student, arrives for her second day of clinical practice. She had developed a good relationship working with her patient the day before and was looking forward to continuing with the plan of care. However, when she arrives on the unit, she learns that her assignment has changed. She is now caring for an elderly Chinese man admitted yesterday whose first language is Cantonese. The team thought Julie would be in an excellent position to care for this patient as she is also of Chinese background (second generation). Julie tries to explain to her instructor that she does not speak the language, but is instead encouraged to "do her best."

- What is the impact of this change on Julie? On the patient? On the team?
- What assumptions have been made in making these changes to Julie's assignments by the team? How might they be addressed?

The myth of sameness also denies the preferences and needs of patients. The author's practice experience indicates that there are many instances where patients will prefer *not* to seek a provider of the same culture for reasons of confidentiality, social distance, and perceived cultural bias on the part of the provider. Cultural communities are often small and close-knit, and patients sometimes express concerns about the potential for breaches in confidentiality when they expect to encounter their health care providers in social situations. In addition, if conditions, diseases, or treatment are considered culturally unacceptable or carry a stigma, patients may shy away from seeking a health care provider from that culture.

Cultural Competence In Action

When "Sameness" Is Concerning

Rita was a registered nurse (RN) manager on an acute medical floor. She noted that a patient, Henry, a 38-year-old West Indian male, seemed to have a difficult time developing a relationship with the nursing team. Rita was concerned, as many of her staff were West Indian and she did not understand the potential barrier to the relationship. In addition, Henry made a request that the West Indian nurses not be assigned to him. Upon further inquiry Rita learned that there were no concerns regarding the quality of care; however, Henry was concerned about confidentiality. He was HIV+ and worried that somehow that information would leak out to his community. He understood professional ethics and that health care providers were bound to protecting patient privacy; however, he was still concerned. The situation was addressed by each nurse who cared for him individually reinforcing their commitment to confidentiality. The nurses also advised him that if they ever ran into each other in a community setting, the nurse would not acknowledge knowing Henry unless he initiated the interaction. The nurses wanted to ensure that Henry had control over the situation and that they were not ignoring or disrespecting him in any way.

The myth of sameness presents other challenges. Not only can ethnic matching go against the patient's best interests, it may be contrary to the health care provider's best interests. It is important to be aware of the dynamics and expectations that may be created for the patients. Patients may have different expectations of health care providers who share their own ethnocultural heritage than of other health care providers. Patients may believe that the similarity will translate into increased understanding and an ability to provide something extra or different than routine care. Such expectations can lead to challenges for the health care provider in maintaining professional boundaries. The expectation that certain health care providers work primarily with members of their own communities can often be limiting and affect professional career and growth opportunities for the health care providers. While targeted use of staff resources can be helpful, particularly in the short term, the long-term goal should focus on increasing workforce diversity, as well as the capacity of the individual health care providers and the system to care for patients across cultural groups.

Cultural Considerations In Care

A Special Bond With the Patient

Ms. Singh, a 23-year-old East Indian person, was referred to the nephrology program for chronic renal failure. She needed dialysis until a kidney transplant became available.

The nephrology team consisted of a physician (of British background), a social worker (a White female Canadian), and a female clinical nurse specialist (CNS) of East Indian origin. The patient's first language was Punjabi, but she was able to communicate in English. The CNS was fluent in Hindi and had some familiarity with Punjabi, and the patient had sufficient familiarity with Hindi to be able to communicate with the CNS in a mixture of Hindi and Punjabi; subsequently, the two developed a special bond.

Ms. Singh started to regard the CNS as a big sister, which she even stated on more than one occasion. As a result, the patient started to disclose personal information regarding her marriage and family, but insisted that this information not be shared with other members of the health care team. The social worker was involved in Ms. Singh's health care with respect to assisting with financial support and planning for dialysis supplies. The patient did not share the marital and family concerns with the social worker, as she did not feel comfortable talking about her personal affairs with strangers,

Continued

and she also feared that issues would be taken out of cultural context and create difficulties for her family members.

Friction occurred within the team. The social worker became frustrated and felt that she was being underutilized by the patient and that the CNS was undermining her role. Subsequently, the patient received a transplant; however, she was unwilling to let go of the CNS and continued to direct questions and concerns toward the CNS instead of the transplantation team. Ms. Singh would frequently leave messages for the CNS, which led to delays in the overall response to patient issues and interfered with the communication and relationship with the transplantation team. The CNS also felt torn: on the one hand, she wanted to provide continuity in care and support for the patient, but on the other, the relationship was creating difficulties.

- Discuss this scenario from the perspective of the patient, the CNS, and the other team members.
- Identify strategies that could best make use of the diversity within the team and prevent some of the difficulties encountered.

MYTH #4: THE MYTH OF CULTURE AS A BARRIER

Within health care, issues of culture and diversity have largely been viewed from a negative standpoint, with a focus on cultural differences and the resulting problems. Culture is frequently regarded as a barrier to be overcome. It is true that differences in cultural values may, at times, lead to conflict, but it is important to remember that values and beliefs play significant positive roles in people's lives. The difficulties and challenges are attributed to the patient's culture rather than to an inability of the system to respond to cultural issues and needs. The view of culture as a barrier or a problem can limit the health care provider's ability to understand the positive aspects of beliefs and values, particularly when they are different from those of the health care provider.

Seeing culture as a barrier often leads to a response of avoidance. Consider what most people do when they encounter a barrier: they tend to go around it or over it, with the hopes of getting to the other side as quickly and efficiently as possible. When culture is regarded as a barrier to be overcome, the health care provider is likely to focus on ways of getting the patient to accept predetermined goals or solutions. However, experience shows that people will ultimately choose what they think is right for them. While a health care provider may be successful in minimizing the influence of cultural values and beliefs in the short term, cultural issues are likely to resurface in the long run.

It would be more effective to recognize that the barriers do not result from the patient's culture, but rather from the values and beliefs inherent in the biomedical culture, insufficient professional training, as well as social and structural barriers within the health care system. An alternative perspective is to view culture not as problem to be overcome, but as a leverage point— a point that can affect the outcome significantly if energy is focused on it. While many of us may be marginalized on the basis of certain aspects of our identity (e.g., sexual orientation, race, gender, religion, [dis]abilities, or ethnicity), it is generally those same aspects that can serve as a source of strength or community. Cultural traditions and approaches often provide comfort and guidance, particularly in times of illness, and serve as a source of strength for the patient and family. Similarly, a lack of cultural support can be a barrier to recovery. Studies on Indigenous people health experiences show that for Indigenous people, health is understood in a holistic way that includes physical, mental, emotional, and spiritual components; only focusing on one aspect (physical), or leaving cultural values and needs unrecognized, can lead to feelings of impersonal, inappropriate, and culturally unsafe care (Auger, 2019). Focusing on culture as a strength and resource and integrating culture into care, can be a powerful strategy in providing high-quality, patient-centred care.

MYTH #5: THE MYTH OF "EVERYTHING MUST BE ACCEPTABLE—OR NOT"

Many health care providers struggle with the boundaries of what is acceptable when it comes to cultural issues. There is a perception that if something is a *cultural value*, it must be accepted. This is simply not true and context is key to understanding. Respect must not be confused with acceptance. Health care must be provided within the parameters of legal and professional boundaries. Patients need to be informed about unacceptable behaviour and its consequences. However, whenever possible, this needs to be done in ways that continue to acknowledge respect and support the health care provider–patient relationship for future interactions (see the example of female genital cutting in Chapter 12).

As well, providers need to understand practices in the context of cultural and social issues. Viero et al. (2019) and Killion (2017) use the example of child abuse to illustrate this misconception. Cultural practices such as "scratching the wind"—where bruises are caused by cupping and scratches are created by running a coin on the skin for the purpose of relieving fever or illness—are considered a healing technique in some cultures but may be misinterpreted as child abuse. Child abuse is clearly unacceptable in our society; however, it is important that health care providers make an accurate assessment based on awareness of specific belief systems before labelling something as abuse. Of course, health care providers must explore concerns of possible abuse; however, the need to understand one's biases, lack of knowledge, and cultural context of such practices is essential.

Another example is that of bed sharing. The practice of parent(s) and child sharing a bed is regarded as harmful in North American society, largely due to concerns regarding sudden infant death syndrome (SIDS) (Ball, 2017). However, this practice is common to many and viewed as a natural, nurturing aspect of family life (Mileva-Seitz et al., 2017). It is important for health providers to recognize this as a controversial issue, understand the evidence, and work with families in a manner that supports informed decision making.

MYTH #6: MYTH OF ALL GENERALIZATIONS AS UNACCEPTABLE

Many professionals claim that generalizations about any cultural group are inappropriate because they ignore variations within a cultural group and therefore stereotype individuals. The term *culture* refers to shared values, beliefs, norms, and patterns; shared values do not preclude individual differences. Generalizations are sometimes necessary to understand groups, but they should not be imposed on individuals within the groups and require caution in use.

It is important to differentiate between generalizations and stereotypes. **Generalizations** can be a helpful beginning point, indicating trends and patterns that require additional information as to their appropriateness and applicability to specific individuals and situations; **stereotypes** are an "end point" at which complexities are not explored and assumptions are imposed (Galanti, 2019). Generalizations are often useful in helping health care providers begin a conversation with some understanding of common traits that may be relatively consistent within and across populations. Stereotypes close conversations and knowledge development and impose specific characteristics on individuals. As Beagan et al. (2012) remind us, "generalizations are a starting point for understanding a person. Practitioners cannot understand an individual from generalizations, but generalities can sensitize nurses to probable patterns, issues of social difference, leading them toward particular kinds of questions" (p. 60). For example, knowing the dietary restrictions associated with a particular religion can be helpful information when it is used to inquire about meal planning; however, an assumption that an individual will follow a particular diet and ordering it for them is practising a stereotype, even when it is done with a positive intent. Stereotyping and lack of individualized assessment are two key reasons why health care providers need to exercise caution about generalizations. However, the need for caution must not be confused with inappropriateness. Learning about the needs of patients with cancer does not mean stereotyping all cancer patients as having the same needs, nor does it preclude individualized care. Health care providers do not impose the knowledge or the predetermined intervention on the patient without validating need and appropriateness. Similarly, learning about communities based on shared characteristics other than illness or diagnosis should not be considered problematic.

MYTH #7: THE MYTH OF FAMILIARITY AS COMPETENCE

Globalization and increased diversity across societies mean increasing familiarity with many cultures and countries. This may make us complacent and overconfident about our understanding of cultures and diversity. Frequently, students and health care providers will state that they are comfortable with diversity since their education has been in a very multicultural environment or a diverse clientele is a regular feature of their practice. However, practice experience indicates that many providers are unable to describe the impact that diversity has on their care, especially with respect to how they engage with the patient and the health care and treatment that is offered (Srivastava, 2008). Familiarity with difference paradoxically makes the difference invisible. Similarly, international exposure through travel may be helpful, but it is not the same as systematic development of cultural knowledge and understanding. Cultural competence requires a desire and a commitment to learn both about and from the cultures to which one is exposed locally, nationally, and internationally.

Multiculturalism: The Social and Legislative Context

Multiculturalism in Canada is a sociological fact, an ideology, and policy (Brosseau & Dewing, 2018). As a sociological fact, the term refers to "the preservation of different cultures or cultural identities within a unified society" (Dictionary.com, 2020). Census data from 2016 show that Canada's population comprises over 250 ethnic origins, with nearly 22% of the population born outside of Canada and almost 20% of Canadians speaking more than one language at home (Brosseau & Dewing, 2018; Statistics Canada, 2017).

Ideologically, multiculturalism has focused on the values of compassion, love, and understanding; celebrating the country's diversity; tolerating and respecting cultural differences; and creating a social space for minority cultures to identify with the language and culture of their choice while promoting citizenship. Over time, multiculturalism has become synonymous with the Canadian identity (Paris, 2018).

As policy, multiculturalism refers to management of cultural diversity through formal initiatives at national, provincial, territorial, and local municipal levels (Brosseau & Dewing, 2018). The origins of multiculturalism in Canada can be traced back to the Lester B. Pearson government's Royal Commission on Bilingualism and Biculturalism. The mid-1960s were a time of increasingly troubled relations between French and English Canadians. Although the Royal Commission was established to look at biculturalism and bilingualism, what it heard went beyond French and English relations. The result was a new model of citizenship based on public acceptance of difference and support of pluralism (existence of many cultures). Unlike the melting-pot model of the United States, which promoted **assimilation** (a process whereby a minority group gradually adopts the customs and attitudes of the dominant culture), Canada preferred the idea of integration and a **cultural mosaic**,[3] in which the various cultures were encouraged to preserve and celebrate their heritage. The term *cultural mosaic* describes a social fabric of multi-ethnic communities as part of Canadian identity. The policy of multiculturalism was introduced by Prime Minister Pierre Trudeau within a framework of "two official languages … [but] no official culture" (Jedwab, 2020).

---

[3]The term *cultural mosaic* can be attributed to travel writer Victoria Hayward, as discussed by McKenney, R. and Bryce, B. (2016). *Creating the Canadian mosaic.* https://activehistory.ca/2016/05/creating-the-canadian-mosaic/.

Multiculturalism was adopted as a national policy in Canada in 1971 with a goal of promoting integration through a) retention and fostering of identity; b) overcoming barriers to participation; c) promoting exchanges and sharing between communities; and d) encouraging minority groups to acquire at least one official language (Griffith, 2017). Since that time, the policy has evolved through several phases, each reflecting on and influencing the social climate of the time. Table 2.1

TABLE 2.1 ■ Canadian Multicultural Milestones

1867: Confederation
- English and French accorded official constitutional status

1960: *Canadian Bill of Rights*
- Barred discrimination by federal agencies on the grounds of race, national origin, skin colour, religion, or sex

1962: Changes to Canada's *Immigration Act*
- As a consequence, immigration became less European and the mix of source countries shifted to nations in southern Europe, Asia, and the West Indies

1969: *Official Languages Act*
- Protected minority language rights

1971: Multiculturalism Adopted as an Official Policy
- Recognized the reality of cultural pluralism in Canada
- Acted to reverse the earlier attempt to have immigrants assimilate
- Confirmed the rights of Indigenous people and the status of two official languages
- Provided for programs and services to support ethnocultural associations and to help individuals overcome barriers to their full participation in Canadian society

1982: *Canadian Charter of Rights and Freedoms*
- Multiculturalism considered to be constitutional
- Equality rights without discrimination (in particular based on race, national or ethnic origin, skin colour, religion, sex, age, or mental/physical disability)
- Section 27 explicitly states that this Charter shall be interpreted in a manner consistent with the preservation and enhancement of the multicultural heritage of Canadians; by virtue of this section of the Charter, Canada became a constitutional multicultural state

1986: *Employment Equity Act*
- Established to achieve equality in the workplace so that no person would be denied employment opportunities or benefits for reasons unrelated to ability
- Established the principle that employment equity means more than treating persons in the same way but also requires special measures and the accommodation of differences
- Identified four designated groups thought to experience disadvantage in employment: women, Indigenous people, persons with disabilities, and persons in a visible-minority group

1988: *Canadian Multiculturalism Act*
- Acknowledged multiculturalism as a fundamental characteristic of Canadian society and specified the right of all persons to identify with the cultural heritage of their choice, yet retain "full and equitable participation… in the… shaping of all aspects of Canadian society"

1996: Creation of the Canada Race Relations Foundation (CRRF)
- Established as one part of the 1988 Japanese Canadian Redress Agreement to combat all forms of racial discrimination in Canada, with special emphasis on systemic discrimination in education and employment

2005:
- Government released *A Canada for All: Canada's Action Plan Against Racism* with the objectives of strengthening social cohesion and demonstrating federal leadership in the fight against racism and hate-motivated crime
- Canada became the first country to adopt the United Nations Educational, Scientific and Cultural Organization (UNESCO) *Convention on the Protection and Promotion of the Diversity of Cultural Expressions*

Modified from Brosseau, L., & Dewing, M. (2018). *Canadian multiculturalism*. Library of Parliament, Ottawa. Publication No. 2009-20-E. https://lop.parl.ca/sites/PublicWebsite/default/en_CA/ResearchPublications/200920E.

TABLE 2.2 ■ **Evolution of Canadian Multiculturalism**

	Focus	Reference Point	Mandate	Problem Source	Solution	Metaphor
Ethnicity (1970s)	Celebrating difference	Culture	Ethnicity	Prejudice	Cultural sensitivity	Mosaic
Equity (1980s)	Managing diversity	Structure	Race relations	Systemic discrimination	Employment equity	Level playing field
Civic (1990s)	Constructive engagement	Society building	Citizenship	Exclusion	Inclusivity	Belonging
Integrative (2000s)	Inclusive citizenship	Canadian identity	Integration	Clash of cultures	Dialogue/mutual understanding	Harmony
Cohesion (2006–2015)	Social cohesion	Canadian values	Cohesion	Faith and culture clashes	Harmony	Conforming
Inclusion (2016–)	Social inclusion	Inclusive citizenship	Inclusivity	Barriers	Shared values, universalist	Embracing

Adapted from Griffith, A. (2017). *Multiculturalism: Evolution & challenges*. http://www.thepearsoncentre.
ca/platform/multiculturalism-in-canada-evolution-effectiveness-and-challenges/. Original source: Adapted
from Fleras, A., & Kunz, J. L. (2001). *Media and minorities: Representing diversity in a multicultural Canada*.
Thompson Education Publishing.

shows Canadian multicultural milestones with respect to official policy and legislation. Table 2.2
describes the evolution of multiculturalism with respect to focus, context, and evolving priorities.
A brief description of key phases follows.

ETHNICITY MULTICULTURALISM

The early 1970s has been described as the first phase of the multicultural policy—that of cultural
preservation and reinforcement reflecting the metaphor of cultural mosaic. Although the policy was
initially established to meet the needs of mainly European immigrant groups, as Canada became
more diverse, support was extended to other ethnic minority communities (Jedwab, 2020). While
the underlying notion that "everyone has a culture" was inherent in the definition of multiculturalism, culture was generally seen to belong to minorities or to the various ethnic groups. During this
time, ethnocultural groups, who may have previously struggled to preserve their cultural values
and lifeways, were able to celebrate them in public through funding and legislative support. Thus
culture became synonymous with ethnicity. With a focus on cultural celebrations, ethnocultural
communities were able to affirm their religious and ethnic identities, and for many Canadians
multiculturalism came to be viewed as the four D's: **d**ress, **d**ance, **d**ialect, and **d**iet. Although the
ethnocultural communities lived side by side, there was nothing that specifically encouraged interaction or understanding between them, and a potential fifth D, for **d**ialogue, remained unrealized.

EQUITY MULTICULTURALISM

Toward the late 1970s and early 1980s, Canadian immigration patterns began to experience a
considerable shift with more new immigrants coming from Asia, Africa, and the West Indies
and being more "visible." As the ethnic mix of the country shifted, multiculturalism policy
was forced to deal with the concerns of the increasing numbers of visible minorities.[4] The new

---

[4]The term *visible minority* is uniquely Canadian and has been used in Canada since the 1980s. It is defined
in the *Employment Equity Act* as "persons, other than Indigenous people, who are non-Caucasian in race or
non-white in colour." It is commonly used by Statistics Canada (https://www23.statcan.gc.ca/imdb/p3Var.
pl?Function=DEC&Id=45152).

and emerging communities were more concerned about equity and discrimination issues than about recognition and preservation of their heritage. Multiculturalism needed to move beyond support of cultural enrichment to elimination of racial prejudice and discrimination. Race relations became part of the official agenda. With the passage of the *Canadian Charter of Rights and Freedoms* in 1982, multiculturalism was viewed as a constitutional right. The law protected equality, ensured freedom from discrimination, and recognized a need to address systemic discrimination—the metaphor shifted to ensuring a "level playing field" for all (Brosseau & Dewing, 2018; see Table 2.2).

The period of the late 1980s and 1990s can be characterized as the anti-racist and anti-oppression phase of multiculturalism. Federal multiculturalism policies and programs emphasized elimination of barriers to economic and social participation of immigrants and designated minority groups to promote inclusivity and belonging (Jedwab, 2020). This period is also known as the civic era of multiculturalism, with emphasis on social cohesion.

INTEGRATIVE MULTICULTURALISM

In the early twenty-first century, multiculturalism entered an era that integrated the previous phases. The 9/11 terrorist attacks that occurred in the United States in 2001 led to increased concerns of security throughout the United States and Canada, recognizing a need to strengthen integration through inclusivity. Responsibilities were added to the rights discourse of multiculturalism to reduce threats of extremism and radicalization (Brosseau & Dewing, 2018). In the past two decades, academic and social discourses have shifted more toward inclusion through the promotion of social justice and a shift from tolerance and acceptance to embracing diversity. Movements such as Black Lives Matter (BLM) have gained support and solidarity from non-Black individuals as well as institutions and organizations (both private and public), leading to acknowledgement of systemic racism and a need for both individuals and institutions to reflect, learn, advocate, and change (see Canadian Nurses Association [2020] as an example). The language of multiculturalism has largely been replaced by calls for social justice and equity. As we head into the next decade, Fleras (2019) notes that Canadians are shifting from a multicultural to a post-multicultural society that is "complexly diverse." Within a multicultural context, inclusion means not excluding anyone by trying to fit them into existing systems, whereas in a post-multicultural world, **inclusivity** calls for the system to adjust "precisely because of … difference-based needs, realities, or values" (p. 42).

Indigenous Relations in Canada

As a nation, Canada is founded on Indigenous lands. The relationship between the Indigenous people and **settlers** (people from different lands who came to live here) was initially based on mutual interests; however, that changed in the late 1800s when Indigenous people were labelled as "culturally inferior" and a "problem" that needed to be controlled or eradicated. Intensive efforts to "civilize the Indian" and assimilate First Nations people into Christianity and British society led to legislation such as the *Indian Act* (1867) and subsequent establishment of residential schools. It is ironic that while Canadian multicultural policy was promoting notions of respect for all cultures and a cultural mosaic rather than assimilation, the approach toward Indigenous people in Canada was the opposite.

Residential schools were established in the 1870s with the specific objective of assimilating Indigenous children into the dominant culture by forcibly removing and isolating children from their homes, communities, and culture. The residential schools started to close in the 1970s, with the last federally operated school finally closing in 1996 (Indigenous and Northern Affairs Canada, 2018). Of the various colonial policies, the residential school policy has been particularly damaging to the health and well-being of Indigenous people, significantly impacting "every level of experience from individual identity and mental health, to the structure and integrity of families, communities, bands and nations" (Kirmayer et al., 2003, p. 4.). Wilk et al. (2017) conducted a scoping review on the negative health effects of residential schooling among former residential school attendees and subsequent generations. Based on 61 studies, the researchers showed negative health effects (physical, mental, and emotional) of residential schooling, both among former residential school attendees and in subsequent generations (Wilk et al., 2017). Most recently, in 2021, there have been discoveries of unmarked graves of children and adults on residential school properties that have reignited the trauma of residential schools and led to calls for stronger commitment and actions toward reconciliation (Migdal, 2021). The impact of residential schools on Indigenous families and intergenerational trauma is explored further in Chapter 7. Table 2.3 provides a brief snapshot of some key events in Indigenous relations from the 1960s to the current era.

TABLE 2.3 ■ Indigenous Relations in Canada

Indigenous Relations in Canada: A Brief Snapshot of Key Events

1960s	The Sixties Scoop, in which thousands of Indigenous children and babies were forcibly taken from their homes and placed in boarding schools or foster homes of Euro-Canadian families
1970s	Most residential schools cease operation by mid-1970s
1982	The Assembly of First Nations is formed to promote the interests of First Nations in the realm of self-government and respect
	Canadian Constitution Act, 1982: Indigenous and treaty rights entrenched in the supreme law of Canada
1990s	Inquiry into residential schools
	The Royal Commission on Indigenous people: report initiated in 1991, recommended a public inquiry into the effects of residential schools in 1996
	Last federally operated residential school closes in 1996
2007	Indian Residential Schools Settlement Agreement, which included the establishment of the Truth and Reconciliation Commission with a mandate to learn the truth about what happened in the residential schools and to inform all Canadians about what happened in the schools
2008	Formal apology from Prime Minister Stephen Harper to residential school survivors and their families
2012	Idle No More movement, which started as a protest against the Canadian government's dismantling of environmental protection laws, quickly became a social movement of Indigenous and non-Indigenous people as a way to draw attention to and fight for Indigenous rights
2015	*Truth and Reconciliation Commission of Canada Report* published, with 94 calls to action across all sectors of society, including education and health care
2016	Canada supports the UN Declaration on Indigenous Rights. The declaration recognizes a wide range of Indigenous rights, from basic human rights to land, language, and self-determination rights
2019	*Missing and Murdered Indigenous Women and Girls National Inquiry* report published
2021	Discoveries of unmarked graves of children and adults on residential school properties in *a number of provinces*, leading to renewed calls for action on release of historical records, continued search for unmarked graves across all resdential schools, recognition of intergenerational trauma, and meaningful action toward reconciliation and transformative healing. September 30th is declared a federal statutory holiday called the National Day of Truth and Reconciliation.

Adapted from https://www.ictinc.ca/blog/a-brief-timeline-of-the-history-of-indigenous-relations-in-canada; https://www.thecanadianencyclopedia.ca/en/timeline/first-nations; http://www.trc.ca/about-us.html; https://www.cbc.ca/news/canada/british-columbia/bc-remains-residential-school-interior-1.6085990.

Perspectives on Culture in Nursing and Health Care

The need for culturally sensitive and culturally appropriate health care has long been recognized in both Canadian society and the health care literature since the 1970s. Since then, the understanding of what is meant by culture and the approach to integrating culture into care has evolved and gone through transformation as the health care community argued about the "correct" approach to addressing the needs. Over the years, the language of *difference*, *diversity*, *equity*, and *intersectionality of multiple oppressions* has replaced the language of *culture*, *multiculturalism*, and *cultural pluralism*. The evolutionary perspectives can be broadly grouped into three major categories: cultural literacy, relational, and the anti-racism/anti-oppression approach.[5] The integrative social realist approach, a fourth, more integrative perspective that focuses on social justice and health equity, has recently emerged as the way forward. Table 2.4 briefly summarizes these approaches. It is important to note that each of the three approaches has strengths and has contributed to the current integrative approach.

CULTURAL LITERACY

Early models of understanding culture reflected the anthropological perspective and focused on learning about variations in values and beliefs regarding illness, health, and health care of different cultures. Known as the **cultural literacy**, culture-specific, or multicultural approach, this perspective encouraged health care providers to learn about the *cultural strangers* with respect to values, beliefs, lifestyles, and culturally determined health beliefs and behaviours (Azzopardi & McNeill, 2016; Jongen et al., 2018). At the individual level, cultural literacy encouraged health care providers to focus on knowledge of other cultures, and such efforts were often supported by the creation of cultural profiles for commonly served groups. Such resources usually group people by country of origin (e.g., Cambodians) or region (Central and South America) and provide information on that group with respect to health and illness beliefs, family roles, and other issues that may affect health and illness decision making (see Kongnetiman & Eskow, 2009, as an example).

TABLE 2.4 ■ Approaches to Culture and Diversity

Approach	Focus of Approach and Intervention	Learning Strategy	Goal
Cultural literacy	Individual	Learn about others	Reduce cultural barriers by adapting interventions
Relational	Individual	Learn from others	Avoid stereotyping and cultural imposition
Anti-racism/ anti-oppression	Organization or system	Challenge power and hierarchy and racist attitudes at personal and institutional level	Deconstruct barriers to promote equity, access, and social justice
Integrative social realist	Individual and system	Recognize the impact of colonialism Intersectional understanding of culture, race, and diversity	Health equity and inclusivity Honouring Indigenous ways of knowing and being Respect for cultural traditions

---

[5]This categorization has been done by the author for ease of discourse.

Critics came to view the cultural literacy path as a "cookbook" approach to health care, with values and beliefs as the identified ingredients. Inherent in the cultural literacy approach is the assumption that culture is static and "out there" to be discovered. Depending on how culture was defined, there was inevitably an overemphasis on a singular aspect of culture (e.g., religion or ethnicity) without consideration of variations within the group or issues related to acculturation or generational or regional differences. There was considerable concern that knowledge of cultural values would lead to increased stereotyping by the health care provider (Azzopardi & McNeill, 2016; Blanchet Garneau & Pepin, 2015; Jongen et al., 2018). Although many proponents of cultural literacy, including Madeline Leininger (1991), articulated the concept of professional cultures and the need to understand the beliefs that the nurse or health care provider brings to the interaction, the focus was on discovering the health care values and patterns of expression related to the health and illness of specific cultural groups. Thus, Leninger's work is often equated with cultural literacy and an essentialist view of culture. Despite calls for critical thinking and thoughtful use of cultural knowledge, it was easy for health care providers, who were struggling to understand culture in care and wishing to add to their repertoire of knowledge, to focus on information-seeking as an answer to their struggles. It was also difficult for providers, whose care largely reflected a dominant perspective, to "see" their culture (personal or professional); thus the focus remained on the patient's culture and how to "overcome" any challenges that arose in the interacions (Shepherd et al., 2019; Watt et al., 2016). The cultural literacy perspective also fails to acknowledge or address issues of discrimination, oppression, and racism (Srivastava & Srivastava, 2019).

RELATIONAL APPROACH

Increasing recognition of the limitations associated with the traditional cultural literacy approach and the fear of stereotyping gave rise to an alternative perspective that highlighted the relational nature of cultural interactions. The contribution and criticism of the cultural literacy approach raised important questions about cultural differences. Should cultural differences between people be highlighted or minimized? As health care providers wrestled with how to apply the knowledge of a cultural group to an individual patient without encountering the challenges of stereotyping, the emphasis shifted to meaning and communication. The language shifted from *culture* to *difference*, and the health care provider's culture and role also gained recognition.

The relational approach is based on the belief that culture is individually and socially constructed, rather than a static entity to be discovered. The focus of this approach is on the structure and content of the clinical encounter between the health care provider and the patient. This view highlighted the continually changing and evolving nature of culture(s) and challenged the health care provider's *culture knowledge*. Rather than having superior knowledge or preconceived notions about the patient, the health care provider is expected to approach the patient from a position of not knowing, with a curiosity and desire to learn from them (Azzopardi & McNeill, 2016). The stance of "not knowing" was seen as a buffer against essentialism and stereotyping (Danso, 2018). The relational approach emphasizes development of shared meanings by recognizing and respecting differences between the health care provider and the patient. In the cultural literacy approach, it is the health care provider's task to understand the cultural stranger; in the relational approach, the onus is on health care providers to consider themselves the stranger, recognize their own biases, and respect differences. Communication becomes the fundamental process through which cultural values are understood and acknowledged in the plan of care. Culture is viewed not as something that is possessed by individuals, but rather as a dynamic process of engagement that is subject to many influences (Blanchet Garneau & Pepin, 2015).

Promoting Holistic Care

Within nursing and other disciplines, there have been calls for strengthening relational practice (Doane & Varcoe, 2007), using strengths-based practice (Gottlieb, 2014), and adopting a caring science philosophy (Watson, 2008) as a way to promote caring (vs. curing) in a holistic way. Culture was implicit in the holistic focus of these approaches. Jean Watson's caring science approach posits a "deeply relational worldview that includes human-to-human relationships as well as human-to-environment relationships" and honours the paradox of differences and similarities (Watson, 2008, p. 58). The holistic approach to caring and healing is guided by caring actions that include creative and authentic use of self to practise loving kindness and co-create a healing environment that cultivates health, healing, and holism (Goldberg et al., 2018). Goldberg et al. (2018) identified three processes that link self-awareness with social justice: *reflexivity* (deep examination of self-knowledge and self-bias), *compassion* (practice of loving kindness), and *politicization* (understanding the political-historical positioning of others) that may lead to inequities in care.

Doane and Varcoe (2007) contend that nurse-patient relationships need to expand beyond caring and being present and recognize the unique cultural, social, political, and historical context that "shape(s) that person's identity" (p. 198). Relational practice recognizes three key, interconnected nursing obligations: (a) to be reflexive and intentional, (b) to open the relational space for difficulty, and (c) to act at all levels to impact health and healing (Doane & Varcoe, 2007). Strengths-based nursing (SBN) is described as a value-driven approach for nursing, built on principles of empowerment, self-efficacy, and hope (Gottlieb, 2014). Gottlieb and Gottlieb (2017) note that SBN is similar to other interprofessional approaches, such as the recovery model in mental health (Jacob, 2015), solutions-focused approach (Cockburn et al., 1997), and positive psychology (Seligman & Csikszentmihalyi, 2000). SBN recognizes the integral relationship between the person and their environment, past and present; it appreciates the uniqueness of each person; and it values self-determination and collaborative partnerships (Gottlieb & Gottlieb, 2017).

Although the relational model focuses on understanding the patient's uniqueness, it has been criticized for imposing an additional burden on the patient—that of "educating" the health care provider (Srivastava & Srivastava, 2019). The inherent assumption is that the patient and the health care provider have a reciprocal relationship and can mutually communicate and understand each other's perspectives. In reality, the assumption that all health care providers have the desire and the ability to be aware of their own biases is false. In a review of the literature to understand the relationship between caring science as described in the European frameworks and culture, Albarran et al. (2011) note that while there may be "a tacit assumption that the cultural aspects of caring are central and integral to the philosophical values and beliefs" of caring science, there was no explicit mention of culture in any of the 22 papers reviewed (Albarran et al., 2011). Similarly, Pashaeypoor et al. (2019) explored barriers to implementation of Watson's caring model in Iran and identified lack of familiarity with cultures and language barriers as challenges to attaining the goals of caring science. As a proposed solution, the authors encourage developing an appreciation for diversity and familiarity with patients' cultural care patterns (or some cultural literacy).

In addition to the limitations in health care providers' abilities to develop cultural understanding, barriers may also exist from the patient perspective. Practice experience indicates that often patients are unwilling or unable to share information about their cultural needs and values, especially when they are already challenged by illness and may be particularly vulnerable. Issues of stigma and concerns of racism can further impact information sharing and disclosure. In addition, when the relationship with health care providers is characterized by deep respect for professional expertise, the patient's own preferences may not be articulated and realized. Even when beliefs are expressed by the patient, they are subject to interpretation by the health care provider. As physicist Robert Shaw noted, "You don't see something until you have the right metaphor to perceive it" (see: https://quotefancy.com/quote/1679670/Robert-Shaw-You-don-t-see-something-until-you-have-the-right-metaphor-to-perceive-it). Thus, without the contextual knowledge of the culture, the chances of misinterpreting patients' health issues increase significantly. A focus on individualizing problems further obscures the social context of illness to the detriment of the provision of good health care (see Myth #5, earlier).

Understanding Explanatory Models of Illness

Despite the challenges, the emphasis on learning from the patient is an important concept, consistent with contemporary views on patient-centred care. In the late 1970s, researchers such as Katon and Kleinman (1980) noted that sociocultural factors exert a major influence on the construction of illness and made a case for applying social science to medical practice. Illness was recognized as both a social and a biological phenomenon. Recognizing that the illness experience is greater than the disease experience, and that the biomedical model of health care is considerably narrower than the bio-psychosocial approach, Katon and Kleinman (1980) proposed a clinical method consisting of three main steps:

1. Determining the patient's perception of illness
2. Determining the illness problems
3. Negotiating the care and treatment

The first step of determining the patient's perception of illness elicits the patient's **explanatory model of illness**. The explanatory model of illness includes not just perceptions of the cause of illness but also perceptions of the severity of illness the expected treatment, and the prognosis. The explanatory model thus determines the meanings and expectations associated with the illness. Step 2 is to determine the additional problems that arise because of the illness experience (e.g., the experiential, family, economic, interpersonal, occupational, and daily life problems caused by the disease). Step 3 involves negotiation between the patient's preferences for health care and the health care provider's recommendations. However, Katon and Kleinman (1980) point out that negotiations between health care providers and patients are based on unequal power relations and variables such as social class. Determining patient preferences is a critical aspect of the negotiation process, as is the determination of who (patient or key family member[s]) is regarded as the appropriate party to negotiate with. The authors caution, however, that although this broader sociocultural approach allows for consideration of a wider range of treatment options, most health care providers have their own preference regarding the therapeutic approach and thus run the risk of constructing symptoms in such a way as to justify their preferred intervention. The patient's symptoms are made to fit the theory (Katon & Kleinman, 1980). While Katon and Kleinman's work is largely based in psychiatry, it has been widely adopted across health disciplines. Although their approach relies on learning from the patient rather than on preformed knowledge of cultures, it is much more than simply listening to the patient. The approach calls for intentional effort to elicit specific types of information about the illness and illness experience from the patient and involves a complex awareness and understanding of sociocultural issues (Jongen et al., 2018). Athough Kanton and Kleinman's approach is patient centred and creates an opportunity to learn from the patient, it is grounded in an illness or problem-based approach and eliciting strengths is an implicit rather than explicit part of the approach.

Anti-Racism/Anti-Oppression Approach

In the late 1980s and early 1990s, many authors emphasized that the real challenge facing health care patients and the wider society was not culture, but the racialization or oppression that existed in society. The so-called "different-ness of minority groups" began to be recognized as the oppression of minority groups. Behaviour was seen to be influenced less by traditions and more by the way in which the group and individuals within the group were treated in the larger society. The perspective shifted from promoting cultural diversity toward challenging the power and privilege associated with dominance, all of which was synonymous with "Whiteness" (Yee & Dumbrill, 2003).

Although anti-racism and anti-oppression are not the same, they have overarchingly similar frameworks. For some, the focus on race as a starting point can be limiting, and anti-oppression is viewed as a broader approach that recognizes the intersection of race with other forms of oppression including gender, class, and sexuality (Corneau & Stergiopoulos, 2012). **Anti-racism/anti-oppression** frameworks move away from the individual and instead focus on the institutional and social structures within which people live their lives and health care is delivered. The language of culture is often regarded as an excuse and as coded logic for racism, and emphasizing cultural differences is seen as glossing over the patient's self-identity or social reality.

Within the anti-racism perspective, the definition of culture was expanded beyond ethnic boundaries and started to highlight the influence of "nonethnic" variables such as race, class, gender, sexual orientation, and physical ability. The terms *multicultural* and *transcultural* were replaced by terms such as *ethno-racial* and *diversity*. Multicultural communities were referred to as *ethnoracial* or *diverse* communities, and ultimately the idea of culture was replaced by the language of power, inequity, and difference.

The anti-racism perspective clearly highlighted that the concept of power had been missing from the cultural perspective. The perspective shifted from promoting cultural diversity toward challenging the power and privilege associated with dominance. Although the anti-racism perspective made major contributions to the cultural perspectives, it also has limitations. The anti-racism approach is harder to translate into clinical practice because it is generally applied at a systemic or organizational level, not an individual level. Even when we understand health issues by placing them in the broader context of the need for systemic change, it is unclear exactly how the health care provider should act to make a difference for a particular patient. This is despite health care providers being aware of the differences in values, beliefs, and expectations and being concerned about potential miscommunication, misdiagnosis, and inappropriate care. Corneau and Stergiopoulos (2012) offer three broad strategies to address these challenges: empowerment, education, and building alliances.

In addition to the challenges of clinical application, the anti-racism approach has also been criticized for being a form of "professional knowledge" that is derived from people in a dominant position, who "… may not be the best to judge what counts as oppression," silencing the voices who "do not fit into the Black/White dichotomy" and potentially reinforcing a stereotype or paternalistic approach that racialized individuals and groups need to be taken care of (Corneau & Stergiopoulos, 2012, p. 275). Despite the criticisms, the anti-oppression discourse continues to make a major contribution toward the goals of social justice and equity.

Integrative Social Realist Approach

The 1990s also witnessed the emergence of the discourse on cultural safety. The term originated in New Zealand as an approach to address the needs of the Indigenous Māori population (Churchill et al., 2020). As an approach, **cultural safety** calls attention to the devastating negative impact of colonization on Indigenous people with respect to all aspects of life and culture, including health. The integrative social realist approach is similar to the anti-racism and anti-oppression approach in that there is explicit recognition of power imbalances along with institutional and cultural discrimination. With growing attention to Canada's relations with Indigenous people and a recognition of Indigenous ways of knowing and being, there is greater emphasis on the concept of equity as a key concept in understanding the impact of colonization, discrimination, racism, and exclusion. Globalization and increasing diversity in society have led to a sociocultural environment where there is increasing mix of national origin, race, ethnicity, and other traits of identity. With growing recognition of the intersectional nature of diversity, culture and cultural identity are seen as dynamic and multidimensional concepts, where salient aspects of identity change over time and place. Cultural identity can thus be understood as a negotiated reality based on context and social power.

As is evident from the above discussions, the perspectives on diversity have themselves evolved over time, with each approach highlighting aspects of culture and diversity, and each contributing toward an increasingly sophisticated understanding of culture and its role in illness, health, and health care. For too long, health care providers have struggled to find the "right" language and approach to effectively address issues of culture and diversity in health care. The evolutionary perspectives have led to a more sophisticated understanding of cultural issues as well as the dynamics associated with the broader social environment. There also is an increased call to examine health outcomes, not just approaches to health care. Concepts of social justice, health equity, power and privilege, intersectionality, and inclusivity need to be understood and included in any approach aimed at improving health outcomes for a culturally diverse population.

Cultural Paradoxes and Complexity Thinking

The varied perspectives, myths, and misconceptions about culture clearly reveal that cultural issues are dynamic, complex, and often paradoxical phenomena. Culture is about groups in a system as well as about individuals, where the individual is simultaneously part of and separate from the group. Within a group, cultural patterns are both universal and diverse. The paradoxical nature of cultural issues can be understood through the principles of complexity thinking—a way of thinking that simultaneously seeks to distinguish (but not separate) and to connect. "Complexity is recognized as an attribute of a system that renders it dynamic, unpredictable, and greater than the sum of its parts" (Bird & Strachan, 2020, p. 50). Complexity thinking is characterized by three key principles: (1) dialogic principle, (2) the principle of recursivity, and (3) the hologrammic principle.

The term *dialogic* means that two logics can exist together without the dual nature being lost. The dialogic principle allows for contradictory notions to exist together. Complexity thinking supports the post-modernist view of "multiple realities based on individuals' perspectives which are influenced by beliefs, experience, and worldview" (Bird & Strachan, 2020, p. 51).

The principle of recursivity challenges the linear notion of cause and effect and recognizes that causes lead to effects but are simultaneously shaped by effects (Cruz et al., 2017). Culture is created by individuals in a group or society, and in turn, influences the behaviour of individuals and society. In the hologrammic principle, parts and wholes coexist simultaneously. It is like the dialogic principle in that the parts are present in the whole; the difference is, the whole is also reflected in the parts. The culture of a group is best understood through the individuals within the group who reflect the various attributes of the culture; at the same time, each individual is a part of the cultural group. Culture is reflected in the individual, and the individuals collectively determine the culture.

Complexity thinking teaches us to embrace uncertainty and the existence of multiple realities and worldviews while seeking to understand the apparent contradictions. It also recognizes that health care interactions are "permeated with unpredictable connections" and built on relationships within the care processes (Cruz et al., 2017, p. 225). The interactions between the patient and care provider can impact both the relationship as well as the environment itself. How we approach and come to understand a situation will influence what is conceptualized as a problem and its possible resolution.

Cultural Competence In Action

Defensiveness and Invalidation Reinforces Racism

Simon, a racialized male, makes his first visit to a specialist's office for assessment. While in the waiting room he notices a number of pamphlets on arthritis and he decides to pick up three to four pamphlets for an elderly relative who has arthritis. The next day Simon is stunned to receive a message on his work voicemail from an unidentified caller that includes statements such as "I don't understand how you people can just help yourself to someone else's property … you ought to be ashamed of yourself." He realizes that the voice sounds very similar to a previous message on his voicemail from the health care provider's office reminding him of the appointment. After processing this event and consulting with others, he decides to contact the health care provider directly, asking them to call him on an urgent issue. The provider calls him back that day. As Simon relays the events, he plays the voice recording of the message and asks if he did something wrong in taking the pamphlets. The health care provider reassures Simon that he did nothing wrong in taking the pamphlets—they are patient education materials; however, the health care provider inquires if Simon had permission to record the voicemail message.

- What factors are at play here from Simon's perspective?
- How did the health care provider frame the issue? Since the message was left on Simon's voice mail, by choice, why is permission an issue?
- What is the potential impact of this event and the health care provider's approach on Simon's trust in the health care system overall, and in future interactions?
- How could this issue be managed differently by the health care provider?

Viewing culture and cultural competence through the prism of complexity means that the development of cultural competence is an approach or a strategy, not a program full of specific content and information. The approach recognizes the need for understanding context along with interactions, reflection, self-knowledge, a willingness to discover, and "flexibility in actions of care" (Cruz et al., 2017, p. 226).

The Culture Care Framework described in Chapter 3 is presented as an approach to develop cultural competence. It is a strategy that can be applied by health care providers to develop their understanding of cultures and to apply the principles in their clinical encounters. There are no universal methods that work in all circumstances or across all cultures. The framework will guide the health care provider in exploring the uncertain world of cultures and navigating the complexities to allow new discoveries and ultimately improve health outcomes.

Summary

This chapter has presented the evolution of thinking on culture and diversity. Common myths and misconceptions that can hinder the development of cultural competence were examined. In addition to discussing the Canadian multicultural policy and a history of Indigenous relations in Canada, three major perspectives on and approaches to culture and health care with respect to their strengths, limitations, and contributions to current thinking on cultural competence were examined: (1) The traditional approach of cultural literacy helps us to recognize there are different worldviews and ways of being that are critical to the patient's health experience. This perspective highlights the need to negotiate care on the basis of the patient's values and recognize that the values of the health care provider may be different. (2) The relational approach holds that cultures need to be understood in context and has helped alert health care providers to potential miscommunication, inaccurate diagnosis, and ineffective care. The approach also recognizes the importance of partnerships with patients and eliciting strengths. (3) The anti-racism/ anti-oppression approach helps identify the need to examine power, the inherent barriers within the health care system, and the impact of multiple factors and oppressions on the expression and experience of illness and health. The evolution in policy and discourses has led to a more complex and deep understanding of issues and recognizes the value of cultural traditions as well as the need to address social structures and systems to achieve culturally appropriate, equitable care. Lastly, the principles of complexity thinking illustrate the paradoxes of cultural issues and call for cultural competence to be recognized as an approach to care rather than a program of knowledge.

Questions for Review and Discussion

1. Explain the difference between equity and equality and why it is important to understand the distinction.
2. Reflect on your own experiences of receiving care from practitioners who were "different" from yourself in some way—did you experience any positives or hesitation based on this difference?
3. What does it mean to think of culture as a "leverage" point? Think of an example that illustrates this.
4. "Culture is created by individuals in a group or society, and in turn, influences the behaviour of individuals and society." Briefly discuss what this statement means to you. How do you see the relationship between an individual and their culture(s)?

Group Experiential/Reflection Activity

Reflect on the myth of "reverse racism." Consider the context in which you may have heard this term before. Discuss the myth of reverse racism with your peers from the perspectives of someone with a socially dominant identity and someone who is from an equity deserving group.

 http://evolve.elsevier.com/Srivastava/culturalcompetence/.

References

Albarran, J., Rosser, E., Bach, S., et al. (2011). Exploring the development of a cultural care framework for European caring science. *International Journal of Qualitative Studies on Health and Well-being, 6*(4). https://doi.org/10.3402/qhw.v6i4.11457.

Alberta Civil Liberties Association. (n.d.). *The myth of reverse racism.* http://www.aclrc.com/myth-of-reverse-racism

Auger, M. D. (2019). 'We need to not be footnotes anymore': Understanding Métis people's experiences with mental health and wellness in British Columbia, Canada. *Public Health, 176*, 92–97.

Azzopardi, C., & McNeill, T. (2016). From cultural competence to cultural consciousness: Transitioning to a critical approach to working across differences in social work. *Journal of Ethnic & Cultural Diversity in Social Work, 25*(4), 282–299.

Ball, H. (2017). The Atlantic divide: Contrasting U.K. and U.S. recommendations on cosleeping and bedsharing. *Journal of Human Lactation, 33*(4), 765–769. https://doi.org/10.1177/0890334417713943.

Beagan, B., Fredericks, E., & Goldberg, L. (2012). Nurses' work with LGBTQ clients: "They're just like everybody else, so what's the difference?". *The Canadian Journal of Nursing Research, 44*(3), 44–63.

Bird, M., & Strachan, P. H. (2020). Complexity science education for clinical nurse researchers. *Journal of Professional Nursing, 36*(2), 50–55.

Blanchet Garneau, A., & Pepin, J. (2015). Cultural competence: A constructivist definition. *Journal of Transcultural Nursing, 26*(1), 9–15.

Brosseau, L., & Dewing, M. (2018). *Canadian multiculturalism.* Ottawa: Library of Parliament. Publication No. 2009-20-E. https://lop.parl.ca/sites/PublicWebsite/default/en_CA/ResearchPublications/200920E

Canadian Nurses Association. (2020). *CNA's key messages on anti-Black racism in nursing and health*. https://www.canadian-nurse.com/en/policy-advocacy/advocacy-priorities/racism-in-health-care

Churchill, M. E., Smylie, J. K., Wolfe, S. H., et al. (2020). Conceptualising cultural safety at an Indigenous-focused midwifery practice in Toronto, Canada: Qualitative interviews with Indigenous and non-Indigenous clients. *BMJ Open*, *10*(9), e038168. https://doi.org/10.1136/bmjopen-2020-038168.

Cockburn, J. T., Thomas, F. N., & Cockburn, O. J. (1997). Solution-focused therapy and psychosocial adjustment to orthopedic rehabilitation in a work hardening program. *Journal Occupational Rehabilitation*, *7*, 97–106. https://doi.org/10.1007/BF02765880.

Corneau, S., & Stergiopoulos, V. (2012). More than being against it: Anti-racism and anti-oppression in mental health services. *Transcultural Psychiatry*, *49*(2), 261–282.

Cruz, R. A. O., Araujo, E. L. M., Nascimento, N. M., et al. (2017). Reflections in the light of the complexity theory and nursing education. *Revista Brasileira de Enfermagem*, *70*(1), 224–227.

Danso, R. (2018). Cultural competence and cultural humility: A critical reflection on key cultural diversity concepts. *Journal of Social Work*, *18*(4), 410–430.

Dictionary.com. (2020). *Multiculturalism*. https://www.dictionary.com/browse/multiculturalism?s=t

Doane, G. H., & Varcoe, C. (2007). Relational practice and nursing obligations. *Advances in Nursing Science*, *30*(3), 192–205.

Federation of Ethnic Communities' Councils of Australia. (2019). *Cultural competence in Australia: A guide*. http://fecca.org.au/wp-content/uploads/2019/05/Cultural-Competence-in-Australia-A-Guide.pdf

Fleras, A. (2019). 50 Years of Canadian multiculturalism: Accounting for its durability, theorizing the crisis, anticipating the future. *Canadian Ethnic Studies*, *51*(2), 19–59.

Galanti, G-A. (2019). *Concepts – understanding cultural diversity in healthcare*. https://www.ggalanti.org/basic-concepts-key-variations/

Goldberg, L., Rosenburg, N., & Watson, J. (2018). Rendering LGBTQ+ visible in nursing: Embodying the philosophy of caring science. *Journal of Holistic Nursing*, *36*(3), 262–271. https://doi.org/10.1177/0898010117715141.

Gottlieb, L. N. (2014). Strengths based nursing. *AJN*, *114*(8), 24–32.

Gottlieb, L. N., & Gottlieb, B. (2017). Strengths based nursing: A process for implementing a philosophy into practice. *Journal of Family Nursing*, *23*(3), 319–340.

Griffith, A. (2017). *Multiculturalism: Evolution & challenges*. http://www.thepearsoncentre.ca/platform/multiculturalism-in-canada-evolution-effectiveness-and-challenges/

Indigenous and Northern Affairs Canada. (2018). *Indigenous history in Canada*. https://www.aadnc-aandc.gc.ca/eng/1100100013778/1100100013779

Jacob, K. S. (2015). Recovery model of mental illness: A complementary approach to psychiatric care. *Indian Journal of Psychological Medicine*, *37*, 117–119. https://doi.org/10.4103/0253-7176.155605.

Jedwab, J. (2020). *Multiculturalism*. The Canadian Encyclopedia. https://www.thecanadianencyclopedia.ca/en/article/multiculturalism

Jongen, C., McCalman, J., & Bainbridge, R. (2018). Health workforce cultural competency interventions: A systematic scoping review. *BMC Health Services Research*, *18*, 232.

Katon, W., & Kleinman, A. (1980). Doctor–patient negotiation and other social science strategies in patient care. In L. Eisenberg & S. Klimidis (Eds.), *The relevance of social science for medicine* (pp. 253–279). D. Reidel Publishing.

Khambhaita, P., Willis, R., Pathak, P., et al. (2017). *Recruitment of South Asian research participants and the challenges of Khambhaita ethnic matching: Age, gender and migration history*. Centre for Research on Ageing, Faculty of Social Human and Mathematical Sciences, University of Southampton. https://eprints.soton.ac.uk/408510/

Khanlou, N., Haque, N., Skinner, A., et al. (2017). Scoping review on maternal health among immigrant and refugee women in Canada: Prenatal, intrapartum, and postnatal care. *Journal of Pregnancy*, *2017*, 8783294.

Killion, C. M. (2017). Cultural healing practices that mimic child abuse. *Annals of Forensic Research and Analysis*, *4*(2), 1042.

Kirmayer, L., & Jarvis, G. E. (2019). Culturally responsive services as a path to equity in mental healthcare. *HealthcarePapers*, *18*(2), 11–23.

Kirmayer, L., Simpson, C., & Cargo, M. (2003). Healing traditions: Culture, community and mental health promotion with Canadian Indigenous people. *Australasian Psychiatry*, *11*(Supplement). https://doi.org/10.1046/j.1038-5282.2003.02010.x.

Kongnetiman, L., & Eskow, E. (2009). *Enhancing cultural competency: A resource kit for health care professionals.* Alberta Health Services.

Leininger, M. (1991). The theory of culture care diversity and universality. In M. Leininger (Ed.), *Culture care diversity and universality: A theory of nursing* (pp. 5–72). National League for Nursing.

McCalman, J., Jongen, C., & Bainbridge, R. (2017). Organisational systems' approaches to improving cultural competence in healthcare: A systematic scoping review of the literature. *International Journal for Equity in Health*, *16*, 78. https://doi.org/10.1186/s12939-017-0571-5.

Migdal, A. (2021). *182 unmarked graves discovered near residential school in B.C.'s Interior, First Nation says.* https://www.cbc.ca/news/canada/british-columbia/bc-remains-residential-school-interior-1.6085990

Mileva-Seitz, V. R., Bakermans-Kraneburg, M. J., Battaini, C., et al. (2017). Parent-child bed sharing: The good, the bad, and the burden of evidence. *Sleep Medicine Reviews*, *32*, 4–27. https://doi.org/10.1016/j.smrv.2016.03.003.

Mukhtar, M., Dean, J., Wilson, K., et al. (2016). "But many of these problems are about funds…": The challenges immigrant settlement agencies (ISAs) encounter in a suburban setting in Ontario, Canada. *International Migration & Integration*, *17*, 389–408. https://doi.org/10.1007/s12134-015-0421-5.

Paris, E. (2018). Canada's multiculturalism is our identity. *The Globe and Mail.* https://www.theglobeandmail.com/opinion/article-canadas-multiculturalism-is-our-identity/

Pashaeypoor, S., Baumann, S. L., Hoseini, A. S., et al. (2019). Identifying and overcoming barriers for implementing Watson's human caring science. *Nursing Science Quarterly*, *32*(3), 239–244. https://doi.org/10.1177/0894318419845396.

Radermacher, H., Feldman, S., & Browning, C. (2009). Mainstream versus ethno-specific community nity aged care services: It's not an 'either or'. *Australasian Journal on Ageing*, *28*(2), 58–63. https://doi.org/10.1111/j.1741-6612.2008.00342.x.

Seligman, M. E., & Csikszentmihalyi, M. (2000). Positive psychology: An introduction. *American Psychologist*, *55*, 5–14. https://doi.org/10.1037/0003-066X.55.1.5.

Shepherd, S. M., Willis-Esqueda, C., Newton, D., et al. (2019). The challenge of cultural competence in the workplace: Perspectives of healthcare providers. *BMC Health Services Research*, *19*, 135.

Srivastava, R. (2008). *Influence of organizational factors on clinical cultural competence.* University of Toronto: Institute of Medical Sciences. Unpublished doctoral dissertation.

Srivastava, R., & Srivastava, R. (2019). Impact of cultural identity on mental health in post-secondary students. *International Journal of Mental Health and Addiction*, *17*, 520–530.

Statistics Canada. (2017). *Linguistic diversity and multilingualism in Canadian homes.* Statistics Canada Catalogue no. 98-200-X2016010.

Steinfeldt, J. A., Clay, S. L., & Priester, P. E. (2020). Prevalence and perceived importance of racial matching in the psychotherapeutic dyad: A national survey of addictions treatment clinical practices. *Substance Abuse Treatment, Prevention, and Policy*, *15*, 76. https://doi.org/10.1186/s13011-020-00318-x.

Suiter, T. (2016). Reverse racism: A discursive history. In Y. Kiuchi (Ed.), *Race still matters: The reality of African American lives and the myth of postracial society* (pp. 3–40). State University of New York Press.

Truth and Reconciliation Commission. (2015). *Truth and Reconciliation Commission of Canada: Calls to action.* http://trc.ca/assets/pdf/Calls_to_Action_English2.pdf

Viero, A., Amadasi, A., Blandino, A., et al. (2019). Skin lesions and traditional folk practices: A medico-legal perspective. *Forensic Science, Medicine and Pathology*, *15*, 580–590.

Watson, J. (2008). Social justice and human caring: A model of caring science as a hopeful paradigm moral justice for humanity. *Creative Nursing*, *14*(2), 54–61.

Watt, K., Abbott, P., & Reath, J. (2016). Developing cultural competence in general practitioners: An integrative review of the literature. *BMC Family Practice*, *17*, 158.

Wilk, P., Maltby, A., & Cooke, M. (2017). Residential schools and the effects on Indigenous health and well-being in Canada—a scoping review. *Public Health Reviews*, *38*, 8. https://doi.org/10.1186/s40985-017-0055-6.

Yee, J. Y., & Dumbrill, G. (2003). Whiteout: Looking for race in Canadian social work practice. In A. Al-Krenaw & J. R. Graham (Eds.), *Multicultural social work in Canada* (pp. 98–121). Oxford University Press.

CHAPTER 3

The Culture Care Framework

Rani H. Srivastava

LEARNING OBJECTIVES

At the end of this chapter, the learner will be able to:
- Describe the main features of the Culture Care Framework
- Discuss how cultural sensitivity, cultural knowledge, and cultural resources work together to foster cultural competence in health care
- Discuss factors that can contribute positively and negatively to the dynamics of difference
- Examine the two dimensions of cultural knowledge: generic and specific knowledge
- Identify cultural resources at the individual, organizational, and professional level
- Apply the Culture Care Framework to facilitate personal development of cultural competence

KEY TERMS

Cultural awareness	Equity	Power distance
Cultural identity	Explanatory model of	Privilege
Cultural knowledge	illness	Self-reflexivity
Cultural resources	Generic cultural	Specific cultural
Cultural sensitivity	knowledge	knowledge
Culturally congruent	Holding knowledge	Trust
care	Layers	Unlearning
Culture care	Legacies	White privilege
Culture Care Framework	Meritocracy	

This chapter describes the **Culture Care Framework** (CCF) as an approach that facilitates development and application of cultural understanding. The aim of the CCF is to make culture visible and to give health care providers a way to understand and work with cultural complexities and influences on health and health care. Based on the core concepts in Madeleine Leininger's Theory of Culture Care Diversity and Universality (Leininger, 1978), the framework is an integrative and practical approach, reflecting the issues of power as well as cultural patterns. For an overview of Leininger's theory, from a historical as well as developmental perspective, readers are referred to McFarland and Wehbe-Alamah (2019) and Busher Betancourt (2015). This chapter introduces and describes the core elements of the framework. These are further discussed with respect to application in Chapter 4.

The key elements from Leininger's theory (Leininger, 1978; McFarland & Wehbe-Alamah, 2019) that are embedded in the CCF are (1) the concept of universality and diversity of culture and care—Leininger noted that there were both similarities *and* differences among populations with respect to values, beliefs, meanings, and patterns; (2) recognizing that culture care values, beliefs, and practices are influenced by worldview and social factors such as religion, spirituality, environment, and politics; (3) appreciating that cultural groups have their own knowledge and values of health care (*emic* or insider, local perspective) and work with professional knowledge of others (*etic* perspective, such as that of health care providers); and (4) three modes of decisions and actions that can be used to provide care that integrates cultural values and knowledge into care.

The CCF was initially developed by the author in 1996 as an attempt to apply and teach cultural understanding in clinical situations. It offers an integrative and practical approach that focuses on applying key concepts of Leininger's theory within a multicultural and diverse care context, where health care providers are likely to care for patients and families from many cultures within a day. The framework evolved from practice with theory guiding exploration, understanding, and articulation of concepts and meaning. It continues to be refined through dialogue with patients, families, and health care providers across a variety of disciplines; feedback from educators and students; and research and practice-based initiatives and literature. Health care providers practising in a diverse society are acutely aware of the need to provide care that is consistent with patients' cultural values; however, application to practice, particularly in fast-paced environments, is more difficult to achieve. Fig. 3.1 presents the guiding principles underlying the framework. Leininger's theory defined care as "assistive, supportive, and enabling experiences or ideas toward others" (McFarland & Wehbe-Alamah, 2019); similarly, in the CCF "care" is interpreted broadly and includes service. Developing a relationship or engaging people is a fundamental aspect of care or service, regardless of the role one may play within health care.

Leininger (1995) defined **culture care** as "subjectively and objectively learned and transmitted values, beliefs, and patterned lifeways that assist, support, facilitate, or enable another individual or group to maintain well-being and health, to improve the human condition and lifeway, or to deal with illness, handicaps, and death" (p. 105). Simply put, the term *culture care* reflects the goal of integrating the issues of culture into all aspects of health care. The ongoing evidence of health inequities experienced by many populations has made this need more urgent. Table 3.1 highlights the main features of the CCF.

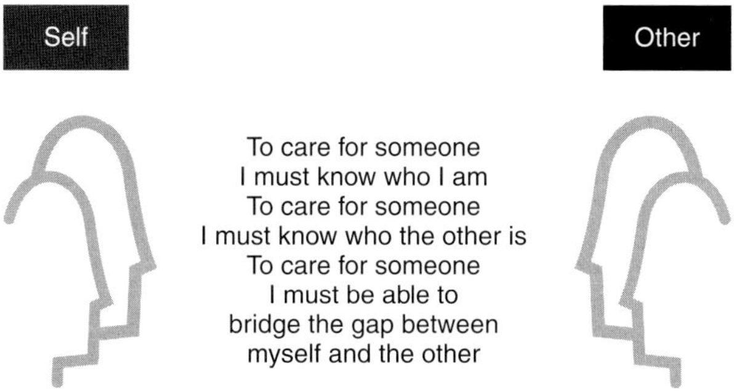

| Self | | Other |

To care for someone
I must know who I am
To care for someone
I must know who the other is
To care for someone
I must be able to
bridge the gap between
myself and the other

Fig. 3.1 Guiding Principle Behind the Culture Care Framework. (Data from Anderson J. [1987]. The cultural context of caring. *Canadian Critical Care Nursing Journal, 4*[4], 7–13.)

TABLE 3.1 ■ **Salient Features of the Culture Care Framework**

- Integrates patterns and power perspectives of cultural diversity
- Focuses on self-awareness
- Provides a way of "knowing the other"
- Recognizes the interactions between the individual and context (past and present)
- Suggests strategies for bridging the gap between self and other
- Provides a way of moving beyond understanding and awareness to application

Overview of the Culture Care Framework (CCF)

A framework is essentially a mental model or map that can be used to identify core concepts, facilitate understanding between concepts, and guide actions and decisions. There is general agreement among scholars and practitioners that cultural competence requires development in the areas of awareness (affective domain), knowledge (cognitive domain), and skills (behavioural domain) (see Hall & Theriot, 2016; Shen, 2015; Shepherd et al., 2019; Sue et al., 2009). There is less clarity and agreement, however, on what is included in each domain. It is also critical to recognize that complexities of cultural competence require a deep and broad understanding of concepts such as the dynamics of difference and equity. The CCF recognizes culture in terms of patterns (worldviews) as well as power (the dynamics of difference, various-isms, and inequities). An overview of the CCF appears in Fig. 3.2. The framework consists of three broad elements—cultural sensitivity, cultural knowledge, and cultural resources—and contends that all three elements are needed to provide effective, culturally appropriate care. Development of cultural competence by health care providers requires intentional learning in each of the three areas. The modes of action serve as useful approaches to translate awareness and knowledge into care. These are discussed in Chapter 4.

Cultural sensitivity refers to awareness, understanding, and a respect for culture and its influence on people and processes. Cultural sensitivity places the focus on self. **Cultural knowledge** recognizes that cultural competence is knowledge-based care. Cultural knowledge has two components: **generic cultural knowledge** or fundamental knowledge that can be applied across cultural and clinical populations, and **specific cultural knowledge** that is focused on specific cultural populations and the care they may require, or the processes of care associated with specific clinical populations that may be particularly impacted by differences in values and worldviews. Specific cultural knowledge is further influenced by context of care. The third element,

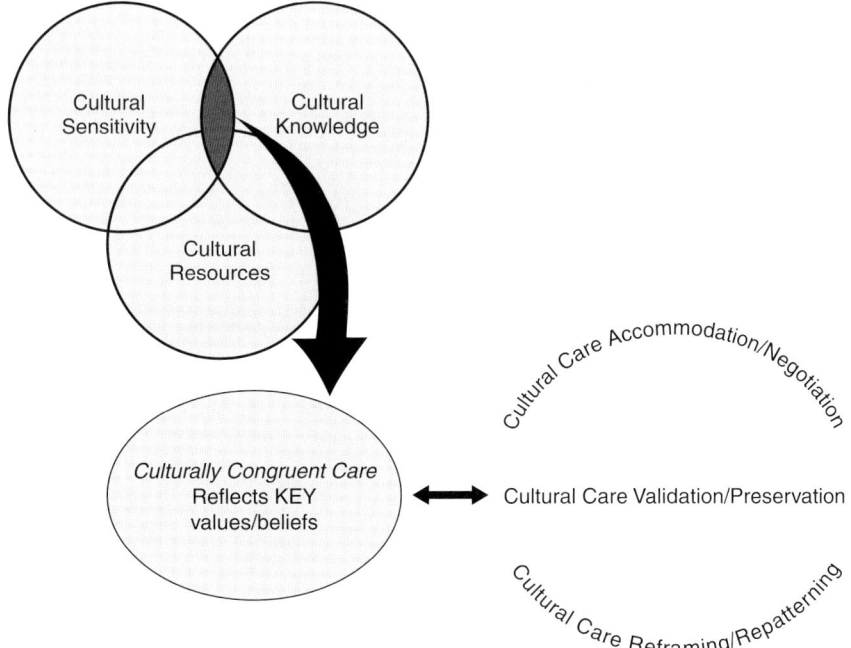

Fig. 3.2 Overview of the Culture Care Framework. For a complete discussion of the terms *accommodation/negotiation, validation/preservation*, and *reframing/repatterning*, please refer to Chapter 4.

cultural resources, recognizes that what happens in a particular clinical interaction depends not only on the cultural competence of the health care provider but also on the context of care and resources available to providers in their personal and professional environment. The elements of the framework are interconnected: sensitivity and awareness are also aspects of knowledge; cultural competence requires learning from self as well as learning from others; and, most importantly, cultural competence requires the need for unlearning. **Unlearning** refers to making a conscious choice to discard an old belief or mental model and adopt a different one (Bonchek, 2016). A famous quote often attributed to Mark Twain states, "It ain't what you know that gets you into trouble. It's what you know for sure that just ain't so" (Young, 2018). In many ways, unlearning can be harder than learning new things.

The CCF is action oriented. Acquisition of cultural knowledge, understanding, and skills need to be applied to make a difference. Change is often not readily visible. Enhanced sensitivity and awareness may begin with simply seeing or hearing things differently, or thinking differently by challenging assumptions. The new perspectives lead to doing things differently (Fig. 3.3). Strategies for navigating differences and bridging the gap across cultures are discussed in Chapter 4.

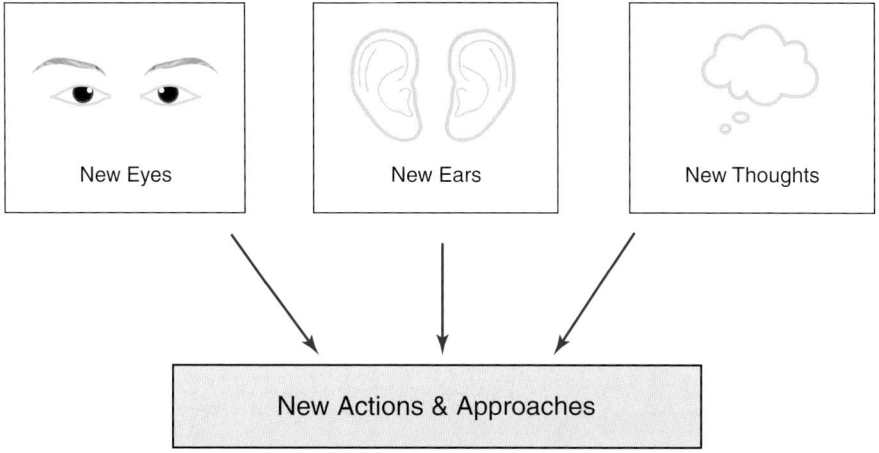

Fig. 3.3 New Eyes + New Ears + New Thoughts = New Actions.

Cultural Competence In Action

Unlearning Grammar to Promote Inclusion

Martha, a medical radiation and imaging technologist, understood that to show respect and inclusivity meant to use preferred pronouns, but it was hard for her to do so. A colleague preferred the pronoun "they"—and Martha had difficulty with this. From the time she was a child, Martha had learned that the pronoun "they" was used in reference to more than one individual. It was plural, not singular. Now gender-neutral language was challenging her knowledge of English grammar!

However, Martha continued to reflect on her discomfort, and began to notice other respected colleagues, including her manager, using the preferred pronoun. She came to understand that using the pronoun "they" for an individual did not mean she was not knowledgeable about grammar; rather it was to show respect and create an inclusive environment for her colleague and others. Martha decided to make an intentional commitment to herself to pay attention and use this pronoun where appropriate, recognizing that while it may initially feel awkward to her it would be more comfortable for others.

One of the difficulties associated with translating cultural awareness into practice, particularly in health care, is uncertainty about the exact goal or what success looks like. In the CCF, the goal of care is identified as culturally congruent, equitable care. The notion of congruence is important because it suggests a "fit" between two or more parties. Leininger described culturally congruent care as care that reflected appropriate and sensitive use of cultural knowledge to provide care that fit with patients' cultural values, beliefs, and lifeways (McFarland & Wehbe-Alamah, 2019). In simple terms, **culturally congruent care** can be described as care that incorporates key values and beliefs of the patient in the situation. Health care providers are not expected to be familiar with all aspects of a patient's culture; rather, the intent is to identify salient patient and provider values that may be affecting the situation. The goal of cultural congruence serves as a reminder for providers to ensure that these values are made explicit and care reflects patient goals along with goals established by the clinical team. Providers can use this criterion to audit their own practice for cultural competence.

Integrating culture into care is complex and challenging. In a doctoral study, interprofessional clinicians (nurses, social workers, physicians) were asked to describe what culturally competent care looked like in their practice. Results showed that despite recognizing the importance of integrating culture into care, it was hard for participants to describe what cultural competence looked like in their practice. Even with acknowledgement that they served a very diverse population in terms of race, ethnicity, sexual orientation, and gender identity, most clinicians still defaulted to the standard approach or protocols for care, unless issues or difficulties surfaced (Srivastava, 2008). Shepherd et al. (2019) noted similar findings in a study of health care workers, where 80% ($n = 56$) sometimes or often found it difficult to engage with or treat patients from cultures different than their own, yet 95% believed they always or often attended to cultural needs. This incongruence can be attributed to unawareness, overconfidence, or "entrenched dominant culture norms" (Shepherd et al., 2019, p. 8).

There are different approaches that can be taken to elicit patient values and goals and to achieve congruence; these will be further discussed in the next chapter, on bridging the gap across cultures. Culturally congruent care recognizes the importance of honouring these values and goals. Equitable care promotes best possible outcomes, by recognizing and reducing barriers to access (to information, care, and supports) and strengthening opportunities for participation and self-determination.

Cultural Considerations In Care

Knowing Yourself

Refer to the exercise in Table 1.4 (Chapter 1). Where are your strengths? What areas of knowledge do you want to explore further? How much do you know about resources that can support culturally diverse communities?

Alternatively, reflect on a recent interaction with a patient who is culturally different from yourself and the mainstream culture. How do you know that interaction reflected cultural sensitivity? Did the patient's cultural beliefs, values, or goals come up in the interaction? If they did not, how could you have modified your approach?

CULTURAL SENSITIVITY

The concept of cultural sensitivity is broad and includes the notion of cultural awareness. "Cultural awareness refers to the development of the consciousness of nurses [and other health care providers] of the different values, beliefs, norms, and lifeways of clients" (Cai, 2016, p. 270). Cultural awareness includes self-awareness, awareness of the impact of culture on identity and behaviour, awareness of and respect for different worldviews and ways of being, as well as awareness of the broader sociopolitical structures on experiences of marginalization and oppression (Danso, 2018; Federation of Ethnic Communities' Councils of Australia [FECCA], 2019).

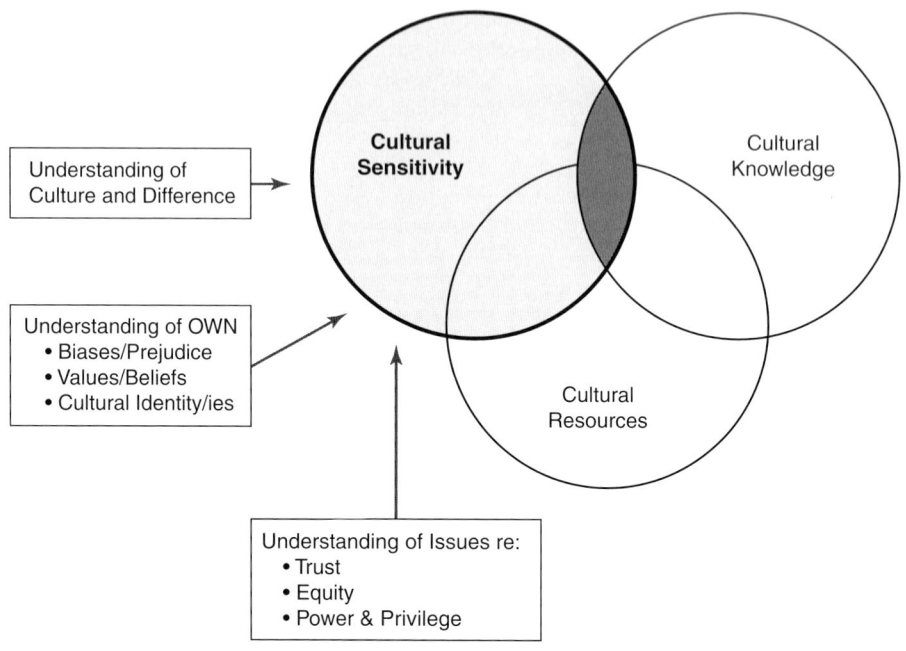

Fig. 3.4 Cultural Sensitivity.

In the CCF, **cultural awareness** is seen as a complex set of perceptions and realizations about culture and about oneself, and the dynamics associated with issues of difference. Although cultural awareness can be considered as "knowing that," sensitivity requires a greater degree of proficiency and includes "knowing how." The concepts of "knowing that" and "knowing how" have been discussed by authors such as Patricia Benner (1984) in the context of nursing skill development from novice to expert. "Knowing that" is described as theoretical knowledge acquired through systematically examining a phenomenon, whereas "knowing how" is viewed as practical knowledge and skills acquired through experience and practice. Cultural sensitivity includes *demonstrated ability* to embrace difference and examine how one's culture affects practice (Danso, 2018).

As shown in Fig. 3.4, cultural sensitivity requires developing insight with respect to

- Understanding the concepts of diversity, culture, and difference in terms of their impact on health
- Understanding one's own culture and cultural identity in terms of patterns and power
- Understanding the dynamics of difference and how to engage with issues of privilege, trust, and equity

UNDERSTANDING CULTURE AND CULTURAL IDENTITY

As discussed in previous chapters, culture is a difficult concept to grasp. As a concept, culture is dynamic: it can be complex, elusive, and at times paradoxical. Culture includes, but is more than, ethnicity, race, and social location. Culture exists at the level of individual, group, organization, and society and serves a dual function, with the integrative values and beliefs giving an individual the rules of engagement with the surrounding world as well as a sense of identity (Srivastava & Srivastava, 2019).

Culture as Identity

Culture refers to shared identities based on values, beliefs, norms, and other characteristics. The extent to which specific traits are shared varies across individuals within a cultural group; thus, although culture is shared, no two people within a culture are identical. Culture is both individual and collective. To understand an individual's culture, we must understand the concept of identity.

There are many types of identities, each reflecting a different set of criteria that may be used to differentiate among individuals or to reinforce sameness. Almost daily all of us negotiate and navigate multiple identities, such as parent, student, doctor, nurse, social worker, immigrant, or person of colour. Key features to note about identity include the following:

1. Different identities are prominent under different circumstances.
2. Intersections of identities can significantly influence experience (e.g., a health care provider who identifies as Indigenous or person of colour may experience a situation differently than another health care provider from a different background or person of colour who is not a health care provider).
3. Identities are often ascribed by others and may have different meanings for others than for the individuals being appraised or labelled. Labels are inherently problematic, and it is important to determine how individuals see and describe themselves.
4. Cultural identity, like culture, is also dynamic and can shift over time and place.

Fig. 3.5 illustrates how individuals are simultaneously unique and similar. Fig. 3.6 presents a visual image of culture as being composed of multiple dimensions of identity.

How does one begin to understand an individual's culture? The recognition that multiple identities exist within the individual allows health care providers to explore the various identities potentially impacting a situation. Thus it becomes possible to identify the cultures and the associated key values and beliefs that might be influencing the interaction. Cultural sensitivity is not about understanding a cultural label or one aspect of identity (e.g., race); rather, it requires

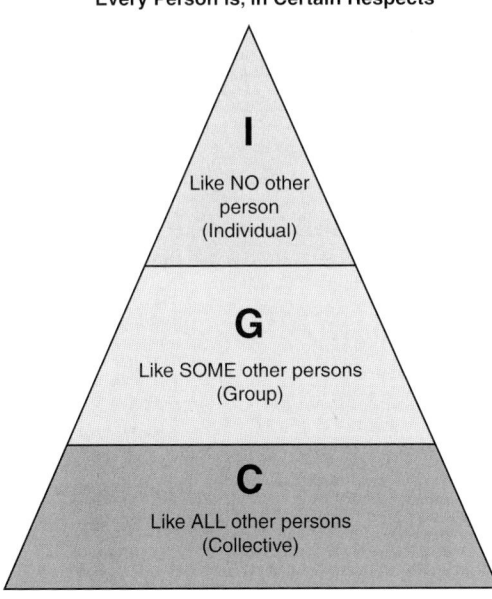

Fig. 3.5   Identity: Simultaneously Unique and Collective. (Adapted from Kluckhohn, C., & Murray, H. A. [1962]. *Personality in nature, society and culture.* Alfred A Knopf.)

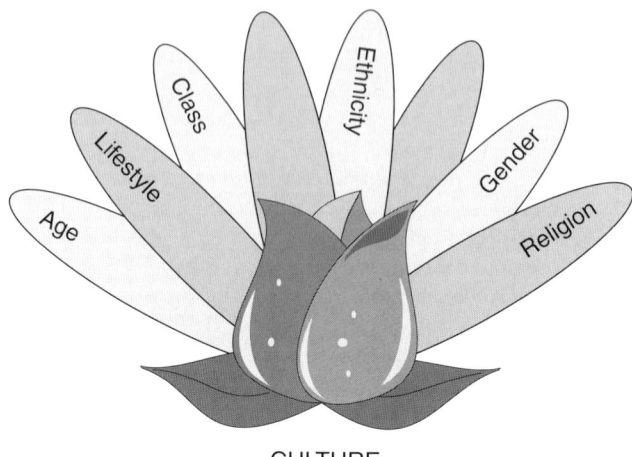

CULTURE

Fig. 3.6 Conceptualization of Culture as Multidimensional Identities (Culture as Patterns).

recognition and an intersectional understanding of various identities and how they influence a given interaction. For example, it is important to assess how various identities of age, gender, race, ethnicity, sexual orientation, etc., impact a situation. Some identities may take on a greater significance in the current health context than others. Sometimes challenges and opportunities arise from the combination of identities; therefore, it becomes essential to consider not just which identity or identities are most important, but also the potential impact of the combination(s).

Cultural Competence In Action

Understanding My Culture

How would you describe your cultural identity? What groups are you like? Consider gender, age, professional role, family status, immigration status, sexual orientation, race, ethnicity, acculturation, and so on.

If you were to discuss your answers in a group, are there some identities that you would be comfortable talking about and others that you would not be comfortable talking about? Why might they be?

Pick two identities and discuss some of the characteristics associated with them. During the discussion, note the degree to which different people have similar or differing beliefs about identities. Why do you think that is?

Cultural identity can be understood in terms of a sense of self that is self-created, ascribed by others, and formed through social forces, past and present (Anderson-Lain, 2017), that may be unique to the individual's experience or perception of their situation (Groen et al., 2018). "Cultural identity focuses on norms and values that constitute an image an individual holds of [self], which urges an individual to decide what is right or wrong, what kind of behaviour is appropriate or not; as well as on norms and values that are negotiated within the (ethnic or ethnoreligious) group the individual belongs to, and within local society" (Groen et al., 2018, p. 70). In other words, cultural identity is a composite of how aspects of various identities manifest in individuals and the meanings attached to those manifestations (Srivastava & Srivastava, 2019). Accordingly, cultural identity is shaped, not prescribed, by heritage as well as experiences. Experiences of prejudice and discrimination can lead to a denial or silencing of one's cultural identity for some, while others may experience stronger identification with their cultural group and seek out a sense of belonging. Cultural experiences of social power can strengthen identification with cultural group(s) (Srivastava & Srivastava, 2019).

Cultural identity influences interpretation of events and interactions with others and is associated with experiences of marginalization or privilege depending on the social power or importance associated with that identity. Fig. 3.7 illustrates the concept of cultural identity as a flower: the centre refers to the dominant norm in society, and each petal is an identity category where one can be placed—either close to the centre or further away depending on how similar or different it is from what is regarded as the "norm" with respect to social power.

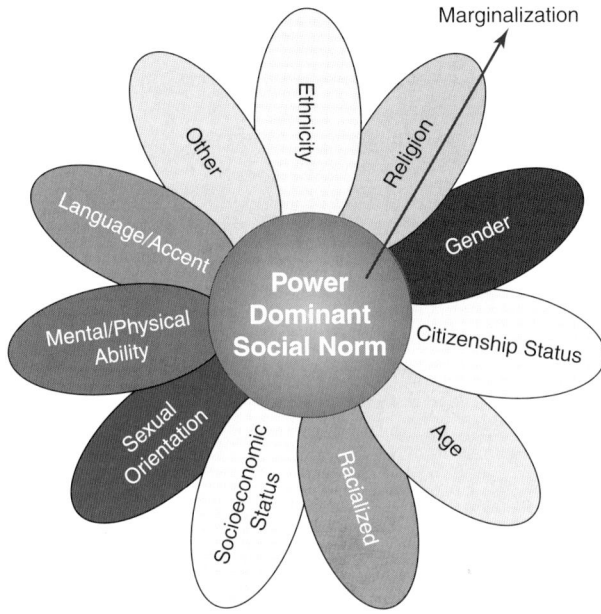

Fig. 3.7 Cultural Identity with Respect to Social Location (Culture as Power).

Cultural Considerations In Care

Reflection on Racial Autobiography

The questions below are meant to promote reflection. Jot down answers for yourself. Also note any thoughts these might generate—you can go back to them later. Feel free to discuss your responses with colleagues or friends you feel comfortable with.

- When was the first time you realized you were _____(fill in your racial or ethnic identity)?
- When was the first time you realized you might be treated differently because of your skin colour?
- When was the first time you realized people of other racialized identities were treated differently in certain circumstances?
- Look at the group of people you usually socialize with—to which racial/ethnic group(s) do they belong? How has that influenced your understanding of racial/ethnic identity and experiences in society?
- When you read this activity did you think this included or excluded White readers? Do you consider being Caucasian or White as a racial identity? Why or why not?

Adapted from Whites for Racial Equality. (2019). *Awareness activities: Racial autobiography and reflection.* https://whitesforracialequity.org/1-awareness-activity-reflection-questions/.

Understanding Your Own Values, Biases, Prejudices, and Privilege

Self-awareness is a critical component of cultural competence. Cultural dynamics are part of all interactions, whether they are recognized or not. Our perspectives are informed by "single stories"—a phrase used by author Chimamanda Adichie (2009) to describe false perceptions and stereotypes that are formed on the basis of our experiences. These perceptions can be about people or processes. When Adichie, a Nigerian-born writer, started to write as a child, all her stories included snow, eating apples, drinking ginger beer, and characters that were White and blue-eyed, because those were the stories she was reading. As she states, "this despite the fact that I lived in Nigeria. I had never been outside Nigeria. We didn't have snow. We ate mangoes." She talks about how her own perceptions of Mexican people were shaped by the stories of Mexicans, portrayed as "abject immigrants," and she carried this bias until she visited Mexico and saw a different reality. Single stories show people in one way only, leading to tunnel vision, and as the story is repeated in our minds the stereotype becomes fact. By recognizing their own cultural values and biases, health care providers can better understand and mitigate unintentional influences.

It is important for health care providers to understand not only what they value, but also what they dislike, fear, or are otherwise biased against. Everyone has biases and prejudices. One way for health care providers to check their own biases is to ask themselves: "Why do I believe or think what I do in this situation? Would someone else looking at this situation come to the same conclusion, or could they come up with a different interpretation?" The answers can be illuminating and may reveal implicit assumptions and biases that are influencing the perception of the situation. Researchers at Harvard University have developed the Implicit Association Test (IAT), which can be taken by individuals to better understand their own biases on a variety of dimensions (see https://implicit.harvard.edu/implicit/canada/takeatest.html).

Legacies and Layers

Our perception of the world is influenced by our own history (what we have learned and experienced) as well as the history of our ancestors and predecessors. **Legacies** are powerful historical events experienced by our ancestors, family, and community of origin that continue to have ripple effects in our lives today. Examples of legacies include colonization, slavery, trauma, capture and redistribution of land, the Holocaust, and the Civil Rights Movement. Even though these events may have happened decades ago, the impact was so powerful that the influence extends across time and generations. Legacies can be a powerful influence on how individuals view themselves and subsequent interactions.

In an article examining Erik Erickson's influence on culture, race, and ethnicity, Syed and Fish (2018) situate legacies of slavery and colonialism "not just as factors in the past that have residual input, but rather as ongoing oppressive forces that shape opportunities for positive development" (p. 278). They note that the historical context of slavery for African Americans can lead to a lack of identity or a negative identity, thus identifying a need for assertion of personhood, value, and agency as part of identity development and well-being—a task made more challenging by ongoing experiences of racism and domination by the White majority. While the legacy of colonialism is one of *cultural loss* for Indigenous people, for African American (or some Black) people, there can be a sense of "never was" when it comes to ancestry and culture. Legacies can also come with strengths that highlight survival and the ability to create social change through leadership and collective action (Schwartz & Sánchez, 2016).

Layers are akin to the notion of intersectionality and can be described as the various aspects of our identity and life experiences that shape perception. As suggested earlier, they can include race, ethnicity, gender, age, marital status, education level, socioeconomic status, religion, sexual orientation, and profession. Layers and legacies are dynamically intertwined, and they contribute to our ideas and beliefs about a variety of issues, including those related to culture, diversity, and health. For health care providers, it is critical to consider all the layers of identity as well as the legacies that lead to assumptions and biases on the part of everyone involved.

As discussed in Chapter 2, a common misconception surrounding cultural competence is that we must accept everything. This is simply not true. Respecting the choices of others does not mean endorsing those choices or the values involved. Nor does it mean forsaking our own values. In fact, self-awareness and personal insight can strengthen appreciation for our own culture while developing respect for other cultures. Cultural clashes often are less about differing values than about how the differences are treated. Consider the difference between having discriminatory tastes and being discriminatory: the first is generally regarded positively and often is a desired trait, whereas the second is usually regarded in a negative light and deemed unacceptable. The difference is in the *impact* of the choices. Having discriminatory tastes usually is associated with being selective and having high or unique expectations or standards. The impact is largely on oneself. However, being discriminatory has an impact on others. It is an imposition of personal choices on others, is associated with exclusion, and has an adverse effect on the ability of others to participate fully in their environment.

Understanding our culture goes beyond being clear about our own values and beliefs. It also is critical to understand the historical legacies and the current layers of power, privilege, and social position. Syed and Fish (2018) point out that the historical context may be "the most fundamental aspect" of identities when it comes to Native Americans, African Americans, and, likely, other groups (p. 278). Health care providers must recognize when and how their personal and professional views can, consciously and unconsciously, negatively affect others, and challenge themselves and others accordingly.

Understanding the Dynamics of Difference

As human beings, we often respond to the unusual and unfamiliar with vigilance and suspicion. Reactions to differences are generally automatic, often subconscious, and based on inherent cultural assumptions. Fear and lack of familiarity or experience with something are the most common barriers to providing culturally sensitive care. Fear often involves the fear of losing something, such as control, power, values, or traditions. In clinical situations, there may be a fear of losing control over the care delivery process or losing personal status as the expert health care provider. Familiarity may decrease fear but does not necessarily promote understanding.

Identifying and understanding the dynamics of difference is the first step to managing the dynamics in ways that minimize the negative and optimize the positive opportunities associated with cultural diversity. It is important to remember that difference is about different worldview as well as about judgement of the difference as inferior. Health care providers need to understand the dynamics of difference at multiple levels. As discussed in Chapters 1 and 2, loss of culture and marginalization in society can lead to increased health risks for both patients and communities. It is equally important for health care providers to recognize the dynamics of difference within the health care provider–patient relationship that can lead to patient values and choices being ignored or excluded in the health care provided.

Consider the following quotation by Ralph Waldo Emerson: "Who you are speaks so loudly, I can't hear what you're saying." Several interpretations are possible, including the following:

- Actions speak louder than words.
- What you do determines who you are.
- Our beliefs (stereotypes) about people determine our judgements regarding their ability and credibility; it is not necessarily about words or actions but rather about the interpretation or meaning ascribed to the words or actions by others.

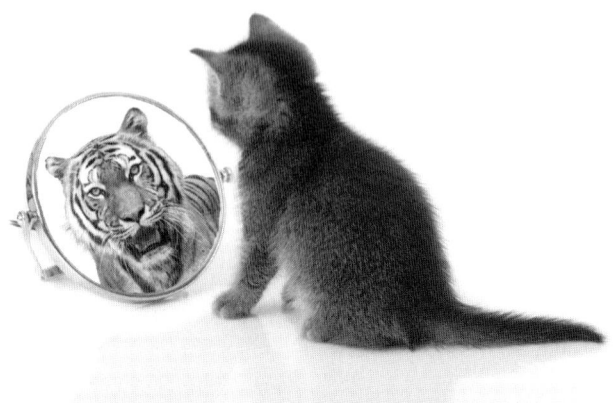

Fig. 3.8   How Do Others See You? (Courtesy iStock.com/ewastudio.)

Cultural sensitivity requires that health care providers become aware of their own assumptions and avoid labelling and judging people. It also requires that providers become aware of the assumptions that others might have or make about them. As illustrated in Fig. 3.8, health care providers may view themselves as a comforting kitten—trustworthy, with positive intentions and expertise; however, our patients and clients may see something else and respond with fear or concern.

When health care providers know how they might come across to others in particular situations, they can better understand and manage the dynamics proactively, thus minimizing or avoiding misinterpretations or unintentional influences. For example, when we are aware that some patients may say "yes" simply to show respect for the health care provider's authority and not ask questions, additional questions can be used to elicit patient views and concerns. This is further discussed in Chapter 4.

Many factors influence the dynamics of an interaction. The CCF focuses on three: privilege, trust, and equity, which are all important in health care interactions and affect provider–patient relationships. An understanding of dynamics of difference needs to be applied throughout the processes of care—from assessment and intervention to outcomes and evaluation.

Privilege

Privilege can be defined as a right or benefit available to specific person(s) or a restricted group that exceeds the advantages available to others (dictionary.com, 2020). Privilege is ubiquitous and a difficult concept to make visible and acknowledge. It is often described in terms of feeling natural, having choices, a warm fuzzy blanket of comfort, or something that facilitates the path forward. **White privilege** can be described as unearned power that is grounded in values of the dominant White society and allocated to White people without a specific request by individuals (Teelucksingh, 2018). It is associated with economic, social, and environmental advantage and an absence of consequences of systemic racism (Dudzinski, 2018; Funnell et al., 2020; Russell, 2020). One of the defining characteristics of White privilege is the ability not to engage in conversations of privilege, equity, and discrimination. Privilege is often unearned (e.g., White privilege or male privilege); however, at times it may be based on hard work (e.g., post-secondary education). Even in the example of education privilege that is earned because of hard work, it is important to recognize other factors that aided in accessing education and remember that the benefits it confers become invisible and can be easily taken for granted.

Cultural Competence In Action

Exploring Privilege and Marginality

Refer to Fig. 3.7. In each petal, mark an "X" at a point where your social location is reflected.[1] For example, in the citizenship status petal a Canadian citizen by birth would be close to the centre; a naturalized Canadian citizen would be a little farther away; a permanent resident—still farther; on a temporary visa (student visa) still farther; and a refugee claimant or on an expired visa—at the very tip of the petal. Do this for all other petals. Once finished, join all the X's together with a line.

What do you notice with regard to the shape of the line—is it a circle, oval, or jagged? What emotions surfaced for you as you were doing this activity?

For most people the connecting line across identities is jagged, in that they are closer to the centre and thus privileged along some identities and farther away or marginalized along others. It is often surprising for individuals to recognize that privilege and marginalization can coexist and to "see" the privilege they may have. For some individuals (usually White males/females), the line is smoother and closer to the centre, indicating a great deal of privilege, which can also lead to feelings of guilt that can be paralyzing or seen as an "undue burden" (Dudzinski, 2018, p. 4). Neither response is helpful—what is important is to recognize and embrace the privilege and think about how it can be used in a positive way to challenge inequities, racism, and discrimination. (Also see discussion on allyship in Chapter 4.)

It is important to note that White privilege, like privilege across other identities, is experienced differently by individuals. For example, White privilege experienced by a White single mother in a low-income neighbourhood will be experienced differently than a middle-class family living in an affluent neighbourhood. For the single mom it is easier to recognize the marginalization that may be associated with the neighbourhood and income rather than the White privilege. Like culture, privilege is also invisible and often hidden from those who have it. **Self-reflexivity** refers to processes of critical self-examination, on an ongoing basis. Accepting the notion of privilege means giving up the notion of **meritocracy** (a belief that individual success is solely based on merit, hard work, ability, and accomplishment). This can be particularly difficult for a society that values individual success, freedom, opportunity, and equality—yet a critical step in developing cultural competence. Cultural competence requires an examination of our own reality, the assumptions on which it is based, and a commitment to using privilege to achieve the goal of equity.

Trust

Trust is an everyday concept with an implied meaning. It is fundamental to helping all relationships across health disciplines and is associated with positive patient outcomes (Chandra et al., 2018; Hawley & Morris, 2017). Within health care, patient trust is based on expectations that the health care provider will be knowledgeable, compassionate, and dependable; will take responsibility for the care that is needed; and the care will lead to good outcomes (Chandra et al., 2018). Providers may feel that their professional role and status automatically makes them deserve or be entitled to trust. This assumption is erroneous. Legacies of past abuse and ongoing racism and discrimination, at both the individual and societal level, make it very difficult for many populations to trust the health care system (Hawley & Morris, 2017; Turpel-Lafond, 2020). The cultural mistrust can carry over to the individual provider(s) that are part of the system (Baker, 2020; Johnstone et al., 2018; Khullar et al., 2020; Wesson et al., 2019).

---

[1] It is important to do the activity with respect to how you are located in society overall, not your own sense of empowerment related to the particular identity.

TABLE 3.2 ■ **Key Characteristics of Trust**

---

1. Trust requires conscious intention and effort to build and maintain it.
2. Trust is built on knowing the patient in a holistic and unique way, requiring acknowledgement of cultural legacies and respect for cultural layers and individual preferences.
3. Trust and good communication are inextricably linked. Trust requires good listening and empathic engagement.
4. Trust requires faith in provider credibility and commitment to providing safe care.
5. Trust requires collaborative partnerships with a commitment to co-learning.

Adapted from Johnstone, M. J., Rawson, H., Hutchinson, A. M., et al. (2018). Fostering trusting relationships with older immigrants hospitalised for end-of-life care. *Nursing Ethics*, 25(6), 760–772.

The health care system expects patients to disclose a great deal of information, some of which the patient may not feel is relevant, at least during the initial visit. Trust influences what patients disclose, as well as when and to whom. Patients may have difficulty trusting an unfamiliar system that they cannot interact with effectively and that does not seem to understand them.

Although trust often takes time to develop, the impact of first impressions cannot be underestimated. Experience with non–English-speaking patients indicates that these patients tend to determine trustworthiness of the provider very early in the interaction. It is important to "get it right from the start" (Johnstone et al., 2018, p. 765). Ensuring that sufficient time and effort are spent early in the relationship to gain (or confirm) a patient's trust is critical, instead of taking the trust for granted. In addition to being earned, trust must be cultivated and sustained (Chandra et al., 2018; Wesson et al., 2019). Key steps in building trust may include acknowledging the patient's potential mistrust of the health care system; being aware of variations in patient preferences and priorities; developing a relationship that is respectful and nonjudgemental; and developing partnerships with humility and a commitment to co-learning (Hawley & Morris, 2017; Johnstone et al., 2018; Wesson et al., 2019). Table 3.2 summarizes key themes on trust.

Cultural Competence In Action

Managing Others' Perceptions

A. Evelyn

Evelyn is a nurse of Asian background. She has become aware that individuals with her background often do not differentiate between the gendered pronouns "he" and "she" in the way that lifelong English speakers do. The pronoun difference led to communication difficulties with colleagues when she talked about her patients during rounds, as well as difficulties with families when she inadvertently used the wrong gendered pronoun (e.g., referring to the daughter as "he").

Since Evelyn became aware of how her culture can have an adverse impact on the effectiveness of her communication, she has developed two strategies to minimize any negative impact:
1. She tries to avoid pronoun problems by referring to patients by name (or by relationship, such as "your mother") when speaking to families.
2. She has acknowledged this difficulty with her colleagues and asked them to let her know if they are not certain whom she is talking about (previously, colleagues were reluctant to appear rude).

B. Saira

Saira is a health educator who is passionate about her work and animated in her discussions. However, she has recognized that her animation can be misinterpreted as anger and may be intimidating to others. Her "loudness" can be a barrier that prevents others from hearing the message she intends to convey.

Continued

> This was becoming a challenge in her personal life as well because her partner's "cultural expectations" require women to be soft spoken. Saira now manages this potential for miscommunication by monitoring two areas of behaviour:
>
> 1. Her own behaviour
> 2. Other people's response to her
>
> Previously, when she saw someone withdrawing from her, she assumed they did not understand or were uninterested; thus her natural response was to become more animated. Now she takes more cues from others and tries a softer style of engagement. Although she has explained to her partner that her "loudness" is passion, not anger, she recognizes that cultural reactions often are unconscious and hard to change. Therefore the couple worked out a system whereby he can give her feedback without it interfering with the communication. Now, when Saira and her partner have a passionate, animated discussion that becomes "too loud" for him, he simply reminds her that they are in the same room and next to each other. The loudness is addressed in a nonthreatening way so that they can each hear what the other is truly saying. Saira has been able to apply this understanding to her clinical work by explaining to her patients that she can get really animated and asking them to let her know when that starts to interfere with the clarity of the message. As well, she intentionally focuses on patients' verbal and nonverbal responses and uses them as cues to guide her own behaviour.

Equity: Barriers and Building Blocks

The concept of equity has been discussed in Chapters 1 and 2. Equality is rooted in the concept of equal opportunity, a cherished value within North American society, and focuses on *equality in the process*. By contrast, **equity**, also rooted in equal opportunity, focuses on *equality of outcomes*. Cultural sensitivity requires that providers comprehend the difference between equity and equality in a way that they can recognize cultural strengths and address barriers to equity. Within health care, there is ample evidence that "equal" or "same treatment for all" results in inequitable health outcomes for some (see Chapter 1). To ensure equal access to health care for all individuals, we must examine the barriers to equity more closely.

In the early 1990s, the Ontario anti-racism secretariat identified five barriers to equity that can transform barriers into building blocks (Ontario Ministry of Citizenship, 1995). These barriers or potential building blocks include the following:

1. Information
2. Connections
3. Experience and expertise
4. Resources
5. Decision making

The building blocks also can be considered as elements or sources of power.

Information. Most of us would agree that information is power. Health care providers need to consider not only issues involving access to information (e.g., language and literacy) but also the kind of information that people access, the sources of information or knowledge, and the kind of information that is considered legitimate or relevant (e.g., teaching nutrition using the typical Canadian diet may not be helpful to someone who recently moved here from Jamaica and eats different foods). It is also important to remember that patients with nondominant racial, ethnic, or cultural backgrounds are less likely to be heard and are disadvantaged with respect to being able to advocate for themselves (Hawley & Morris, 2017).

The information barrier can be transformed into a building block when its influence is recognized and purposefully used to improve the following:

- *Accessibility* (e.g., when information is conveyed in the patient's language and appropriate literacy level and in a manner that assesses understanding and invites questions; widespread health promotion communication through ethnic media may also be helpful)

- *Credibility* (i.e., the information comes from sources that are deemed to be credible and trusted, such as community leaders and healers)
- *Relevance* (i.e., the information uses and builds on concepts that are familiar and important to the patient; patient perspectives and needs are recognized with respect to issues and priorities)

Connections. A great deal of communication happens informally through networks. Groups that are excluded from dominant networks are at risk for missing information or opportunities. Connections can be critical to gaining access to information and resources and for developing credibility. Connections also serve to reinforce thoughts and can thus help to reinforce the status quo or dominant ideas or challenge perspectives. Health care providers must consider the connections that a patient has and the potential influences of those connections. For example, a patient whose community stigmatizes mental illness may have difficulty seeking and accepting help, as well as integrating back into society. Recognizing the strengths and limitations of connections also helps us identify perspectives that may be missing from our day-to-day interactions. For example, patients unfamiliar with a particular treatment option may find comfort in connecting with members of their own community who have had experience with this type of treatment.

Health care providers also need to reflect on their own connections. Discussing situations with like-minded individuals will probably result in a high degree of agreement. However, seeking out individuals who could have a different perspective is likely to result in a broader range of interpretations and possibilities. Purposeful development and use of connections can broaden the worldview of both the health care provider and the patient. Health care providers who seek out information about a particular community and cultural influences on care are better able to enhance their own assessment skills, develop credibility, and provide more effective care to diverse populations.

Experience/Expertise. In any health interaction, it is critical to recognize what expertise is being valued and what may be discarded by the patient, the health care provider, or both. For example, health care providers may ask about a patient's experience with a particular medication or treatment, but might not think about posing similar questions about herbal or other nonpharmacological agents or other forms of treatment. Patients' stories often remain unheard because health care providers are looking only for specific information and the patient's other perceptions or beliefs are not considered valid or legitimate. Patients may place greater value on whether a health care provider seems trustworthy and less on professional credentials.

Cultural Competence In Action

Patients Can Be Experts Too

Gcina visited her family physician with her daughter, Thoka, and provided a history in the following manner: "For the past 4 days, my daughter has had a low-grade fever during the day and it spikes in the evening." At this point the doctor interrupted and asked Gcina if she had measured the temperature with a thermometer and recorded it on paper to see the trend she was describing. Gcina's response was "no." The doctor responded by saying, "So you can tell temperature by touch, can you?" Gcina was embarrassed and perceived this as a dismissive response. She did not know how to respond further and said little throughout the rest of the interaction.

Consider this situation from the physician's point of view: is the physician's expectation of temperature measurement and record appropriate and legitimate? How might Gcina have contributed to this expectation? Does it make a difference to know that Gcina is a nurse and has considerable experience in the pediatric setting?

How could the physician handle such an interaction differently to benefit from a mother's expert knowledge of her child and meet the need for specific data on which to base a diagnosis and intervention? What if the doctor had asked for more information on what helped distinguish between no fever, low-grade fever, and spike in a nonjudgemental way?

Cultural Considerations In Care

Keeping Written Records Doesn't Thrill Everyone

Mainstream North American society relies heavily on data and trends as noted by graphs. For self-care management, patients are often asked to maintain a diary or record of their symptoms or response to treatment (e.g., documenting blood pressure, blood sugar, fluid intake, or temperature). However, people vary as to their preference for and value of written documentation. There is a real possibility that patients will come for follow-up appointments with incomplete records or, worse, with records that have been completed to please the health care provider and may be inaccurate.

Decision Making. Health care decisions and health behaviours are influenced by cultural values (Levin-Zamir et al., 2017). To achieve equity it is important to reflect on how decisions are made. Who has input and who is at the table when various options are being considered? The role of consultations in the ultimate decision also needs to be clear. Is the consultation or input being sought simply to inform someone else's decision, or is it expected that the input will be reflected in the outcome? It is also important to consider the decision maker and the basis on which decisions are made. Often, the context significantly influences people's ability to participate effectively in decision making (Khanlou et al., 2017). A patient who does not speak English and cannot access an interpreter is unable to participate effectively in decisions regarding health care. Similarly, if a patient cannot relate to the treatment being proposed, the cultural barrier remains and informed decision making is compromised, even if an interpreter is used to address the linguistic barrier. Patients may also wish to consult others before decisions are made, and while some consultations may be recognized and supported by the health care setting (e.g., consultations with immediate family), others may not (e.g., consultations with extended family, community healers, or Elders).

Cultural Considerations In Care

Decisions: Needs and Consequences

Consider the situation of a patient who chooses not to take medications during a period of fasting. What decision is being made here: to honour the fast or to disregard the medication? What are the consequences of this decision for the patient's physical and spiritual health and for the patient's relationship with the health care team, particularly if some members of the team perceive the refusal to take medications as "nonadherence"?

Resources. Resources are fundamental to achieving equity, and providers need to consider how resources are accessed and allocated. For example, if interpreter services are available to health care providers but no clear mechanism exists to inform patients that they can request or arrange for an interpreter, access is still compromised.

In some instances, health care providers feel that if a patient seeks help through an emergency room or walk-in clinic, the patient is willingly accepting the treatment offered. This assumption is erroneous. The patient may not know in advance what to expect or may be unfamiliar with the treatment that is offered. Even if patients know that a medical approach is different from what they are used to, they simply may not know what else to do or may not have access to any other resources. Thus, patients access what they can, even if it is with a combination of fear, trepidation, and hope.

In summary, culture sensitivity focuses on the first part of the guiding principles; knowing "who I am" (see Fig. 3.1) and self-awareness includes how one is situated in a broader personal and professional context. It also requires humility and the ability to develop relationships across difference to serve as the foundation for collaborative partnerships and engagement with patients, families, and communities.

Cultural Knowledge

Cultural knowledge is widely recognized as a critical element of cultural competence, but exactly what makes up the base of that knowledge is murky. What, for example, do we mean by *knowledge*? The term can be defined as "familiarity, awareness, or understanding gained through experience or study" (American Heritage Dictionaries, 2020). Frequently, health care providers' views are perceived as professional knowledge that reflects the culmination of what has been learned through professional education and socialization and built on by clinical experience. Conversely, when it comes to patients, their views are referred to as cultural beliefs. A *belief* is defined as a mental acceptance of, and conviction in, the truth, actuality, or validity of something (American Heritage Dictionaries, 2020). The implication is the knowledge that health care providers possess is superior to the beliefs that patients hold. While a reasonable assertion for clinical knowledge, it is important for health care providers to closely examine their own sources of knowledge and to accept patient cultural knowledge as legitimate, even when it is not part of the health care provider's own worldview. Health care also privileges "evidence" as garnered through research, whereas many patients and communities prefer knowledge and wisdom that has been passed down from generations or is grounded in lived experience.

Cultural knowledge is a key domain of cultural competence; however, the literature is unclear on how cultural knowledge is defined and understood. Implied definitions of cultural knowledge often limit it to information about cultures—understanding of different beliefs, values, worldviews, etiquettes (including do's and don'ts), cultural aspects of disease incidence, and biocultural variation (Alizadeh & Chavan, 2016; Cai, 2016; Khanlou et al., 2017; Rising, 2017; Yu et al., 2020). However, there are also expanded conceptualizations that include culture of biomedicine (Almutairi et al., 2017), knowledge about processes of marginalization (Wesp et al., 2018), and recognition of the dynamic nature of complex social identities as well as similarities and differences across cultural groups (Higginbottom et al., 2011).

Cultural generalities should not be used to obscure individual differences, but the generalities are helpful in recognizing and understanding cultural patterns. Consider the saying by Thomas Khun, "You don't see something until you have the right metaphor to perceive it" (Gleick, 1987, p. 262). Cultural knowledge is about understanding a variety of worldviews so that we can expand our own repertoire of metaphors. Pattern recognition is easier when the pattern is familiar and meaningful. Leininger (1995) refers to this understanding of cultural patterns as **holding knowledge**—knowledge of cultural patterns that is held by the health care provider and used to reflect on ideas and experiences, not to make stereotypical judgements. This is like the notion of "informed not knowing," described in the social work literature as knowledge of groups which "can be helpful to sensitize social workers to potential cultural practices and experiences of individuals without essentializing them" (Azzopardi & McNeill, 2016, p. 288). Health care providers have always studied facets of groups (e.g., psychosocial concerns of cardiac patients) and patterns (e.g., stages of grieving) without the expectation that all patients who fall into the general group (e.g., cardiac patients and those experiencing grief) will exhibit identical behaviours; instead, this knowledge is "held" by providers and used in care selectively when it is relevant. Similarly, cultural knowledge is knowledge of populations that needs to be used selectively to better understand and manage the clinical encounter.

It is important to consider how cultural knowledge is developed. Knowledge development is often attributed to personal and professional encounters; however, these can be limiting. Intentional seeking and critical examination of information are important to understand applicability. Most importantly, it is essential to validate the applicability of information to individual patients and encounters. The vast variety and quantity of cultural information can be overwhelming. The CCF provides a streamlined approach that allows health care providers to focus on two broad areas of cultural knowledge:

1. *Generic cultural knowledge:* basic knowledge about cultural domains and processes that apply across a wide variety of cultural groups. Examples of generic cultural knowledge include an understanding of historical legacies such as colonialism, enslavement, and holocaust; systemic and structural barriers that perpetuate health inequities; cross-cultural communication; care processes that are shaped by culture; and cultural issues related to families. Generic cultural knowledge applies across cultural environments and enables providers to see nuanced similarities and differences across groups. This, in turn, can lead to greater insights across cultural environments (Stadler, 2017).

2. *Specific cultural knowledge:* knowledge that focuses on the specific cultural groups, or aspects of care that are influenced by culture. Specific cultural knowledge is often desired as it is focused and frequently more concrete; however, indiscriminate use of specific cultural knowledge risks missing key contextual information and stereotyping (Stadler, 2017). Examples of specific cultural knowledge could involve focusing on the values and beliefs of specific cultural groups such as an Indigenous nation or the Muslim community in a particular part of the country, the health issues faced by particular populations such as immigrants and refugees, or pain management across cultures.

In a critical review of culture-specific versus culture-general intercultural competence development in a global world, Stadler (2017) notes that both approaches have their strengths and limitations and argues for an integrated, combined approach. Similarly, the CCF contends that both types of knowledge are necessary for the development of cultural competence in health care (Fig. 3.9). The generic and specific areas work hand in hand because a strong grasp of generic cultural knowledge alerts the health care provider to potential issues that should be explored and to information that may be required in specific clinical situations.

GENERIC CULTURAL KNOWLEDGE

Different authors have identified different domains of culture as important components for health care providers to understand (see Alizadeh & Chavan, 2016; Cai, 2016; Olaussen & Renzaho, 2016; Yu et al., 2020). *Generic cultural knowledge* is understanding how culture shapes key processes, as noted in Table 3.3. Such culturalaaaaaa knowledge (i.e., for understanding a variety of health care processes from communication through rituals or customs like diet and prayer) is more commonly applicable across clinical populations and health care settings. The knowledge required to understand cultural variations in incidence, prevalence, physiology, and pharmacology varies considerably depending on the clinical setting; however, it is important for all health care providers to have a basic understanding that these processes may be susceptible to cultural variations.

The discussion that follows offers a brief explanation of how cross-cultural variations may affect these processes. (We look at the issue in more depth in Sections II and III of the book.)

Dimensions of Individualism and Collectivism

In the 1970s Hofstede began studying value systems across different countries and identified differences along cultural dimensions,[1] including those of individualism, collectivism, and power distance. The original and subsequent work by Hofstede also identified the dimensions

---

[1]*Dimension* is described as an aspect of a culture that can be measured relative to other cultures (Hofstede, G. [2011]. Dimensionalizing cultures: The Hofstede Model in context. *Online Readings in Psychology and Culture, 2*[1]. https://doi.org/10.9707/2307-0919.1014).

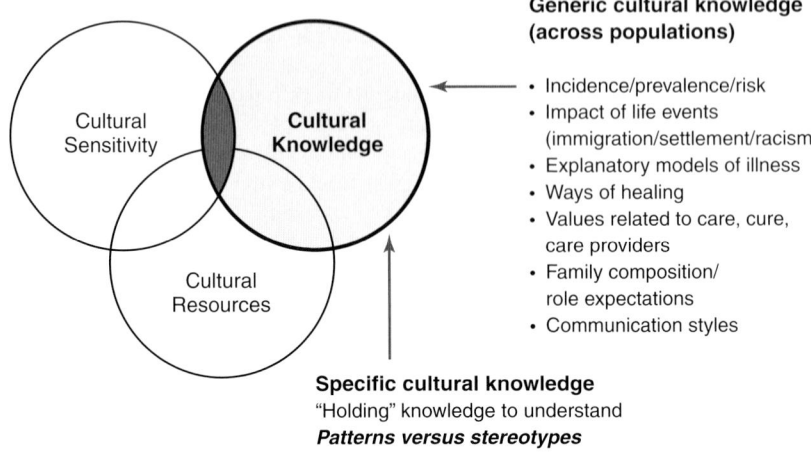

Generic cultural knowledge (across populations)

- Incidence/prevalence/risk
- Impact of life events (immigration/settlement/racism)
- Explanatory models of illness
- Ways of healing
- Values related to care, cure, care providers
- Family composition/ role expectations
- Communication styles

Specific cultural knowledge
"Holding" knowledge to understand
Patterns versus stereotypes

Fig. 3.9   Cultural Knowledge.

TABLE 3.3 ■ **Health Care Processes Shaped by Culture**

Dimensions of culture such individualism and collectivism and power distance
Communication: high context versus low context
Incidence, prevalence, physiology, and pharmacology
Personal space (public/private; what is disclosed)
Views toward care, cure, and caregivers
Rituals/customs related to treatment, including diet and prayer
Models of illness and systems of healing
Time orientation

---

of uncertainty, avoidance, masculinity/femininity, long-term versus short-term orientation, and indulgence versus restraint (see Hofstede, 2011). All of the dimensions have potential implications for health care; however, the discussion that follows is mainly limited to individualism/collectivism. Although the concepts are presented in a dichotomous manner, they exist on a continuum with most cultures having a range of characteristics.

The dimension of individualism and collectivism describes patterns of group integration in a society (i.e., the balance between individual goals and dependence on the broader social unit). Individualistic culture views the individual as the central unit with loose ties between people. For example, there is a focus on "I" as evident in language, the family usually includes the nuclear family, decisions are based on what is good for the person, opinion and questioning is expected, and privacy is a cherished value. Conversely, collectivist cultures have more interdependence between the individual and their community. Language is "we" focused, families are extended as opposed to immediate, decisions are made in the interest of the collective rather than the individual, and belonging is favoured over privacy (Table 3.4). Individualism is associated with Eurocentric values and is predominant in Western countries such as the United States and Canada, while collectivism is more prevalent in Eastern countries and among Indigenous people in Canada (Hofstede, 2011).

The impact of individualism is evident throughout the Canadian health care system where individual autonomy and rights prevail with respect to privacy, access to information, and decision making. There is high regard for self-care and independence and services are largely oriented

TABLE 3.4 ■ **Differences Between Individualistic and Collectivist Societies**

Individualistic Society	Collectivist Society
Core element is the individual	Core element is the group
"I" consciousness	"We" consciousness
Right to privacy	Stresses belonging
Self-care/self-reliance	Family caregiving/reliance
Task over relationship	Relationship over task
Individual rights, confrontations can be healthy	Collective harmony
Low-context communication (everything must be specified)	High-context communication (many things are obvious)
Low power distance	High power distance

Hofstede, G. (2011). Dimensionalizing cultures: The Hofstede model in context. *Online Readings in Psychology and Culture, 2*(1). https://doi.org/10.9707/2307-0919.1014.

toward the individual, with family as contextual. In collectivist cultures, individualism may be seen as self-centred and uncaring behaviour, and caring for family members is considered a moral obligation to maintain family honour. In collectivist cultures, seeking professional care and institutionalization may be associated with personal shame and family dishonour, and consequently individuals may be reluctant to seek help with caregiving, even when they experience difficulties in coping (Hanssen & Tran, 2019).

Cultural Considerations In Care

We Take Care of Our Own

Mrs. Chen is a 55-year-old first-generation Chinese immigrant who lives with her husband. Mr. Chen has had chronic health issues, and over the last year his mobility has declined considerably. He was recently hospitalized for cardiac issues, and as the team engages in discharge planning, Mrs. Chen mentions to you she is having a very difficult time at home and is uncertain how she can care for him. She is very tearful during this conversation. When you mention this to Dr. Wong at the team meeting, he is very surprised, as he just had a conversation with Mrs. Chen the evening before and she did not mention anything. He also makes a comment that "Chinese people take care of their own."

- Why do you think Mrs. Chen is giving different messages to different team members?
- How can you advocate for the family with regard to the supports needed?

An option to consider is to point out to Dr. Wong that she might be uncomfortable letting him know her difficulty because she might be feeling sad or ashamed at not being able to care for her husband. The doctor is also Chinese; thus she may think he will be disappointed if she cannot continue to be the caregiver. In such a situation, it will be helpful if Dr. Wong can initiate a discussion of options including additional supports or potential institutional care. He can use his authority and Chinese ancestry in a positive way by giving her permission to discuss what she might be ashamed of. Mrs. Chen can then feel comfortable to explore the needs and options that are required.

Individualism/collectivism dimensions can also have a significant impact on health care communication. For example, when a person from an individualistic culture makes a statement such as "you need to …," it is considered a simple and direct communication of need. This may be regarded by a collectivist as rude or disrespectful because the statement may be interpreted as a personalized directive. Similarly, a collectivist may approach a situation with "what should we do?" as a way of respecting relationships. This could be misjudged as a lack of personal ability or responsibility, and indirect communication styles can be readily misconstrued as incompetence (Ong-Flaherty, 2015).

Power distance describes the extent to which power is expected to be distributed equally (or not) within the family and society. Individualism is associated with low power distance, reflected by a greater likelihood of consultation, questions, and expressions of disagreements; whereas collectivism is associated with high power distance, reflecting less expectation of consultation and greater expectation that those in authority can tell others what to do. In high power distance cultures, society's level of inequality is endorsed by the followers as much as by the leaders (Hofstede, 2011). This has potential implications for how patients might engage with providers with respect to questions and engagement in care decisions. Patients with a collectivist orientation may be hesitant to express disagreement with a proposed plan of care and treatment and have greater expectations for the provider to determine treatment goals and interventions.

Communication

Effective communication is critical for good clinical care. Culture and diversity affect many aspects of communication, the most obvious being language, whether verbal or nonverbal, including eye contact, hand gestures, facial expressions, and tone of voice. Communication affects not only what is said, but also how it is said, to whom it is said, and what remains unsaid.

American anthropologist and cross-cultural researcher Edward Hall described the relationship between culture and communication as inseparable and described two types of communication characterized by the degree to which the message was explicit (verbal) or implicit (nonverbal). These differences in communication styles can have an impact on relationship building and negotiations (Manrai et al., 2019). Low-context communication is associated with individualistic cultures, where tasks are prioritized and there is a focus on being direct and efficient. The focus is on the words that are used to convey the message. Conversely, high-context communication is associated with collectivist cultures, where the message is not just in the words but rather in contextual factors such as who, why, when, where, and to whom (Manrai et al., 2019). In high-context communication, tone and nonverbal demeanor as well as *what is not said* can be just as important as what is said. Cross-cultural communication skills are fundamental to cultural competence because without effective communication, every phase of the clinical encounter can be compromised—from establishing the therapeutic relationship to making an assessment and following through with interventions. Cross-cultural communication issues and working effectively with interpreters are discussed in greater depth in Chapters 5 and 6.

Time Orientation

The high-/low-context orientation is also associated with time orientation. Low-context cultures such as Canada and the United States are associated with monochromatic time (M-time), which are characterized by schedules, structure, logic, linear thinking, and rationality. In contrast, high-context cultures are associated with polychromatic time (P-time), where schedules are less important than relationships, multiple tasks may be done at once, and circular (nonlinear) patterns of thinking are accompanied by a view that truth emerges through a process of discovery without explicit application of rationality (Manrai et al., 2019).

Health care agencies and providers frequently note that they experience challenging variations in patient punctuality for appointments and in the value that patients place on time generally. Health care systems, particularly hospitals, are highly dependent on appointments and schedules, with little flexibility to accommodate people who appear at nonscheduled times. Mainstream North American society is highly oriented toward the 24-hour clock: punctuality is a cherished value, and a lack of adherence to schedules is interpreted as disrespectful or associated with a lack of engagement. However, patients with P-time cultural orientation may value time differently. In some cultures, schedules may be perceived as guidelines rather than strict rules, and being late, especially when there is a good reason, is considered appropriate. In addition to cultural orientation, there are numerous other reasons that may cause or compound patients' ability to meet appointment times. These include:

- Issues related to transportation and accessibility
- Issues related to work
- Inability to find child care
- Requiring more time to find a friend or family member to accompany for support and system navigation
- Issues related to religious or inauspicious (unfavourable/unlucky) days

Rather than simply giving an appointment time, it is important to take a few minutes to verify that the time is suitable, offering alternatives if it is not and providing the information necessary to change the appointment if needed. Other helpful steps include anticipating potential challenges and assisting patients with planning and accessing the necessary support systems and resources.

Time orientation also can affect a patient's medication habits, particularly with respect to the interval between doses. Health care providers can teach patients the optimum times for taking medicine, ask when exactly they see themselves being able to take it, explain how much latitude exists in the schedule, and discuss issues involving skipped doses (e.g., fasting). It is important to approach such issues in a supportive, nonjudgemental manner. Despite the explanations and coaching, some patients may still have difficulty with time management issues or following instructions that are dictated by the clock.

Personal Space

The amount of personal space we are comfortable with varies across cultures (Marin et al., 2018); the same is true for what we consider to be private and what activities we are comfortable with in the presence of others. Many health care processes require close physical contact and discussions of an intimate nature; thus personal boundaries can be particularly significant with respect to patient disclosure and co-operation with activities. Issues concerning personal space and gender often surface during activities involving physical assessment and personal care. Health care providers need to use sensitivity and to talk with patients to find approaches that best fit the patients' health care needs and personal preferences. In the author's personal and professional experience, it has become very evident that cultural rules for personal and intimate activities can vary greatly across cultures. For example, individuals may feel uncomfortable undressing in front of others, including people of their own gender, yet be totally comfortable sharing a bed with same-gender family members. In many cultures, it is normal for infants and children to share a bed with their parents or other relatives every night. This is in sharp contrast with North American society, where parents and children have separate sleeping quarters, only intimate partners share a bed night at night, and in a locker-room setting some degree of nudity in front of members of the same gender is not regarded as inappropriate.

Incidence, Prevalence, Physiology, Pharmacology

In recent years, research has acknowledged differences in incidence, prevalence, illness expression, and medication efficacy based on gender, race, and ethnicity. The reasons for such differences should be explored. For example, Schofield et al. (2019) note high rates of psychosis in the Black community and attribute it to stressors such as discrimination, socioeconomic deprivation, lack of social support, internalized stigma, and "inequitable treatment from mental health services and a tendency to over-diagnose ethnic minorities" (p. 970). Research has also identified a higher risk of cardiac disease in South Asian population. South Asians are more likely to develop heart disease at a younger age, with some evidence of higher risk for cardiovascular death as compared to other ethnic groups (Fernando et al., 2015). This population also has a higher risk for diabetes, which can be attributed to changes in diet and lifestyle post-migration and potential genetic factors. Understanding the disease-specific implications for cultural groups, including genetic and environmental factors, will allow for better assessment and treatment and could reduce the illness burden.

Ethnicity and gender have also been noted to influence responses to certain medications (Ramamoorthy et al., 2015; Tamargo et al., 2017). The differential response can be attributed to the rate of metabolization, which in turn leads to different dosage requirements for certain populations. Drugs such as codeine, antipsychotics, antihypertensives, and anticoagulants have been associated with differential responses. People from Japan, China, Thailand, and Malaysia may require lower doses of drugs such as codeine; people with an Asian background may require lower dosages of antipsychotic agents; and Black people can have a less favourable response to antihypertensives (Abuatiq, 2018). Mak et al. (2019) demonstrated difference in the dosage for anticoagulants such as warfarin among Whites, Hispanics, and Asians, and Cazzola et al. (2018) noted less responsiveness for asthma medications in African American and Hispanic populations (as compared to white people). Gender differences have been noted for cardiovascular drugs and analgesics (Pieretti et al., 2016; Tamargo et al., 2017). Overall, these differences are generally attributed to a combination of genetic and environmental influences. It is important for health care providers to always assess for individual dosage response and adverse effects to medications; however, knowing patterns of ethnocultural variations associated with major classifications of medications can also lead to better monitoring.

Care/Cure/Caregivers

Cultural norms influence our personal preferences regarding who provides care and what kind of care or treatment is involved. The roles of various family members in health care decisions and interventions also vary across cultures. North American society focuses strongly on individuals' abilities to maintain or achieve independence and be able to take care of themselves (Hofstede, 2011). In many cultures, the concept of being sick means dependence and being taken care of, and taking care of others is part of the family role. Some elders may expect to be taken care of and see it as the children's duty. Parents often view "doing for" as an expression of love and support; others, particularly health care providers, may interpret the same behaviour as fostering dependence (Manrai et al., 2019). Conflict can occur when there are discrepancies between family members and between the family and health care providers. It is important that health care providers determine and explain the reasons behind the desired behaviours and strive to maintain a balance between patients' achieving independence and feeling they are being cared for.

Cultural Considerations In Care

Dialysis Training—With a Thoughtful Twist

North American society places a high value on independence. Often, treatments are geared toward helping individuals gain as much as independence as possible. Consider what happens when we encounter an individual who attaches a different significance to independence.

A home dialysis program was teaching patients how to maintain themselves on continuous ambulatory peritoneal dialysis. One of the biggest advantages of this therapy over other types of dialysis is that it allows patients to do the dialysis themselves and thus be completely independent. However, the staff soon realized that many of the older patients, particularly those from Eastern backgrounds, were relying on their spouses or children to do the procedure. This was of concern since the spouses and children had not received the training on how to do the procedure safely.

Initially, the team's response was to emphasize the need for the patient to do the procedure and express disapproval when this was not being done. Some patients continued to rely on other family members for the procedure. As the team took time to reflect on what was happening, team members understood the issue differently and they built greater flexibility into the program to allow for training not just the patient but also the key family member(s) who might be doing the procedure. The concern for patient safety was addressed, along with the family's need to care for their sick family member.

Consulting professional caregivers is commonplace in some cultures; relying only on one's family or community is the norm in others. Understanding how to work effectively with families across cultures is a key aspect of generic cultural knowledge and will be discussed in greater depth in Chapter 7.

With respect to cure, patients may have different expectations about the type of care or treatment they expect to receive. Desired treatment will vary depending on the preferred health goal(s), which can include the following:

- Strengthening the body's capacity to fight illness
- Maintaining the balance among physical, spiritual, and emotional health
- Addressing the symptoms of illness
- Addressing the root cause of the illness

Consider common treatments for a cold: while some people prefer hot liquids (e.g., tea or chicken soup), others advocate citrus juices (usually served cold in North America), and still others seek out medications to either boost their immune system or control the symptoms related to the cold.

When it comes to the caregivers themselves, Canadian and American health care systems are based on a team approach, with different members of the team having different roles, often with clear boundaries in terms of who does what. Many cultures, however, are used to a single caregiver, who may be a spiritual healer, medical doctor, or trusted elder. Patients may therefore be unfamiliar with the kinds of roles that comprise a team, or their perceptions of specific roles may be at odds with the reality they now face. For example, in some cultures nurses are regarded as assistants to doctors, and social workers may be viewed as representatives of the state rather than as advocates for patients. It is critical that health care providers not assume that the patient knows what they do and instead take the time to discuss their role in a way that is relevant to the patient.

Cultural Competence In Action

Opposite Practices Have a Common Thread

During your childhood, how did your family react when a child had a fever? Did they put on additional layers of clothing or take layers off? How was the practice explained?

The two responses may seem completely opposite, yet ultimately, they serve a similar purpose. The stated purpose behind adding layers is to encourage the body to break into a sweat, which cools the body as it evaporates. Advocates of taking layers off are also trying to promote body cooling through heat loss. Interestingly, the practice that is most familiar to you is also likely the one that makes you feel more comfortable, both physically and emotionally.

Systems of Health Care and Models of Illness

An **explanatory model of illness** is the way a patient conceptualizes a sickness episode (Abitz, 2016; Kleinman et al., 1978) (see Chapter 2). Explanatory models are influenced by cultural concepts, beliefs, and values. Beliefs about etiology or cause of illness are likely to determine the type of care or therapy that is sought. If illness is attributed to bacteria, virus, or abnormal cell growth (i.e., internal or external invasion of the body), the approach will likely be to attack and conquer, through mechanical or chemical means. Alternatively, if illness is seen as punishment for deeds, the remedy may be penance and the symptoms are tolerated and accepted.

The biomedical system of health care in North America (also called *allopathy*) is frequently referred to as the conventional treatment; however, it is only one of several scientifically based systems of healing. Some other systems of healing that are based on philosophical and scientific approaches include Indigenous medicine, traditional Chinese medicine, Ayurveda (a form of traditional Hindu medicine), and naturopathy. Although it is impossible for a health care provider to have expertise in all the healing systems, awareness of major systems and the associated key concepts can be helpful. It is important to have respect for the foundations on which they are built and the therapies they entail (this is discussed in greater detail in Chapter 8). Individuals often make use of more than one source of care during an episode of illness. While seeking care from biomedical health care providers, patients may simultaneously be consulting traditional healers and using herbal remedies or other complementary therapies.

SPECIFIC CULTURAL KNOWLEDGE

In keeping with the CCF's two-step approach to developing cultural knowledge, the preceding discussion focused on core issues that health providers need to be able to recognize and explore further. However, it is also important to develop more in-depth knowledge about populations and issues specific to one's practice. The two types of knowledge are intertwined: knowledge of specific cultures and issues allows us to reflect on generic processes, and understanding generic processes provides a context in which we can recognize the specific (Stadler, 2017). Being able to recognize the two types of cultural knowledge also promotes a critical-thinking approach. Health care providers always need to assess situations to identify the extent to which the issues involved can be categorized as (1) unique to the individual, (2) reflective of the broader culture or cultures, and/or (3) reflective of cultural processes in general.

Specific cultural knowledge refers to in-depth knowledge about groups or populations (Stadler, 2017). In the CCF the term also includes specific knowledge of care processes that can be affected by culture. Populations may be defined by clinical specialty (e.g., mental health), cultural group based on ethnic identity (e.g., Indigenous people), nondominant social group (e.g., transgendered people), or location where health care is accessed (e.g., hospital or community). Each population has issues that are of particular importance for health care providers to understand.

Section III of this book offers a range of population-specific examples. The population-specific knowledge should also be used with caution. It is important to understand that specific cultural knowledge is context sensitive and continues to change over time and place; thus it is critical to understand the specific context, history, issues, needs, and strengths associated with the particular group(s) that one is working with.

In summary, cultural knowledge begins to address the second half of the guiding principle behind the CCF: "To care for someone I must know who the other is" (see Fig. 3.1). Both generic and specific cultural knowledge can help us know the other, but only with respect to whom the other *might* be. Cultural knowledge also requires understanding the professional culture and the processes of care that are impacted by variations in worldviews as well as processes of marginalization. A critical step in knowing the other is to apply this cultural knowledge to individual assessments. This will be discussed further in Chapter 4.

Cultural Resources

Cultural resources are the third element in the CCF. Understanding and developing such resources is a critical part of the cultural competence journey. No health care provider is expected to have all the answers. Cultural competence requires the ability to seek out and develop resources and supports within the practice environment to provide timely, appropriate, and effective care. While it is essential for health care providers to develop their own sensitivity, knowledge, and cultural skills, no individual can do it alone. Cultural competence requires the ability to seek out and develop resources and supports within the practice environment to deliver quality care. Cultural resources exist at the personal, organizational, professional, and social domains and can provide invaluable guidance (Fig. 3.10).

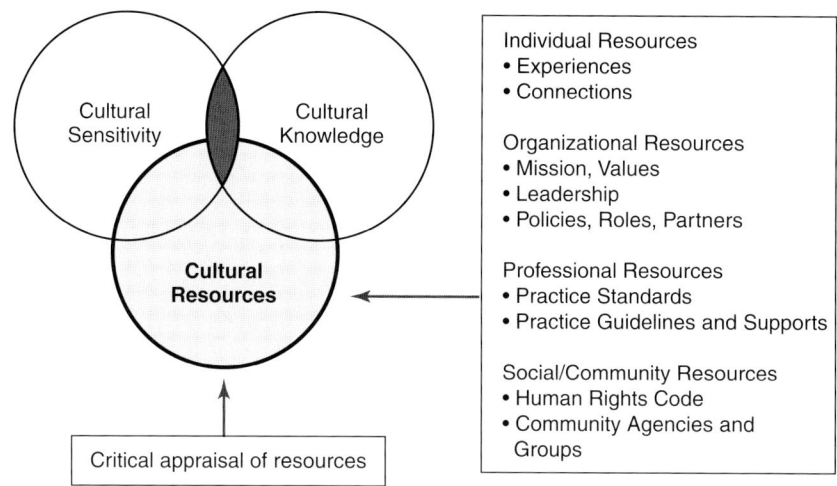

Fig. 3.10 Cultural Resources.

INDIVIDUAL-LEVEL RESOURCES

Individual health care providers can develop cultural competence in several ways:

- By seeking information
- By reflecting on experiences
- By developing diverse connections

Relevant experiences and connections are essential to developing the confidence and competence necessary to provide good care across populations. The first requirement is a genuine desire to learn *from* the other, not just *about* the other—in other words, to engage in cultural networking. Like other personal networks, cultural networks develop over time. Seeking out opportunities to interact with people (including colleagues) from different cultural communities is a good beginning; it is important, though, to go beyond dance, dialect, dress, and diet to engage in dialogue with people and learn about different worldviews and approaches to health, illness, caring, and healing. This requires taking the risk of being unwelcome and not being offended or discouraged should that occur. Being able to examine the reasons and processes behind a lack of welcome provides a unique learning opportunity.

Other ways of strengthening an individual's capacity to connect with diverse groups include learning a second language, learning about legacies and history of different groups, and continuously reflecting on what needs to be unlearned so that new learning can occur. Films, books, and other media are also rich sources of cultural knowledge. Health care providers can access a variety of informational resources that are made available on the Internet through various associations and interest groups (Table 3.5). Canada is indeed a diverse country, and that diversity has the potential to enrich our personal and professional knowledge and networks in countless ways. The key is how we choose to engage and learn from the diversity that surrounds us.

ORGANIZATIONAL-LEVEL RESOURCES

Even though resources developed by individuals (such as personal contacts) can be invaluable, over-reliance on those resources can be counterproductive. Imagine a health care system in which referrals to other agencies, communities, or specialty services cannot take place until individual

TABLE 3.5 ■ Selected Websites Providing Cultural Resources

This list is based on an online search with the term *cultural competence* and then *country*. These
  websites are a good beginning and readers are encouraged to look at resources at the provincial
  level, through the professional and regulatory associations and major health authorities and health
  services organizations.

https://www.kidsnewtocanada.ca/culture/competence

Developed by the Canadian Paediatric Society, this website is for health care providers caring for
  immigrant and refugee children, youth, and families.

https://www.nccih.ca/en/

The National Collaborating Centre for Indigenous Health (NCCIH) is a national Indigenous organization
  funded through the Public Health Agency of Canada (PHAC) to support First Nations, Inuit, and
  Métis public health renewal and health equity through knowledge translation and exchange. The
  mandate of the organization is to foster links between evidence, knowledge, practice, and policy
  while advancing self-determination and Indigenous knowledge in support of optimal health and
  well-being. The approach utilizes a holistic, co-ordinated, and strengths-based approach to health.

https://thinkculturalhealth.hhs.gov/resources

Sponsored by the US Department of Health & Human Services, Office of Minority Health, this website
  provides information and continuing education opportunities for health care providers to learn more
  about CLAS (culturally and linguistically appropriate services).

https://nacchocommunique.files.wordpress.com/2016/12/cultural_respect_framework_1december
  2016_1.pdf

The Cultural Respect Framework (CRF) 2016–2026 was developed for the Australian Health Minister's
  Advisory Council (AHMAC) by the National Aboriginal and Torres Strait Islander Health Standing
  Committee (NATSIHSC). The framework is intended for use by the health sector, to guide strategies
  to improve culturally respectful services.

https://www.healthnavigator.org.nz/clinicians/c/cultural-competence/

Health Navigator is a nonprofit community initiative combining the efforts of a wide range of partner
  and supporter organizations. The link provides information and education resources for health care
  providers on cultural competence and cultural safety.

team members have initiated searches for the services or for the specialists needed to make the
referrals. Not only would this lead to patient delays in accessing services, but it also causes duplica-
tion of effort and inappropriate referrals, which compromises the efficiency and effectiveness of
health care. Cultural resources need to be considered in a similar light. Organizational cultural
competence is discussed further in Chapter 4.

Organizational resources may be both internal and external to the organization. Internal
resources include policies and guidelines that create an expectation for cultural competence in
clinical care. Internal organizational resources also include support from a diverse workforce, as
well as interpreter services, multi-faith religious and spiritual care, and services that offer complementary therapies. Although it is important to have the resources, it is equally important to consider how to make good use of them. Having a diverse workforce may increase an organization's
potential capacity to meet the needs of a diverse population (FECCA, 2019), but, in practice,
it can also increase the potential for conflict. Without recognizing this potential, and without
introducing effective processes to manage the conflict, an organization might have a diverse
workforce that remains an untapped resource. Health care providers need to be able to tap into
this expertise and develop an environment that encourages learning from others. As discussed in
Chapter 1, developing team-level cultural competence is important, but that can occur only when
individuals within the team make the commitment and provide leadership and support for each
other. Patients and families can also be excellent resources for health care providers to learn from,
provided the health care provider recognizes and values their experience and expertise.

External organizational resources may include services noted above (e.g., interpreter services or religious support) and a variety of partnerships (e.g., with community leaders and groups, non-mainstream health care agencies, and alternative therapy providers). Strategies to develop such partnerships are like strategies for developing personal networks. It is important to identify the potential resources that are in the community—particularly individuals and groups who may not be connected to the health care agency—and to explore opportunities to partner with them. Such engagement must be accompanied by humility and reciprocal exchange where mainstream organizations can share their resources and expertise in return for the wisdom and services of the cultural and community groups and organizations.

When we work with resources such as culture-specific services, one issue that often arises is the balance between referring to a service and seeking advice from a service. While ethno-specific services may be preferred because of their ability to better understand and address the cultural context, they often have limited capacity, and mainstream agencies need to develop greater responsiveness as well as effective partnerships with cultural and community groups (Radermacher et al., 2009). It is critical that health care providers view such services as learning resources to help develop their own abilities as well as a resource that patients can use to receive care.

PROFESSIONAL AND SOCIAL RESOURCES

The recognition for cultural competence and health equity across health professions has led to the development of tools and resources from various health discipline regulatory bodies and professional associations at the provincial and national level. There is also guidance available from specialty associations, hospitals and health authorities, research funding agencies, and various communities and Indigenous nations. Social resources also include community groups and agencies as well as documents such as the provincial *Human Rights Codes* and the Truth and Reconciliation Commission (TRC) report and its calls to action. New information is constantly being generated, and readers are encouraged to develop their own lists of information sources based on their interests and focus.

Critical Appraisal and Use of Resources

Having access to resources is essential for the provision of culturally appropriate care; however, health care providers also need to use critical-thinking skills to assess how applicable the resource is. In the technologically enriched twenty-first century, with a variety of Internet search engines offering information from numerous sources, the challenge is assessing the quality, adequacy, and applicability of the information. When we use a cultural resource, no matter what the form—printed, electronic, human, or experiential—we need to practise ongoing individualized assessment. A single experience with a culture tells us only about that encounter; the experience may or may not be typical of or like other experiences with that culture. A single individual from a culture can be a valuable informant, but no individual represents all aspects of a culture. Culture is about possible patterns, not universal truths. Resources can help us recognize patterns, interpret information, or generate hypotheses, but ultimately the interpretation needs to be validated with the patient and refined for the specific situation.

Summary

This chapter presents the CCF as an approach to developing cultural competence. The three elements of cultural sensitivity, cultural knowledge, and cultural resources are needed to assist health care providers in identifying key cultural values that affect the clinical encounter. Cultural sensitivity requires an understanding of culture, as patterns and as power, and recognizes that learning "who I am" is the first step toward developing cultural competence. Cultural sensitivity focuses on respect, humility, awareness, and understanding—not only about our own values and reactions to difference, but also how we might be perceived by others. The framework also describes the dynamics of difference created by systemic barriers to equity. Culturally sensitive health care providers have both theoretical knowledge ("knowing that") and practical knowledge ("knowing how"). They value diversity in all individuals, understand the dynamics of difference, and can use their knowledge and understanding to turn barriers into building blocks.

Cultural knowledge is both knowledge of other cultures and knowledge of legacies, structures, and systems that continue to perpetuate health inequities. It is important for health care providers to develop generic cultural knowledge that applies across populations and knowledge that is focused on specific cultures or clinical populations. Cultural resources need to be developed at the individual as well as the organizational level. The various exercises and reflections presented in this chapter are intended to foster critical self-reflection. Students and health care providers can continue to develop their own cultural sensitivity, knowledge, and resources through ongoing reflection and dialogue with themselves and with others within their community.

Thus far, the discussion of the CCF has focused on the three elements of sensitivity, knowledge, and resources. However, success lies in applying the awareness and knowledge into practice to effectively navigate differences and bridge gaps that might exist between cultures. This will be discussed in Chapter 4.

ⓔ http://evolve.elsevier.com/Srivastava/culturalcompetence/.

Questions for Review and Discussion

1. Reflecting on the culture you grew up in, identify two values, traditions, and ways of knowing that were/are important to you and your family but may not be understood by outsiders looking into your culture. What is it that you wish others understood about who you are and what you practise? If possible, discuss with a peer or reflect on how such an interaction can occur in a positive learning way.
2. List some strategies that you apply to get to know person(s) from other cultural groups. Consider observation, questions and conversation, reading, and so on. How do you determine if your understanding is unique to the individual or situation or could be applied more broadly to the group?
3. Reflect on the new eyes, new ears, new thoughts, new actions approach. As you complete this and previous chapters, how has your thinking changed? What are you now noticing that was not so obvious before? Was there something that you have "unlearned" as a result of new knowledge?
4. Refer back to Fig. 3.8. When you think of yourself in your professional capacity, how do you see yourself? What words would you use to describe yourself? How do you think others may see you?
5. Where do you see yourself on the individualism–collectivism continuum? Is it similar to or different from your peers? How does that affect your interactions?

Group Experiential/Reflection Activity

In a small group select a cultural group you would like to learn more about. How do you go about seeking information? How do you critically appraise what you learn? What did you learn about the worldviews or cultural patterns of this group? What did you learn about the sociopolitical power dynamics experienced by this group as a whole? How can your learning be applied in your practice?

References

Abitz, T. L. (2016). Cultural congruence and infusion nursing practice. *Journal of Infusion Nursing, 39*(2), 75–79.

Abuatiq, A. (2018). Cultural competency in ethno pharmacology. *Chronicles of Pharmaceutical Science, 2*(4), 617–621.

Adichie, C. N. (2009). *The dangers of a single story.* TEDGlobal 2009. https://www.ted.com/talks/chimamanda_ngozi_adichie_the_danger_of_a_single_story

Alizadeh, S., & Chavan, M. (2016). Cultural competence dimensions and outcomes: A systematic review of the literature. *Health & Social Care in the Community, 24*(6), e117–e130.

Almutairi, A. F., Adlan, A. A., & Nasim, M. (2017). Perceptions of the critical cultural competence of registered nurses in Canada. *BMC Nursing, 16*, 47.

American Heritage Dictionaries. (2020). *The American heritage dictionary of the English language.* Houghton Mifflin Harcourt. https://ahdictionary.com/

Anderson-Lain, K. (2017). Enacting the self-awareness imperative in intercultural communication. *Communication Teacher, 31*(3), 131–136. https://doi.org/10.1080/17404622.2017.1314529.

Azzopardi, C., & McNeill, T. (2016). From cultural competence to cultural consciousness: Transitioning to a critical approach to working across differences in social work. *Journal of Ethnic & Cultural Diversity in Social Work, 25*(4), 282–299.

Baker, D. W. (2020). Trust in health care in the time of COVID-19. *JAMA, 324*(23), 2373–2375.

Benner, P. (1984). *From novice to expert.* Addison Wesley.

Bonchek, M. (2016). Why the problem with learning is unlearning. *Harvard Business Review*, 2–4. Digital Articles.

Busher Betancourt, D. A. (2015). Madeleine Leininger and the transcultural theory of nursing. *The Downtown Review, 2*(1). https://engagedscholarship.csuohio.edu/tdr/vol2/iss1/1

Cai, D.-Y. (2016). A concept analysis of cultural competence. *International Journal of Nursing Sciences, 3*(3), 268–273.

Cazzola, M., Calzetta, L., Matera, M. G., et al. (2018). How does race/ethnicity influence pharmacological response to asthma therapies? *Expert Opinion on Drug Metabolism & Toxicology, 14*(4), 435–446.

Chandra, S., Ward, P. R., & Mohammadnezhad, M. (2018). Trust and communication in a doctor-patient relationship: A literature review. *Journal of Healthcare Communications, 3*(3), 36.

Danso, R. (2018). Cultural competence and cultural humility: A critical reflection on key cultural diversity concepts. *Journal of Social Work, 18*(4), 410–430.

Dictionary.com. (2020). *Privilege.* https://www.dictionary.com/browse/privilege

Dudzinski, D. M. (2018). White privilege and playing it safe. *The American Journal of Bioethics, 18*(6), 4–5.

Federation of Ethnic Communities' Councils of Australia (FECCA). (2019). *Cultural competence in Australia— A guide.* https://ethniccouncilshepparton.com.au/wp-content/uploads/2019/05/Cultural-Competence-in-Australia-A-Guide.pdf

Fernando, E., Razak, F., Lear, S. A., et al. (2015). Cardiovascular disease in South Asian migrants. *The Canadian Journal of Cardiology, 31*(9), 1139–1150.

Funnell, S., Kitty, D., & Schipper, S. (2020). Moving toward anti-racism. *Canadian Family Physician, 66*(8), 617.

Gleick, J. (1987). *Chaos.* Viking Books.

Groen, S. P., Richters, A., Laban, C. J., et al. (2018). Cultural identity among Afghan and Iraqi traumatized refugees: Towards a conceptual framework for mental health care professionals. *Culture, Medicine and Psychiatry, 42*(1), 69–91. https://doi.org/10.1007/s11013-016-9514-7.

Hall, J. C., & Theriot, M. T. (2016). Developing multicultural awareness, knowledge, and skills: Diversity training makes a difference? *Multicultural Perspectives, 18*(1), 35–41. https://doi.org/10.1080/15210960.2016.1125742.

Hanssen, I., & Tran, P. T. M. (2019). The influence of individualistic and collectivistic morality on dementia care choices. *Nursing Ethics, 26*(7–8), 2047–2057.

Hawley, S. T., & Morris, A. M. (2017). Cultural challenges to engaging patients in shared decision making. *Patient Education and Counseling, 100*(1), 18–24.

Higginbottom, G. M., Richter, M. S., Mogale, R. S., et al. (2011). Identification of nursing assessment models/tools validated in clinical practice for use with diverse ethno-cultural groups: an integrative review of the literature. *BMC Nursing, 10*, 16.

Hofstede, G. (2011). Dimensionalizing cultures: The Hofstede Model in context. *Online Readings in Psychology and Culture, 2*(1). https://doi.org/10.9707/2307-0919.1014.

Johnstone, M. J., Rawson, H., Hutchinson, A. M., et al. (2018). Fostering trusting relationships with older immigrants hospitalised for end-of-life care. *Nursing Ethics, 25*(6), 760–772.

Khanlou, N., Haque, N., Skinner, A., et al. (2017). Scoping review on prenatal health among immigrant and refugee women in Canada: Prenatal, intrapartum, and postnatal care. *Journal of Pregnancy*, 8783294. https://doi.org/10.1155/2017/8783294.

Khullar, D., Darien, G., & Ness, D. L. (2020). Patient consumerism, healing relationships, and rebuilding trust in health care. *JAMA, 324*(23), 2359–2360.

Kleinman, A., Eisenberg, L., & Good, B. (1978). Culture, illness, and care: Clinical lessons from anthropologic and cross-cultural research. *Annals of Internal Medicine, 88*(2), 251–258.

Leininger, M. (1978). *Transcultural nursing: Concepts, theories, and practices.* John Wiley and Sons.

Leininger, M. (1995). Overview of Leininger's culture care theory. In M. Leininger & M. R. McFarland (Eds.), *Transcultural nursing: concepts, theories, research and practice* (2nd ed., pp. 93–114). McGraw Hill.

Levin-Zamir, D., Leung, A., Dodson, S., et al. (2017). Health literacy in selected populations: Individuals, families, and communities from the international and cultural perspective. *Information Services & Use, 37*, 131–151. https://doi.org/10.3233/ISU-170834.

Mak, M., Lam, C., Pineda, S. J., et al. (2019). Pharmacogenetics of warfarin in a diverse patient population. *Journal of Cardiovascular Pharmacology and Therapeutics, 24*(6), 521–533.

Marin, C. R., Gasparino, R. C., & Puggina, A. C. (2018). The perception of territory and personal space invasion among hospitalized patients. *PLoS ONE, 13*(6), e0198989. https://doi.org/10.1371/journal.pone.0198989.

Manrai, L. A., Manrai, A. K., Lascu, D., et al. (2019). Determinants and effects of cultural context: a review, conceptual model, and propositions. *Journal of Global Marketing, 32*(2), 67–82.

McFarland, M. R., & Wehbe-Alamah, H. B. (2019). Leininger's theory of culture care diversity and universality: an overview with a historical retrospective and a view toward the future. *Journal of Transcultural Nursing, 30*(6), 540–557. https://doi.org/10.1177/1043659619867134.

Ong-Flaherty, C. (2015). Critical cultural awareness and diversity in nursing: A minority perspective. *Nurse Leader, 13*(5), 58–62.

Ontario Ministry of Citizenship. (1995). *Building blocks to equity.* Author.

Olaussen, S. J., & Renzaho, A. (2016). Establishing components of cultural competence healthcare models to better cater for the needs of migrants with disability: A systematic review. *Australian Journal of Primary Health, 22*, 100–112. https://doi.org/10.1071/PY14114.

Pieretti, S., Di Giannuario, A., Di Giovannandrea, R., et al. (2016). Gender differences in pain and its relief. *Annali dell'Istituto Superiore di Sanita, 52*(2), 184–189.

Radermacher, H., Feldman, S., & Browning, C. (2009). Mainstream versus ethno-specific community aged care services: it's not an 'either or'. *Australasian Journal on Ageing, 28*(2), 58–63. https://doi.org/10.1111/j.1741-6612.2008.00342.x.

Ramamoorthy, A., Pacanowski, M. A., Bull, J., et al. (2015). Racial/ethnic differences in drug disposition and response: Review of recently approved drugs. *Clinical Pharmacology and Therapeutics, 97*(3), 263–273.

Rising, M. L. (2017). Truth telling as an element of culturally competent care at end of life. *Journal of Transcultural Nursing, 28*(1), 48–55.

Russell, G. (2020). Reflecting on a way of being: anchor principles of cultural competence. In J. Frawley, G. Russell, & J. Sherwood (Eds.), *Cultural competence and the higher education sector.* Springer.

Schofield, P., Kordowicz, M., Pennycooke, E., et al. (2019). Ethnic differences in psychosis-Lay epidemiology explanations. *Health Expectations: An International Journal of Public Participation in Health Care and Health Policy, 22*(5), 965–973.

Schwartz, M., & Sánchez, E. (2016). *Social movement and their leaders that changed our world.* https://www.globalcitizen.org/en/content/movements-social-change-apartheid-civil-rights-suf/

Shen, Z. (2015). Cultural competence models and cultural competence assessment instruments in nursing: a literature review. *Journal of Transcultural Nursing, 26*(3), 308–321. https://doi.org/10.1177/1043659614524790.

Shepherd, S. M., Willis-Esqueda, C., Newton, D., et al. (2019). The challenge of cultural competence in the workplace: Perspectives of healthcare providers. *BMC Health Services Research, 19*, 135.

Srivastava, R. (2008). *Influence of organizational factors on clinical cultural competence.* Unpublished doctoral dissertation. Institute of Medical Sciences, University of Toronto.

Srivastava, R., & Srivastava, R. (2019). Impact of cultural identity on mental health in post-secondary students. *International Journal of Mental Health and Addiction, 17,* 520–530.

Stadler, S. (2017). Which competence? A comparative analysis of culture-specific vs. culture-generic intercultural competence development. *Advances in Economics and Business, 5*(8), 448–455. https://doi.org/10.13189/aeb.2017.050803.

Sue, S., Zane, G., Nagayama, H., et al. (2009). The case for cultural competency in psychotherapeutic interventions. *Annual Review of Psychology, 60,* 525–548. https://doi.org/10.1146/annurev.psych.60.110707.163651.

Syed, M., & Fish, J. (2018). Revisiting Erik Erikson's legacy on culture, race, and ethnicity. *Identity, 18*(4), 274–283.

Tamargo, J., Rosano, G., Walther, T., et al. (2017). Gender differences in the effects of cardiovascular drugs. *European Heart Journal-Cardiovascular Pharmacotherapy, 3*(3), 163–182.

Teelucksingh, C. (2018). Dismantling white privilege: The Black Lives Matter movement and environmental justice in Canada. *Kalfou: A Journal of Comparative and Relational Ethnic Studies, 5*(2), 304.

Turpel-Lafond, M. E. (2020). *In plain sight: Addressing Indigenous-specific racism and discrimination in B.C. health care.* Government of British Columbia. https://engage.gov.bc.ca/app/uploads/sites/613/2020/11/In-Plain-Sight-Full-Report.pdf

Wesp, L. M., Scheer, V., Ruiz, A., et al. (2018). An emancipatory approach to cultural competency: The application of critical race, postcolonial, and intersectionality theories. *Advances in Nursing Science, 41*(4), 316–326.

Wesson, D. E., Lucey, C. R., & Cooper, L. A. (2019). Building trust in health systems to eliminate health disparities. *JAMA, 322*(2), 111–112.

Young, S. H. (2018). The art of unlearning. https://www.scottyoung.com/blog/2018/04/12/the-art-of-unlearning/?fbclid=IwAR2EM4a8zlRyJvQVabE6Whb2N8V3URzHrhRZeCvaCBUS0xXvEmipA1KwIO8

Yu, Z., Steenbeek, A., Biderman, M., et al. (2020). Characteristics of Indigenous healing strategies in Canada: A scoping review. *JBI Evidence Synthesis, 18*(12), 2512–2555.

CHAPTER 4

Navigating Difference

Rani H. Srivastava and Janet Mawhinney

LEARNING OBJECTIVES

At the end of this chapter, the learner will be able to:
- Recognize the individual (micro), team (meso), and organizational or system (macro) domains of navigating difference
- Identify the significance of unconscious bias and unlearning in the design and implementation of cultural competence strategies
- Discuss how the strategies of cultural care preservation, cultural care accommodation and negotiation, and cultural care reframing can be used to bridge the gap across cultures
- Describe the LEARN framework as an approach to promote cultural congruence in care
- Recognize how to be an effective ally
- Differentiate between being an ally, an advocate, and an activist
- Identify priority areas for the development of organizational cultural competence

KEY TERMS

Activist	Cultural care reframing/ repatterning	Explanatory model of illness
Advocate		
Ally	Cultural care validation/ preservation	Two-eyed seeing
Allyship		Unconscious bias
Cultural care accommodation/ negotiation	Emic knowledge	Unconscious privilege
	Etic knowledge	Unequal risk

The Culture Care Framework (CCF) identifies the need to go beyond knowing oneself and the other to address cultural gaps between the health provider and patient. Previous chapters have discussed key concepts that are important to bridge the gap (e.g., humility, respect, and negotiation); however, practical interpretations and behavioural guidelines are important for the application of these concepts in health care practice.

Navigating difference begins with a recognition of unconscious bias at the individual level, along with an appreciation of the dynamics of difference that exist within a team, and extends to addressing the hidden bias that exists in our systems and processes. **Unconscious bias** refers to attitudes, beliefs, and perceptions that affect behaviour, interactions, and decision making (Marcelin et al., 2019; also see Chapter 1). The flip side of unconscious bias is **unconscious privilege**. Privilege by its very nature is invisible and hidden most from those who have it. "Privilege is hard for the privileged to identify and then to know what to do about it" (Russell, 2020, p. 34). Privilege provides access to opportunities, connections, and resources. It creates a sense of belonging, a seat at the table, and immunity from day-to-day challenges of navigating one's social environment.

There are many forms of privilege and intersectional systems of dominance and supremacy. The most critical forms of unconscious bias and privilege are manifestations of structural and systemic inequities, and their impact resonates beyond the individual and local environment to society as a whole. White privilege can be described in terms of how it presents (e.g., "blanket of power that envelopes everything we know like a snowy day") (Russell, 2020, p. 34) as well as by the absences it affords. Having White privilege means having an ability to ignore the consequences of racism, such as a lack of opportunity, over-scrutiny and interrogation with respect to belonging, subtle acts of exclusion, or violence. Unconscious and unrecognized privilege makes it difficult for those who have privilege to recognize that others do not have the same advantages and opportunities (Holm et al., 2017; Nixon, 2019).

As discussed in previous chapters, culture can be described in terms of both patterns *and* power. Patterns are the variation in worldviews and traditions. Power takes many different forms, including status and position/authority, but is also understood as the ever-present manifestations of historical and current legacies of systemic inequities, including those based on race, ethnicity, sex, gender identity, class, and ability. Culture exists at the level of the individual (micro), group (meso), as well as the broader institution and society (macro); it is therefore important to understand and work with the dynamics of difference at the various levels and recognize the interaction between levels. In practice, navigating difference builds on and integrates the clinical, leadership, and practice skills that providers already have or are developing. Like any competency, cultural competence requires knowledge, skill, judgement, and opportunities for application and is not a mysterious or separate domain of expertise.

This chapter explicates some of the core domains of navigating difference in practice, anchored within professional and existing knowledge and skills. We discuss issues and strategies that can assist health care providers in navigating differences and bridging the cultural divide across the individual, team, and organizational levels. Removal of barriers requires actions that address the cause of exclusion and shift power in ways that have a sustainable impact. The discussion that follows is organized into three major sections: navigating difference at the individual level, at the team level, and at the organizational level. Given that the barriers and challenges to cultural safety and equity are longstanding, structural, and systemic, the work ahead requires direct intervention as well as indirect support to others through the roles of an ally and advocate.

We are writing this in a time of heightened activism and awareness on many fronts, including movements focused on anti-Black racism[1] (e.g., Black Lives Matter [BLM]); First Nations, Inuit, and Métis reconciliation work[2]; and #Me Too and Time's Up,[3] in addition to the robust evidence of health disparities (see Chapter 1). With these social and political movements, we are seeing heightened expectations and enhanced commitments to create change in service design, delivery, leadership, and outcomes for communities and populations that have been marginalized and experience poorer health outcomes. There is increased commitment to "getting it right," but often that simply translates into seeking information and education without the associated efforts of changes that are needed at the team and organizational level. It is important to remember that development of cultural competence and equity awareness (knowledge and skills) is not only achievable but also a core requirement for practice across professional and ethical standards of practice. The truism is often heard that no one is born racist, sexist, homophobic, or ableist but that it is taught and learned; thus unlearning is necessary to see things in a different, even paradoxical way (see Chapter 2 for complexity thinking). While the heightened commitment and focus is promising,

---

[1] https://www.bcg.com/en-ca/publications/2020/reality-of-anti-black-racism-in-canada
[2] https://www.cihi.ca/en/about-cihi/first-nations-inuit-and-metis
[3] #Me Too and #Time's Up movements are similar in that they call attention to sexual violence and harassment, largely against women, and have similar goals of strengthening voice and empowerment. Time's Up aims to create concrete change leading to workplace safety and equity and thus can be regarded as an action-oriented next step to #Me Too (Langone, 2018).

TABLE 4.1 ■ Key Principles for Navigating Difference

- Commit to ongoing learning and unlearning
- Approach differences with humility and intentionality to learn *what matters most*
- Appreciate the need for unlearning as well as new learning that may be unique to the situation
- Realize the existence of uneven knowledge, understanding, and privilege across individuals, within groups, and in organizations
- Balance inquiry with critical reflection and self-interrogation
- Recognize unequal risks in the creation of safer spaces for individuals and groups
- Understand that there is no checklist; the approach must be contextual and relational
- Develop and draw on resources within self, patients, profession, and community
- Understand that barriers can also be building blocks (see Chapter 3)

---

superficial responses in words without committed actions will not be effective or lead to change. Navigating difference at all levels requires competencies that are inherently developmental and require commitment, guidance, and practise. Cultural competence is as much a way of being as it is a way of doing (Russell, 2020) and requires always embracing a learner's mindset. Table 4.1 identifies key principles that are fundamental guides for this work.

Navigating Difference at the Individual Level

The first step in bridging cultural divide is to understand the similarities and differences between the patient's and the health care provider's interpretation of the situation. Leininger's Theory of Culture Care Diversity and Universality explicitly recognizes the interactions between patients' generic folk-care (emic) practices and health care providers' care-cure (etic) practices (Leininger, 1995). Leininger (1995) notes that it is important to obtain a patient's **emic knowledge** (local, insider, or Indigenous cultural knowledge) before reflecting on **etic knowledge** (outsider's or stranger's, including health provider's, knowledge). This allows the health care provider to "discover" care meanings and proceed in ways that avoid imposing the values of the health care provider (Leininger, 1995). While this may seem like an unrealistic expectation in a busy health care environment, eliciting and understanding the patient's perspective and priorities is fundamental to patient-centred care and leads to improved efficiency and efficacy in the long run.

Kleinman et al. (1978) refer to the understanding of patient perspectives as understanding patient "agendas" and offer a framework for drawing out patients' **explanatory models of illness** and care through a series of questions that can be readily incorporated into various assessment approaches (see Table 4.2).

The questions in Table 4.2 are adaptable and can focus on the illness as well as specific aspects of the treatment, along with hopes and fears. They are open ended, begin with the current issue, and expand outward to what else may be significant. The open-ended nature of the questions allows for a broader, holistic perspective beyond the illness orientation and reinforces the need to value patient expertise in the interaction. The questions are a tool and serve as a guide that can be selectively used by providers, modifying the words and tone as needed to fit the setting and the relationship. A useful strategy is to listen to the words that the patient uses and reflect them in the questions. For example, the patient may refer to the problem as a problem, illness, sickness, or condition; the health care provider can use the same word as a way of acknowledging the patient's expertise and building mutual understanding. The order of questioning is not critical, and not all the information needs to be collected during the first interaction. Sometimes it is useful to depersonalize the questions. In some circumstances, patients may be reluctant to disclose their own beliefs but may be more willing to share beliefs held by the community in general or some individuals within the community. In such circumstances, questions can be phrased so to ask how

TABLE 4.2 ■ Understanding the Patient's Explanatory Models of Illness and Care

1. What do you think has caused the problem?
2. Why do you think it started when it did?
3. What do you think the sickness does to you? How does it work?
4. How severe is the sickness? Will it have a short or long course?
5. What are the major problems or difficulties that the sickness has caused in your life?
6. What have you done for this problem up to now?
7. Who else should be consulted or involved in care?
8. What are the most important results you hope to achieve from this treatment?
9. What do you fear most about the sickness or the treatment?

Adapted from Kleinman, A., Eisenberg, L., & Good, D. (1978). Culture, illness, and care: Clinical lessons from anthropologists and cross cultural research. *Annals of Internal Medicine, 88*, 251–258.

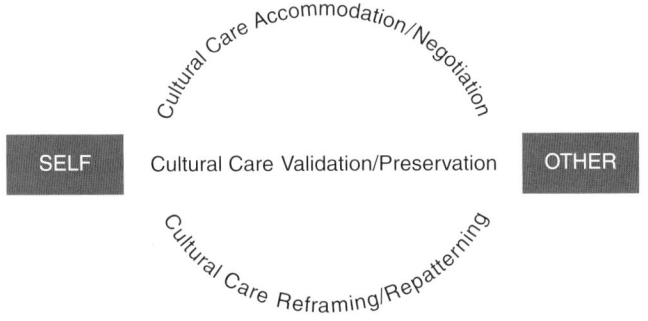

Fig. 4.1   Strategies to Bridge the Gap.

the problem would be treated in the family or community, or what the patient thinks others fear about the illness or treatment. Similarly, when working with family members, the questions can be modified to elicit perspectives of various family members. Using the list of questions with different family members can alert the health care provider to conflicting viewpoints within the family, which in turn may influence acceptance of the suggested interventions.

Exploring the patient's explanatory model of illness is a useful way to identify key values and issues that may be influencing the health care encounter and should be included in the plan of care. For example, if illness is seen as an imbalance in the environment, then an effective plan of care needs to include strategies to restore the balance; alternatively, if illness is seen as punishment from God or an outcome of past deeds, interventions need to include spiritual/religious support, not just care of the body. The questions also create a space where the provider can demonstrate humility and invite patient expertise and engage in both unlearning and new learning.

Modes of Action and Decision

The modes of action identified in the CCF are based on Leininger's original work and focus on **cultural care validation/preservation, cultural care accommodation/negotiation**, and **cultural care reframing/repatterning** (Leininger, 1995; see Fig. 4.1). The chosen mode(s) needs to fit the patient's worldviews (emic knowledge) as well as incorporate provider expertise (etic knowledge) that may benefit the patient. Leininger's theory does not explicitly reference power, privilege, or the dynamics of difference (as discussed in Chapter 3); however, the approach to these modes of actions is one of respect, humility, and inclusion.

CULTURAL CARE VALIDATION/PRESERVATION

Cultural care *preservation* refers to actions and decisions that help patients retain their meaningful care values and lifeways (Leininger, 1995). This approach means making efforts to integrate a patient's preferences into the plan of care when these preferences are important to the patient's physical, spiritual, or emotional health. The CCF uses the additional term *validation* to emphasize the need for patient values to be explicitly recognized as legitimate preferences and not just idiosyncratic beliefs. With the acceptance of the Truth and Reconciliation Commission (TRC, 2015a,b) recommendations and commitment to attain equitable health care for Indigenous people, recognizing and preserving cultural traditions and values is now regarded as a basic requirement for care. TRC Recommendation 22 specifically calls for the need to "recognize the value of Indigenous healing practices and use them in the treatment of Indigenous patients in collaboration with Indigenous healers and Elders where requested by Indigenous patients" (TRC, 2015a ,p. 3). The importance of validation extends across cultural populations (Churchill et al., 2020).

It should be noted that acknowledging and supporting others in preserving their values, traditions, or practices does not mean that the health care provider must agree with or endorse those practices. Cultural care validation/preservation encourages health care providers to find the values and practices that are important to the patient and, where possible, work with these values and practices as a foundation for mutual goal setting. Where preservation or support for particular practices or preferences is not possible, it still important to convey respect for the values and the reasons why they cannot be supported. It is critical that this is done in nonjudgemental ways that do not compromise respect for the patient and the patient–provider relationship. Cultural validation/preservation occurs when health care providers present information in ways and places that are acceptable and valued in the patient's culture. This could include respecting the role of particular family members or recognizing the importance of spiritual practices as part of care.

Even though acknowledging patient preferences is a foundation for good practise, health care providers generally underutilize this approach, particularly when the values in question are not problematic and thus remain invisible. However, acknowledging or validating care values that are important for patients can have extremely positive effects with respect to the relationship. It also signals to the patient that the health care provider understands and respects their culture, which increases the likelihood of subsequent disclosure on issues that may be more personal or controversial. Similarly, a lack of acknowledgement and validation can have a significantly negative impact on the patient and family. Validation thus serves to infuse respect and safety (to disclose concerns and perspectives) in the interactional space.

Cultural Considerations in Care

Exorcism as Part of the Plan of Care

Within the mental health setting, patients and families may have concepts of illness that are vastly different from those of the health care providers.

In eliciting one patient's and family's explanatory model of illness, it became apparent that the patient and family believed that supernatural forces were behind the illness and wished to have an exorcism performed by a spiritual leader. Although the psychiatrist did not believe in exorcism or subscribe to this explanatory model, he recognized that the current situation was at an impasse with the family refusing proposed treatment (medications). He understood the family's need for a spiritual intervention and negotiated with them time away from the hospital so they could have the treatment performed outside the hospital. He outlined his concerns about the ongoing lack of treatment and asked the family to come back and let the team know of the progress after such an intervention. By doing so, he was able to maintain a trusting relationship with the family and keep them engaged in care.

This approach demonstrates respect for patient values and should not be taken as the team or the psychiatrist's acceptance or endorsement of a particular treatment; rather, it means respecting patient choices even when they are not understood or sanctioned by the health care provider.

> ### Cultural Competence in Action
>
> #### *Religious Insight Goes a Long Way*
>
> An 18-year-old patient arrived in the emergency room after a motor vehicle accident. From the admission sheet, the nurse noted that the patient's stated religion was Islam. During the nutritional assessment, the nurse sought out the patient's food preferences and asked him whether he was fasting during Ramadan and how that might affect the care he could receive while in hospital.
>
> The patient reacted with considerable surprise that not only was the nurse aware of the Islamic tradition of fasting during Ramadan, a special month of the year when keeping fasts is obligatory for many Muslims, but, more importantly, was willing to consider how this practice could be incorporated into the care schedule. This initial question enhanced trust within the nurse–patient relationship and allowed the patient to be more comfortable in discussing his nutritional, spiritual, and other needs.

CULTURAL CARE ACCOMMODATION/NEGOTIATION

The term *accommodation* means to make suitable or adapt. It can, however, also imply doing a favour or obliging someone. It is important to recognize that cultural care accommodation is not about obliging; rather, it is about assisting patients and health care providers in adapting their ways to include courses of action that may have been previously unfamiliar or inaccessible to the patient. In this mode of action, providers are encouraged to explore ways to support patient choice and access by minimizing barriers, risks, and concerns. Common examples of accommodation include using interpreters to support patient participation in care, allowing different or multiple family members to visit and/or participate in care, and scheduling procedures and tests around times of prayer or significant events or visits.

Like validation, the act of negotiation itself can be very useful in decreasing the power imbalance in the health care provider–patient relationship by signalling that patient values, preferences, and perspectives are important. The first step in clinical negotiation is to develop trust in the therapeutic relationship (Kleinman et al., 1978). Negotiation implies a balancing of competing priorities and occurs when there are differences between the patient's and the health care provider's preferences, and the health care provider feels strongly that their medical interventions are essential to the patient's care. This means first making those preferences and priorities explicit by eliciting the patient's explanatory model of illness. If the health care provider does not understand the patient's explanatory model, negotiation can occur on parallel paths, with the health care provider focusing on one problem and the patient focusing on other illness-related issues. Information sharing and education are critical for accomplishing informed choices and a successful negotiation. Negotiation often occurs around therapies such as medications that the patient may be reluctant to accept because of a preference for herbal or other kinds of treatments or fear of adverse effects. It is important that health care providers both learn about and provide information on the various therapies under consideration. For further discussion of complementary and alternative therapy see Chapter 8.

When considering the mode of cultural care accommodation/negotiation, health care providers should avoid seeing the strategies as "either/or" and should explore the "this and …" approach instead. A useful question to ask is, "What would it take to ____?"; the blank can be filled in with the patient's preferences and values. The answer may, in turn, generate another "What would it take" question. Consider the example of a Middle Eastern family requesting that their father not be cared for by female nurses. If one uses the "What would it take" question, the first answer would obviously be a male nurse. However, if there were no male nurses scheduled on that shift, accommodation in the short term would not be possible. It then becomes important to negotiate with the family about the care needs that need to be performed and who can perform it. The question might then become, "What would it take to provide the care in a culturally acceptable manner?" In some instances, male family members may be willing to take on some responsibility while female nurses carry out other medical interventions. Other answers to "What would it take" questions could be to request a male nurse as a temporary member of the staff. However, that might not be possible because of either budgetary limitations (in this instance, the family may be willing to bear the cost of private-duty nurses if the hospital agrees) or lack of availability (all nurses who are qualified are female). Even if the request is not accommodated successfully, the family is likely to be more accepting of the limitation when they believe that genuine attempts have been made to accommodate them; the health care providers and family would then work together to determine the appropriate actions given the circumstances. Sometimes "What would it take" requires a change in policy or necessitates the development or expansion of a resource. Raising the issue becomes the first step in addressing the need, and although the change may not occur in time to be beneficial to the patient who instigated the question, it may benefit other patients in the future.

Cultural Competence in Action

Organizing Family Visits

Mrs. Porkapolos is an older Greek woman who often has many family members visiting her, even though signs are posted that clearly restrict the number of visitors per patient. The family often becomes very loud and disturbs the other patient in the room. Nursing staff are unsure how to deal with this situation.

Some staff members allow the extra visitors to accommodate the patient's cultural needs. They recognize that close family in this culture includes members of the extended family and that the role of family is significant in care. Other health care providers, however, are concerned about the needs of the other patient and the disruption that the family causes. The inconsistency leads to frustration for both the family and the hospital staff.

How would you handle this situation? Several strategies can be tried. The most important consideration is to have a consistent plan of care, developed collaboratively with the patient, so that individual health care providers are not required to make decisions independently or arbitrarily. Recognizing and involving the family is critical but can be done in ways that avoid allowing multiple visitors. Staff can acknowledge the value of family support while raising their own concerns and limitations. Potential solutions can include assisting Mrs. Porkapolos to the lounge area during visiting hours to minimize the impact on the other patient, encouraging the family to take turns rather than visiting all at once, and determining whether one or two family members could serve as spokespersons and coordinators of the family activities.

CULTURAL CARE REFRAMING/REPATTERNING

Cultural care repatterning helps patients to reorder, change, or modify their lifeways to discover new possibilities and ways of achieving health goals. The mode of action is about reframing preconceived ideas to discover new meanings and new patterns, hence the term reframing. *Reframing* is about seeing something differently; *repatterning* is about changing our patterns to do things differently. Cultural care reframing/repatterning must be differentiated from cultural imposition, in which the health care provider's viewpoint is assumed to be somehow superior and efforts are made to convince the patient to accept that viewpoint.

Reframing offers the patient alternative ways of understanding behaviour and discovering new patterns and meanings if the patient chooses to try it. For example, Western society is heavily focused on the individual and the value of taking care of oneself. As noted previously, in many other cultures, the comparable value is to care for others. In these cultures, putting oneself first is not considered a priority and may even be regarded as selfish behaviour, especially by the women.

Women of Eastern cultures often are unwilling to seek health care for complaints perceived to be minor or take time for self-care to improve their own health and well-being. Health care providers working within this context must acknowledge the value of taking care of others but offer the alternative explanation that being healthy is a prerequisite to being able to take care of others. An analogy of airline safety practices can be used to illustrate the point. In the safety instructions on all flights, passengers are advised that if oxygen masks become necessary, adults should put on their masks before assisting children or others needing assistance.

Another example is when inaction occurs due to an understanding of illness reflecting God's will. In such instances it may be helpful to engage external colleagues, such as community and religious leaders (e.g., Christian chaplain, Muslim imam, Jewish rabbi, or Hindu priest). Religious leaders are often considered instruments of God and interpreters of the scriptures and are trusted guides for the community (Almukhaini et al., 2020; Lewis Hall & Hill, 2019; McEvoy et al., 2017).

The mode of cultural care reframing and repatterning is not limited to patients; it can apply equally to health care providers. In many cultures, speaking explicitly about terminal illness and death is said to hasten death (Rising, 2017). As a result, families may request that news of this nature not be communicated directly to the patient. Some health care providers regard compliance with such a request as withholding the truth and may feel obligated to disregard family wishes and provide such information to the patient. However, others consider that going against family wishes would constitute imposing the truth. Recognizing different ways of framing a situation may allow both parties to consider a third option, that of offering the truth as asked and allowing the patient to determine how much and what kind of information they wish to have in order to make decisions about their care. Cochran et al. (2017) present a case where a Pakistani father requests that the medical team hold off on conveying their child's fatal prognosis to his wife, as he knows her best and believes she will not be able to handle such news in her present circumstances. The case is presented from multiple perspectives (including the father's), including questioning the assumption that every parent wants to know everything. The authors note that "[c]ultural factors that may be initially perceived as barriers may be better understood as opportunities for enhanced, personalized treatment" (Cochran et al., 2017, p. 4). The discussion reinforces the need for commitment, active engagement, and ongoing learning. The reframing/repatterning mode is based on the need for continually challenging old assumptions and creating new possibilities and options for patients, health care providers, and the health care system.

In summary, the modes of decision making offer concrete strategies that can be explored to provide culturally congruent care. As noted by Jeffreys and Zoucha (2018), while there is growing recognition regarding the need for cultural competence, "culturally congruent action strategies for creating change and making a positive difference within one's spheres of influence [remain] obscure" (p. 120). The authors provide several case examples of both culturally incongruent and culturally congruent care to illustrate their point (Jeffreys & Zoucha, 2018). Strategies for validation, accommodation/negotiation, and reframing provide concrete guidance on actions that can be taken by health care providers with and across cultures.

Cultural Competence in Action

When Male Partners Do the Talking

Nancy is a nurse who works in the women's outpatient program in a hospital that serves a large number of refugees and recent immigrants to Canada. In her practice, Nancy frequently encounters situations in which the male partner accompanies the woman to her appointment, answers the questions on her behalf, and essentially does not allow the woman to interact directly with the health care providers.

Continued

Nancy has found this extremely frustrating. Although she recognizes that many cultures have different gender roles and behaviours, she feels that because the women are now in Canada, the health care providers need to empower them to claim equal status. Nancy is also concerned from a practice perspective. She is aware of the increased potential for domestic violence in immigrant communities that has been associated with the stress of migration, underemployment, and changing family roles, and she finds it difficult to assess for this risk without an opportunity to interact with the woman alone.

In a discussion about cultural competence, Nancy realizes that much of her reaction has been influenced by her own feminist background, beliefs related to gender roles, and the associated history of women's rights in society. However, she still finds this situation extremely challenging to deal with.

What advice would you give Nancy in working through this situation? Would you agree that the male partner's behaviour is oppressive and its influence needs to be minimized? Would any other explanations account for the male partner's behaviour?

In your discussion, imagine the following scenario: you have travelled to a strange country with someone you care for very much (e.g., spouse, child, sibling, or parent). Your significant other becomes ill and needs health care; however, the language as well as the health care system are unfamiliar. When seeking health care, would you accompany your significant other? Are there circumstances under which you might speak for them (bearing in mind that many native-born Canadians do that when they think their significant others will not be clear or complete about their symptoms)? How would you react if you felt that people were trying very hard to separate you from your significant other?

This scenario illustrates that what may be labelled as oppressive behaviour could in fact be an expression of caring. Nancy's attempts to ignore or distance the male partner are likely to have the opposite effect, by increasing distrust. The alternative explanation does not mean that the first hypothesis was incorrect, but it does caution against premature judgement and suggests the need for additional data. Nancy's desire to empower women (or at least to set the tone) on their initial visits is reflective of her priority and not necessarily that of her patient. If, however, Nancy is successful in developing a relationship with both the woman and the male partner, the woman is likely to feel safer and in subsequent interactions may share any concerns she has related to her partner and/or domestic stress and abuse.

The earlier discussion on modes of action and decision offers a practical approach to addressing gaps that cultural differences may have created. The modes we have discussed can serve as the bridge across the cultural divide. It is important to recognize that there are no clear answers or strategies that work in all circumstances. Instead, multiple strategies will need to be used simultaneously to validate, accommodate, and reframe the values and meanings that underlie behaviour. Successful interactions will result in positive learning experiences for *both* the patient and the health care provider. These strategies have applicability across all levels of cultural competence.

A useful tip to guide the implementation of the above strategies can be summarized by the acronym LEARN (**L**isten, **E**xplain, **A**cknowledge, **R**ecommend, **N**egotiate) (Berlin & Fowkes, 1983). In busy health care environments, there is pressure to ensure that the issues providers believe to be important are attended to first, and then they can take time to listen to any other concerns patients may have. Explanations are viewed as prerequisites to informed questioning by patients. However, the LEARN framework reminds us to listen first, to understand patient priorities, and then explanations can be responsive to the issues discerned. It is also important to acknowledge the patient's values as well as differences and gaps that may exist between care that is desired and what is available. In the spirit of being patient-centred and cautious about imposing their own views, providers often hesitate to share their own recommendations; however, it is important to acknowledge and share provider experience and expertise. Providing such explanations as alternatives to consider can be a great opportunity to expand the patient's worldview and options available to them.

Navigating Difference at the Group Level

Navigating difference at the team level means recognizing the dynamics of difference that may exist within a team with respect to varied cultural identities and the associated worldviews and levels of privilege or marginalization. It is important to recognize the dynamics and the impact of varied identities on group functioning. The inherent power dynamics within a group lead to not only unequal opportunity but also **unequal risk** for individuals. For example, an individual who is new to a team, is racialized, or reflects a different age bracket from that of most of the team will face a higher level of risk when challenging a norm or providing an alternate perspective, because of the unconscious biases, stereotypes, and other expressions of inequity they are already subjected to. In other words, unequal risk occurs because people are more vulnerable and less likely to have the protection of systemic privilege.

Navigating Difference as a Minority "Other"

Increasing workforce diversity is a frequently identified strategy in developing organizational cultural competence, building organizational capacity, and effectively navigating issues of culture and discrimination in health care (Handtke et al., 2019; McCalman et al., 2017). The TRC recommendations also call for an "increase [in] the number of Indigenous professionals working in the health-care field" (TRC, 2015a, 23.i, p. 3). While in theory such individuals bring critical, diverse, and much needed strengths and perspectives to a system that needs to change, they are also at risk for experiencing the racism and exclusion that exist in the system (Hunter & Cook, 2020; Turpel-Lafond, 2020).

The scenario below was shared by a nursing student as part of a project on culturally responsive therapeutic relationships that involved small-group discussions over time. Unfortunately, similar experiences continue to be a reality across health disciplines.

Cultural Considerations in Care

Being the Minority Other

When I first came to Toronto [to study] about 3 years ago, I was excited and impressed by the diversity of culture, ethnicity, and languages. However, the excitement of being in a different cultural environment was soon replaced by feelings of frustration and vulnerability because of communication barriers. My self-esteem was seriously shaken by the negative feedback from my interactions with some people. I did not understand the cause of it. For example, there was a preceptor who displayed unwillingness in teaching me; he was treating other students differently. When this pattern appeared constantly, I realized that there was something wrong. However, I did not [realize] that I was involved in a cultural issue. In another example from a different clinical setting, a preceptor often put me down by saying "you are hopeless because you are a foreign student… People will never accept you because 'there is a big cultural gap'." I felt deeply insulted and helpless. I questioned my competence as a student nurse; therefore, I avoided seeking supports. At that time, my understanding of being culturally competent was simply about my relationship with patients, such as respecting my patients' culture, ethnicity, and values, because I understood their vulnerability and my obligations as a student nurse. I was satisfied with my interactions with patients; however, I was not aware of my own vulnerability of being a nondominant student nurse and the potential impact on my nursing practice. My confidence of becoming a competent nurse was shaken over and over by these situations, even though professors and clinical instructors recognized my academic and clinical performances.

Through the education sessions, my understanding of being culturally competent has broadened and deepened. I recognize that being culturally competent means much more than respecting patients' values and dignity [and includes] being able to deal with culture-related issues in many other situations, such as culturally incompetent staff mentors.

In a 2020 report that documents Indigenous-specific racism in British Columbia, a key finding was that "Indigenous health care workers face significant racism and discrimination in their work and study environments" (Turpel-Lafond, 2020, p. 91) and that "the racism experienced by Indigenous health care students and workers has a negative impact on their health and well-being. It is career-limiting to voice concern about racism and can bring negative professional impacts and lead to decisions to leave their profession. Those who do raise concerns are often traumatized by the experience" (p. 91). While the report documents stories of racism and discrimination from students and practitioners in medicine and nursing, the experiences likely resonate across all professions. The challenges include a lack of cultural supports, direct experiences of racism and discrimination, additional trauma associated with witnessing such behaviour, and the burden of advocacy—which often lead to negative repercussions.

Similarly, in a qualitative inquiry of experiences of Māori nurses, Hunter and Cook (2020) described the experiences under four themes: te tuakiri Māori—cultural identity; kawenga taumaha—bearing the burden; te kaikiritanga—racism; and tauutuutu—reciprocity. The nurses described how their cultural identity shaped their approach to professional practice, although at times this created conflict with Westernized professional boundaries. Cultural identity also influenced opportunities for professional growth. The nurses reported witnessing "routinized everyday practices that diminished, demeaned, and disempowered the unique identity and wellbeing of Māori and yet were not recognized as culturally unsafe" (p. 15). They also experienced a deep sense of obligation and the emotional burden of advocacy. The theme of reciprocity was described by interactions in which their advocacy was embraced and led to better patient care outcomes or change at the system level (Hunter & Cook, 2020). Similar findings of discrimination, including microaggressions from patients, peers, and faculty, have been reported in US research with minority nurses and nursing students (Graham et al., 2016; Iheduru-Anderson et al., 2021) as well minority resident physicians (Osseo-Asare et al., 2018). A thorough discussion of provider experiences of racism in health care is beyond the scope of this chapter; however, it is important to recognize this as an issue for *all* health care providers. Understanding is the first step to empowerment and ability to challenge the system.

Strengthening workforce diversity is an important strategy, but its strength and effectiveness will not be realized until those in the health care system begin to truly value and support a diverse workforce. The necessary changes will come when dominant and nondominant groups learn to "see," understand, and address culture, discrimination, and inequities that exist within health care teams. Currently, in Canada, and across other countries, considerable effort and initiatives are underway in health care organizations and educational settings to better inform and support health care practitioners of all cultural identities. It is important for all individuals to engage in genuine, albeit at times uncomfortable, dialogue, for the unlearning and new learning required to ensure success toward inclusion and equity. Making racism visible and ending the silence on racism (Iheduru-Anderson et al., 2021) are critical steps to supporting and benefitting from a diverse workforce.

Accountability, Allyship, and Advocacy

Anicha et al. (2018) recognize three "big ideas" that are central to achieving equity and social justice: advocacy, allyship, and accountability. They note that "accountability to/with marginalized 'others' is identified as crucial because clear understandings about the behaviors and systems that perpetuate social (in)justices rarely emerge spontaneously in the minds of privileged individuals. Rather, persons directly experiencing unearned disadvantages become cartographers of the privilege landscape" (p. 157). The authors contend that such accountability requires both allyship and advocacy.

An **ally** is defined and described as "a person, group, or nation that is associated with another or others for some common cause or purpose" (Dictionary.com, 2020). "**Allyship** is the active, consistent, and arduous practise of unlearning and re-evaluating, in which a person in a position of privilege and power seeks to operate in solidarity with a marginalized group" (The Anti-Oppression Network, n.d.). It is an active and strategic engagement practice that is rooted in the recognition of structural inequality and of specific histories of oppression and domination that one is standing in opposition to and in solidarity with those who are marginalized. Given that in different contexts the salient political issue(s) will vary, the identities of those in allyship will also vary. For example, a racialized person may be an ally to a White person on issues of disability, poverty, or gender identity.

In a social justice context, an ally is a member of a dominant group who uses their privilege to support members of the oppressed or marginalized group(s). The privilege can come from one or more aspects of their identity and social location that are part of the dominant group(s). The support can take many forms. It might be active and visible in the form of speaking out in public to challenge the status quo and attempt to alter the dynamics of a given situation; it may be private in the form of advocacy behind the scenes in support of individuals and groups; or it may be working to dismantle or change the structures and processes that perpetuate inequities (Juntanamalaga et al., 2019; Melton, 2018; Zuzelo, 2020). The key characteristic is that allies use their understanding and the power associated with their identity to support individuals who are marginalized and issues related to marginalization (Melton, 2018). It is important to note that allies do not do for others; rather, they support others to gain power and exercise power (Juntanamalaga et al., 2019). In this perspective, allies are facilitators who help others with access to information, connections, resources, decision-making tables, and the ability to tap into internal wisdom and voice. Allies can also take on the role of sponsors, champions, and amplifiers. The following was shared by a consumer speaking on behalf of an ally for the consumer movement in mental health: "And she *coached me and supported me* [emphasis added] to be able to do that. And very often, in a meeting, she would say, 'And what about you? *What's your idea on this?*' … So then I'd share my experience and how that related to the situation. And … *because it meant so much to her to have my voice there, … because of her senior role, others picked up on that* [emphasis added] and started to listen as well and started paying attention" (Juntanamalaga et al., 2019, p. 861). This example illustrates the strategies of empowering support, amplifying voice, and using one's role and privilege to set expectations.

Being an effective ally is context dependent; therefore, there is no simple checklist. Table 4.3 provides a concise description of an ally, and Table 4.4 provides tips on being an effective ally.

Being an ally requires a commitment and vulnerability. Actions such as expressions of outrage on social media, feeling guilty, shaming others, and speaking for others are not ally behaviour as they shift the focus to oneself (Phillips, 2020); rather, allies always put the interests of the groups they are supporting over self-interest. Being an ally also does not mean being infallible; allies will make mistakes, and it is important that criticism be accepted with grace and an ongoing commitment to learning.

Cultural Competence in Action

From Awareness to Action in Becoming an Ally

Nadia, a White student, noticed that one of her peers, Toya, who is racialized, was often quiet in clinical group discussion. This was surprising to her as she had great conversations with Toya and always appreciated her insights. Upon reflection she began to notice that often Toya would say something, but it was not heard or acknowledged by others (even by her). Someone else would make a similar point and receive positive recognition. Nadia felt that the group's behaviour was continuing to marginalize Toya and she began to look for opportunities to acknowledge Toya's contribution and even encourage her to share her perspective and insights.

What else can Nadia do to support Toya in a way that is respectful and effective?

TABLE 4.3 ■ A Succinct Description of an Ally

Always centre the impacted person(s), let them define the issues.
Listen, learn from, and engage with those who live in the oppression.
Leverage your privilege, acknowledge the issues.
Yield the floor and provide support—it's not about you!

Adapted from Reed, K. (2021, March 11). *A succinct description of an ally* [Tweet]. Twitter. https://twitter.com/iKaylaReed/status/742243143030972416.

TABLE 4.4 ■ Tips for Being an Effective Ally

1. Recognize that being an ally is not a label, it's a process.
2. Identify your power and privilege to act as an effective ally.
3. Follow and support those from marginalized groups as much as possible.
4. When you make a mistake, apologize, correct yourself, and move on.
5. Spend time educating yourself and use the knowledge to help.
6. Take time to think and analyze the situation.
7. Try to understand perception versus reality.
8. Take a stand.
9. Work to change the systemwide issues.
10. Leverage other powers of authority.

From Axner, M. (n.d). *Learning to be an ally for people from diverse groups and backgrounds*. https://ctb.ku.edu/en/table-of-contents/culture/cultural-competence/be-an-ally/main. University of Nevada Library. (2021). *Becoming an ally.* https://guides.library.unlv.edu/c.php?g=604186&p=4187428.

While allies are usually from outside the community they are supporting, advocates may be insiders or outsiders. **Advocates** have all the characteristics of allies and are usually more public with their activities. Where allies focus on centring the voices of those impacted and may interrupt or intervene in discriminatory or exclusionary situations, advocates take on the role of lobbying for change in solidarity with others. In current times, advocacy has shifted from a sociopolitical focus to the use of social media power "on behalf of vulnerable others" to call attention to issues and call out behaviour of individuals and groups. While social media has the power to have broad and significant impact, it also poses a risk of superficiality and making it about the so-called advocate rather than the issue or the individuals who experience the inequities or injustice (Anicha et al., 2018).

An **activist** is someone who works to bring about social or political change, often through activities that agitate and create tension with the intention of "alert[ing] masses to ignored suffering" of others (Melton, 2018, p. 3). To be productive and not simply reactionary, health care activism needs to be framed within a social justice framework (Cabrera et al., 2017). Musolino et al. (2020) describe health activism as consisting of the following themes: movement building to tap into others beyond one's workplace; capacity building through building relationships with others to develop a shared culture and purpose; campaigning through advocacy and policy dialogue; and knowledge generation and dissemination to inform public policy. The roles of ally, advocate, and activist overlap and can be seen as a continuum of activity, agitation, and power (Zuzelo, 2020). Being an ally requires moving beyond awareness and knowledge to leveraging social identity and power to act in support of cultural safety and equity. While an advocate can champion issues on behalf of others and societal change, an activist may extend advocacy into a campaign that includes agitation and demands for righting the wrongs of the past through political or social change (Melton, 2018).

Zuzelo (2020) notes that "many nurses likely feel unprepared to lead or participate as militant agents rocking the status" (p. 191). However, being an ally and advocate should not be seen as militant action; rather, it is simply speaking up for care that is person-centred and equitable *for all*—an expectation and aspiration of health care providers regardless of their role or discipline. Using knowledge to inform practice and policy is an expected aspect of practice. Goldberg et al. (2017) further remind us that through self-reflexive and compassionate practices, nurses have the ability to "more deeply understand the relevance of sociocultural-political and historical positioning of self, others, and the broader global community" (p. 270). This provides better opportunities to care for and with historically and currently under-represented communities and aligns nursing practice with the profession's mandate of providing equitable care for all (Goldberg et al., 2017).

As noted earlier in the chapter, the work of bringing equity and cultural competence into practice operates at the individual (micro), team (meso), and broader organizational and system (macro) levels. An understanding of the integral relationship between the three levels is critical to success. Fig. 4.2 presents a four-part or quadripartite model that illustrates how to understand and navigate the core dimensions of cultural competence. Fig. 4.2A presents the elements of the CCF in a different format: cultural sensitivity, knowledge, and skills are augmented by explicitly creating a dimension of application in practice. This highlights our belief that without application, knowledge and understanding are incomplete. In our experience, interventions often focus on awareness or knowledge acquisition at the individual or team level, but without conscious effort to translate this knowledge into skills and apply it to practice, the work is merely edifying, with no impact on outcomes. The difficulties in application can be better understood in Fig. 4.2B, which identifies the domains of personal, professional, organizational, and society. Embedded in each domain are strengths as well as barriers that need to be challenged and leveraged to achieve the goal of equity. The domains intersect and have a cumulative impact on what happens in practice. Since practice functions at all these levels, each of the core domains must be strategically engaged for efficacy. For example, while personal biases and lack of knowledge can be a barrier, a commitment to change

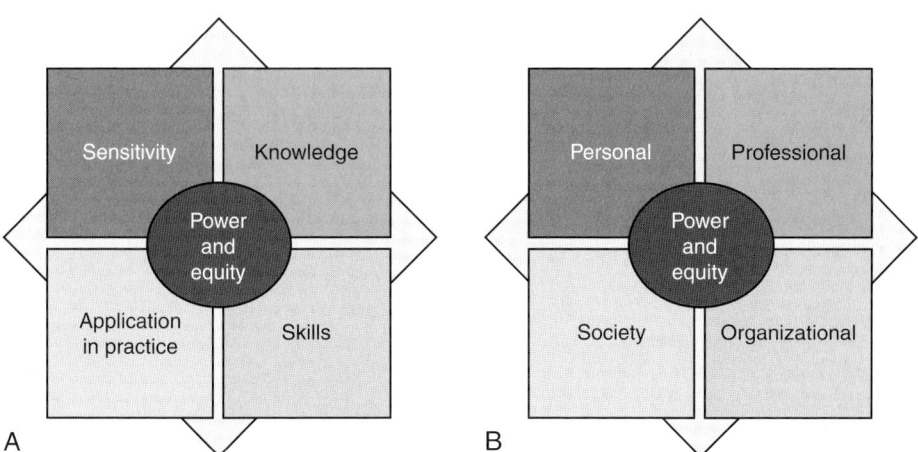

Fig. 4.2 A four-part or quadripartite model illustrates how to understand and navigate the core dimensions of cultural competence. (A) Cultural sensitivity, knowledge, and skills are augmented by explicitly creating a dimension of application in practice. (B) The domains of personal, professional, organizational, and society are shown. Application in practice requires an understanding of resources and barriers in each of these four domains.

and ability to seek knowledge is a resource. While all health care professions have their legacies intertwined with colonialism and oppression, there are practice guidelines, resources, and tools that can support practitioners in better understanding and applying their knowledge toward the goal of health equity. Similarly, organizations have mission statements and mandates along with accountability for equitable service, and while society is full of "-isms," there is optimism as well as opportunity in diversity along with commitments of cultural pluralism and guidance from works such as the TRC report. Crucially, we see the centring of power as ever-present (as discussed in Chapter 3) and with equity as the recognized goal.

Cultural Competence in Action

Challenging Racism with Understanding

You work in an interdisciplinary team that provides services to patients and communities who are diverse and marginalized[4] in many ways. Your program is effective overall; however, you have noticed that when things "go wrong," individuals and the interdisciplinary team as a whole do not deal with the issues well. A recent example has you thinking that this needs to change.

In running a nutrition and food budgeting group for people with low income and diabetes you witnessed a patient shouting at Mahreen, a racialized colleague. The patient (an older White man) raised his voice and kept repeating, "I don't want to talk to you, I want to talk to a real nurse." Then he yelled at her, "Don't touch me you XXXXX." Your colleague Mahreen is a nurse, born in Canada, whose parents originate from Bangladesh. Another team member, Clara, a social worker (who is White and also born in Canada) spoke up at this point and firmly said to the patient that Mahreen was fully qualified and that his outburst was not acceptable. The patient then said, "She [Mahreen] should go back home." Both colleagues were visibly upset.

Consider what is the role of both clinicians in this scenario? Should Clara have spoken up? Why or why not? What could be done at the team level to develop approaches to this issue? Who else in this scenario might need some support? How do the concepts of team accountability, allyship, and empowerment impact potential responses?

Navigating Difference at the Organization/System Level

The invisibility of privilege extends into our teams and systems and structures where written and unwritten rules reinforce some norms and create barriers for others, thereby reinforcing inequities (Nixon, 2019). The culture of the organization affects the individual patient and provider experience. In a US study of LGBTQ nurses' experiences in the workplace, Eliason et al. (2011) illustrated the connection between individual experiences and broader organizational policies. Study participants spoke to place in terms of the city they were located in as being liberal or conservative, religious affiliation of the organization, and organizational policies and practices that were discriminatory (partner benefits) or inclusive (diversity statements and inclusive language in policies). Of note, in this study participant reference to friendly environment meant not hostile as opposed to an inclusive environment (Eliason et al., 2011).

---

[4]As noted earlier, terminology is evolving and subject to interpretation. We are comfortable with the term *marginalization* as it continues to remind us of the need to pay attention to those on the periphery and centre their voices. More recently the terms *equity deserving* and *equity priority* groups have come into the discourse. The challenge with "equity deserving" when used in a global way is the notion that all groups should be equity deserving. "Equity priority" recognizes where the biggest need may be.

Recognizing the barriers and enablers that exist within an organization and system is essential for transformational change. For example, systems of higher education privilege Western knowledge in ways that result in unfair and unsafe environments for others, including Indigenous people (Russell, 2020). The Canadian health care system privileges the biomedical approach to illness and "evidence-informed medicine" for treatment; anything else is considered less legitimate (see Chapter 8). At the same time, many health authorities and agencies are actively engaged in broadening the services offered to include Indigenous healing (for example, see www.camh.ca/en/driving-change/shkaabe-makwa) or cultural adaptation of evidence-informed treatments such as cognitive behavioural therapy (Naeem et al., 2019). It is important to recognize that the goal of health equity cannot be achieved without change at the organizational level through providing services that are culturally appropriate and accessible to all.

The organizational journey toward equity needs be understood from the perspective of practice change as well as organizational change—with associated standards, tools, models, and frameworks to support that work. McEvoy et al. (2017) discuss an initiative aimed at improving access to mental health care in an Orthodox Jewish community in the United Kingdom. Their critical reflection points to the importance of relationship building, dialogic engagement, and distributed leadership as key elements. The process allowed for the uncovering and examination of assumptions, new insights, and the importance of respecting the other's autonomy, even if that meant a "full alignment of the goals of different constituencies may not always be possible" (p. 12).

Different jurisdictions, regions, and counties have varied approaches to models of health system and care delivery. This extends to the extent to which there are formal standards or professional practice guidelines. In the domain of health equity and cultural competence we are seeing an increase in legal frameworks, health policy statements, and, in some cases, standards and guidelines. This is an example of the "system" component of the quadripartite model (see Fig. 4.2B) and can be used to impact and enable work at the organizational level.

In health care, the United States has developed national standards for culturally and linguistically appropriate services (CLAS) that provide expectations, guidance, and support to organizations in their journey toward cultural competence. The standards are organized in four broad categories: (1) principal standard; (2) governance, leadership and workforce; (3) communication and language support; and (4) engagement, continuous improvement, and accountability. This model demonstrates a robust mapping of health system measurement and accountability to a specific set of equity issues—in this case, culture and language. Note that culture here does not include sexual and gender minorities.

In Canada, guidance comes from a variety of sources. Within the Canadian context there is increasing reference to equity a being a core dimension of quality care (BC Patient Safety and Quality Council, 2020; Ontario Ministry of Health and Long Term Care, 2018). There is also guidance in the form of focused recommendations from the TRC. These recommendations call on government to provide sustainable funding for Indigenous healing centres, call for change within the health care system to recognize the value of Indigenous healing practice and support their use in collaboration with Indigenous healers and Elders, and support recruitment and retention of Indigenous professionals in health care and providing cultural care training for all health care providers (TRC, 2015). These calls to action are slowly leading to greater availability and acceptance of Indigenous healing traditions. Guidance is also available from organizations such as Accreditation Canada and other accrediting bodies, as well as regulatory and professional bodies that set out standards of practice and provide guidelines for care. See Table 4.5 for selected examples. It is important to note that resources with respect to guidance and standards is continuing to evolve.

In Canada, there is no legislated requirement for language support for patients, except for required interpretation for deaf patients as a result of a Supreme Court ruling in 1997 (Stradiotto, 1998). Despite Canada being a bilingual nation, the requirement for French language support

TABLE 4.5 ■ Selected Resources for Organizational Cultural Competence

Australia
Cultural Respect Framework:
https://apo.org.au/sites/default/files/resource-files/2016-01/apo-nid256721.pdf

Canada
Building a Foundation for Change: Canada's Anti-Racism Strategy 2019–2022:
https://www.canada.ca/en/canadian-heritage/campaigns/anti-racism-engagement/anti-racism-
strategy.html#a
Equity, Diversity, Inclusion in the Research System:
https://cihr-irsc.gc.ca/e/52543.html
Health Equity for People with Disabilities:
https://www.cdc.gov/ncbddd/humandevelopment/health-equity.html
Truth and Reconciliation Commission of Canada: Calls to Action:
https://ehprnh2mwo3.exactdn.com/wp-content/uploads/2021/01/Calls_to_Action_English2.pdf

New Zealand
Guidelines for Cultural Safety, the Treaty of Waitangi and Māori Health in Nursing Education and
Practice:
https://www.nccih.ca/634/Guidelines_for_Cultural_Safety,_the_Treaty_of_Waitangi_and_Maori_
Health_in_Nursing_Education_and_Pra....nccih?id=1141
Health Quality and Safety New Zealand:
https://www.hqsc.govt.nz/our-programmes/patient-safety-day/previous-psw-campaigns/psw-2019/
cultural-safety-and-cultural-competence

United Kingdom
The Equality and Health Inequalities Hub:
https://www.england.nhs.uk/about/equality/equality-hub

United States
CLAS Standards
https://thinkculturalhealth.hhs.gov/clas
Institute for Health Improvement: *Achieving Health Equity: A Guide for Health Care Organizations:*
http://www.ihi.org/resources/Pages/IHIWhitePapers/Achieving-Health-Equity.aspx

World Health Organization
Women's Health:
https://www.who.int/health-topics/women-s-health

---

applies to only designated organizations. However, most health care organizations across Canada recognize the importance of language support and provide access to interpreters in most major languages (also see Chapter 6).

Canadian literature on organizational cultural competence is limited. There is recognition of key organizational dimensions that need to be addressed to achieve success on this journey. These include organizational values and norms; leadership; recruitment and retention; training and education for all staff; accessible program and services including language support, community partnerships, and collaboration; adaptation of physical and social environment; data that make progress (or lack of it) visible; and focused roles that support navigation and patient advocacy (culture brokering) (Cherner et al., 2014; Fung et al. 2012; Handtke et al., 2019). In our experience in working with health care and educational institutions, the critical elements for organizational cultural competence include leadership, community engagement and partnerships, workforce development strategy that is inclusive of recruitment and staff education, and the use of data. When these four elements exist, other changes follow.

Leaders, at all levels of the organization, have a key role in translating intent and commitment into strategy and action to deliver on the stated goals. They create expectations and can infuse the necessary principles into the institutional structure with respect to policy, culture, environment, and other aspects of the organization. Cultural competence is both a way of being and a way of doing. In addition to changing hearts and minds, it is also about changing behaviour and practice; practice expectations are set, monitored, and reinforced by leadership. The journey toward organizational cultural competence requires collaborative partnerships with diverse communities and groups. Such partnerships are critical to augment service provision as well as support development of accessible programs and services needed to achieve the equity goals. Workforce development is another key organizational strategy. However, recruitment and education will not be successful without ongoing support and organizational commitment to expand and transform the care and services delivered. Finally, we advocate the use of data, both quantitative and qualitative, that can document and make visible the change and progression from an organization that is culturally blind and treats everyone the same way to an organization that is culturally proficient with partnerships, has an ability to provide care based on identified needs, builds on its own and others' expertise, and measures the progress toward the goal of health equity.

In addition to the identification of areas of change, it is also important to consider *how* the change is initiated, supported, and maintained. The aforementioned dimensions provide guidance on the priority areas for action, and frameworks of organizational change can guide how the change occurs in ways that are effective and sustainable. It is beyond the scope of this chapter to discuss organizational change frameworks, and most frameworks are not equity based; however, wisdom from this field about what supports meaningful change can be an added tool for cultural competence work. An example is offered by McEvoy et al. (2017). The key is to develop an approach that focuses on learning as well as unlearning at the individual and organizational level and embraces a both/and approach that values professional expertise along with patient, family, and community expertise. There is much to learn from the Indigenous wisdom of **two-eyed seeing**,[5] which recognizes the strengths of both Western and Indigenous ways of knowing and uses both together to provide effective care for all (Bartlett et al., 2012).

Summary

This chapter highlights issues, approaches, and strategies for navigating difference at the individual, team, and organizational levels. The micro, meso, and macro levels of this work are a reality of practice, and our approach needs to recognize the interdependencies between the levels and enable us to strategically plan and operate within these complexities. Cultural competence is a practice strategy to reach health equity goals, informed by an understanding of culture as both patterns and power; thus our strategies need to intentionally address both dimensions of difference and its contextual impact on individuals, groups, and communities.

Recognition of privilege and unconscious bias at individual and systems levels is a foundational aspect of working effectively across cultures. The CCF presents three broad approaches to bridge the gap across cultures. Cultural care preservation/validation, cultural care accommodation/negotiation, and cultural care reframing are approaches that can be intentionally utilized to enhance trust, collaborate with patients and families, and tap into both provider and patient expertise. A key aspect of cultural competence is to make the invisible visible—to explicitly identify values,

---

[5] The principle of two-eyed seeing was brought forward by Elder Albert Marshall, a Mi'kmaw Elder in Unama'ki-Cape Breton.

beliefs, and agendas that may be influencing decisions in particular contexts, or policies and processes that can be exclusionary and unfavourable to specific individuals and groups. Thus while the work of navigating difference begins as an individual, it requires extension to groups and system transformation. Allyship and advocacy are key processes that can support this journey and the desired goals.

At the organizational level we identify key domains and priority areas (leadership, collaborative partnerships, workforce development, and use of data to monitor progress toward goals) requiring attention to facilitate and support the development of cultural competence. We maintain that cultural competence and equity work can be integrated within the models and toolkits for practice development as well as frameworks and approaches for organizational developmental and change, to achieve the needed transformation for care that is culturally congruent and equitable.

ⓔ http://evolve.elsevier.com/Srivastava/culturalcompetence/.

Questions for Review and Discussion

1. Provide one example of each of the modes of decision making that you could apply in a clinical setting.
2. Reflect on your own upbringing—are there "explanatory" models of health and illness that you heard from your family that may be different from your professional knowledge? How do you reconcile the two?
3. Reflect on the terms *marginalized, equity deserving,* and *equity priority*. What do they mean to you? Is there one term you prefer over others—why or why not?
4. Briefly describe two strategies that can be implemented by organizational leaders to support health care providers in the delivery of culturally competent equitable care.

Group Experiential/Reflection Activity

Think of an example or situation that you encountered in which there were cultural differences and experiences of actual or potential inequitable outcomes. Using the quadripartite model in Figs. 4.2A and 4.2B, assess the strengths and challenges in each domain for your scenario. Where are the barriers? Where are the opportunities? Do this exercise individually first and then discuss as a group. Compare responses and discuss as a group. Note the similarities, differences, and collaborative opportunities for learning. Strategize approaches for similar situations in the future.

References

Almukhaini, S., Goldberg, L., & Watson, J. (2020). Embodying caring science as Islamic philosophy of care: Implications for nursing practice. *Advances in Nursing Science, 43*(1), 62–74. https://doi.org/10.1097/ANS.0000000000000300.

Anicha, C., Bilen-Green, C., & Burnett, A. (2018). Advocates and allies: The succession of a good idea or what's in a meme? *Studies in Social Justice, 12*(1), 152–164.

Bartlett, C., Marshall, M., & Marshall, A. (2012). Two-eyed seeing and other lessons learned within a co-learning of bringing together Indigenous and mainstream knowledge and ways of knowing. *Journal of Environmental Studies and Sciences, 2*(4), 331–340.

BC Patient Safety and Quality Council. (2020). *What is quality?* https://bcpsqc.ca/what-is-quality.

Berlin, E. A., & Fowkes, W. A., Jr. (1983). A teaching framework for cross-cultural health care. Application in family practice. *The Western Journal of Medicine, 139*(6), 934–938. https://www.ncbi.nlm.nih.gov/pmc/articles/PMC1011028/.

Cabrera, N. L., Matias, C. E., & Montoya, R. (2017). Activism or slacktivism? The potential and pitfalls of social media in contemporary student activism. *Journal of Diversity in Higher Education*. https://doi.org/10.1037/dhe0000061.

Cherner, R., Olavarria, M., Young, M., et al. (2014). Evaluation of the organizational cultural competence of a community health center: A multimethod approach. *Health Promotion Practice*, *15*(5), 675–684. https://doi.org/10.1177/1524839914532650.

Churchill, M. E., Smylie, J. K., Wolfe, S. H., et al. (2020). Conceptualising cultural safety at an Indigenous-focused midwifery practice in Toronto, Canada: Qualitative interviews with Indigenous and non-Indigenous clients. *BMJ Open*, *10*(9), e038168. https://doi.org/10.1136/bmjopen-2020-038168.

Cochran, D., Saleem, S., Khowaja-Punjwani, S., et al. (2017). Cross-cultural differences in communication about a dying child. *Pediatrics*, *140*(5), e20170690.

Dictionary.com. (2020). *Ally*. Dictionary.com, LLC. https://www.dictionary.com/browse/ally?s=t

Eliason, M. J., Dejoseph, J., Dibble, S., et al. (2011). Lesbian, gay, bisexual, transgender, and queer/questioning nurses' experiences in the workplace. *Journal of Professional Nursing*, *27*(4), 237–244. https://doi.org/10.1016/j.profnurs.2011.03.003.

Fung, K., Lo, H. T., Srivastava, R., et al. (2012). Organizational cultural competence consultation to a mental health institution. *Transcultural Psychiatry*, *49*, 165–184.

Goldberg, L., Rosenburg, N., & Watson, J. (2017). Rendering LGBTQ+ visible in nursing: Embodying the philosophy of caring science in nursing. *Journal of Holistic Nursing*, *36*(3), 262–271. https://doi.org/10.1177/0898010117715141.

Graham, C. L., Phillips, S. M., Newman, S. D., et al. (2016). Baccalaureate minority nursing students perceived barriers and facilitators to clinical education practices: An integrative review. *Nursing Education Perspectives*, *37*(3), 130–137. https://doi.org/10.1097/01.NEP.0000000000000003.

Handtke, O., Schilgen, B., & Mösko, M. (2019). Culturally competent healthcare – a scoping review of strategies implemented in healthcare organizations and a model of culturally competent healthcare provision. *PLoS ONE*, *14*(7), e0219971. https://doi.org/10.1371/journal.pone.0219971.

Holm, A. L., Gorosh, M. R., Brady, M., et al. (2017). Recognizing privilege and bias: An interactive exercise to expand health care providers' personal awareness. *Academic Medicine*, *92*, 360–364. https://doi.org/10.1097/ACM.0000000000001290.

Hunter, K., & Cook, C. M. (2020). Cultural and clinical practice realities of Māori nurses in Aotearoa New Zealand: The emotional labour of Indigenous nurses. *Nursing Praxis in Aotearoa New Zealand*, *36*(3), 7–23. https://doi.org/10.36951/27034542.2020.011.

Iheduru-Anderson, K., Shingles, R. R., & Akanegbu, C. (2021). Discourse of race and racism in nursing: An integrative review of literature. *Public Health Nursing*, *38*, 115–130. https://doi.org/10.1111/phn.12828.

Jeffreys, M. R., & Zoucha, R. (2018). Cultural congruence in the workplace, health care, and academic settings for multiracial and multiheritage individuals. *Journal of Cultural Diversity*, *25*(4), 113–126.

Juntanamalaga, P., Scholz, B., Roper, C., et al. (2019). 'They can't empower us': The role of allies in the consumer movement. *International Journal of Mental Health Nursing*, *28*(4), 857–866.

Kleinman, A., Eisenberg, L., & Good, D. (1978). Culture, illness, and care: Clinical lessons from anthropologists and cross cultural research. *Annals of Internal Medicine*, *88*, 251–258.

Langone, A. (2018). #MeToo and Time's Up founders explain the difference between the 2 movements — and how they're alike. *Time Magazine*. https://time.com/5189945/whats-the-difference-between-the-metoo-and-times-up-movements

Leininger. M. (1995). Overview of Leininger's theory of culture care. In M. Leininger (Ed.), *Transcultural nursing: Concepts, theories, research and practice* (2nd ed, pp. 93–114). John Wiley & Sons.

Lewis Hall, M. E., & Hill, P. (2019). Meaning-making, suffering, and religion: A worldview conception. *Mental Health, Religion & Culture*, *22*(5), 467–479. https://doi.org/10.1080/13674676.2019.1625037.

Marcelin, J. R., Siraj, D. S., Victor, R., et al. (2019). The impact of unconscious bias in healthcare: How to recognize and mitigate it. *The Journal of Infectious Diseases*, *220*(2), S62–S73.

McCalman, J., Jongen, C., & Bainbridge, R. (2017). Organisational systems' approaches to improving cultural competence in healthcare: A systematic scoping review of the literature. *International Journal for Equity in Health*, *16*, 78. https://doi.org/10.1186/s12939-017-0571-5.

McEvoy, P., Williamson, T., Kada, R., et al. (2017). Improving access to mental health care in an Orthodox Jewish community: A critical reflection upon the accommodation of otherness. *BMC Health Services Research*, *17*, 557. https://doi.org/10.1186/s12913-017-2509-4.

Melton, M. L. (2018). Ally, activist, advocate: Addressing role complexities for the multiculturally competent psychologist. *Professional Psychology: Research and Practice*, *49*(1), 83–89.

Musolino, C., Baum, F., Freeman, T., et al. (2020). Global health activists' lessons on building social movements for Health for All. *International Journal for Equity in Health*, *19*, 116. https://doi.org/10.1186/s12939-020-01232-1.

Naeem, F., Phiri, P., Rathod, S., et al. (2019). Cultural adaptation of cognitive behaviour therapy. *BJPsych Advances*, *25*, 387–395. https://doi.org/10.1192/bja.2019.15.

Nixon, S. A. (2019). The coin model of privilege and critical allyship: Implications for health. *BMC Public Health*, *19*, 1637. https://doi.org/10.1186/s12889-019-7884-9.

Ontario Ministry of Health and Long Term Care. (2018). *About the Excellent Care for All Act*. https://www.health.gov.on.ca/en/pro/programs/ecfa/legislation/act.aspx

Osseo-Asare, A., Balasuriya, L., Huot, S. J., et al. (2018). Minority resident physicians' views on the role of race/ethnicity in their training experiences in the workplace. *JAMA Network Open*, *1*(5), e182723. https://doi.org/10.1001/jamanetworkopen.2018.2723.

Phillips, H. (2020). *Outrage isn't allyship*. https://forge.medium.com/outrage-isnt-allyship-ed7d3f874790.

Reed, K. (June 12, 2016). https://twitter.com/iKaylaReed/status/742243143030972416

Rising, M. L. (2017). Truth telling as an element of culturally competent care at end of life. *Journal of Transcultural Nursing*, *28*(1), 48–55.

Russell, G. (2020). Reflecting on a way of being: Anchor principles of cultural competence. In J. Frawley, G. Russell, & J. Sherwood (Eds.), *Cultural competence and the higher education sector* (pp. 31–42). Springer. https://doi.org/10.1007/978-981-15-5362-2.

Stradiotto, R. A. (1998). Supreme court determines failure to provide sign language interpretation during medical care unconstitutional. *Hospital Quarterly*, *1*(3), 74–76.

The Anti-Oppression Network (n.d.). *Allyship*. https://theantioppressionnetwork.com/allyship

Truth and Reconciliation Commission of Canada (TRC). (2015a). *Truth and Reconciliation Commission of Canada: Calls to action*. Author.

Truth and Reconciliation Commission of Canada (TRC). (2015b). *Truth and Reconciliation Commission of Canada: Honouring the truth, reconciling for the future*. Author.

Turpel-Lafond, M. E. (2020). *In plain sight: Addressing Indigenous-specific racism and discrimination in B.C. Health Care*. Government of British Columbia. https://engage.gov.bc.ca/app/uploads/sites/613/2020/11/In-Plain-Sight-Full-Report.pdf

Zuzelo, P. R. (2020). Ally, advocate, activist, and adversary: Rocking the status quo. *Holistic Nursing Practice*, *34*(3), 190–192.

Universally Applicable Cultural Knowledge

Rani H. Srivastava

Section Outline

This section presents seven chapters that systematically examine communication, interpretation, family, illness beliefs, and ways of healing. Section II also addresses issues encountered by Indigenous people, immigrant and refugee populations, and people considered to be a sexual minority or non-binary. The issues and strategies discussed are considered to be generic cultural knowledge (a fundamental requirement for cultural competence), regardless of the specific cultural or clinical population that a health care provider may work with. While people who identify as Indigenous, as immigrants or refugees, and as having a nondominant sexual orientation or gender identity can be considered specific cultural groups, the reality of our diverse society is that every health care provider, regardless of geography or clinical specialty, must be equipped to provide respectful, effective care to people from these communities. References to specific ethnoracial cultural groups appear throughout the chapters for illustrative purposes only, and readers are reminded to remain alert to individual variations when working with patients, in order to avoid stereotyping. It is also important for readers to constantly remain self-aware regarding the issues presented in each discussion.

Chapter 5 examines cross-cultural communication and the complexity of communication within health care. Effective communication is essential to the delivery of quality patient care. This chapter discusses issues in communication in health care generally and more specifically with respect to linguistic and cultural differences. Communication styles, both verbal and nonverbal, differences in values and approaches, kinds of communication and with whom the communication takes place, and communication barriers are discussed. The chapter ends with an exploration of the influence of digital technology and presents strategies that can be utilized for effective cross-cultural interactions.

Chapter 6 discusses language barriers that can lead to negative health experiences and outcomes, the difference between translation and interpretation, and five fundamental steps to identifying the need for interpretation and working effectively with interpreters. Different modes of interpreting, roles of interpreters, and effective strategies for communication between patients, health care providers, and interpreters are discussed. While the chapter focuses mainly on spoken-language interpretation, many of the issues and strategies apply equally to working with clients who depend on sign language.

Chapter 7 looks at the influence of culture on families, their role in health and illness, and their ability and potential to achieve equitable health outcomes. It begins with an exploration of diversity within family structures, roles, and worldviews and how these may be affected by processes such as migration and acculturation. The chapter discusses the significant impact of colonization on Indigenous families. Intergenerational trauma is explored with respect to Indigenous people and others, including refugee and racialized communities. The chapter concludes by presenting guidelines for family assessment and working effectively with diverse families.

Chapter 8 explores the impact of culture, religion, and spirituality on health and well-being. It presents an overview of the major healing traditions of allopathic medicine, Ayurveda, Indigenous medicine, and traditional Chinese medicine. The chapter includes discussion of complementary therapies, including naturopathy and chiropractic medicine, and the challenges and opportunities that exist with integrative care. The chapter promotes expanded understanding of holistic care, one that extends to the spiritual, intergenerational, and natural world.

Chapter 9 explores how health care providers may develop knowledge and skills for cultural safety with Indigenous people. This chapter discusses key concepts of constructivist, anti-colonial knowledge, and relationality with Indigenous people that are foundational to understanding the historical and sociopolitical impacts of colonialism. An overview of Indigenous people health in Canada highlights the need for engaging in anti-oppressive practices and advocacy, individually and within systems, to advance health equity. Cultural humility, relational practice, and trauma-informed care are critical to promoting cultural competence and cultural safety in Indigenous communities.

Chapter 10 explores common health disparities and health care needs of sexually and gender diverse people. It reviews common terms used in discussions surrounding sexual and gender diversity (SGD) and familiarizes readers with language, cultural context, and many actionable changes critical to making health care more inclusive of SGD people. The chapter focuses on how health care providers can improve experiences for SGD people in specific health care settings and at particular stages of life. The chapter outlines key principles that can be used by health care providers to guide interactions for more effective and equitable care.

Chapter 11 discusses determinants of immigrant and refugee health. It provides an overview of different categories of immigrants and refugees to Canada and examines multiple interacting factors influencing the health and well-being of immigrants and refugees to Canada. The healthy immigrant effect and post-migration factors, such as income, education, employment, social exclusion, access to health care services, culture, language, and intersecting identities, that influence immigrant and refugee health are examined. The implications for policymakers, program planners, and health care service providers are highlighted.

CHAPTER 5

Cross-Cultural Communication

Karima Karmali, Karen Sappleton, and Rani H. Srivastava

LEARNING OBJECTIVES

At the end of this chapter, the learner will be able to:
- Identify the influence of culture on verbal and nonverbal communication
- Distinguish between high-context and low-context communication styles and identify strategies to work with each of them
- Identify the impact of power and authority on communication
- Acquire practical skills for enhancing communication with patients who have limited English proficiency
- Describe the characteristics of effective conversations
- Differentiate between inquiring and dismissive responses
- Recognize the impact of digital technology on cross-cultural communication

KEY TERMS

Active listening	High-context communication	Masculinity—femininity
Bidirectional conversations	Idioms	Monochronic time (M-time)
Collectivism	Individualism	Polychronic time (P-time)
Face	Inquiring responses	Power distance
Health literacy	Low-context communication	Uncertainty avoidance

Communication is critical in health care and is essential to the delivery of quality patient care. Health care communication is complex. At the most basic level, communication requires a bidirectional exchange of information between the patient and the health care provider. Patients and families must be able to convey their concerns and complaints; health care providers must be able to understand and interpret the information accurately to determine appropriate treatment; and providers must be able to convey appropriate information to ensure successful follow-through with respect to treatment and preventive measures for future health management (Ratna, 2019).

Communication can be described as a set of processes that result in an "exchange of information and meaning between persons" (Chichirez & Purcărea, 2018). However, it is anything but a simple process, as the sending and receiving of messages happen simultaneously, with the two processes influencing each other (Ruben, 2016). Interpersonal communication consists of several components, including verbal forms (words language), nonverbal forms (gestures, posture), and paraverbal forms (tone, rhythm, intonation, verbal flow), that occur in an integrated manner (Chichirez & Purcărea, 2018). Culture affects all of these components.

Health care communication is further complicated by its context. There is a strong interdependence between the content (the "what") and the process (the "how") of communication (Cox & Li, 2020). Also, the interactions often occur in environments that may be unfamiliar, have varying degrees of privacy, and are full of activity that can be distracting or distressing for patients and family. Communication is also influenced by the relationship between the health care provider and the patient, and while the importance of the relationship is readily acknowledged, in our current health care system the processes of care are structured in ways that can compromise the relationship. Team-based care means that patients and families receive care from multiple health care providers working in varying degrees of alignment and time constraints. Differences also exist in patient perspectives ("voice of the lifeworld" or everyday concerns) and the more dominant health care provider perspectives ("voice of medicine") reflecting the medical agenda and reasoning (Cox & Li, 2020). It is important to recognize that the inherent power dynamic associated with the roles of the health care provider (expert authority) and the patient (seeking help) can influence all aspects of communication.

This chapter begins with a brief discussion of the vital role that communication plays in health care and the influence of culture on health care communication. Knowledge of cross-cultural communication can be seen as generic knowledge that is important for all health care providers to have in order to ensure quality care. Differences in communication norms and styles across cultures are examined in terms of cultural characteristics and values. Language issues, including those associated with limited proficiency in the dominant language, are also presented; these are discussed in greater depth in Chapter 6. For the purposes of this chapter, the dominant language is assumed to be English. The influence of digital technology on cross-cultural communication is explored briefly. The chapter ends with a discussion on strategies for effective cross-cultural or intercultural conversations.

Culture, Communication, and Health Care

Health care communication is complex even when both the patient and health care provider speak the same language. Misunderstanding and miscommunication are not uncommon in health encounters, and this likelihood is compounded by cultural and linguistic differences (Bowen, 2015). To provide quality, culturally competent care, health care providers must take steps to navigate language and cultural differences and improve cross-cultural communication. Health care involves **bidirectional** conversations since information flows from and to both patient and health care provider and is therefore affected by the attributes of both. A key patient factor that impacts communication in health care is health literacy. **Health literacy** can be defined as "the patient's ability to obtain, comprehend, communicate and understand basic health care information and services" (Ratna, 2019, p. 2). Health literacy is further thwarted by the complexity of the health care system and a care context often filled with uncertainty and vulnerability of illness and treatment trajectories (Ratna, 2019).

The Institute of Medicine's influential report, *Crossing the Quality Chasm: A New Health Care System for the 21ˢᵗ Century,* identified six key aims of quality that have been widely adopted by health care organizations and are considered fundamental to the provision of quality care. According to the report, to deliver quality health care, care must be safe, timely, efficient, effective, equitable, and patient centred. The report defines patient-centred care as "care that is respectful of and responsive to the individual patient preferences, needs, and values and ensuring that patient values guide all decisions" (Institute of Medicine Committee on Quality of Health Care in America, 2001, p. 40); thus patient-centred care is "highly customized and incorporates cultural competence" (p. 49). Good communication skills are essential for patient-centred care and associated with improved health outcomes, improved patient satisfaction and experience of care, as well as safer work environments (Merlino, 2017).

The ability of the health care provider to communicate effectively with the patient is key to providing patient- and family-centred care (SickKids Centre for Innovation & Excellence in Child and Family-Centred Care, 2021). Evidence suggests that patient perceptions of the quality of health care received are influenced by the quality of their interactions with the health care provider and the health care team (Bowen, 2015; Ruben, 2016). Furthermore, a positive experience and quality interactions can improve patient engagement, adherence to treatment, and self-management (Golda et al., 2018; Paternotte et al., 2015).

Communication is critical to processes of establishing trust and engagement (Brooks et al. 2019; Habadi et al., 2019; Ladha et al., 2018; Loriéa et al., 2017), decision making (Ruben, 2016), and self-management of chronic illnesses (Ratna, 2019). The health care provider must be able to must use their communication skills to elicit information about the patient's key health problem and convey a diagnosis; understand the impact of the problem on the patient's life and well-being; discuss treatment options; provide relevant information to get informed consent for treatment; and provide information that the patient can use to manage their health condition. Studies show that effective and empathetic communication has a positive impact on building trust and a therapeutic relationship between the patient and health care provider (Merlino, 2017).

Several factors can have a detrimental effect on the patient's ability to understand what is communicated to them. These include patient anxiety and stress levels, health care provider use of medical jargon, and rushed provider–patient encounters due to time pressures. Poor communication is recognized as a leading cause of adverse events (The Joint Commission, 2015). The Canadian Patient Safety Institute (CPSI) identifies communication as one of six domains of patient safety and maintains that it is "beneficial to patients [and] health care providers, builds trust, and is a precondition of obtaining patient consent" (CPSI, 2020, p. 15). It is important to recognize that patient safety is more than preventing or reducing adverse events; it also includes use of best practices to optimize patient outcomes (de Moissac & Bowen, 2019). Communication challenges, including language barriers, can lead to more cautious treatment—resulting in additional investigations that ultimately increase the demand on the patient and the system (Bowen, 2015).

Language and cultural differences between patient and health care provider can further compound the issues associated with ineffective and poor communication in health care (Al Shamsi et al., 2020). Research suggests that in Canada and the United States, patients with limited English proficiency (LEP) are more likely than English-speaking patients to experience adverse safety events caused by communication errors (de Moissac & Bowen, 2019). Even though Canada is a bilingual nation, these difficulties extend to the French-speaking population across most of Canada. Language and cultural barriers between patients and health care providers can lead to gaps in assessment, diagnosis, informed consent, and health care teaching (Bowen, 2015; de Moissac & Bowen, 2019; Terui, 2017).

Although language is an obvious and frequently cited challenge to cross-cultural communication, it is important to remember that communication is a multidimensional concept and involves much more than the spoken word. Challenges in intercultural communication can be attributed to several factors, including different understandings and expectations of the interaction, nonverbal cues, and different styles of communication. In a review of the literature on intercultural doctor–patient communication, Paternotte et al. (2015) identified four mechanisms or themes surrounding communication challenges: language differences, differences in perception of illness and disease, social component of communication (includes the role of family and emotion), and prejudices and assumptions. Differences in communication patterns and styles are often attributed to differences in cultural values, perspectives, and social patterns (Barker, 2016).

Differences in Communication Style

Communication takes place at varying levels of awareness. Many interactions occur at very low levels of awareness—these are things we do automatically without a great deal of conscious thought. Although we vary our communication approaches based on the situation, patterns and unconscious biases tend to surface unless we make intentional efforts to understand and act differently. The discussion that follows examines the patterns associated with key dimensions of cultural variability. It is important to stress that there are many factors that influence communication, and individual differences exist within these patterns. Significant among these is the impact of social location and experiences (past or present) of racism and discrimination that influence the degree to which individuals may raise concerns, express disagreements, or engage in any interaction that can potentially be seen as conflictual or lead to reprisal.

HIGH- AND LOW-CONTEXT COMMUNICATION

In the 1950s, anthropologist and cross-cultural researcher Edward Hall developed a theoretical model of cultural variability—ways in which cultures differ—based on the concepts of information processing, time orientation, and the interaction patterns used by particular cultures. Identifying these dimensions as "silent languages" and their impact on communication, Hall noted that culture and communication were inextricably linked and that context was critical to understanding the meaning of information (Hall, 1959; Manraia et al., 2019). The most commonly referenced patterns of cultural variability are the dimensions of low–high context of communication and the values of individualism and collectivism (Gudykunst, 2004).

Although each culture has its own unique cultural patterns and communication styles, there are "systematic similarities and differences" (Gudykunst, 2004). Based on observations that people from different cultures use different information-processing systems for the information they take in, Hall proposed a continuum of low- and high-context–oriented styles of communication. The two styles differ as follows:

1. **Low-context communication:** the focus is on the content or the "what" of the message (Manraia et al., 2019). The assumption is that the listener's knowledge is limited or immaterial and the message should include everything. The message is in the spoken word and must be explicit (Gudykunst, 2004). The characterizing phrase might be "listen to my words."

2. **High-context communication:** reflects an acknowledgement of contextual factors that include the "who, why, when, where, to whom, and how" along with nonverbal cues (Manraia et al., 2019). The assumption is that the listener understands the relevant circumstances and therefore has the necessary background information to understand the concerns and key messages. The message is not as much in the spoken word as it is embedded in the context (Gudykunst, 2004). The characterizing phrase might be "it's not what is said that is the most important, but the how it is said, including what is not said."

An example of high-context communication is the everyday conversation between partners (life or professional) who share so much history that they understand each other without having to say very much. Teaching–learning situations, in which every detail is made explicit, provide an example of low-context communication; teachers start out by defining what will be reviewed, then they review the content, and in concluding they repeat key points. High- and low-context communication patterns are seen as a continuum, with different countries and cultures being placed on the continuum according to the predominant communication pattern in that group. For example, countries such as Canada, the United States, Australia, New Zealand, and the United Kingdom are associated with low-context communication, whereas countries in Asia (Japan, China, India, Korea), South America (Brazil, Argentina), and the

Middle East (Saudi Arabia) are associated with high-context cultures (Gudykunst, 2004). Being aware of these patterns and associations can be helpful; however, it is important to recognize that globalization and acculturation means that all forms of communication patterns will be evident in our society. Indigenous people in Canada are more likely to exhibit high-context communication patterns. Table 5.1 presents characteristics of high- and low-context cultures. Health care providers need to be aware of these patterns and take an intentional approach to communication that includes a greater emphasis on listening and being attentive to both verbal and the nonverbal cues.

In general, high-context cultures tend to be more concerned with the overall emotional quality of the interaction than with the meaning of particular words and sentences. How something is said and what is not said are just as important as what is said. People in this group are more likely to give an agreeable and pleasant answer to a question if the factual answer is seen to be embarrassing or unpleasant. Expressions of agreement such as "Yes" can range in meaning from "I understand what you are saying," with no agreement or commitment to follow through, to "I agree," with the patient following through. This can be particularly challenging in health care, where mutual goal setting and a negotiated plan of care are important elements of the services provided. Subsequent lack of follow-through may be viewed as breach of contract and lead to frustration and labels of nonadherence. High-context cultures also make use of silence more than low-context cultures. The pause is necessary for meaning making. It is critical that health care providers recognize the valuable that role silence plays in high-context communication by promoting reflection, and that they not interrupt the silence with questions or comments.

Given that Canadian and American societies have low-context communication as the predominant communication style, it follows that social norms favour low-context, direct communication. There is a propensity to regard low context as the "correct" or superior approach and assume that high-context communication is ineffective or inferior. Common expressions such as "say what you mean and mean what you say" or "get to the point" are valued. However, "indirect messages can be very effective in collectivistic cultures because members of the cultures understand how to interpret the contextual cues that tell them what the indirect messages mean" (Gudykunst, 2004, p. 59). Difficulties arise when contextual cues are not effectively interpreted because of unfamiliarity with the cultural context or inability to recognize or appreciate the communication pattern. The key is not to judge the style of communication but work with the preferred style to ensure clear and accurate understanding (Gudykunst, 2004).

TABLE 5.1 ■ Characteristics of High- and Low-Context Communication

High-Context Communication	Low-Context Communication
■ Most of the message is in the physical context or internalized in the person, and less is explicit.	■ Most of the information is made explicit in the language used.
■ More emphasis on what is left unspoken; more likely to "read into" the interactions	■ Information often is repeated for emphasis to ensure there is no misunderstanding (if it is relevant and important, it must be stated; if it is not stated, it is not relevant).
■ Less reliance on verbal communication—the obvious does not need to be stated	■ The responsibility for communication clearly lies with the speaker; it is better to over-communicate and be clear than to leave things unsaid.
■ More responsibility on the listener—to hear, to interpret, and then to act	
■ More need for silence; longer pauses (to reflect, understand the context, and process the message)	■ Silence and pauses are often misunderstood as signs of agreement or a lack of interest.

Time Orientation

High- and low-context orientation is also related to the view of time, which can vary from linear or **monochronic time (M-time)** to circular or **polychronic time (P-time)** (Hall, 1976, cited in Manraia et al., 2019). M-time is associated with low-context cultures and emphasizes schedules, appointments, promptness, and doing things in a structured manner with a "one at a time" focus. People on P-time (associated with high-context culture and Indigenous cultures) are more apt to do several things at once and value involvement with others over schedules and appointments (Gudykunst, 2004; Manraia et al., 2019). As a result, P-time people may come to appointments late or change schedules frequently, much to the frustration of their M-time colleagues or health care providers, who may view this as a sign of disrespect, disorganization, or a lack of interest in participation. High-context cultures are also associated with greater formality and may equate the formal form of address (e.g., Dr., Mr., Mrs., Ms.) with respect; low-context cultures may view informality as a sign of closeness and friendship.

Cultural Competence in Action

Preferred Forms of Address

Health care providers are taught to respect patient wishes with respect to preferred forms of address.

Rita, a registered nurse, worked on a unit with several older patients and always referred to the patients by their titles and last names (e.g., Mr. X or Mrs. Y). One patient, Robert Smith, indicated that he preferred to be called Bob and shared this preference with Rita directly. Rita was from a South Asian background and had grown up in a culture where elders were rarely referred to by first names, and thus had difficulty using first names for her older patients. However, she respected the patient's preference and agreed to use his first name, only to slip back into calling him Mr. Smith.

After Bob's third request that she use his first name, Rita decided to explain her difficulty and shared with him her background and the subsequent challenge in using first names for patients who reminded her of her elders. To Rita, the formality of address was a form of respect and not meant to introduce distance into the relationship or to disregard the patient's preference. Once Bob became aware of the meaning of the address for Rita, he said, "Oh, in that case, you call me Mr. Smith—I kind of like that."

This scenario illustrates the influence of the health care provider's personal culture, the dilemma it can create, and the importance of developing shared meanings.

INDIVIDUALISM AND COLLECTIVISM

First described by Harry Triandis in the 1980s, individualism/collectivism is a major dimension of cultural variability that influences many aspects of behaviour, including communication (Gudykunst, 2004). **Individualism** is a social pattern in which individuals are primarily motivated by their own preferences, needs, rights, and desires and view themselves largely as being independent of the larger collective. Individualistic cultures place greater emphasis on individual goals and achievements and promote self-realization for their members (Gudykunst, 2004; Manraia et al., 2019). The language in individualistic cultures features "I." In **collectivism**, individuals see themselves as parts of one or more collective and are motivated primarily by group norms (versus individual pleasures) and by collectively imposed duties and expectations (versus individual preferences and desires). The language in collectivist cultures is "we," even when the person may only be referring to themselves. Table 5.2 highlights the contrasting characteristics associated with individualism and collectivism. Individualism is associated with low-context cultures and collectivist cultures, are predominately associated with high-context communication.

TABLE 5.2 ■ **Characteristics Associated With Individualism and Collectivism**

Individualism Focus on the "I"	Collectivism Focus on the "We"
Emphasize	*Emphasize*
■ Goals, needs, views of the individual	■ Goals, needs, views of the group
■ Individual preferences, rights, and pleasure	■ Shared in-group beliefs
■ Individual initiatives and outcomes	■ Co-operation with in-group members
Reward individual initiative and achievement	■ Harmony
	Reward support of the collective and collective achievement
Universalistic approach, where same values are applied to all	*Pluralistic approach*, where different value standards are applied to members of "in-group" and "out-group"
Influence of group views and values on the individual is limited in intensity and scope (group norms affect individual behaviour in very specific circumstances)	*Influence* of group views and values is greater in intensity and scope (group norms affect behaviour in many different aspects of an individual's life)

It is important to note that individualistic and collectivist values do not always conflict and that promoting the one form of values does not have to be at the expense of the other. Although individuals and societies can have both individualistic and collectivist tendencies, one style tends to predominate. In Canada and the United States, individualism predominates, whereas many Asian, South American, and African cultures are collectivist, where the focus is on the group (Gudykunst, 2004; Manraia et al., 2019). Indigenous communities in Canada also reflect a collectivist orientation.

In health care, the influence of individualism and collectivism is evident in areas such as family involvement in care and decision making. For people with a collectivist orientation, the family is an important part of the individual's care, and decision-making is a more consultative and time-consuming process. Individualistic cultures often will make decisions on the basis of the patient's best interests, whereas collectivist cultures may consider the needs of other family members or the family as a unit when making major decisions. It is not uncommon for the decision maker to be an authority figure in the immediate or extended family. When health care providers understand a family's decision-making processes and ensure that the appropriate members are involved in care discussions early, timely and informed decisions are more likely (see Chapter 7 for more information on working with families).

Members of collectivist, high-context cultures are likely to adopt an indirect style of communication that includes hesitancy even when positive sentiments are being expressed, thus making it hard for health care providers to determine the degree to which something is desired or valued. When working with patients and families who use the indirect approach of communication, health care providers may need to establish ties to the patients at the outset through community members and friends. Such patients may be reluctant to ask questions directly and are more likely to involve intermediaries in care; questions may not elicit immediate responses.

The direct/indirect communication style becomes particularly important in health promotion activities involving patient, family, or community education. Where indirect communication style predominates, it is critical to first listen and then explain (see Chapter 4 for the LEARN framework discussion). Another approach is to offer messages or perspectives in ways that invite consideration and dialogue, not as an imposition or a directive. Examples of the two approaches to framing messages are as follows:
■ "Someone who has such a problem might do this" (consideration approach)
■ "Here's what you must do" (directive approach)

Cultural values influence how conflict is viewed and addressed. Some cultures view conflict as a positive factor, while others see it as undesirable and something that must be avoided. Canadian, American, and European cultures often prefer to deal with conflict directly, via face-to-face meetings, and directly with the individuals involved. In contrast, in many Eastern cultures, open conflict is perceived as embarrassing or demeaning. The preferred style of conflict management is embedded in the larger cultural values of individualism, collectivism, and power distance and requires one to bear in mind the concept of face (see later) during negotiation.

Cultural Competence in Action

Cross-Cultural Communication Style Inventory

Directions:

Use Table 5.3 (Cross-Cultural Communication Style Inventory) to complete this exercise.

a) Consider your own style of communicating at work (school) and indicate your preferences on the items below by placing an *X* on each line. Then connect your Xs, forming a profile.

b) Now think of an individual from a different culture with whom you have had some interaction (maybe a patient or a colleague). Put a second checkmark on each line representing the other person's style. You may wish to use a different colour ink to highlight the difference. Draw a dotted line to connect the checkmarks to form the other person's profile. Where does your profile help or hinder you as a communicator?

Compare the profiles to analyze the interaction of your two styles. Are there areas of similarity or differences? Can you reflect on your past interactions and consider the impact of communication style differences on your relationship? What style shifts can you make to reconcile differences and communicate more effectively with this person?

From Gardenswartz, L., Rowe, A., Digh, P., et al. (2003). *The global diversity desk reference: Managing an international workforce* (p. 152). John Wiley & Sons Inc./Pfeiffer. Reprinted with permission.

TABLE 5.3 ■ Cross-Cultural Communication Style Inventory

Verbal	
Directness: Implicit, indirect	Explicit, direct
Topics: Personal, considerable self-disclosure	Impersonal, little self-disclosure
Formality: Formal	Informal
Nonverbal	
Gestures: Considerable facial and physical expression	Little facial and physical expression
Eye contact: Direct, sustained	Not direct or sustained
Proximity: Close	Distant
Touch: Considerable touch	No touch
Pace: Slow	Rapid
Pitch/tone: High (loud)	Low (soft)
Silence: Frequent pauses, considerable silence	Few pauses, little silence

From Gardenswartz, L., Rowe, A., Digh, P., et al. (2003). *The global diversity desk reference: Managing an international workforce* (p. 152). John Wiley & Sons Inc./Pfeiffer.

Face

The concept of face may also be of significance in collectivistic cultures. The term **face** refers to the projected image of oneself in a relational situation involving two or more parties and is associated with honour as well as related emotions such as respect, shame, pride, dignity, and guilt (Xu & Davidhizar, 2004). In collectivist cultures, face concerns not only individuals but also the family, work unit, and community; in individualistic cultures, face tends to be limited to the individuals and the situation. The notion of face varies in importance across cultures, and thus preserving, maintaining, or saving face becomes a key communication principle. Face is a critical concept in many Asian cultures where saving, maintaining, and preserving face is of extreme importance and may even be greater in importance than the substantive issues in the conflict situation (Xu & Davidhizar, 2004). Understanding that conflict situations may contain both an issue of conflict and a face orientation is important for health care providers because there is always the potential for conflict within a team and with students, patients, and families.

Uncertainty Avoidance

Uncertainty avoidance refers to a tolerance for ambiguity. People in high uncertainty avoidance cultures prefer structures and rules in all situations including interactions. There is greater desire for formal rules and for absolute truth with respect to what is right, and less tolerance for behaviour that is outside the norm and therefore considered deviant (whether that be positive or negative). Uncertainty avoidance is not the same as risk avoidance—in fact, as Gudykunst (2004) notes, people may engage in riskier behaviour to decrease uncertainty (e.g., "pick a fight" vs. "see how things unfold") (p. 61). This can have significant implications in health care environments characterized by uncertainty and an often "wait and see" approach to treatment efficacy. High uncertainty avoidance is also associated with greater emotional expression (which could be misinterpreted as anxiety), bigger generation gaps, and a hesitancy in interacting with strangers until the expectations of how the interaction might unfold are clearer (Gudykunst, 2004).

Power Distance

Power distance refers to the degree to which there is an acceptance of equal distribution of power across the group, particularly by powerful members of the group (Gudykunst, 2004; Manraia et al., 2019). Individuals with a high power distance orientation perceive themselves as being responsible for actions of others, such as subordinates or younger people within the group. High power distance is also associated with a greater valuing of expertise, so who conveys the message (i.e., the source) is important. This may also affect the degree to which an individual or family may feel comfortable in shared decision making, particularly for decisions that are perceived as better in the hands of experts or persons of authority. High power distances are usually associated with high-context cultures.

Masculinity–Femininity[1]

The dimension of **masculinity—femininity** is associated with the degree of competitiveness and defined gender roles. Masculine cultures are associated with assertiveness, competitiveness, and independence and focus on material rewards, whereas feminine cultures focus on consensus, cooperation, modesty, interdependence, and nurturance (Gudykunst, 2004; Manraia et al., 2019). The implication of this characteristic is potentially evident in interactions across genders within a family or with strangers and may also influence decision making. Like other dimensions, this also exists on a continuum.

---

[1] The terms are used as a descriptive characteristic, albeit stereotypical, as per the original work. It is not meant to reflect gender assignment or identity of individuals.

Cultural Competence in Action

Direct Communication and Feedback

One area of practice in which the differences in direct/indirect communication and the concept of face often are evident is that of feedback. In developing clinical cultural competence, feedback is therefore an important area for health care providers to focus on.

The usual Western assumption is that the best approach to providing feedback is immediate and direct. Verbal feedback is thought to be less intimidating than written feedback since the latter often is associated with progressive discipline. However, individuals—whether they are patients or part of the health care system—do not all perceive direct, verbal feedback in the same way. Individuals may prefer an email or note as it allows them control over when to engage with the message and to react in private. Where possible, it is important to determine preferred ways of communication or give people options of how they wish to engage and receive feedback.

NONVERBAL COMMUNICATION

People all over the world use their hands, heads, and eyes to communicate expressively. Often, the nonverbal aspects of communication are thought to convey stronger messages than the verbal ones, by reinforcing or contradicting the verbal message. For instance, when a manager indicates verbally that they have time to talk to a staff member and yet uses the nonverbal gesture of checking their watch constantly, they are likely to indicate to the staff that they do not have time, and the verbal response is interpreted to be polite but untrue. In another situation, a wave of the hand may suffice as a greeting, with no words needed. Facial expressions, eye contact, gestures, and touch are common nonverbal methods of communication.

Touch

While all human beings have a need to be touched, cultural norms and contexts determine what is considered an appropriate amount of touching. The amount of personal space we need also is strongly influenced by culture. Many cultures use touch as part of a greeting (e.g., handshakes, hugs, and kisses), whereas other cultures express respect and emotion through less direct contact. In cultures with greater personal distance, non-touch greeting gestures are used (e.g., bowing and/or using folded hands to indicate a greeting). Many cultures frown on public displays of affection, especially across genders.

Touch is also used to convey respect and power. Examples of differentiations in power as a message in body language are the friendly shoulder pat, the stroke over the head, the arm around the shoulder, and the bowing down and touching of feet. Gender and age rules also may dictate the circumstances under which "power-related" gestures or close physical contact (such as a hug or kiss) can occur. For example, some cultures interpret the stroke over the head as a blessing given by elders to young people (thus it is inappropriate for young people to do it to elders), while younger members may convey respect by touching elders' feet.

Physical touch is a major part of health care for diagnostic and treatment purposes. Experiences of touch vary depending on gender, age, parts of the body that are touched, and how the message of touch is interpreted. Although most patients interpret a health care provider's touch as a caring gesture, physical touch (including a firm handshake) may also be interpreted as control or exercise of power. Touch can also play a positive role in conveying warmth, respect, and developing trust (Loriéa et al., 2017). Understanding both the provider's and the patient's cultural norms around touch will not only help health care providers to ensure respect and caring, but can also aid in gaining insight into the patient's relationships with others.

TABLE 5.4 ■ **Behaviours**

Behaviour	Column A: What It Means to Me	Column B: What It Might Mean to Another Person
1. Not making eye contact		
2. Saying "yes" or nodding when they don't understand		
3. Giving a soft handshake		
4. Standing very close when talking		
5. Spending time on small talk instead of getting to the reason for coming		
6. Arriving late for an appointment		
7. Bringing family members to an appointment		
8. Addressing you as Dr./Mr./Mrs./Ms./Nurse rather than by your first name		
9. Giving inaccurate or vague information		
10. Not making a decision without consulting other family members who are not present		

Reproduced with permission, copyright 2004 Centre for Addiction and Mental Health; no unauthorized copying, distribution or amendment without the written permission of Centre for Addiction and Mental Health.

Cultural Competence in Action

Culture, Communication, and Interpretations

Table 5.4 lists some behaviours that are frequently encountered in a variety of health care settings. In the middle column (A), write down what the behaviour means to you. After reflecting on your knowledge of other cultures, write down what the same behaviour might mean to someone of a different culture or background.

At the end of this exercise, discuss your answers with a colleague or in a small group. Did you have similar interpretations? Did you discover interpretations that you had not considered before?

From Diversity level II: Clinical Cultural Competence Education, Workshop I, 2005, presented by Centre for Addiction and Mental Health, March 23, 2004.

DISCLOSURE

Cultural variations exist with respect to disclosure of personal and intimate information. From our own lived experience and practice, we have noted that prerequisites for disclosure include an element of trust and the establishment of both a relationship and shared values. Even when there is a safe relationship, patients have been hesitant to discuss specific issues because of the provider's age, gender, and/or authority. Public health nurses and social workers may be regarded as representatives of the state, for example, and thus viewed with suspicion. Patients with uncertain residency status (refugees, visitors, or those who are undocumented) often hesitate to disclose information for fear that doing so would affect their residency. In addition, disclosure may be limited in situations involving emotions, intimacy, and conflict. Providing selective information to preserve face is often viewed as a cultural expectation and norm; therefore, it is not regarded as lying by omission or being untruthful. Patients from cultures with indirect styles of communication may feel uncomfortable during direct questioning or consider the practice rude and not worthy of a complete response.

Within cross-cultural encounters, challenges frequently arise with respect to disclosing bad news to patients. Many cultures believe that speaking of future illnesses and consequences will bring them to pass, and others prioritize withholding truth as a way of preventing further distress to the patient. Even though the preference for nondisclosure is a caring and protective gesture, it conflicts with the norms of our health care practices. It is important to take a moment to reflect on the language that emerges on this issue. Within health care, we have noted that the discourse may be framed as "truth telling," "withholding truth," or "family collusion"—terminology that is clearly value laden, potentially inflammatory and judgemental. It is important for health care providers to reflect on their own understanding of the issue and consider use of more neutral terminology, such as "disclosure," where possible.

Rosenberg et al. (2017) explored truth-telling across cultures in the context of incurable pediatric illness and noted that within the medical profession in the United States (and Canada is no different), there is a strong value and expectation of disclosure as a professional and moral imperative. However, the authors point out that this has evolved over time. In the 1960s most physicians believed that "disclosing a cancer diagnosis could be overly distressing and potentially harmful to patients, with 90% preferring nondisclosure" (p. 1115). However, there was a significant reversal by the late 1970s with physicians favouring complete disclosure, and by the 1980s, the concept of honesty was embedded into professional codes of conduct. The authors point out that it is important to recognize that the change was not due to shift in values but rather evidence. The value of "patient best interest" is still paramount; however, the shift can be attributed to evidence showing that most patients "(1) were already aware of their serious diagnosis; (2) imagined the worst in the absence of specific details; and (3) were denied both opportunities to make plans for the future as well as an open and honest environment to explore their fears and hope" (p. 1115). It is critical for health care providers to be informed by such evidence when negotiating with families around disclosure.

Zolkefli (2018) explicates three values that underpin the ethics of truth-telling. These include (1) truth-telling as a show of respect for informed decision making; (2) truth-telling as upholding duty and trust; and (3) truth-telling to promote patient engagement in care, leading to better physical and psychological health. However, the author raises the question of health care provider obligations to support patient autonomy and the "right to not know" (Zolkefli, 2018, p. 137). Although nondisclosure can be "counter-productive" to informed decision making, there is also a question about the obligation of the health care provider not to cause distress by "imposing truth" (Faith, 2018; Rosenberg et al., 2017; Zolkefli, 2018). Health care providers constantly balance the amount of information that is shared to support informed decision making without overwhelming patients and families or causing information overload that can be paralyzing.

Ultimately, the approach to disclosure is one where, rather than relying on assumptions, providers take the time to understand the patient and family values and preferences and act in a way that aligns with their professional obligations. Actively engaging in dialogue with families will allow for exploration of both patient–family and provider perspectives and developing a mutually acceptable approach. For many people, life-and-death decisions are attributed only to a higher power, and withdrawal of treatment by health care providers, for example, is not acceptable.

Communicating Through Language

Unfamiliarity with the language is perhaps the most identified communication barrier in a multicultural society. In Canada, four population groups face barriers to health care access due to language: Indigenous peoples, immigrants, people who use sign language, and people who speak one of Canada's official languages but live in an area where the other language is prominent (e.g., French-speaking people living in a predominantly English-speaking environment, and vice versa) (Bowen, 2015). In the following paragraphs, we will consider issues and strategies for working with patients who have limited proficiency in the dominant language. Chapter 6 focuses on working with interpreters.

Language issues, particularly in the health care context, are far more complex than whether we can speak a particular language or not. In every culture, many expressions and phrases that are commonly understood by members of the cultural group can be ambiguous or confusing for others. For example, health care providers often use expressions such as "you are stable," "you are treading water," or "you are out of the woods," all of which may be misinterpreted by patients. Familiarity with language does not ensure familiarity with associated meanings and behaviours.

SECOND-LANGUAGE ISSUES

There is limited research on the impact of second-language issues in health care. Although individuals may be proficient in a second language for day-to-day interactions, additional challenges arise within the health care context because of potential lack of fluency in medical and health terminology and the need to express nuanced or deeper feelings and concepts, often under stressful conditions. Research indicates that older patients may revert to their first language under conditions of stress or cognitive impairments (Bowen, 2015).

In our practice we have observed that often times of crisis or stress can compromise fluency in a second language. In the emergency room, health care providers often are frustrated with patients who are unable to communicate in English, even though they can convey and understand basic information at other times. It is also important to remember that limited fluency in a second language often means individuals need more time to respond because they must first translate the question from English into their own language, prepare an answer in their own language, and then translate the answer back into English. Unfortunately, such individuals are at risk of being labelled as not being engaged or unable to provide the desired information.

Karuthan et al. (2020) studied nurse–patient interactions with nurses in Malaysia using English as a second language. To accommodate, nurses used strategies such as speaking slower, enunciating carefully, repeating phrases or words, avoiding colloquial jargon, and relying on nonverbal gestures and written cue cards. The researchers noted that accommodation was required on the part of nurses and patients to enhance clarity of communication; however, not all patients were willing to do so—perhaps due to personal biases or negative stereotypes. Given the diversity of Canadian society, it is likely that English is a second language for many patients, providers, or both. Careful assessment and attention are needed in such circumstances to ensure effective communication for patient safety and quality care.

Cultural Considerations in Care

When Providing Instructions Is Not Enough

A young Tamil couple brought their 18-month-old son to the hospital emergency room with complaints of fever and irritability. The child was also tugging on his ear. Both parents had limited English proficiency, and interpreter services were neither requested nor offered.

Following an assessment, the parents were informed that the child had an ear infection in his right ear, and they were given a prescription for an oral antibiotic that they were instructed to give to the child every 6 hours. The parents were repeatedly asked if they understood the instructions, and each time they

Continued

responded with a "yes." Two days later, the parents returned to the emergency room in greater distress. They said they had followed the instructions carefully, but the child was getting worse. The triage nurse noted a yellowish discharge from the right ear.

The parents had followed the instructions, as they understood them. They had taken the prescription to a pharmacy and received a bottle of liquid medicine with a dropper to administer the medication. While the physician had emphasized instructions to administer 2.5 mL every 6 hours, the route of administration was not communicated explicitly. The parents used the dropper to administer the 2.5 mL directly into the child's right ear instead of orally.

In this scenario, the communication concern was not what was said, but rather what was assumed and not said. Health care providers were not explicit that the medication had to be taken orally, and the parents assumed that the medicine was to be applied to the affected area, as was often the practice in their home country.

Influence of Digital Media in Health Care Communication

Social media and digital technology are changing the way people receive and share information. The world is more connected with increased access to information and exposure to different cultures through the popular media, including television and movies. Lifintsev and Wellbrock (2019) looked at the opportunities provided via digitalization to facilitate cross-cultural communication processes. The results indicate that cross-cultural communication skills are highly desired by the younger generation and digitalization facilitates cross-cultural communication. Digital tools can simplify the process by avoiding direct face-to-face communication; instead, online communication can be supported by translation software, "auto correct" for spelling, and even support for grammar, and can lead to a greater sense of confidence in such interactions. Digital interactions also have their limitations. The lack of face-to-face contact alters the nature of the relationship and may compromise trust. As well, even though digital communication appears more polished, words are only one component of "meaning-making," thus individuals may have different interpretations of what is being said, and without the nonverbal cues or the interactional opportunity to verify meaning, the smoother communication may be a miscommunication (Lifintsev & Wellbrock, 2019). Nevertheless, increased access to cultures and language support through digital means is a definite asset for cross-cultural communication. Health care providers and organizations are also using digital media to raise awareness of services, increase access through virtual care, and support health literacy—often in multiple languages.

Communication and the Global Pandemic

We are writing this chapter at an unprecedented time in history, when the world is experiencing a global pandemic of unimagined proportion. As a result, individuals, families, and communities are experiencing isolation and increased virtual care in an environment characterized by uncertainty, anxiety, and tragedy of small and large proportions. The impact will be evident in months and years to come; however, two areas are highlighted here. First, limits to physical contact have led to a loss of touch for many individuals, particularly those who live alone and have been severely limited in interactions with friends and families. While virtual interactions have become the norm, they are challenging for many and can accentuate already existing barriers. Second, the requirements to wear a mask in interactions can challenge verbal communication; the mask interferes with the clarity of communication—particularly for those with hearing difficulties and language barriers. While the pandemic will come to an end, the use of masks has always been part of health care, thus it is important for health care providers to reflect on the impact of this practice on communication—particularly cross-cultural communication.

Cultural Competence in Action

Safety Issues Can "Mask" Communication

John, a practical nursing student, is excited to begin a practicum in a long-term care setting. He is a little nervous going into a health care facility during a global pandemic but is also eager to complete his studies and join the workforce. John is an international student in Canada and English is not his first language. He sometimes has difficulty understanding others and making himself understood; however, he does not see this as a major obstacle.

In his second week in the practice setting John is looking after Mr. Wallace, a 75-year-old patient. John goes into the room to assist Mr. Wallace with his bath and states to Mr. Wallace that it is "bath day." John is shocked that he is met with anger from Mr. Wallace, who declares, in a loud voice, it is not his birthday today and then wonders if John has read up on his care plan and understands his needs.

- What are the factors contributing to the miscommunication?
- What suggestions do you have for John?

Strategies for Effective Cross-Cultural Communication

The approach to effective cross-cultural communication is a combination of cultural sensitivity, knowledge, and resources. When health care providers value communication and the expression of the patient's voice, they are more likely to use additional strategies to ensure meaningful, accurate communication. It is not enough for health care providers to feel that they understand the contexts of their patients; empathic and effective communication requires that such understanding be communicated back to patients and verified. Cultural competence requires that health care providers develop both individual and systemic knowledge to address the complexities and inequities associated with culture and difference.

COMMITMENT

Effective conversations begin with an intentional focus on and commitment to ensuring that messages sent are received and understood in ways they are intended. In a concept analysis of culturally sensitive communication, Brooks et al. (2019) identified the following antecedents of culturally sensitive communication: the environment and culture of the ward; organizational structures and policies; education and communication experience of clinicians; sociocultural characteristics of patients, families, and health care providers; and personal characteristics and professional experiences of health care providers. Thus it is important to note that while communication barriers may be attributed to the patient, multiple factors within the system lead to biases and challenges; health care providers need to take responsibility individually and collectively for addressing these challenges to ensure delivery of quality care.

Commitment to effective communications also requires that health care providers understand the issues from patient and family perspectives. Literature reveals that health care providers often overestimate their skills and ability for culturally responsive communication. In a review of literature on culturally responsive communication, Minnican and O'Toole (2020) note that despite reporting a lack of confidence in culturally responsive communication and adopting "a generic one size fits all" approach, health care providers still felt they achieved culturally responsive care; the perceptions of service users, however, were different and described communication as patronizing, using excessive jargon, and lacking in cultural sensitivity. It is important that health care providers challenge their own ethnocentrism, seek feedback, and understand communication needs from the patient and family perspective. The key health care provider characteristics for culturally responsive communication include reflexivity, flexibility, self/other awareness, honesty and transparency, trustworthiness, and a willingness to learn (Minnican & O'Toole, 2020).

Cultural Competence in Action

Inquiry or Assumption

Janice worked in a pediatric outpatient clinic that served many new immigrant families and people of lower socioeconomic status. Over time, Janice had learned to develop authentic partnerships with parents and always tried to see the illness experience through the parent's eyes. The team had been working with a new immigrant family whose child was on a strict schedule of taking medications three times a day (breakfast, lunch, and dinner). However, despite repeated attempts at explanations with the parents, the routine was not followed (the evening dose was often missed or delayed, thus affecting the next day's schedule), and the child's health was being compromised. The physician was very frustrated and suggested that Janice involve the Children's Aid Society (CAS) for intervention. However, Janice advocated on the family's behalf and convinced the team to have a family meeting where she took the lead and began by first acknowledging the family's concern for their child and then began with an inquiring question.

Janice began with: "Can you tell me what your daily routine looks like?" Through the family's response the team learned that the family always waited for dad to come home in the evening before having dinner. This was variable and often happened around 8 or 9 p.m. and sometimes later. Mom understood that the medication was to be taken at dinner, but for the family this was not a fixed time. The physician realized that the problem was not neglect or disregard but rather an assumption that children ate dinner around 6 pm.

- How could this misunderstanding have been prevented?
- What factors may have been at play in the suggestion of involving CAS?
- How do Janice's actions demonstrate cultural competence?

SELF-AWARENESS

Awareness of strengths and limitations of one's own preferred communication style is another critical step in the development of culturally responsive communication. Observing patient–family interactions with each other and the health care team will allow health care providers to understand patient–family communication patterns and pick up on cues regarding communication norms. It is important to remember that communication across cultures is affected by how messages are framed and delivered, as well as by the relationship between the health care provider and the patient (Baker et al., 2017). Habadi et al. (2019) identify three goals in effective health care provider–patient communication: good interpersonal relationship, exchange of information, and patient engagement in decision making. Thus it is important to attend to the relationship along with the information that needs to be sought or conveyed. By recognizing and using their privilege and expertise, providers can create a safe and inclusive space for patients and families to express their questions and concerns that lead to informed decision making.

Table 5.5 lists some strategies of culturally responsive communication. Treating all views and communication styles with respect, regardless of how one feels about them, is foundational. Other key strategies include ensuring bidirectionality, utilizing inquiring responses, acknowledging and balancing (where possible) the power dynamics, and verifying understanding.

BIDIRECTIONALITY AND ACTIVE LISTENING

Bidirectionality means that information flows both ways—from provider to patient–family and vice versa. Bidirectional conversations require health care providers to further develop their listening skills and use their minds as well as their hearts to understand not just what is being said but also what it means to patients, and what it reflects about the patients' views of who or what they are. All these views and meanings need to be heard, acknowledged, and acted on as appropriate.

TABLE 5.5 ■ Strategies for Effective Cross-Cultural Conversations

- Understand your values and communication style and develop comfort with alternate communication approaches.
- Observe and adopt, as appropriate, the patient's general communication style; pay attention to verbal and nonverbal cues.
- Use open-ended questions and inquiring responses.
- Use your privilege and authority to raise issues that may be hard for patients to raise.
- Balance or acknowledge the "power" in the relationship by acknowledging patient–family expertise.
- Earn trust by answering questions directly, providing explanations, and providing information about care coordination and system navigation, anticipating difficulties and suggesting options.
- Acknowledge perspectives and challenges and discuss alternatives.
- Manage expectations and ensure the working relationship is built on trust and a partnership relationship.

Bidirectionality is enhanced through utilization of inquiring responses and open-ended questions. **Inquiring responses** are responses that inquire into the patient's perspectives and invite further conversation. Often, what we ask and how we ask a question can prematurely end conversations. Patients may not continue talking if they perceive that their story is not being heard or understood, or if they are afraid that their views will be judged, trivialized, or ignored.

Listening is a powerful skill that often is underused. Rivers (2015) states, "listening to others helps others to listen." Patients are better able to listen to health care providers once they have shared their concerns. **Active listening** can be described as careful and intentional listening to hear the verbal and nonverbal messages in an engaged way. Active listening is associated with empathy and fosters self-awareness (Haley et al., 2017). Table 5.6 provides some tips for active listening.

NAVIGATING POWER AND PRIVILEGE

Recognition of power differences between the patient and the health care provider is important. Strategies to balance the power include attention to physical and interpersonal context. It is important to assess for privacy to promote comfort and safety. When communicating with children, many adults automatically bend down to be at the same level as the child or use age-appropriate language; with adults it is better to sit with than to stand over a person (Golda et al., 2018).

Balancing power can also mean using privilege and authority to raise issues that are hard for a patient to broach. For example, when the patient has disclosed an aspect of a cultural identity, the health care provider can follow up with statements along the line of, "You indicated that you are Buddhist. Can you tell me what I need to know about the religion and how it could influence your care?" or "Many of my patients use herbal or other remedies. Is there anything you are using or want to use that might be of help?" The key is not to stereotype or impose particular characteristics to a given identity, but rather to use the knowledge of patterns to assess for individual applicability and relevance. These statements are inquiring but also reflect an indication of interest and acceptance and the use of the provider's authority to legitimize the issues. Avoiding medical jargon, acknowledging patient–family expertise, and an invitation to collaborate are useful strategies to balance the power in the patient–provider relationship and foster engagement. Statements such as "I have expertise as a dietician, but you and your family will know what works best for you;

TABLE 5.6 ■ Tips for Active Listening

- Always focus on the sender and do not get distracted or sidetracked. Remember "listening to others helps others listen."
- Listen to the message (not what you want or expect to hear), with the intent to understand.
- Be mindful of judgement bias—pay attention to the sender's body language as well as your own.
- Acknowledge what you hear by summarizing it back in your own words. Acknowledging is not the same as agreement or approval and is particularly important if there are differences in viewpoints.
- Ask clarification questions to ensure accurate understanding. If you are unsure of the sentiment expressed, make a tentative guess and invite correction (e.g., "It sounds like you are angry/frustrated/sad...; am I understanding that correctly?")
- Do not start formulating a response before you have heard, understood, and verified the message.

From Rivers, D. (2015). *Cooperative communication skills for success at home and at work*. https://newconversations.net/sevenchallenges.pdf; Tennant, K., Long, A., & Toney-Butler, T. J. (2020). Active listening. In *StatPearls* [Internet]. StatPearls Publishing.

it is important for me to understand that ..." can be used to promote engagement and informed decision making. Finally, it is important for health care providers to be honest and acknowledge their own limitations or challenges. For example, when faced with multiple family members asking questions, rather than getting frustrated or dismissive, health care providers can acknowledge the difficulty and suggest alternatives. Statements such as "I recognize that you are a close family, and everyone is engaged; however, it is difficult for me to communicate regularly with multiple people. Is it possible to ..." can be helpful.

Cultural Considerations in Care

Relationship and Trust Matter

Jasmine, a social worker, worked in a pediatric metabolic clinic and engaged with families on a variety of issues, including building skills in children and youth for self-management, to facilitate a smooth transition from children to adult services. Two years after she left this role, she met a family she had cared for at another hospital 200 km away. She was excited to see them and inquired how they were doing, wondering what brought them out so far. She was stunned to learn that shortly after she left her role, the family also stopped going to that hospital and sought care at another hospital. To get there, they had to drive for over 2 hours, often in adverse weather conditions. The family, a young Indigenous couple, faced multiple challenges in the big city trying to care for a child with chronic illness and also establish themselves as working adults. Jasmine had found them to be very caring and hardworking. They also had support from an Indigenous community agency to assist with services such as transportation and cultural support. She was pleased to see that they were doing well but could not understand what caused the family to seek care so far away from home. What happened to the relationship the family had with the health care team in the original hospital?

Jasmine remembered that in a course on cultural safety, she had learned the great importance that Indigenous people place on relationship and trust, particularly given the historical injustices and inequities they have experienced. She thought she had been thoughtful in her handover to her successor, but the family had not developed a trusting relationship with the new person. Although they continued to receive excellent support from the Indigenous community agency, the over-reliance on the agency by the hospital team may have led to a failed relationship with the family. As such, the burden of illness was magnified for this family, especially with having to drive 2 hours each way to another hospital for their ongoing appointments.

WORKING WITH PATIENTS WHO HAVE LIMITED ENGLISH PROFICIENCY (LEP)

When working with patients with LEP, it is important to assess for and seek resources such as interpretation services. Other strategies include speaking slowly (not loudly), using short, simple sentences, avoiding the use of jargon and idioms, repeating information, and seeking patient understanding and interpretations of information presented. Table 5.7 presents some strategies for communicating with patients with LEP in the absence of language interpretation. It is recommended that interpreters be engaged for interactions in which information that can impact assessment and diagnosis is shared by the patient, or when members of the health care team need to convey important medical information or provide teaching.

There is growing evidence that language barriers, when not addressed through the engagement of interpreters, can pose a risk to patient safety when medical information needs to be conveyed to the patient, including through teaching and counselling. Chapter 6 further expounds on these risks and the benefits of working with interpreters.

TABLE 5.7 ■ Cultural Competence in Action: Strategies for Improving Direct Communication With Limited English Proficiency (LEP) Patients

1. *Speak slowly, not loudly*. A loud voice implies anger; and in most cultures, the health care provider holds a high position of respect and authority. When patients feel that the "authority figure" is angry, they tend to become anxious or feel intimidated and begin to answer questions in the way that they think will please that person rather than give the true picture of the complaint. Speaking slowly does not mean exaggerating the enunciation of words, as that is often more confusing than helpful.
2. *Face the person and use nonverbal communication* such as gestures, pictures, and facial expressions. By the same token, watch the patient's face, eyes, and other nonverbal communications carefully. When these don't agree with the patient's words, inquire further. Don't assume that the nonverbal communication used in your culture is the same as that in the patient's culture.
3. *Avoid difficult and uncommon words* and idiomatic expressions. **Idioms** are phrases or expressions that are based on culture rather than the sum of the meanings of each individual word. North American English is full of idioms, such as "right on target" or "kill two birds with one stone."
4. *Be aware of frequently misunderstood words*, such as "anxiety," "depression," "dizziness," and words that describe sensations (e.g., "pins and needles").
5. *Don't complicate communication* with unnecessary words or information. More is not better in this situation. Keep what you say simple.
6. *Organize what you say for easy access*. Use short, simple sentences, starting with the subject and following it as closely as possible with the verb and a simple object. A good rule of thumb is that people tend to remember information in an inverted bell curve—what is said at the beginning and end is remembered best, while information in the middle is missed or quickly forgotten.
7. *Repeat when you have not been understood*. If something has been said as simply as possible, try repeating the same sentence again first; changing words may confuse the patient.
8. *Rephrase and summarize often*. Summarize what you understand the person is saying, and check with the patient to see if your understanding is correct. When giving information, ask questions, and try to say the same thing or ask the same question in at least two or three different ways.
9. *Don't ask questions that can be answered with a "yes" or "no."* The person's answer will only tell you whether or not the question has been heard—not whether it has been understood. If you phrase questions in a way that requires the person to respond with information (what, where, when, why, and how), they can only reply sensibly if they have understood the question. Use such phrases as "tell me about."
10. *Greet the client in the client's own language* to establish a rapport.

From Breen, L. (1999). What should I do if my patient does not speak English? *Journal of the American Medical Association, 282*(9), 819; McPhee, S. (2002). Caring for a 70-year-old Vietnamese woman. *Journal of the American Medical Association, 287*(4), 495–503; Putsch, R. W. (1985). Cross-cultural communication. The special case of interpreters in health care. *Journal of the American Medical Association, 254*(23), 3344–3348.

Summary

Effective communication is critical for quality care. This chapter discussed issues in communication in health care generally and more specifically with respect to linguistic and cultural differences. Within the health care environment, communication can be compromised by patient physical and emotional distress as well as by health care providers' professional jargon and time constraints. Communication differences can lead to ineffective communication, which, in turn, contributes to misdiagnosis, inadequate health teaching, failure to obtain informed consent, compromised health care provider–patient relationship, dissatisfaction with care, and adverse safety events.

Cross-cultural communication is characterized not only by differences in communication styles (verbal and nonverbal) but also by fundamental differences in values and approach that influence how communication happens, what kind of communication happens, and with whom. The major elements of cross-cultural communication include an understanding of the role of context and power, as well as values related to individualism or collectivism and disclosure.

Barriers related to LEP can be addressed by health care providers by being intentional and using deliberate strategies. The characteristics of effective cross-cultural conversations remain the same across cultures and include a focus on respect, listening, empathy, inquiring responses, and, most important, recognition that effective communication is essential for quality, safety, equity, and patient-centred care. Health care providers must also recognize the importance of valuing the perspectives of their patients.

Questions for Review and Discussion

1. "Communication is more than a verbal exchange." Reflect on this statement and identify nonverbal factors that influence communication.
2. Consider the scenario presented in the box "Cultural Consideration in Care: When Providing Instructions Is Not Enough." Describe three strategies that could have been used by health care providers to ensure that the care instructions given to the parents were understood and that there was no misunderstanding.
3. Identify two differences between high-context and low-context communication styles and identify strategies to work with each of them.
4. Briefly describe three barriers to effective communication.
5. List two ways that digital communication can enhance quality care.

Group Experiential/Reflection Activity

1. Working in small groups, discuss strategies to communicate more effectively with patients in cross-cultural situations. How will you commit to improving communication with patients and families in cross-cultural situations? Using Table 5.7 "Cultural Competence in Action: Strategies for Improving Direct Communication with Limited English Proficiency (LEP) Patients" as a reference, discuss practical skills for enhancing communication with patients who have limited English-language proficiency.
2. Working in small groups, discuss behaviours and gestures you've encountered in cross-cultural situations. Looking back, are there situations that you may have misunderstood because of the gestures used in communication? Are there gestures and behaviours that you use that could be misunderstood by others?

References

Al Shamsi, H., Almutairi, A. G., Al Mashrafi, S., et al. (2020). Implications of language barriers for healthcare: A systematic review. *Oman Medical Journal, 35*(2), e122. https://doi.org/10.5001/omj.2020.40.

Baker, S. C., Watson, B. M., & Gallois, C. (2017). Exploring intercultural communication problems in health care with a communication accommodation competence approach. In L. Chen (Ed.), *Intercultural communication*. De Gruyter Mouton. http://doi.org/10.1515/9781501500060-022.

Barker, G. (2016). Cross-cultural perspectives on intercultural communication competence. *Journal of Intercultural Communication Research*, 45(1), 13–30. https://doi.org/10.1080/17475759.2015.1104376.

Bowen, S. (2015). *The impact of language barriers on patient safety and quality of care. Final report prepared for the Société Santé en français* (pp. 1–46). http://www.santefrancais.ca/wp-content/uploads/2018/11/SSF-Bowen-S.-Language-Barriers-Study-1.pdf

Breen, L. (1999). What should I do if my patient does not speak English? *Journal of the American Medical Association*, 282(9), 819.

Brooks, L. A., Manias, E., & Bloomer, M. J. (2019). Culturally sensitive communication in health care: A concept analysis. *Collegian*, 26, 383–391.

Canadian Patient Safety Institute (CPSI). (2020). *The safety competencies* (2nd ed.). https://www.patientsafetyinstitute.ca/en/toolsResources/safetyCompetencies/Documents/CPSI-SafetyCompetencies_EN_Digital.pdf

Centre for Addiction and Mental Health. (2005). Diversity level II: Clinical cultural competence education, Workshop I. Toronto, presented March 23, 2004.

Chichirez, C. M., & Purcărea, V. L. (2018). Interpersonal communication in healthcare. *Journal of Medicine and Life*, 11(2), 119–122.

Cox, A., & Li, C. (2020). The medical consultation through the lenses of language and social interaction theory. *Advances in Health Sciences Education*, 25, 241–257. https://doi.org/10.1007/s10459-018-09873-2.

de Moissac, D., & Bowen, S. (2019). Impact of language barriers on quality of care and patient safety for official language minority francophones in Canada. *Journal of Patient Experience*, 6(1), 24–32. https://doi.org/10.1177/2374373518769008.

Faith, K. (2018). Truth telling. *Rehab and Community Care Medicine*, 27(1), 20–23. https://www.rehabmagazine.ca/ethics/truth-telling/

Golda, N., Beeson, S., Kohli, N., et al. (2018). Recommendations for improving the patient experience in specialty encounters. *Journal of the American Academy of Dermatology*, 78(4), 653–659.

Gudykunst, W. B. (Ed.). (2004). Understanding cultural differences. In W. B. Gudykunst (Ed.), *Bridging difference: Effective intergroup communication* (pp. 41–73). Sage.

Habadi, M. I., Mahanash, F. A., Alkhudidi, A. J., et al. (2019). Patient-physician communication: Challenges and skills. *EC Microbiology*, 15(12), 1–10.

Haley, B., Heob, S., Wright, P., et al. (2017). Relationships among active listening, self-awareness, empathy, and patient-centered care in associate and baccalaureate degree nursing students. *NursingPlus Open*, 3, 11–16.

Hall, E. (1959). *The silent language*. Doubleday.

Hall, E. (1976). *Beyond cultures*. Anchor Press.

Institute of Medicine Committee on Quality of Health Care in America. (2001). *Crossing the chasm: A new health system for the 21st century*. National Academies Press. https://pubmed.ncbi.nlm.nih.gov/25057539/.

Karuthan, A., Kaur, S., Krishnan, K., et al. (2020). Communication accommodation: Do nurses and patients speak the same language?. *ASM Science Journal*, 13(5), 175–182. https://www.akademisains.gov.my/asmsj/article/communication-accommodation-do-nurses-and-patients-speak-the-same-language/

Ladha, T., Zubairi, M., Hunter, A., et al. (2018). Cross-cultural communication: Tools for working with families and children. *Paediatrics & Child Health*, 23(1), 66–69.

Lifintsev, D., & Wellbrock, W. (2019). Cross-cultural communication in the digital age. *Estudos em Comunicação*, 28(1), 93–104. https://doi.org/10.25768/fal.ec.n28.a05.

Loriéa, A., Reineroa, D. A., Phillips, M., et al. (2017). Culture and nonverbal expressions of empathy in clinical settings: A systematic review. *Patient Education and Counseling*, 100, 411–424.

Manraia, L. A., Manraia, A. K., Lascub, D., et al. (2019). Determinants and effects of cultural context: A review, conceptual model, and propositions. *Journal of Global Marketing*, 32(2), 67–82.

McPhee, S. (2002). Caring for a 70-year-old Vietnamese woman. *Journal of the American Medical Association*, 287(4), 495–503.

Merlino, J. (2017). Communication: A critical competency. *Patient Safety & Quality Health Care*. https://www.psqh.com/analysis/communication-critical-healthcare-competency/

Minnican, C., & O'Toole, G. (2020). Exploring the incidence of culturally responsive communication in Australian healthcare: The first rapid review on this concept. *BMC Health Services Research*, *20*, 20. https://doi.org/10.1186/s12913-019-4859-6.

Paternotte, E., van Dulme, S., & van der Lee, N. (2015). Factors influencing intercultural doctor–patient communication: A realist review. *Patient Education and Counseling*, *98*, 420–445.

Putsch, R. (1985). Cross cultural communication: The special case of interpreters in health care. *JAMA*, *254*(23), 3344–3348.

Ratna, H. (2019). The importance of effective communication in healthcare practices. *Harvard Public Health Review*, *23*, 1–6. https://www.jstor.org/stable/48546767

Rivers, D. (2015). *Cooperative communication skills for success at home and at work*. https://newconversations.net/sevenchallenges.pdf

Rosenberg, A. R., Starks, H. S., Unguru, Y., et al. (2017). Truth telling in the setting of cultural differences and incurable pediatric illness. *AMA Pediatrics*, *171*(11), 1113–1119. https://doi.org/10.1001/jamapediatrics.2017.2568.

Ruben, B. D. (2016). Communication theory and health communication practice: The more things change, the more they stay the same. *Health Communication*, *31*, 1–11.

SickKids Centre for Innovation & Excellence in Child and Family-Centred Care. (2021). *Our care philosophy*. https://www.sickkids.ca/en/patients-visitors/care-philosophy/

Tennant, K., Long, A., & Toney-Butler, T. J. (2020). Active listening. In *StatPearls* [Internet]. StatPearls Publishing. https://www.ncbi.nlm.nih.gov/books/NB442015/

Terui, S. (2017). Conceptualizing the pathways and processes between language barriers and health disparities: Review, synthesis, and extension. *Journal of Immigrant and Minority Health*, *19*, 215–224. https://doi.org/10.1007/s10903-015-0322-x.

The Joint Commission. (2015). Human factor analysis in patient safety systems. *The Source*, *13*(4). https://store.jcrinc.com/human-factors-analysis-in-patient-safety-systems/?_ga=2.71205400.966402193.1620788044-1068379720.1620788044

Xu, Y., & Davidhizar, R. (2004). Conflict management styles of Asian and Asian American nurses: Implications for nurse managers. *The Health Care Manager*, *23*(1), 46–53.

Zolkefli, Y. (2018). The ethics of truth-telling in health-care settings. *Malaysian Journal of Medical Science*, *25*(3), 135–139. https://doi.org/10.21315/mjms2018.25.3.14.

CHAPTER 6

Working With Interpreters in Health Care Settings

Karen Sappleton, Karima Karmali, and Rani H. Srivastava

LEARNING OBJECTIVES

At the end of this chapter, the learner will be able to:
- Recognize interpretation and translation services as integral aspects of equity in quality health care services
- Distinguish between linguistic interpretation, translation, and cultural interpretation
- Explain the value of trained, medical interpreters for health care settings
- Describe situations in which untrained individuals may be appropriate for health care delivery
- Describe techniques required to work effectively with professional interpreters or a bilingual person of a language of lower diffusion (rare languages)
- Discuss common interpretation errors and appropriate strategies that can be utilized to overcome them

KEY TERMS

Ad hoc interpreters	Interpretation	Sight translation
Back translation	Language concordance	Simultaneous interpreting
Bicultural	Linguistic interpretation	Translation
Bilingual	Medical interpreter	Triadic communication
Consecutive interpreting	Pre-session	Whispered simultaneous interpreting
Cultural interpretation	Remote interpreting	

Working with interpreters in health care requires knowledge of issues and standards in interpretation and organizational commitment for language support to ensure that all patients and families with limited English proficiency (LEP) receive quality and equitable care. In 2001 the Institute of Medicine introduced their quality framework that includes equity as one of their six key dimensions to be sure that health systems develop quality health care services (Agency for Healthcare Research and Quality [AHRQ], 2018). The aim was to ensure that, regardless of one's personal characteristics and life circumstances (i.e., social determinants of health), individuals have access to quality health care. After all, access to quality and safe health care is a fundamental aspect of the right to health as set by the Office of the United Nations High Commissioner for Human Rights and the World Health Organization (OHCHR, 2018). However, nearly two decades later, individuals with LEP continue to experience inequitable care as a result of language barriers (Basu et al., 2017; de Moissac & Bowen, 2018; Yeheskel & Rawal, 2019), underutilization of trained and professional interpreters (Brandl et al., 2020; Jacobs et al., 2018; Nápoles et al., 2015; Ryan et al., 2017), and systemic and process issues (Fox et al., 2020; Goenka, 2016; Green & Nze, 2017). The Wellesley Institute in Canada reported that embedding equity into institutional policies and practices between departments within the health sector was an important intersectoral approach to health equity, that is, improving communication, translation services, and interpreting strategies within health systems (Anderson & Um, 2016) so that there is a cohesive, organizational commitment to such services. Ensuring that LEP patients and families can communicate in their preferred language of care allows for equitable access to health care services (Basu et al., 2017). Equitable access is critical to safe and quality care (Green & Nze, 2017), and research shows that language barriers negatively affect patient safety, quality health care, and patient and health care provider satisfaction (Al Shamsi et al., 2020). However, even with organizational commitment to embed interpreter services in health care, there are still safety and quality issues related to language services. Factors such as limited resources, mismatch of supply–demand, challenges with workflow, variable quality of interpretation, and issues with mismanagement of the services can be barriers to improving safety and quality of health care (Fox et al., 2020). Communicating successfully with patients who do not speak the same language as the health care provider requires various levels of planning and dedicated resources and workflow management. This ensures that access to language services is available in advance or on demand, with organizations prioritizing the use of interpreter services for LEP patients and families 24/7.

Language barriers contribute significantly to health disparities for LEP patients and families (Goenka, 2016; Green & Nze, 2017; Lindley et al., 2017), and underutilization of medical interpreters may increase hospitalization (Njeru et al., 2015), and length of stay (Abbato et al., 2019). Interpreters can greatly reduce the language gap; however, being able to find a suitable interpreter when needed and making the most effective use of interpretation services remains an ongoing challenge. This chapter discusses basic steps that are critical to identifying the need for interpretation and essential elements to working effectively with medical interpreters and cultural interpreters. The discussion is largely framed with respect to spoken language interpretation, but many of the issues and strategies also apply to working with patients who depend on sign language. More information about sign language is provided later in the chapter, and readers are referred to the Canadian Hearing Society.

Although Canada's official languages are English and French, 22% of Canadians have a mother tongue other than English or French (Statistics Canada, 2016). The level of bilingualism varies across the country, and given that 215 other languages were spoken in Canada in 2016, it is undeniable that many Canadians may in fact require interpreter services for their health care encounters. Those who speak a language different from the dominant language(s) are best able to relay their thoughts, ideas, and feelings in their mother tongue or first language (Tannenbaum & Har, 2020). Research also shows that when immigrants have experienced trauma, they are best able to describe their emotions in their first language, with more description and rawness, than in their second language (Bailey et al., 2020). This speaks to the need for asking patients and families what their preferred language is for their health care encounters. Many immigrant groups, Indigenous patients, individuals who require sign language, and even those who speak an official language, such as French, in a predominantly English-speaking area experience significant language and communication difficulties (de Moissac & Bowen, 2018). Regardless of language minority group, their experiences with health care and health outcomes are similar because of the language barriers they face (Bowen, 2015).

A significant amount of research has documented the negative impact of language barriers on patient health care (Berdahl & Kirby, 2019; Bowen, 2015; Rawal et al., 2019). In their study specific to Toronto, Ontario, an incredibly linguistically diverse city with over 160 languages spoken by its community members (Statistics Canada, 2016), Rawal et al. (2019) showed that patients who were not proficient in the dominant language of English and had heart failure were more likely to return to the emergency room. Also, those with LEP and who had heart failure or chronic obstructive pulmonary disease were more likely to be readmitted. This further speaks to the need for an intersectoral approach to health equity that recognizes that all aspects of our organizations and health care system must do better to provide quality care to language-diverse populations (Anderson & Um, 2016). As such, cultural competence in health care is one strategy that should be used to elevate and improve health care for language-diverse populations, with communication as a key component of this strategy. Culturally competent care means communicating effectively and working collaboratively to deliver the best health care possible, based on the needs of the individuals (Ladha et al., 2018). Without effective strategies to address linguistic needs of our diverse populations, patient safety and quality are compromised.

Advancing her earlier work regarding language access, Bowen (2015) published a critical analysis of the impact of language barriers on patient safety and quality care. She showed that research in Canada on language barriers and health care is limited, but the research conducted aligns with research done in the United States and elsewhere, as shown by Al Shamsi et al. (2020) in their systematic review of the impact of language barriers. Significant findings of Bowen's (2015) review include that language barriers affect access, which refers "not only to the availability of services, but to service characteristics that make it possible or comfortable for persons in need to utilize such services" (p. 13). Language barriers affect access by limiting the person's capacity with respect to the following:

- Awareness and understanding of conditions and services
- Finding a regular health care provider
- Participation in health promotion and prevention activities
- Participation in cancer screening
- Receiving recommended preventive care
- Access to mental health services
- Access to other or alternate forms of services

Along with language barriers limiting access to health care, patients and families with LEP also experience less patient satisfaction and poor communication with providers, resulting in limited understanding of what was said. A review done by Yeheskel and Rawal (2019) shows how communication and language barriers impact patient experience, a key element of quality in health care. In a review by Aelbrecht et al. (2019), studies showed that those with lower education attainment and limited language proficiency experienced more negative interactions with clinicians. Ultimately, this leads to compromised patient safety and quality of care that results in (Bowen, 2015)

- Inaccurate or incomplete patient assessment
- Poor disease management and outcomes
- Increased risk of medication errors and complications
- Increased risk of adverse events
- Compromised informed consent and confidentiality
- Omission and commission errors

A key finding that Bowen (2015) speaks to is the risk of "illusion of communication" (p. 25). When the patient or family speaks some or limited English, providers assume there is understanding and no need for interpreters. This poses greater risks to the person with LEP as the burden then rests on the LEP patient and family to understand, rather than requiring providers to be better educated and knowledgeable about language barriers and culturally competent communication.

Despite compelling evidence of the need for language support, health care organizations do not have a consistent way of approaching this issue. Consequently, the unmet need of interpreter services is very high, even in traumatic, challenging situations like an emergency room (Taira, 2019).

Cost comes into play for all health care organizations as they attempt to address language barriers and health equity. However, given the potential for exorbitant costs because of poor health outcomes by not offering interpreters, it is in the best interest of health care organizations to provide professional medical interpreters (Brandl et al., 2020), especially as patients with LEP requiring interpreters have a greater number of emergency department (ED) and inpatient visits (Njeru et al., 2015). **Medical interpreters** are trained professionals with skills in interpretation as well as medical terminology. Although language barriers are recognized globally as inequities impacting health experiences and outcomes of patients and families with limited language proficiency (Berdahl & Kirby, 2018; Hilder et al., 2019; Krupic et al., 2017; Tannenbaum & Har, 2020; van Rosse et al., 2016), there is no global standard for expectations, requirements, or resources for how health care organizations should incorporate interpreter services to reduce the disparities experienced by language-diverse populations in all parts of the world.

However, in North America there are examples of national standards, individual health care organizations, and coalitions that promote professionalism of interpreting, as well as limited mandatory government requirements to provide interpretation services. In the United States the Department of Health and Human Services and the Office of Minority Health enhanced the 2000 Culturally and Linguistically Appropriate Services (CLAS) to the National CLAS Standards in 2013. Four out of the fifteen standards focus on communication and language assistance to promote quality of care and health equity (Office of Minority Health, 2018). Federal and state laws, including the 1964 *Civil Rights Act*, mandate that health care organizations provide language access and services for patients with LEP, although compliance is poor (Ollove, 2019). Canada, however (except for interpretation services for deaf patients), has not categorically established the rights of patients to trained health interpretation. There is no overall legislative framework that requires the provision of language access to all language communities, and the different language constituencies (Indigenous communities, immigrants and refugees to Canada, deaf and deaf–blind persons, and official language minorities) often operate in isolation, and rights to access vary for these constituencies. The specific requirements are governed by different legislation and vary depending on the province or territory (Bowen, 2015). Consequently, considerable variation exists in the availability of services and in the development of standards and accountabilities across health care organizations and provincial jurisdictions.

In Canada, a 1997 landmark case of *Eldridge v. British Columbia* highlighted the inequities and discrimination that people who are deaf or hard of hearing experience in the health care system when they are not afforded the same rights as hearing patients that are guaranteed by the Canadian Charter of Rights and Freedoms. Robin Eldridge and John and Linda Warren were the deaf appellants who preferred to communicate through sign language. Prior to 1990 they had received interpretation services through a nonprofit agency, and the government (through neither the *Hospital Insurance Act* nor the *Medical and Health Care Services Act* in BC) would not provide the same services once this nonprofit funding ended. As a result, they were unable to communicate with their doctors, which decreased the quality and safety of the care they received. The Supreme Court ruled that it is unconstitutional to not provide sign language interpreters for deaf persons based on their physical disability, and that the hospitals and the governing bodies of provincial health should ensure that sign language is offered for free for people who are deaf or hard of hearing (Weinstein, 2020). As such, each health authority and the provincial governing bodies have their own acts or laws in place; no deaf or hard-of-hearing person who requires a sign interpreter should be denied or refused such services because of funding issues (lack of interpreters/resources is a different matter). In Ontario, for example, the *Accessibility of Ontarians with Disability Act* governs this mandate to ensure that all Ontarians receive goods and services without necessary accommodations for their disabilities. As Canada is a dual-language country, in Ontario, American Sign Language (ASL) and Langue des signes Québécoise (LSQ) are provided as required through the Canadian Hearing Services/Ontario Interpreting Services program.

Cultural Considerations in Care

Devastating Impact of Language Barriers

Communication barriers because of limited language proficiency in a medical office or an emergency ward could have grave consequences, as the following examples show.

In 1980 Willie Ramirez was an 18-year-old student, baseball player, brother, and son who suddenly fell ill after eating a hamburger at a fast-food restaurant. He was rushed to the emergency department in Southern Florida, and there his family stated that he was "intoxicado," which means "ill due to something one ate" in Spanish. There was no interpreter or Spanish-speaking clinician present. The physician misunderstood what was said to mean that Willie was intoxicated, suffering from a drug overdose. This may be the result of unconscious bias and his assumptions about young Cuban men and drug use, not knowing that Willie was a star baseball player and a very healthy, goal-driven young man. Without an interpreter there was no way to clarify any misunderstandings, and the family and his girlfriend's family were unable to explain to the physician that Willie was not suffering from a drug overdose. As a result, Willie was left in a comatose state for 2 days while his brain hemorrhaged. Consequently, Willie was left a quadriplegic. This case continues to be a prime example of when patients and families with limited English proficiency (LEP) are not provided the necessary language supports, this can result in poor communication, a serious adverse event, and a very large malpractice suit (Price-Wise, 2015).

Fast-forward to September 2020, when Joyce Echaquan suffered maltreatment and died from adverse reactions from morphine. She had attempted to express her concerns about receiving morphine, but was ignored and then berated with racist comments made by hospital employees just prior to her death in a Quebec hospital. She had gone to the emergency room for stomach pain, and because of previous encounters with health care providers whose language she did not fully understand, as well as to document the maltreatment she suffered, she live-streamed her last few moments before she died. In this video that her cousin recorded, a nurse and an orderly are heard saying racist, sexist, and inhumane things to her while disregarding Joyce's concerns about the morphine provided to her. In addition to the video capture of anti-Indigenous racism, there were language and cultural barriers that led to her need to record her fateful encounter. Consequently, there is an ongoing investigation of the two staff members who were fired and of the hospital. This case reminds us that health care systems must do better to end the medical violence that many Indigenous people have experienced for so many generations (Bettache & Shaheen-Hussain, 2020).

Both examples highlight the devastating consequences of inadequate language and cultural supports for health care outcomes. While not all language barriers result in such outcomes, we know that access to many aspects of health care is negatively affected by lack of language services (Bowen, 2015). After all these years of continued inequities, our health care systems know better and should act to implement programs such as interpreter services to ensure that patients and their families feel heard, understood, and communicated with in the way they need.

Translation Versus Interpretation

Language barriers can be addressed via translation as well as interpretation. **Translation** is "the process of transposing the meaning of a written text from one language (source) to the other (target) by producing an equivalent target text that retains the elements of meaning, form and tone" (National Standard Guide for Community Interpreting Services [NSGCIS], 2007). **Interpretation** is done with spoken word—the original message is delivered from the source language into the target language between two or more parties who do not share a common language. Another key aspect of interpreting is sight translation, something that professional interpreters are asked to do in many health care encounters. **Sight translation** is reading written material in one language and reading it out loud verbally in another language.

Generally, interpretation focuses purely on the spoken interaction, without omission, addition, editorializing, or any distortion in meaning (NSGCIS, 2007). However, there are times when understanding the meaning embedded in the words, tone, and gestures is just as important as understanding what is being said. Hence, a distinction needs to be made between the following:

- **Linguistic interpretation**, in which only the spoken word is interpreted
- **Cultural interpretation**, in which an interpreter may offer additional information about the culture

Linguistic interpreters understand the language but may not understand all the subtleties of the cultural context. Cultural interpreters not only understand the spoken language but also understand and communicate the cultural context, including the meanings of looks and gestures. Cultural interpreters can help navigate the conversations. Without leading the conversation, cultural interpreters are able to provide clear, precise interpretations that include nuances in meaning and nonverbal cues (Ladha et al., 2018). The extent to which an interpreter functions (or should function) as a linguistic or cultural interpreter depends on a variety of factors that will be discussed later in the chapter. Keep in mind that cultural interpreters, or cultural brokers as they are sometimes called, exist in the United States and in other provinces of Canada, but in Ontario, the *National Standard Guide for Community Interpreting Services*, published by the Healthcare Interpreting Network (now part of the Ontario Council on Community Interpreting [OCCI]) Services, states that a community interpreter's ethical duty to provide impartial interpretation is compromised when they are asked to be cultural interpreters. More information regarding standards and code of ethics will be provided later in the chapter.

It is important to note that standards that exist for translation services apply to organizations, not the individual translators. Individuals must go through a different set of requirements to become certified translators. Both aspects are important to ensure that health care providers feel confident to use translated materials with their patients. Certified translation agencies provide quality assurance and accuracy via forward translation (from source language to target language), back translation, and reconciliation processes (Language Scientific, 2020). Once the original text has been translated into the target language, **back translation** is performed by taking the translated document and having an independent, separate translator (who does not know anything about the original text) translate it back to the source/original language. Reconciliation is the third step in the process, in which the original document is compared with the back-translated document to determine if meaning and intent are similar or if more work is required. Due to language differences, translations are not always word for word, but meaning and context are vital to ensure translations convey the messages from the original text. An added step to this process could be to then have an interpreter sight translate to provide further consultation and ensure accuracy of meaning, as interpreters automatically consider context and meaning of the message instead of just translating word for word.

Recognizing the Need for an Interpreter

The first step to working effectively with an interpreter is to recognize the need for one. Lack of effective interpretation remains a major access barrier to quality health care for many communities (Bowen, 2015; Taira, 2019; Walji & Flegel, 2017). In most situations the decision as to whether to request an interpreter is frequently left to the individual health care provider (and, to a lesser extent, the patient). Often, the need for an interpreter is clearly indicated, but on many occasions it is not addressed or the need is underestimated. Patients may also assume the service is fee based and may not ask for interpretation support. Depending on health care providers to ask individuals about their preferred language is not enough; posters, bookmarks, and signs in different languages that let patients and clients know that interpretation services are free are important tools to utilize.

Factors that contribute to a health care provider's underestimation of the need for an interpreter include the following:

- Overconfidence in interpretation of nonverbal behaviour
- False fluency or illusion of communication (overestimation of one's abilities at understanding or speaking a second language) on the part of the patient or the health care provider (Bowen, 2015)

Patients and health care providers who have limited proficiency in a language may be able to communicate effectively in social situations but often have greater difficulty in the health care context, which is characterized by jargon, medical terminology, and stress. In such situations, patients may not recognize their own needs or may be hesitant to indicate their difficulties because of high self-expectations or fears of being judged negatively by the system. At the same time, health care providers may assume fluency based on a patient's background and initial presentation. The mere fact that some English words are being spoken should not give the English-speaking health care provider a false sense of security that accurate information transfer has taken place (Bowen, 2015).

It is also important to note that while we can identify the number of patients who may need an interpreter in a study, it is hard to know if such numbers actually show real need when language needs are not assessed and recognized in a systematic way (Blay et al., 2018). Research continues to show the value of language services, but recognizing the need may indeed be a barrier when the right type of questions are not asked (e.g., "What is your preferred language to speak with your health care provider?"). A systematic review showed that LEP parents of sick children who had professional interpreters improved their health literacy, had better communication with health care providers, had an enhanced comprehension of the child's condition, and experienced improved patient satisfaction (Boylen et al., 2020). However, it was interesting to note that LEP parents of pediatric patients felt their quality of care was less than that for English-speaking parents. This is not surprising, especially if language access was a burden placed on them and interpreter services were not readily provided or provided reluctantly.

Even when the need for an interpreter is recognized, health care providers often choose to provide care without a qualified interpreter because of perceptions that working with interpreters takes too long, interpreters are an avoidable expense, or interpreters are potentially problematic in the areas of accuracy and confidentiality (Ahmed et al., 2017; Jungner et al., 2019). Self-overestimation, combined with lack of knowledge regarding the impact of ineffective interpretation on health care experiences and outcome, results in underestimating the need for, and the use of, interpreters.

Standards and Code of Ethics

While it is critical to recognize the need for interpreters, it is also crucial to ensure that interpreters act ethically and follow standards of practice to promote quality, impartiality, and equity. In 2005, the National Council on Interpreting in Health Care established the National Standards of Practice for Interpreters in Health Care, a year after they had created the National Code of Ethics for Interpreters in Health Care (NCIHC, 2005). These standards were created because of an absence of established standards and requirements for interpretation in the United States. Interestingly, the International Medical Interpreters Association (IMIA), also based in the United States, developed Medical Interpreting Standards, of Practice in 1995, revised last in 2007 (IMIA, 2007). They both provide excellent guidelines and standards for practice for medical interpreters in the United States. In 2007, the Healthcare Interpretation Network (now a member of OCCI as their health care branch) developed the *National Standard Guide for Community Interpreting Services,* based on the NCIHC ethics and standards, to advance the professionalism of community interpreters (see definition later in the chapter) in Canada, but more specifically in the province of Ontario (NSGCIS, 2007). The key ethical principles of these standards are noted in Table 6.1.

TABLE 6.1 ■ **Ethical Principles for Interpretation Standards**

1. Accuracy and fidelity
2. Confidentiality
3. Impartiality
4. Respect for persons
5. Maintaining role boundaries
6. Accountability
7. Professionalism
8. Continued competence

TABLE 6.2 ■ **How to Become an Accredited Interpreter in Canada (OCCI)**

To be an accredited community interpreter, one must meet the following criteria:

1. Show English proficiency, such as:

   International English Language Testing System (IELTS), Internet Based Test of English as a Foreign Language (iBT TOEFL), a recognized college language assessment, or Ministry of the Attorney General (MAG) accreditation

2. Provide postsecondary credentials or equivalent

3. Provide a fully passed language interpreter test certificate, such as:

   Community Interpreter Language and Interpreting Skills Assessment Tool (CILISAT), Interpreter Language and Skills Assessment Tool (ILSAT), or Court Interpreter Certification Exam (Corporation of Translators, Terminologists, and Interpreters of Canada (CTTIC)/ Ordre des traducteurs, terminologues et interprètes agréésdu Québec (OTTIAQ)/MAG)

4. Complete post-secondary training in interpreting, for example:

   Certificate of completion of the Language Interpreting Training Program (LITP) or Glendon Graduate Diploma in General Interpreting (GDGI)

5. Have a membership in a professional association of interpreters in North America, such as:

   Association of Professional Language Interpreters (APLI), Association of Translators and Interpreters of Ontario (ATIO), American Translators Association (ATA), International Medical Interpreters Association (IMIA), and so on

Medical interpreters are considered to be specialized and require additional requirements to be an Accredited Medical Interpreter (AMI):

- Accredited Community Interpreter
- Successful completion of a minimum 30-hour medical terminology training course
- 250 hours documented medical interpreting experience

Ontario Council on Community Interpreting. *OCCI categories and requirements for accredited community interpreters*. www.occi.ca, see "Accreditation Framework."

In the United States, the National Board of Certification for Medical Interpreters, an affiliation of the IMIA, currently provides certification for these six languages, requiring the passing of certification exams: Korean, Russian, Vietnamese, Mandarin, Cantonese, and Spanish (The National Board, 2020). While the OCCI, established in 2015 to promote professionalism of interpreting in Canada, supports the accreditation of interpreters, it is not a certifying body; therefore, there is no certified medical interpreter status in Canada. While professional interpreters can practise without OCCI accreditation, having this accreditation further ensures quality and standards of practice in Canada. Table 6.2 shows the requirements for professional interpreters in Canada.

Models of Interpreting

We can overcome language barriers in a variety of ways. Examples of different kinds of interpreters found in health care environments include trained interpreters; multilingual health care providers; and bilingual staff, volunteers, friends, or family members. Interpretation also can take many forms, most notably face-to-face consecutive interpreting, telephonic interpreting, and remote interpreting. It is important for health care providers to be aware of the strengths and limitations of the various approaches.

MODES OF INTERPRETING

Face-to-Face Interpretation

Face-to-face, on-site interpreting is the most frequent and desired mode of interpretation in health care. All modes of interpreting are used for community interpreting—described as the "bidirectional interpreting that takes place in the course of communication among speakers of different languages. The context is the provision of public services such as health care or community services and in settings such as government agencies, community centres, legal settings, educational institutions, and social services" (NSGCIS, 2007, p. 10). The clear advantage of this approach is that it allows for observation and interpretation of verbal as well as nonverbal responses. Face-to-face interpreting can be done remotely, which is discussed later. In-person interpreting, however, can be done in different ways and includes the following types. Most health care encounters are done with consecutive interpreting.

- **Simultaneous interpreting**: nearly instantaneous interpretation of the message from the target language to source language.
- **Consecutive interpreting**: the interpreter listens to chunks of information from the health care provider and then interprets in the patient/family's language. During consecutive interpreting interpreters can take notes, interrupt the speaker, and ask for them to repeat, clarify, or rephrase to ensure accuracy and completeness of the message.
- **Whispered simultaneous interpreting**: the interpreter is seated next to one or more persons with LEP and whispers in the target language the content of the speech. Also called "chuchotage."

Even though face-to-face interpreting is the preferred mode (Taylor et al., 2020), there are many situations where an interpreter is not available in a timely manner. In-person interpretation appointments require advanced booking because of the limited availability of interpreters. **Remote interpreting** refers to situations in which the interpreter is not in the presence of the speakers but may be face-to-face via virtual video interpreting or over the telephone for on-demand or prebooked virtual assignments. Rare languages or languages of lesser diffusion are very challenging to fulfill and often need to be prebooked for remote interpreting. As well, virtual clinical appointments have increased in usage, and video interpreting has proven to be an effective mode of providing language services in health care settings (Kletecka-Pulker et al., 2021). Although on-demand video interpretation sessions are incredibly costly, the availability of such a resource is ideal for urgent situations and last-minute demands.

Telephonic and other remote styles of interpretation, such as using telephone lines, speakerphones, and headsets, rely on technology to provide language support. The most popular service of this nature in Canada and the United States is over-the-phone interpretation, which offers multiple languages, 24-hour access, and interpreters who are trained and certified for the health care context. The clear advantage of telephonic interpretation is that it can provide access to a trained interpreter within minutes, regardless of where (geographically) or when (time of day) the language support is needed, and it is less costly than on-demand video interpretation. Emergency services frequently use such services. Disadvantages to telephonic interpretation include cost (it is more costly than in person assignments) and the lack of ability to assess nonverbal cues and meanings. Interestingly, barriers to language access persist even with remote interpreting available and require more research, as clinicians delay or defer communication when an interpreter is required, affecting the quality of care that patients with LEP receive (Gutman et al., 2020). This may be because of lack of knowledge about the organization's language services; continued information sharing, presentations, and staff meetings for all clinical areas are required to ensure ongoing and appropriate usage of interpretation services.

Other methods of interpretation include using a combination of the following: translated materials, picture cards or cards with key phrases that patients can point to, and key phrases that are learned by the health care provider. As noted earlier, caution is needed when such strategies are employed, as over-reliance on limited pictures, phrases, or gestures can lead to misinterpretation and miscommunication. Although translated documents and materials are important resources and helpful tools for communication, for many patients and families who require interpreter services, the translated documents are not enough. Patients and families want engagement with the providers and need the ability to ask questions, seek clarifications, and confirm understanding. It is vital that clinicians review the documents with an interpreter, as health literacy and literacy in their mother tongue may be an issue as well.

TYPES OF INTERPRETERS

We have already touched on the reality that even though the need for competent, professional health care interpreters is readily recognized in health care, the availability of such resources is frequently limited. Instead, health care providers rely on various other types of interpreters—family, friends, volunteers, as well as professional staff. The volunteers or professional staff may be untrained or trained, and the training they have received may vary from brief workshops to formal training programs lasting several days. It is important that health care providers understand the challenges associated with each category of interpreter to make the most appropriate decision under the circumstances. Understanding these challenges also allows health care providers to develop strategies for minimizing the disadvantages.

Bilingual, Bicultural Health Care Providers

Being **bilingual** and **bicultural** is considered ideal for a health care provider because it means they have familiarity and fluency in language and culture, as well as an understanding of health care terminology, methods, and procedures. When the health care provider is fluent in the patient's language, the need for three-way communication (i.e., involving an interpreter) and the associated dynamics is eliminated. However, many Canadian cities have small numbers of individuals from different linguistic and ethnic groups, and thus it is not feasible to offer even primary care to all communities by a health care provider of the same ethnic or language background (Bowen, 2015). Even when there is support from bilingual health care providers, many of the communication barriers discussed in the previous chapter may still exist. Linguistic similarity cannot be equated with cultural similarity, particularly when we consider the complexity of the various cultural identities and the associated issues of power and authority.

Bilingual Health Care Staff

In the past, many health care organizations had used professional and nonprofessional employees to volunteer as interpreters, but given concerns around liability, privacy, confidentiality, and workload issues, this practice has been discouraged or curtailed in large health care centres. However, health care providers who are within the circle of care of the patient who are bilingual or multilingual and are comfortable speaking in the patient's preferred language (language concordance) are encouraged to do so. This can be problematic if the clinician is actually not bilingual and does not have good medical terminology in both languages. For example, while a physician may feel confident in their ability to speak two or more languages, if their medical training was done in English (their second language), it is possible that they will have limited medical vocabulary in their mother tongue.

> ## Cultural Considerations in Care
>
> ### Being Bilingual Is Not Always Sufficient for Interpretation
>
> An Arabic interpreter at a pediatric centre attended a scheduled appointment for a patient in the critical care unit. A clinical fellow whose mother tongue was Arabic was offended that the interpreter was there. He told her that because he speaks Arabic, he did not need her services. However, because she was booked, the interpreter remained, and ultimately this ensured safety of the patient's care and understanding by parents of the patient's condition. The clinical fellow could not describe the Arabic word for fungus, as he was trying to explain that the patient had a fungal infection in his lungs, causing the breathing issues that the child was having. The interpreter politely offered the Arabic term for fungus, and the fellow in return said, "Thank you. I am glad you stayed."

While **language concordance** (health care provider speaks the same non-English language) is associated with improved physician–patient trust, improved communication between the patient with LEP and the health care provider, and improved health outcomes (Jaramillo et al., 2016), it is important to note that language discordance can be particularly problematic for racialized patients and families with LEP who have endured past and current traumas, resulting in mistrust of health care systems (Molina & Kasper, 2019). However, a challenge of language concordance is that it is difficult to assess language proficiency of the clinician in the patient's preferred language. One way to provide quality language concordance could be to assess or test for language proficiency of medical and nursing students who have the capacity to speak more than one language (Molina & Kasper, 2019).

Ad Hoc Interpreters

Ad hoc interpreters, also known as *informal interpreters*, include family, friends, and community volunteers. While they may be convenient, there are many risks associated with using ad hoc interpreters, including issues related to communication accuracy, privacy, patient safety, confidentiality, disclosure, and errors in interpretation (Paradise et al., 2019). The error rates of ad hoc interpreters are twice that of professional interpreters, with moderate or significant clinical error being much more likely with ad hoc interpreters (Nápoles et al., 2015).

Family and friends continue to be a frequently used type of interpreter, mainly because of easy access and sometimes because of patient preference. Family and friends are appropriate to use when the information involved is factual and nonsensitive, such as personal statistics (e.g., name, age, phone numbers), information about appointments or directions, or simple instructions for procedures. Health care providers should always be sensitive to potential interpersonal dynamics, however, and be alert to any signs of discomfort on the part of either the patient or the interpreter.

Friends and family are frequently unprepared for the complexity or intensity of the health care situation. Confidentiality also is threatened, and in some instances, patients may be reluctant to disclose information of a personal nature, particularly if it implies cultural transgressions. Family members may be reluctant to relay everything the patient says, because of concerns of privacy, shame, or family dynamics. Family members who act as interpreters can readily, often unintentionally, become proxy decision makers, particularly if there are questions regarding the patient's capacity to make their own decisions. Family members also can be selective about what they share with the patient, determining about what and how the patient should be informed of their health care (van Eechoud et al., 2017). Another risk is that health care providers start to favour the family member's perspective, and the patient's voice remains unheard.

In many immigrant families, children become the interpreters for their parents. This practice puts undue burden on the children, potentially creating traumatic situations, and the role reversal can adversely affect the entire family unit. Children as interpreters usurp the parental role of guide and decision maker. This is true regardless of the age of the children, and even parents of adult children who are acting as interpreters may feel their position or status compromised. The patient also may feel that the interpretation is selective, based on the family member's desire to protect the patient and minimize the concerns.

Cultural Competence in Action

Allaying Anxiety With Direct Communication

Mrs. Giovani, a 55-year-old woman of Italian origin, was hospitalized for acute renal failure and started on dialysis. Both the patient and her husband had limited English proficiency, but their 27-year-old daughter was available for regular family meetings.

Over the first week, Mrs. Giovani's condition stabilized, although she continued to experience many symptoms related to the renal failure and dialysis, including fatigue, nausea, and vomiting. The couple's anxiety level continued to increase, as indicated by the husband's constant presence in the hospital room, nonverbal expressions of anxiety and confusion, and loud verbal expressions in Italian.

The clinical team felt that the communication with the patient was good because of regular family meetings, and they tried to address the couple's anxiety through reassuring words in English and through nonverbal communication such as pats on the shoulder. Little attempt was made to communicate fully with the couple in a direct way until a new nurse on the clinical team began meeting with the couple regularly during daily rounds. In response to the couple's obvious distress, this nurse tried to establish a direct relationship with the patient and enlisted the help of an Italian-speaking staff member in the hospital.

The first such interaction resulted in a lengthy conversation during which the husband had many questions about the treatment, medications, prognosis, and progress. After the initial concerns had been addressed, the nurse asked if the information was new to the couple or if they had heard it before through their daughter. The couple looked at each other and then the husband responded, "Of course, our daughter told us all this, about the medicines and that her mother was getting better, but what else could she say? Do you think our daughter would be able to tell us that her mother was dying?"

This clearly illustrates the need for ensuring that the communication between the patient and health care provider is as direct as possible. If family members serve as interpreters, it is important to identify and address the issues around uncomfortable topics such as death and the dynamics around disclosure. Even when direct communication is not possible on a regular basis, attempts should be made to access professional interpreters at periodic intervals to ensure that the patients and providers have the same understanding of the situation and that there are regular opportunities for assessment and clarification of issues.

Professional Interpreters

In contrast to ad hoc interpreters, professional interpreters can interpret with consistency and accuracy and adhere to a code of ethics (NCIHC, 2005; OCCI, 2021). For rare languages or those of lesser diffusion, it is difficult to find trained, professional medical interpreters as defined by NCIHC and OCCI. A study by Hordyk et al. (2017) showed the complexity of being an Inuit interpreter, who must navigate medical information with knowledge of Inuit, French, and English languages while also acting as a cultural navigator. Supporting Indigenous people to become interpreters has been very challenging, with limited access to certain languages and lack of availability of bilingual or multilingual people.

Professional interpreters can generally be counted on to have obtained some form of certification that usually includes language assessment, as well as training related to medical terminology, ethics, and working in health care teams. In Canada, there are no clear credentialing requirements for professional interpreters nationally, but in the province of Ontario, for example, there are requirements fore becoming a professional interpreter (see Table 6.2). A study by Liang et al. (2017) showed how interpreting requires incredible cognitive demands of the person. While simultaneous interpreting is indeed high pressure and requires quick processing, consecutive interpreting requires excellent working memory. This further illustrates the need for using professional interpreters rather than ad hoc interpreters. Providers are encouraged to learn about the requirements in their jurisdiction.

In general, the use of trained professional interpreters has been associated with positive experiences and outcomes for both patients and health care providers (Boylen et al., 2020; Yeheskel & Rawal, 2019).

Cultural Navigators

The standards and ethics of community interpreters, including medical interpreters, requires that the role of the interpreter is to focus on the delivery of just the messages and words between two or more individuals who do not share a common language. They are not to provide cultural interpretation—the cultural differences and nuances of the speakers—nor are they to act as navigators of a system that can often be overwhelming and complex for patients and families with LEP. Therefore, there may be great value to having a separate role of a cultural navigator. As a member of the health care team, partnering with professional interpreters, this may be an ideal strategy to improve access to quality health care and better communication for patients and families with LEP (Hilder et al., 2019).

FACTORS AFFECTING THE QUALITY OF INTERPRETATION

The quality of interpretation is affected by the type of interpreter used. Untrained interpreters are more likely to cause the following errors, although some of these errors occur regardless of the type of interpreter used:

- Omitting information provided by the patient or health provider
- Adding information to what the patient or provider has said
- Substituting words, concepts, or ideas
- Using inaccurate words for anatomy, symptoms, or treatment
- Failing to interpret a message
- False fluency
- Editorializing
- Role exchange (e.g., taking over the interviewing role)

Many errors are made over a short period of time in an encounter and have serious clinical consequences. One study showed that, on average, 29 interpretation errors were made per encounter and that 63% of these errors had clinical impact (Bowen, 2015). However, professional, trained medical interpreters commit fewer errors than ad hoc interpreters (Wu & Rawal, 2017). Another challenge is the lack of linguistic equivalency between any two languages. Many commonly used medical terms may not have an equivalent term in other cultures; similarly, many terms and concepts from other cultures do not have parallel terms in English. In such circumstances, clarification and verification of understanding become critical.

For an interpretation to be effective, all parties need to be knowledgeable about the issues and feel comfortable in the situation. In some instances, patients may be uncomfortable with interpreters because they do not understand the interpreter's role and may be concerned about confidentiality. Explaining the role and the advantages of an interpreter, stressing confidentiality, and obtaining consent are effective strategies to increase patient comfort with a third party in the interaction. It also is critical for health care providers to accurately assess their own biases and skills at working effectively with interpreters. Interpreters should be regarded as resources that provide language support to the patient–provider interaction. Table 6.3 shows five steps to working effectively with interpreters. To use the resources effectively, health care providers need suitable education and experience.

One uncertain experience with interpretation should not be used as the basis for making all future decisions regarding the usefulness of interpreters. It is essential that interpreters be seen as legitimate, valued members of health care teams and that they be provided with some information regarding the context of the situations in which they are asked to interpret. It is equally essential that both the patients' and the interpreters' voices be heard. In health care, cross-cultural communication is frequently challenged by relationships in which the health care providers are dominant; this can be changed by training health care providers and interpreters to maintain a patient-centred approach (Wu & Rawal, 2017).

The potential dynamics between the interpreter and patient also need to be considered. When working with family and friends as interpreters, health care providers need to be aware of the potential influence of both family and interpersonal dynamics. In many cultures, role relationships between generations and genders are extremely structured and defined. There may be strong objections to even mentioning sexual organs or their functions to members of the opposite sex or members of a different generation, and patients may avoid discussing symptoms or concerns. Sometimes, interpreters may revise or omit questions thought to be inappropriate, insulting, or embarrassing. The interpreter's cultural beliefs or superstitions may influence such omissions. For example, in cultures that believe words precipitate deeds, nonprofessional interpreters may omit mentioning complications of surgery or other similar information. Interpreters also may offer their own advice or may selectively interpret what the patient says in order to present the culture in a positive light. It is important to note, however, that addressing language barriers and ensuring quality interpretation should be addressed as an issue of quality and safety, requiring organizational commitment to make necessary changes in their structure or system. Placing the onus on the individual health care provider to determine whether an interpreter is needed or not disregards the significant impact language barriers can have on health care outcomes and patient experiences (Bowen, 2015).

THE STRESS OF INTERPRETING

Interpreters view their role as essential for safe clinical encounters and feel they provide a voice for patients with LEP (Wu & Rawal, 2017). However, when we view interpreters as neutral "language processors," their experiences tend to become invisible. The role of an interpreter is in fact extremely demanding.

Interpreters often report that their role is stressful, because of fear of making mistakes, fear of public speaking, and feeling as though they are in the spotlight (Korpal, 2016). This highlights a need to consider psychological aspects of interpreting and the type of training required

---

TABLE 6.3 ■ Five Steps to Working Effectively With Interpreters

STEP 1: Recognize the need for an interpreter.

STEP 2: Seek out the appropriate type of interpreter.

STEP 3: Clarify the role of the interpreter and that of the health care provider.

STEP 4: Maintain control and engage in direct conversation with the patient.

STEP 5: Be vigilant for errors in interpretation.

as people enter the profession. In addition, interpreters often deal with painful and conflictive communication, which may (particularly in the case of trauma or abuse) affect them personally. In one study in Australia, four in five interpreters reported experiencing some vicarious trauma after an encounter involving traumatic patient material. The majority of these interpreters noted that they were distressed for only a short period of time afterwards, but without the right training and supports, this could affect how they perform during that period of time as well as in future assignments (Lai et al., 2015). A key recommendation from this study was to ensure that interpreters are aware of signs of vicarious trauma and to ensure there is support provided for interpreters through debriefing, counselling, or other forms of organizational support. Peer support is an organizational resource that is available in some hospitals that could also be a great resource for medical interpreters.

TRIADIC INTERVIEWS

Triadic communication involves three parties. A triadic interview involves the following three individuals:

1. Health care provider
2. Interpreter
3. Patient

In triadic communication, attention should be paid to the following (Putsch, 1985):

- Emphasis on shared meaning and understanding, including a desire to learn
- A pre-session
- Physical positioning to encourage direct interaction between the health care provider and patient
- Unobtrusive posturing and eye contact by the interpreter
- Strategies to maximize provider–patient interaction
- Use of first-person voice by the interpreter and health care provider
- Control by the health care provider

Table 6.4 provides guidelines for working with cultural interpreters.

Emphasis on shared meanings requires an appreciation for the scope of the interpreter's role. Neutrality is traditionally emphasized in professional interpreting; in health care, differences in class, culture, expectations, trust, and power require the interpreter to play a more active role. Health care providers need to be open to patient perspectives and value the role an interpreter can play in fostering mutual understanding. A **pre-session** (a brief meeting between the health

---

TABLE 6.4 ■ General Guidelines for Working With Cultural Interpreters

- Allow for extra time for the session.
- Use trained bilingual/bicultural interpreters.
- Never use children as interpreters.
- Consider the gender, ethnicity, language/dialect, and other characteristics of the interpreter.
- Beware of common issues:
  - Words that can't be translated
  - Jargon or terminology
  - Being too rushed
  - Interpreter answering for the patient
  - Conflict between interpreter and patient (if this occurs, stop the session immediately!)
- Verify to avoid misunderstandings, mistakes, and distortions.

care provider and interpreter before the interpreted session) is a useful strategy for reinforcing the role of the interpreter on the team, as well as for clarifying the purpose of the encounter and establishing necessary ground rules and boundaries for the upcoming session (Putsch, 1985).

It is also important to take a few minutes to initiate the session by exchanging pleasantries and building a personal connection to the patient as a person. Such intentional attention to establish the relationship has been shown to strengthen patient engagement (Estrada & Messias, 2018). Throughout interpretation sessions, it is important that health care providers be clear on their accountability for care and that they maintain control over the session. Effective ways to accomplish this goal include the following:

- Ensuring transparency
- Ensuring proper positioning
- Using first-person speech
- Insisting that all conversations be interpreted

Direct health care provider–patient interaction can be maximized in several ways. The health provider's use of the first-person point of view, for example, reinforces that the health care provider's voice should be conveyed to the patient. Rather than talking to the interpreter and saying, "Please tell her that I will be asking questions about her illness," the health care provider needs to say, "I'd like to ask you some questions about your illness." Similarly, the interpreter's use of the first-person perspective conveys the patient's voice to the health care provider. In some instances, interpreters may interject forms of address to communicate respect and honour. For instance, the interpreter may say, "Auntie, the social worker says, please help me understand. . ." This is acceptable because the interaction continues to use the first person.

Positioning also can maximize health care provider–patient interaction. Health care providers should face the patient directly and maintain appropriate eye contact. The interpreter is encouraged to be as unobtrusive as possible, sitting beside or behind the patient, to avoid having the interpreter become the focus of the exchange.

Health care providers frequently become concerned when interpreters give long translations to their shorter questions. It is critical that this gets addressed with the interpreter immediately. Sometimes the long translation is needed to set the cultural context of the question(s), and other times the interpreter may be editorializing. It is therefore important to ask the interpreter to interpret everything as directly as possible. Health care providers need to know about any cultural editorializing so that they can increase their own understanding of cultural issues and assess the quality of interpretations.

Cultural Considerations in Care

Working With Interpreters: The Pre-Session

Whenever possible, take a few minutes to have a pre-session with the interpreter in order to

- Introduce yourself and briefly get to know the interpreter
- Identify the objectives of the interview, topics to be covered, and time available
- Provide a brief summary of the patient
- Ask the interpreter if they have any cautions, concerns, or issues regarding this patient or the situation
- Remind the interpreter to interpret everything using the first person
- Ask the interpreter to share their cultural insights with you as the health care provider, but to differentiate these from the interpretation itself as a medical interpreter
- Encourage clarification
- Reinforce confidentiality

Cultural Considerations in Care

Working With Interpreters: The Interpretation Session

- Face the patient directly.
- Always speak in the first person as if talking directly to the patient.
- Introduce yourself and the interpreter to the patient(s).
- Describe your role and the purpose of the session.
- Speak slowly, clearly, and directly to the patient, not the interpreter.
- While the interpreter is speaking, observe the patient's nonverbal communication.
- Verify interpretations of any nonverbal behaviour ("I notice you are tapping your foot—is this something you do when you are nervous or is there something else. . .?").
- Use simple language and short, straightforward sentences.
- Use plain language and avoid jargon.
- Be patient; remember that the interpreter may require much more time to interpret something than you needed when you spoke in English.
- Ask open-ended questions as needed, to clarify what the patient says or to hear what the patient may wish to convey.
- Observe and evaluate what is going on before interrupting the interpreter.
- Always ask that the patient repeat instructions. Use teach-back to check for understanding.
- Provide written information (preferably in the patient's language) for instructions, appointments, and contact information.
- Provide information as to how the patient may access an interpreter (preferably the same interpreter) in the future.
- Document the name of the medical interpreter or ID number for telephonic interpretation in the patient chart.

Holding a brief post-interview meeting with the interpreter could clarify information and result in discussion of relevant impressions, insights, and issues, including any difficulties that were encountered during the interpretation session. Keep in mind, however, that some medical interpreters are bound to be always impartial and neutral and not act as cultural brokers. In Canada this is especially important with regard to their training, code of ethics, and professionalism, as discussed earlier in the chapter.

It is also important to assess the degree of effectiveness of the interpretation session from the perspective of the patient and family with respect to comfort, degree of engagement, adherence and follow-up, and, ultimately, outcomes of care.

Summary

The chapter began by explaining the language barriers to health care, which, if not recognized, can lead to negative health experiences and outcomes. The chapter discussed the difference between translation and interpretation, and then described five basic steps related to working effectively with interpreters (recognizing the need for interpretation; seeking out the appropriate type of interpreter; clarifying the interpreter role; engaging in direct communication with the patient by maintaining control over the interpretation; and utilizing strategies to minimize errors and miscommunication).

Different modes of interpreting were discussed, most notably face-to-face interpretation and telephonic and other remote interpretation. The types of interpreters encountered in a health care setting may range from untrained, ad hoc interpreters to those who are professionally trained. The role of the interpreter also ranges from message passer to advocate.

It is important that health care providers be aware of the advantages and disadvantages associated with the various types of interpreters and interpreter roles and that they make appropriate choices based on patient need. Interpreters have much to offer in a clinical encounter, and their role needs to be understood and valued for maximum effectiveness. Strategies for enhancing three-way communication between patient, health care provider, and interpreter were explained. Regardless of the role of the interpreter, the health care provider must maintain control and engage in direct communication with the patient. Effective interpretation is vital to effective communication in situations requiring language support.

 http://evolve.elsevier.com/Srivastava/culturalcompetence/.

Questions for Review and Discussion

1. Explain the impact of language barriers for patients with limited English proficiency and families.
2. What is the difference between ad hoc and professional interpreters? Why are professional interpreters used for best practice?
3. What are some of the key aspects of working effectively with an interpreter? What is the first step in working effectively with an interpreter?
4. What is the difference between linguistic interpretation, translation, and cultural interpretation? What type of interpretation is used most in health care encounters?
5. Explain how providing trained, medical interpreters promotes health equity and contributes toward reducing health inequities or disparities.

Group Experiential/Reflection Activity

Working in pairs, read about the *Eldridge v. British Columbia* landmark case from 1997. You can find a good case summary here: https://canliiconnects.org/en/summaries/71876. As you review the case, consider the following questions:

- What were the key aspects or topics of the case?
- Why did the Supreme Court of Canada in its entirety favour the appellants in this case?
- What type of precedent, if any, did this case set for other disabilities or language barriers? Are language barriers (i.e., people speaking nondominant language) considered a disability?
- What are the key points you would make to use this case to argue for or against the provision of interpretation services for *all* nondominant language–speaking patients and families in health care?
- Present and argue your case to the rest of the group.

References

Abbato, S., Greer, R., Ryan, J., et al. (2019). The impact of provision of professional language interpretation on length of stay and readmission rates in an acute care hospital setting. *Journal of Immigrant Minority Health, 21*, 965–970.

Aelbrecht, K., Hanssens, L., Detollenaere, J., et al. (2019). Determinants of physician-patient communication: The role of language, education and ethnicity. *Patient Education and Counseling, 102*(4), 776–781.

Agency for Healthcare Research and Quality. (2018). *Six domains of health care quality.* https://www.ahrq.gov/talkingquality/measures/six-domains.html

Ahmed, S., Lee, S., Shommu, N., et al. (2017). Experiences of communication barriers between physicians and immigrant patients: A systematic review and thematic synthesis. *Patient Experience Journal, 4*(1), 122–140.

Al Shamsi, H., Almutairi, A. G., Al Mashrafi, S., et al. (2020). Implications of language barriers for healthcare: A systematic review. *Oman Medical Journal, 35*(2), e122. https://doi.org/10.5001/omj.2020.40.

Anderson, L., & Um, S. (2016). *International review of health equity strategies.* Wellesley Institute for Health Quality Ontario, Commissioned Report.

Bailey, C., McIntyre, E., Arreola, A., et al. (2020). What are we missing? How language impacts trauma narratives. *Journal of Child & Adolescent Trauma, 13*, 153–161.

Basu, G., Costa, V. P., & Priyank, J. (2017). Clinicians' obligations to use qualified medical interpreters when caring for patients with limited English proficiency. *AMA Journal of Ethics, 19*(3), 245–252.

Berdahl, T., & Kirby, J. (2019). Patient-provider communication disparities by limited English proficiency (LEP): Trends from the US medical expenditure panel survey, 2006-2015. *Journal of General Internal Medicine, 34*(8), 1434–1440. https://doi.org/10.1007/s11606-018-4757-3.

Bettache, N., & Shaheen-Hussain, S. (2020, Sept 30). Opinion: Joyce Echaquan's treatment wasn't an isolated incident: Systemic racism against indigenous people is endemic within the health-care system. *Montreal Gazette*. https://montrealgazette.com/opinion/opinion-joyce-echaquans-treatment-wasnt-an-isolated-incident

Blay, N., Ioannou, S., Seremetkoska, M., et al. (2018). Healthcare interpreter utilisation: Analysis of health administrative data. *BMC Health Services Research, 18*(1), 348–353.

Bowen, S. (2015). The impact of language barriers on patient safety and quality of care. *Final Report Prepared for the Société Santé en français*, (pp. 1–46). http://www.santefrancais.ca/wp-content/uploads/2018/11/SSF-Bowen-S.-Language-Barriers-Study-1.pdf

Boylen, S., Cherian, S., Gill, F. J., et al. (2020). Impact of professional interpreters on outcomes for hospitalized children from migrant and refugee families with limited English proficiency: A systematic review. *JBI Evidence Synthesis, 18*(7), 1360–1388.

Brandl, E. J., Schreiter, S., & Schouler-Ocak, M. (2020). Are trained medical interpreters worth the cost? A review of the current literature on cost and cost-effectiveness. *Journal of Immigrant and Minority Health, 22*(1), 175–181.

de Moissac, D., & Bowen, S. (2018). Impact of language barriers on quality of care and patient. *Safety for Official Language Minority Francophones in Canada, 6*(1), 24–32.

Estrada, R. D., & Messisas, D. (2018). Language co-construction and collaboration in interpreter-mediated primary care encounters with Hispanic adults. *Journal of Transcultural Nursing, 29*(6), 498–505.

Fox, M. T., Godage, S. K., Kim, J. M., et al. (2020). Moving from knowledge to action: Improving safety and quality of care for patients with limited English proficiency. *Clinical Pediatrics, 59*(3), 266–277.

Goenka, P. K. (2016). Lost in translation: Impact of language barriers on children's healthcare. *Current Opinion in Pediatrics, 28*(5), 659–666.

Green, A. R., & Nze, C. (2017). Language-based inequity in health care: Who is the "poor historian"? *AMA Journal of Ethics, 19*(3), 263–271.

Gutman, C. K., Klein, E. J., Follmer, K., et al. (2020). Deficiencies in provider-reported interpreter use in a clinical trial comparing telephonic and video interpretation in a pediatric emergency department. *Joint Commission Journal on Quality and Patient Safety, 46*(10), 573–580.

Hilder, J., Gray, B., & Stubbe, M. (2019). Health navigation and interpreting services for patients with limited English proficiency: A narrative literature review. *Journal of Primary Health Care, 11*(3), 217–226.

Hordyk, S. R., Macdonald, M. E., & Brassard, P. (2017). Inuit interpreters engaged in end-of-life care in Nunavik, Northern Quebec. *International Journal of Circumpolar Health, 76*(1), 1291868. https://doi.org/10.1080/22423982.2017.1291868.

International Medical Interpreters Association & Education Development Center, Inc. (IMIA). (2007). *Medical Interpreting Standards of Practice*. http://www.imiaweb.org/standards/standards.asp

Jacobs, B., Ryan, A., Henrichs, K., et al. (2018). Medical interpreters in outpatient practice. *Annals of Family Medicine, 16*, 70–76.

Jaramillo, J., Snyder, E., Dunlap, J. L., et al. (2016). The Hispanic clinic for pediatric surgery: A model to improve parent-provider communication for Hispanic pediatric surgery patients. *Journal of Pediatric Surgery, 51*(4), 670–674.

Jungner, J. G., Tiselius, E., Blomgren, K., et al. (2019). Language barriers and the use of professional interpreters: A national multisite cross-sectional survey in pediatric oncology care. *ACTA Oncologica, 58*(7), 1015–1020.

Kletecka-Pulker, M., Parrag, S., Doppler, K., et al. (2021). Enhancing patient safety through the quality assured use of a low-tech video interpreting system to overcome language barriers in healthcare settings. *Wiener Klinische Wochenschrift*. https://doi.org/10.1007/s00508-020-01806-7.

Korpal, P. (2016). Interpreting as a stressful activity: Physiological measures of stress in simultaneous interpreting. *Poznań Studies in Contemporary Linguistics, 52*(2), 297–316.

Krupic, F., Samuelsson, K., Fatahi, N., et al. (2017). Migrant general practitioners' experiences of using interpreters in health-care: A qualitative explorative study. *Medical Archives (Sarajevo, Bosnia and Herzegovina)*, *71*(1), 42–47.

Ladha, T., Zubairi, M., Hunter, A., et al. (2018). Cross-cultural communication: Tools for working with families and children. *Paediatrics & Child Health*, *23*(1), 66–69.

Lai, M., Heydon, G., & Mulayim, S. (2015). Vicarious trauma among interpreters. *International Journal of Interpreter Education*, *7*(1), 3–22.

Language Scientific. (2020). *Translation quality management and certification of translation accuracy*. https://www.languagescientific.com/translation-quality-management-and-certification-of-translation-accuracy/

Liang, J., Fang, Y., Lv, Q., et al. (2017). Dependency distance differences across interpreting types: Implications for cognitive demand. *Frontiers in Psychology*, *8*, 2132. https://doi.org/10.3389/fpsyg.2017.02132.

Lindley, L. C., Held, M. L., Henley, K. M., et al. (2017). Nursing unit environment associated with provision of language services in pediatric hospices. *Journal of Racial and Ethnic Health Disparities*, *4*(2), 252–258.

Molina, R. L., & Kasper, J. (2019). The power of language-concordant care: A call to action for medical schools. *BMC Medical Education*, *19*(1), 378–382.

Nápoles, A., Santoyo-Olsson, J., Karliner, L., et al. (2015). Inaccurate language interpretation and its clinical significance in the medical encounters of Spanish-speaking Latinos. *Medical Care*, *53*(11), 940–947.

National Council on Interpreting in Health Care (NCIHC). (2005). *National Standards of Practice for Interpreters in Health Care*. https:// www.ncihc.org

National Standard Guide for Community Interpreting Services (NSGCIS). (2007). Healthcare Interpretation Network. https://www.occi.ca/_files/ugd/8d6ad0_d427c489a313431b83bf89d4b919edab.pdf

Njeru, J. W., St. Sauver, J. L., Jacobson, D. J., et al. (2015). Emergency department and inpatient health care utilization among patients who require interpreter services. *BMC Health Services Research*, *15*(214). https://doi.org/10.1186/s12913-015-0874-4. 2015.

Office of the High Commissioner of Human Rights (OHCHR). (2018). *The right to health*. https://www.ohchr.org/Documents/Publications/Factsheet31.pdf

Office of Minority Health. (2018). *The National CLAS Standards*. https://minorityhealth.hhs.gov/omh/browse.aspx?lvl=2&lvlid=53

Ollove, M. (2019, August 29). *New Trump rule on medical interpreters could leave immigrants behind*. Stateline Article. The PEW Charitable Trusts. https://www.pewtrusts.org/en/research-and-analysis/blogs/stateline/2019/08/29/new-trump-rule-on-medical-interpreters-could-leave-immigrants-behind

Ontario Council on Community Interpreting (OCCI). (2021). *How to become an accredited interpreter*. https://www.occi.ca/occi-accreditation-framework-details

Paradise, R. K., Hatch, M., Quessa, A., et al. (2019). Reducing the use of ad hoc interpreters at a safety-net health care system. *Joint Commission Journal on Quality and Patient Safety*, *45*(6), 397–405.

Price-Wise, G. (2015). *An intoxicating error, medical malpractice and prejudice* (pp. 1–180). Centre for Cultural Competence, Inc.

Putsch, R. (1985). Cross cultural communication: The special case for interpreters in health care. *JAMA*, *254*(3), 3344–3348.

Rawal, S., Srighanthan, J., Vasantharoopan, A., et al. (2019). Association between limited English proficiency and revisits and readmissions after hospitalization for patients with acute and chronic conditions in Toronto, Ontario, Canada. *JAMA*, *322*(16), 1605–1607.

Ryan, J., Abbato, S., Greer, R., et al. (2017). Rates and predictors of professional interpreting provision for patients with limited English proficiency in the emergency department and inpatient ward. *The Journal of Health Care Organization, Provision, and Financing*, *54*, 1–6.

Statistics Canada. (2016). *Statistics on official languages*. https://www.canada.ca/en/canadian-heritage/services/official-languages-bilingualism/publications/statistics.html

Tannenbaum, M., & Har, E. (2020). Beyond basic communication: The role of the mother tongue in cognitive-behavioral therapy (CBT). *International Journal of Bilingualism*, *24*(4), 881–892.

Taira, B. R., & Orue, A. (2019). Language assistance for limited English proficiency patients in a public ED: Determining the unmet need. *BMC Health Services Research*, *19*(1), 56.

The National Board of Certification for Medical Interpreters. (2020). *Becoming a certified medical interpreter*. https://www.certifiedmedicalinterpreters.org/

Taylor, D. L., Sierra, T., Maheshwari, D., et al. (2020). Satisfaction with telephone versus in-person interpretation services in limited English-proficient urogynecology patients: A randomized controlled trial. *Female Pelvic Medicine & Reconstructive Surgery*, 27(6), 388–392. https://doi:10.1097/SPV.0000000000000880.

van Eechoud, I., Grypdonck, M., Leman, J., et al. (2017). Balancing truth-telling: Relatives acting as translators for older adult cancer patients of Turkish or northwest African origin in Belgium. *European Journal of Cancer Care*, 26(5). doi:10.1111/ecc.12498.

van Rosse, F., de Bruijne, M., Suurmond, J., et al. (2016). Language barriers and patient safety risks in hospital care. A mixed methods study. *International Journal of Nursing Studies*, *54*, 45–53.

Walji, M., & Flegel, K. (2017). Healthy interpretation. *Canadian Medical Association Journal*, *41*(189), 1.

Weinstein, T. (2020, Sept. 30). *Eldridge v. British Columbia (AG), [1997] 3 SCR 624*. https://canliiconnects.org/en/cases/1997canlii327

Wu, R. S., & Rawal, S. (2017). "It's the difference between life and death": The views of professional medical interpreters on their role in the delivery of safe care to patients with limited English proficiency. *PLoS ONE*, *12*(10), e0185659.

Yeheskel, A., & Rawal, S. (2019). Exploring the 'patient experience' of individuals with limited English proficiency: A scoping review. *Journal of Immigrant and Minority Health*, *21*(4), 853–878.

CHAPTER 7

Caring for Diverse Families

Salma Debs-Ivall and Rani H. Srivastava

It is believed that demography is destiny, demographic change is reality, and demographic sensitivity is imperative.
—Giger and Haddad (2021, p. 3)

LEARNING OBJECTIVES

At the end of this chapter, the learner will be able to:
- Describe the family as a system
- Identify the characteristics of family diversity that influence health and illness behaviours
- Discuss individualism and collectivism in terms of the family system
- Examine personal beliefs and assumptions about families
- Describe the impact of colonization on Indigenous people and families
- Discuss the concept of intergenerational trauma
- Know how to assess families and their needs when working with culturally diverse patients

KEY TERMS

Acculturation	Individualism	Nuclear family
Collectivism	Intergenerational trauma	Relational practice
Familism	Joint family	Restorative justice
Filial piety	Lone-parent family	Skip-generation family
Health literacy	Multigenerational family	

Families, defined broadly, are an integral part of the care process with all patients (children, adults, and elders), wherever care is provided (home, hospital, or community settings), and however the care is delivered. The concept of patient- and family-centred care has been recognized as a necessary element for quality care since the late 1980s (Park et al., 2018). While there are different models of family-centred care and how to achieve it in practice, there is generalized consensus on its core concepts of dignity and respect, information sharing, collaboration, and partnerships (Al-Motlaq & Shields, 2017). Each of these concepts is subject to cultural nuances, values, and interpretations.

Health care providers in Western society have learned to attribute most illnesses to biological causes and to uphold Western medicine as the answer to health care needs (Giger & Haddad, 2021), thereby relying heavily on scientific methods and processes as the ways to determine and resolve health problems. This may put them in conflict with cultural perspectives of many patients and families whose definition of health extends beyond the physical to the social, emotional, and spiritual.

Families differ in terms of structure and composition; roles within the family; and expectations, preferences, and abilities to effectively navigate health issues and the health care system. These differences can be attributed to differences in cultural traditions and worldviews as well as social determinants of health, including historical legacies of colonialism. Working with families across cultures requires health care providers to develop sensitivity, knowledge, and resources and apply this understanding in practice to effectively partner with families. Provision of culturally sensitive care requires health care providers to understand the family situation, develop a collaborative relationship, adapt practice to patient situations, and facilitate understanding of illness and treatment (King et al., 2015).

The purpose of this chapter is to explore the influence of culture on families, families' role in health and illness, and their ability and potential to achieve equitable health outcomes. Families, like individuals, are unique, complex, and diverse. At the same time, the concept of family is universal in that it has meaning for all of us. We begin the chapter with an exploration of understanding family diversity with respect to familial worldviews and how families may be affected by the process of acculturation. This is followed by a discussion of family structure, function, rules, and roles. In Canada and other countries, the historical legacy of colonization has had significant impact on Indigenous families, which are highlighted in this chapter. We explore the concept of intergenerational trauma that impacts Indigenous people and others, including refugee and racialized communities. The chapter concludes by presenting some guidelines for family assessment and working with diverse families.

Family Definition and Worldviews

The definition of family varies depending on whether we have a sociological, economic, psychological, legal, or biological perspective (Kaakinen, 2018a). Families can be defined by structure (what they look like) or function (what they do). While countries collect national census data according to slightly different definitions, there is consensus that *family* is often described as two or more people who usually reside in the same household and are related to each other by blood, marriage (registered or not), adoption, step, or fostering (Australian Bureau of Statistics, 2016; Statistics Canada, 2021; US Department of Health and Human Services, 2017). The family may consist of a couple (of same or opposite sex) with or without children, or consist of a lone parent and at least one child (Statistics Canada, 2021). Census data also distinguish between family and household. While family members have a relationship with each other, a *household* refers to a group of people (not necessarily related) who live at the same address and share common space. A household may consist of multiple families or may be a group of unrelated people (Office for National Statistics, 2021). Thus a household is the physical environment, and family is the social environment where individuals come together for different purposes (Tam et al., 2017). The two may or may not be the same.

INFLUENCE OF CULTURE ON FAMILIAL WORLDVIEWS

Children are born into a family and a culture, and it is the family that socializes and teaches (formally or informally) the values, language, rules, and roles of society. These familiar worldviews are based on the cultural context in which the family develops. However, it is important to remember that families are dynamic and change in response to social, economic, and cultural contexts. The relationship between families and society is reciprocal—families influence and are influenced by the sociocultural environment (Coehlo et al., 2018).

Individualism and Collectivism

Much of what we know about family members' closeness and family relatedness in cultural communities comes from research in social and cross-cultural psychology involving adults (Rothbaum et al., 2000). Much of this research, for example the work of Triandis (1995), has focused on individualistic versus collectivist outlooks (first discussed in Chapter 3) that can be applied to family systems. **Individualism** and **collectivism** within the family context should be seen only as a starting point for asking the right questions. *Individualistic cultures* give importance to individual rights, viewing each person as a separate entity from the group. Emphasis is placed on self-expression, personal freedom of choice, individual responsibility, and independence. Autonomy is valued, and the unit of confidentiality is the individual (Rothbaum et al., 2000; Triandis, 2018).

Rothbaum et al. (2000) consider families as interdependent subsystems, with rules and boundaries whose functions cannot be understood in isolation of one another. Interpreting the individualistic culture in view of family systems theory, Rothbaum et al. (2000) labelled it romantic relatedness. They note that "in romantic relatedness, the individual subsystem and the spousal subsystem are prioritized—that is, their boundaries are relatively impermeable" (p. 345). The boundaries around the spousal pair keep the couple together and separate from the children and, thus, keep the family intact. The family will also foster a "growing away" attitude toward the children (see Fig. 7.1).

Collectivist cultures, on the other hand, focus on the family or group as the smallest unit in the society and give importance to social role obligations. Calling it "harmonious relatedness," Rothbaum et al. (2000, p. 345) note that in collectivist cultures the boundaries between the individual and the couple are permeable, and it is the boundary around the larger family unit that is impermeable. Children are expected to "grow within" the family unit. The emphasis is placed on the group interest, propriety, social obligation, and interdependence within the family. Group membership and harmony are valued, and the unit of confidentiality is the family or the group

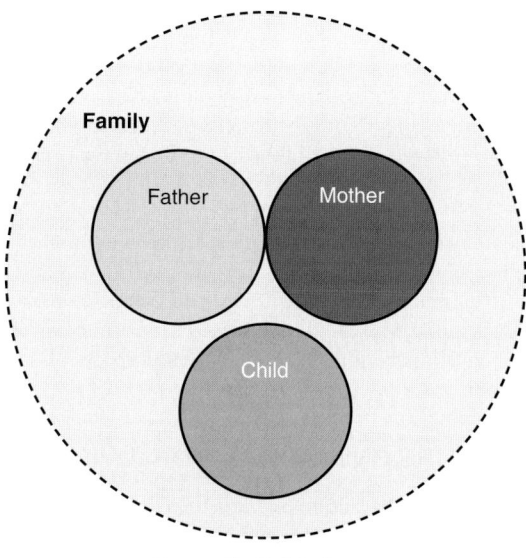

Romantic Relatedness

Fig. 7.1 Individualistic Culture. (Based on Rothbaum, F., Morelli, G., Pott, M., & Liu-Constant, Y. [2000]. Immigrant-Chinese and Euro-American parents' physical closeness with young children: Themes of family relatedness. *Journal of Family Psychology, 14*[3], 334–348.)

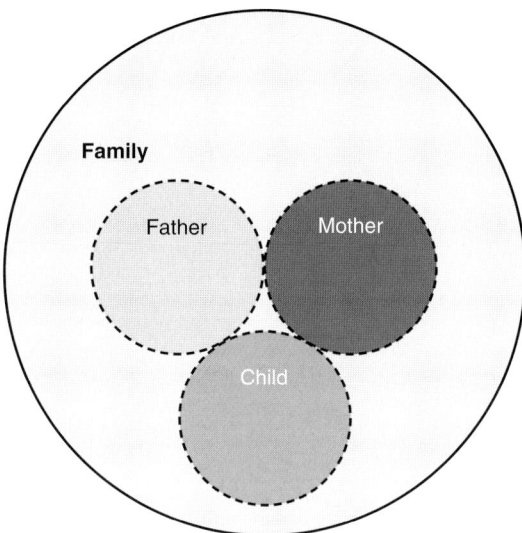

Harmonious Relatedness

Fig. 7.2 Collectivist Culture. (Based on Rothbaum, F., Morelli, G., Pott, M., & Liu-Constant, Y. [2000]. Immigrant-Chinese and Euro-American parents' physical closeness with young children: Themes of family relatedness. *Journal of Family Psychology, 14*[3], 334–348.)

(Rothbaum et al., 2000; Triandis, 2018). Individuals may be very conscious of the obligations toward family members and the role they play in maintaining the good name and honour of the family (see Fig. 7.2).

In many collectivist cultures, decisions are made by consensus, and the family may prefer to filter difficult information to the patient, regardless of age (Alden et al., 2018). Family members, in this case, could be protecting the patient from the harmful effects of losing hope and may also be acting within the context of social obligation and interdependence. In individualistic cultures, autonomy is valued, and the individual makes the decisions. The family in this case will act as a support system and, depending on the dynamics, may not be aware of all the specifics of the illness. Family roles also influence decision making related to care. While one parent may undertake the care of the child in hospital, significant decisions may be made by another, often in consultation with extended family members. Health care providers who value autonomy in decision making may find this a difficult practice to accept. In such circumstances it is important that the family norms be respected and that health care providers allow the family to make informed choices by sharing their experience and expertise. Table 7.1 shows some contrasting beliefs, values, and practices across cultures.

Researchers are becoming ever more aware that elements of individualism and collectivism (also called **familism**) can coexist within immigrant families, as families grow and evolve over time and context. Some aspects of life in these families may resemble those of the community of choice, while others still conform to the community of origin (Rothbaum et al., 2000; Triandis, 2018). When individuals move from one setting to another, such as from rural into urban, there is a shift in their concept of self as dependent or interdependent (McFarland & Wehbe-Alamah, 2015). Depending on the situation, members of a family may act in ways consistent with either a group orientation or an individual orientation. Keeping in mind that family structure differs between cultures, health care providers need to be aware of their own views on family and determine what

TABLE 7.1 ■ Contrasting Family Beliefs, Values, and Practices Across Cultures

Collectivistic Culture	Individualistic Culture
Family as primary unit	Individual as primary unit
Family relationship, solidarity, responsibility, and harmony	Individual pursuit of happiness, fulfillment, and self-expression
Continued interdependence on family is fostered	Early independence is encouraged
Family members strive to fit in	Family members strive to be unique
Hierarchical family roles, ascribed status	Variable roles, achieved status
Parent–child (parental) bond is stressed	Spousal (marital) bond is stressed
Parent provides authority and expects obedience and conformity	Parent provides guidance, support, and explanations, and encourages curiosity and critical/independent thinking
Decisions are made within the family	Autonomous decisions expected
Family makes decisions for the child	Child is given many choices
Parents ask: "What can you do to help the family?"	Parents ask: "What can I do to help you?"
Older children are responsible for the siblings' actions	Each child is responsible for their own actions

Adapted from Chan, S., & Lee, E., (2004). Families with Asian roots. In E. W. Lynch & M. J. Hanson (Eds.), *Developing cross cultural competence: A guide for working with children and their families* (3rd ed., p. 293). Paul Brookes Publishing Co.; Hofstede, G., (2011). Dimensionalizing cultures: The Hofstede model in context. *Online Readings in Psychology and Culture, Unit 2*. http://scholarworks.gvsu.edu/orpc/vol2/iss1/8.

the patient's definition of family is and how the family is to be included in all aspects of the care. Establishing how decisions are made and how to support various family members is essential for collaboration with the family.

Acculturation

Acculturation is "the process in which culture changes and adaptations occur when individuals of different cultures come into contact" (Mao et al., 2018, p. 4). Canada facilitates acculturation through policies that enable the newcomer to retain cultural values from the sending country while embracing Canadian life and values. Canadian policies also enable cultural interactions that facilitate integration in and familiarity with Canadian society. These policies are founded on the underlying belief that individuals may compatibly hold multiple identities and participate in multiple cultures (Berry & Hou, 2016). It is important to note that acculturation is a two-way process in that it can lead to biculturalism or multiculturalism and not just assimilation of the newcomers into the host society. While immigrants may adopt aspects of the host country's culture, they may maintain other aspects of their own culture and cultural identity. Members of the host country are also influenced by the culture of immigrants (Erdem & Safi, 2018).

Acculturation stress refers to the difficulties, challenges, pain, and suffering involved in acculturation. Research with refugees in Australia, Canada, and the United States has identified common areas of acculturation stress to be language, education, employment, discrimination, loss of status, and changes in family roles (Betancourt et al., 2015; Joyce & Liamputtong, 2017).

Language. In 2016, 72.5% of immigrants reported a mother tongue (first language) other than English or French (Statistics Canada, 2017e). The lack of competency in the new culture's language is a major stressor for many immigrant families as it affects education, employment, and overall social integration. Children and young adults may attain language skills much faster than older adults, who may have limited social activities outside their communities.

Education. According to the 2016 census (Turcotte, 2019), first- and second-generation immigrant children in Canada were more likely to complete postsecondary education (43%) than their non-immigrant counterparts (29%). Education is often highly valued as it is seen to be the road to better economic and social status. Interestingly, lack of education of parents in the native culture had less of an impact on the educational attainment of immigrant children than in the case of Canadian-born parents (Turcotte, 2019).

Employment and Economic and Social Status. Despite the educational attainment of first- and second-generation immigrant children, Turcotte (2019) found that, in 2016, immigrant university graduate men who worked part-time or full-time generally earned less than their Canadian counterparts. The gap in employment income is less for female university graduates. Immigrants in all linguistic groups, however, continue to generally have lower earnings than their Canadian counterparts (Houle, 2019). Many immigrants and refugees who may have held professional roles and employment in their country of origin are unable to access those roles in the new country. The challenges may include factors such as language, lack of recognition of professional credentials, and lack of local culture experience. Instead, they find themselves taking on low-paying jobs and starting over in their original or a new career.

Family Life. All aspects of family life are affected when immigrants leave extended families with extensive support networks and come to a new culture where they must function as a nuclear family. Roles change and shift as arrangements are made for child care, meal preparation, and new responsibilities. Both parents may have to work—sometimes at more than one job—to provide for the needs of the family, which prevents them from participating fully in their children's lives. By including the grandparents in the household, the family addresses these needs as well as the requirements for filial piety to parents. **Filial piety** is the value of conveying respect and deference to elders and authority figures. Conflict between the parents, between the parents and the grandparents, or with the children may arise as marital relationships and traditional gender roles are challenged in the new society (Betancourt et al., 2015; Hanna & Ortega, 2016; Joyce & Liamputtong, 2017; Mostoway, 2020). Some parents are able and opt to leave their children behind in their country of origin to facilitate resettlement in the new land; however, this adds another layer of stress (Mostoway, 2020).

Experiences of racism and discrimination related to race, religion, or ethnicity can be another stressor for migrant families. Refugees may have added stressors because they were forced to leave; were victims of physical, emotional, or psychological oppression their homeland; and have precarious health care coverage and residency status in their new country.

Family Structure and Composition

Family is often regarded as a core central unit in society. Every culture has its own views on what a traditional family should look like. In the Western world, the long-standing "stereotypical image" of a traditional family is that of a **nuclear family**, defined as a couple with dependent children. While historically it was understood that the nuclear family consisted of a mother and father, the definition is not restrictive and has been expanded to include same-sex couples. Children in a nuclear family may be biological or adopted. Across the Western world (including Canada, the United States, the United Kingdom, Australia, and New Zealand) the family composition is changing. The nuclear-family type has been on the decline in Canada, dropping from 83% of census families in 1981 to 78.7% in 2016 (Statistics Canada, 2017c).

Statistics on same-sex couples were captured for the first time in 2001, with 34 200 same-sex common-law couples reported, accounting for 0.5% of all couples. Between 2006 and 2016, the number of same-sex couples increased much more (+60.7%) than that of opposite-sex couples (+9.6%). Approximately one-third of same-sex couples in Canada were married and 12% (one in eight couples) had children living with them (Statistics Canada, 2017f).

A **lone-parent family** is a family that has only one parent and child(ren). Lone-parent families in Canada made up 16% of census families in 2016. The majority of these families, 78%, were headed by women (Battams, 2018). Of interest, one-third of Indigenous children under the age of 4 years lived with a lone parent as compared to 17% of non-Indigenous children, and just over 10% shared a household with a grandparent (Statistics Canada, 2017b). In their exploration of the well-being of lone-parent families, Nieuwenhuis and Maldonado (2018) concluded that lone parents faced the triple jeopardy of inadequate resources in terms of finances, time, and care; inadequate employment resulting in gender-wage gaps and in-work poverty; and inadequate policies that could help benefit the well-being of lone parents.

The extended family often is a multigenerational household and includes relatives by birth or adoption. In many cultures, the extended family (also known as "kin") also includes close family friends and community members. When individuals move from one country to another, the loss of extended family often creates a gap in their ability to receive support, including health care advice, and the ability to cope with the demands of an illness. Some cultures also have the concept of a **joint family**, or a family in which parents and adult children and their families live under a single roof. Canadian statistics reflect that in 2017, approximately 9% of adults (aged 25–64) lived with a parent, as compared to 5% in 1995. However, among South Asian and Chinese adults, this number increased to nearly 20% (one in five) living with at least one parent (Statistics Canada, 2019a). **Multigenerational families**, defined as at least three generations of the same family, are the fastest growing household type in Canada, accounting for nearly 3% of households (Statistics Canada, 2017c). This type of living arrangement is common among immigrant populations and Indigenous people (Statistics Canada, 2019a). While culture plays an important role in living arrangements, the statistics may also reflect economic factors, including the high cost of housing in many parts of the country (Statistics Canada, 2019a).

With changing demographics and the increasing numbers of lone-parent and extended families, grandparents have longer and possibly enhanced relationships with children. Many grandparents now find themselves taking care of grandchildren. Elders are highly valued within many populations and share in the raising of grandchildren—as nurturers, family and cultural historians, spiritual guides, child care providers, or caregivers. In 2016, close to 33 000 children under the age of 14 years were living with grandparents, with neither parent present (Battams, 2018), indicating that the grandparent(s) had taken on the dual role of parent and grandparent. This family type is also known as the **skip-generation family**. Grandparent caregiving is more prevalent among racialized and socioeconomically disadvantaged populations, including the Indigenous population (Fuller-Thomson, 2005; Statistics Canada, 2019b). Turner (2016), in an analysis of the 2011 National Household Survey, reported that close to 3% of Indigenous children under the age of 14 lived in a skip-generation household as compared with 0.4% of non-Indigenous children.

Family Function and Roles

The Vanier Institute of the Family (2021) defines family as "any combination of two or more persons who are bound together over time by ties of mutual consent, birth and/or adoption or placement and who, together, assume responsibilities for variant combinations of some of the following: physical maintenance and care of group members, addition of new members through procreation or adoption, socialization of children, social control of members, production, consumption, distribution of goods and services, and affective nurturance—love." This comprehensive definition of family focuses on roles and relationships and is inclusive of the diverse family structures discussed earlier.

Within the context of family-centred health care, it is generally accepted that family is defined by the person and is "who they say they are" (Wright & Leahey [2009], and quoted by

Shajani & Snell [2019, p. 55]). This definition stresses the self-definition of family and is based on the family's perceptions of belonging, rather than on the premise of cohabitation (Stanhope & Lancaster, 2018).

FAMILY FUNCTION

Family function refers to prescribed social and cultural obligations and roles of family in society (Kaakinen, 2018a). As a basic social unit, families take on roles of reproducing, meeting economic and emotional needs of its members, and nurturance and socializing of the younger generation to cultural values and etiquette (Kaakinen, 2018a; Mirabelli, 2018). Individuals within the family system are interconnected, often across generations. This connection can serve as a sense of pride and identity, and can lead to vulnerabilities associated with trauma experienced by ancestors, as discussed later in the chapter.

For many families the ability to meet their social roles and achieve desired outcomes are affected by the social determinants of health such as poverty, racism, and citizenship status, leading to inequitable access to resources. As discussed in earlier chapters, the social determinants of health are interrelated. For example, experiences of racism, discrimination, and poverty can be mutually reinforcing and lead to negative outcomes in housing, education, food security, income, and health (Coehlo et al., 2018).

FAMILY ROLES

Family roles are influenced by family structure as well as sociocultural expectations. Roles are either assigned or acquired, and they define what each member does within the family. Family roles are also dynamic and can shift with time or in response to changes within the internal and external environments. Roles within the family usually complement one another and help preserve equilibrium within the internal environment. A change affecting one member is likely to impact all other members of the family. Family roles can be influenced by factors such as acculturation, age, gender, birth order, or marital relationship.

Gender Roles

While traditionally females were associated with caregiving and nurturing, and males with income generating, these roles have been changing for several decades. However, gender continues to be a social determinant of health and a significant factor shaping roles in family and society. For example, women are more likely than men to be the head of lone-parent households and experience wage gaps, earning on average 20% less than men for the same job (Canadian Women's Foundation, 2019; Coehlo et al., 2018). While caregiving roles are often shared across genders and family members, women often assume a greater share of the caregiving burden in times of need (Kaakinen, 2018a).

The association of caregiving work with women's gender roles is widespread, regardless of whether the societal rules are those of contemporary mainstream Canada or a traditional ethnic community (Beaujot et al., 2017). As the Canadian population ages, and with the trend toward shorter hospital stays, women are increasingly finding themselves caring for family members in the home. The caregiving burden on women has become more evident during the COVID-19 pandemic. With the lockdown measures in the United States, for example, mothers of young children had to reduce their work hours four to five times more than fathers (Collins et al., 2021). This finding was confirmed in Canada by Qian and Fuller (2020), who found that the pre-existing gender inequalities were further exacerbated by the pandemic. Their analysis revealed that the gender employment gap was widened between mothers and fathers of school-aged children as mothers had to reduce their work hours to provide parental care in the home.

For many immigrant families, gender roles may be more defined, at least traditionally, and those values and beliefs add to the complexity of re-establishing family in a new land (Mostoway, 2020). In a Canadian study of refugee new parents from Africa, Stewart et al. (2015) noted gender role conflicts among the challenges faced by the new parents. The changing gendered roles were described by both male and female participants (also see Chapters 11 and 12). Women had to take on paid employment roles for economic reasons and men recognized the need to assist with household chores. Participants also described challenges along the themes of marital conflicts, insufficient time for family, and cultural conflicts in parenting style between Canada and the home country. Parents describe the challenge of preserving the culture of origin while supporting the need for children to function effectively in Canadian society. These challenges were described in a context of diminished social support, loneliness, and war trauma that led to a refugee status in Canada (Stewart et al., 2015).

In a study of family dynamics and the integration of professional immigrants to Canada, Phan et al. (2015) also noted "that traditional gender expectations and the absence of social networks are particularly detrimental to the integration experiences of professional female spouses" (p. 2061). Despite being professionals who worked outside the home in their home country, the integration experience was challenged by gendered role expectations of women being responsible for domestic work. For many men, taking on additional domestic roles is recognized as a necessity; however, it is not without additional stress due to "misaligned cultural gender norms" (Phan et al., 2015, p. 2076). Career aspirations were affected by the high cost of child care and potentially lower wages as newcomers. As well, the family was impacted by an absence of paid or family support experienced in the country of origin. Many couples had paid domestic labour back home who took on chores, which might not be available or affordable in Canada (Phan et al., 2015).

In addition to gender, role responsibilities may be influenced by roles within a family structure. For example, expectations of responsibility, caregiving, and decision making may vary between daughter and daughter-in-law or son and son-in-law. In many South Asian cultures, the daughter-in-law is expected to assume family caregiving responsibilities, while the son-in-law is given a revered status. This can create conflict within the family as some members try to negotiate cultural expectations (own and others) with the realities of what is feasible. In addition to role conflict, women, particularly daughters-in-law in patriarchal cultural groups, may feel silenced and unable to seek psychological support and help for issues such as domestic violence (Banwait, 2019). It is important that health care providers be sensitive to these possibilities and assess for the need for support, without judgement and without imposing their own solutions.

Roles of Children

Socialization and nurturing of children to become well-functioning adults is a key function of families, regardless of culture. Parents use daily routines, examples, praise, and punishment to teach children the cultural values and norms that lead to the development of cultural identity and position them for a successful future (Da & Welch, 2016). These learned behaviours are often maintained throughout life.

Many immigrant families come from cultures that are traditionally considered collectivist, where children are thought of within the context of the family rather than individually. They are kept close, and their individuality is de-emphasized. This may lead to a more authoritarian parenting style characterized by a desire for conformity to cultural norms, parental control, and monitoring of activities (Smetana, 2017). A more controlling or authoritarian parenting style has been associated with many non-Western cultures, including Chinese, Arab, and Middle Eastern, and Mexican (Da & Welch, 2016; Kim et al., 2017; Mostoway, 2020; Smetana, 2017), and can be regarded as serving a protective function for children and limiting perceived negative effects of some host society values (Da & Welch, 2016; Smetana, 2017).

Immigrant parents may vary in their involvement in education. Whereas some parents may be very engaged in educational endevours because of the high value placed on formal education (Da & Welch, 2016), other parents may be minimally engaged in their children's education. The barriers to engagement may be cultural or social and include language barriers in communicating with teachers, inability to make time to attend parent–teacher meetings due to multiple jobs, or deferring to the education system because they believe that education is the teacher's expertise (Mostoway, 2020). Indigenous families may have little trust in the Western education system given the historical legacy of education being a targeted way of assimilation, instead preferring traditional teachings that pass on cultural values and knowledge to the next generation (Grammond & Guay, 2016).

In Western cultures, where independence is valued, children are taught autonomous thinking. Western cultures encourage children's individual expression in the family. Parents emphasize discontinuity of relationships as a way of encouraging the children's independence and their freedom to form new families of their own (Rothbaum et al., 2000). Self-reliance is encouraged and self-esteem is valued. However, Asian cultures value obedience and may view the pursuit of independence as disrespectful, interpreting it as undesirable and as evidence of lack of concern for parents, as well as a threat to traditional family values and beliefs (Da & Welch, 2016; Mostoway, 2020). In Asian cultures, independence is seen as maturing within the family rather than away from it. Children are taught filial piety, or respect for the authority of the parents and the elders in the family. As they mature, children in turn will take care of the parents (Kim et al., 2017).

In 2016, immigrant first- and second-generation children comprised 3 of 10 children in Canada, with the number projected to rise to close to 50% by 2036 (Statistics Canada, 2017a). Immigrant children contribute to the settlement effort and continuing functioning of immigrant families by assuming three specific roles:

1. Language broker: taking on the tasks of teaching, translating, and interpreting for their parents and younger siblings (Bauer, 2016; Valenzuela, 1999)
2. Advocate: intervening or advocating on behalf of their parents and younger siblings (Delgado, 2020; Valenzuela, 1999)
3. Surrogate parent: undertaking the parent-like activities of babysitting, feeding, dressing, caring, and providing for younger siblings (Garcia-Sanchez, 2018; Valenzuela, 1999)

The transition and settlement experience of children and adolescents is both similar to and different from that of their parents. Children are also vulnerable to the impact of discrimination and loneliness; however, these experiences are often not shared with others because of concerns about adding to family burden and a desire to "fit in" with peers. Children are usually faster at learning a new language and new culture and may take on additional support roles in the family. Navigating multiple cultures may also lead to a greater reliance on peers and siblings rather than parents, who are also trying to understand new cultural and social norms (Mostoway, 2020). In addition, children and youth are more likely to maintain closer family ties, out of cultural desire or obligation, and may experience immense pressure to succeed to make up for parental sacrifices.

The parent–child relationship often is challenged by the influence of the new culture's values and beliefs on children and the shift from a collectivist to an individualistic worldview (Albertini et al., 2019). In Canada, immigrant children may become more independent as they follow the cultural norms of Canadian children. Because children acquire language skills faster than adults, English or French will become their primary language and a communication gap may develop between immigrant children and the parents, whose mother tongue remains their primary language. Statistics Canada (2017e) reported that, in 2016, more than one-third of immigrant children spoke one of the two official languages (English or French) at home as compared to less than 10% of the parents. Poor communication and a different pace of acculturation place the children in the role of cultural interpreters to the parents, often eroding the parents' role as socialization agents (Das, 2018). The strained relationship can add to the hardships and stressors families are already facing (Bergnehr, 2018). In some families, however, the experience of migration and discrimination and the loss of social networks may lead to stronger family ties and intergenerational relations (Albertini et al., 2019). Furthermore, family ties are strengthened, and acculturation stress alleviated, when children reciprocate the love and care of the parents, participate in household chores, and succeed academically (Bergnehr, 2018).

In their review of the literature, Albertini and colleagues (2019) highlighted several areas of intergenerational relation differences between the immigrant and the host populations in Europe. First, the expectations of filial piety or responsibility are stronger among the immigrant population. The authors attributed this to the collectivist worldview of most immigrant families. Second, unlike Western norms of parents providing financial support to children and leaving them an inheritance, in the majority of immigrant populations, the expectation is that children provide financial support to the aging parents. This practice could be due to the sparsity of social programs to support older persons in the originating countries. Third, multigenerational households are more prevalent in immigrant populations than in the host population, perhaps due to financial constraints, filial responsibility, and the desire for grandparents' help with child care as women enter the workforce (Albertini et al., 2019).

Health care providers need to be aware of the important roles that children play in the care of immigrant families. It is also important to recognize the issues that children, adolescents, and adults in the family may be experiencing and to identify opportunities and resources both within and outside the family. While the intergenerational issues are not without challenge, familiarity with multiple languages and traditions can be seen as a strength (Da & Welch, 2016) and used to further build capacity and resiliency.

Roles of Elders

Older persons in traditionalist (collectivist) cultures gain generational status as they age. They are accorded respect and deference and receive physical, emotional, and financial support in their old age. Family members within these cultures expect to physically care for their elders; multigenerational households are common (Kim et al., 2017).

Immigration to Canada may result in a disruption of the roles of the older family members as they move into a more Western culture than they are used to. Older persons may have had to immigrate to a new culture, not because they wanted to, but so that they are not left behind when their children settle in a new country. Their acculturation is impacted by their language skills, unfamiliarity with services, limitations in accessing the community outside their immediate family, increased physical and health needs, and loss of social and financial status (Mao et al., 2018). Lack of familiarity with the new culture may make it more challenging to continue in the role of head of the household or advisor. The resulting isolation is likely to affect their physiological and psychological well-being and increase their dependence on family members, impacting the relationships within the household (Mao et al., 2018).

As grandparents, older family members often take on child care activities. However, despite the emotional and practical support that the older immigrant adult(s) provide, relationship, financial, and care strain may occur for the adult child. Grandparents, on the other hand, face conflict as their status of respected, wise elders is challenged. The knowledge they possess may not be of use in the new country. They may become dependent on their children and grandchildren, both to help them navigate through the new culture and to provide for their economic and social needs. They may perceive a loss of cultural identity as both their children's and grandchildren's roles shift to accommodate the new culture (Guo et al., 2015).

Impact of Colonization on Indigenous Families

The impact of colonization on Indigenous people and families is immense. Colonial policies significantly reduced the strength and vitality of Indigenous families through direct genocide, forced assimilation in residential schools, and child apprehension policies of the 1960s and 1970s, by which Indigenous children were taken from their home communities and raised in non-Indigenous foster homes (Menzies, n.d.). The *Indian Act* in Canada also "reinforced a Eurocentric concept of family on First Nations people" (Menzies, n.d.). An individual's legal status as an Indian was defined by the State and the act was particularly discriminatory toward women. An Indian woman would lose legal and ancestral identity (Indian status) if she married a non-status man. Women also lost status if they became widowed or were abandoned by their husband. Losing status also meant expulsion from the community and loss of family and community support. Children in these marriages were also not entitled to have status. For men, however, marriage to a non-status woman meant that the woman and subsequent children would have status (Menzies, n.d.; Wilson, 2018).

Of all the colonial policies, residential schools have been noted to be particularly damaging to Indigenous people in Canada (Wilk et al., 2017). The explicit purpose of the residential school system was to "civilize and Christianize Indigenous children" and wipe out cultural traditions, including language, through forced assimilation. In addition to disconnection from community and family, the children experienced abuse (psychological, physical, and sexual), were subject to poor nutrition and living conditions, and often received limited education (Grade 5) as they were expected to be low-wage earners in society (Wilk et al., 2017; Wilson, 2018). The loss of language, culture, family, and community has had devastating and long-lasting impacts on individuals and family. Parents and grandparents were separated from children who were unable to learn from their elders and grew up with little knowledge and skills of how to be parents and raise their own families (Wilson, 2018). These experiences and impacts are similar to forced-assimilation experiences in Australia and the United States for Indigenous people (Wilk et al., 2017). The concept of intergenerational trauma and its impact is discussed later in this chapter.

Indigenous families today may be characterized by complex family and household structures and kinship systems that are different from Western systems. The family may be multigenerational and include members who are non–blood related but are considered "kin." Indigenous families are more likely to experience multiple caregivers, broad and varied kinship structures, and frequent mobility (Tam et al., 2017). Grandparents may also play a significant role in raising children, often becoming the primary caregivers and taking on the responsibility of passing on traditional cultural wisdom and practices. Within Indigenous culture, grandparents, particularly grandmothers, are highly revered and play a significant role in child rearing. Based on findings from a scoping review of grandparent caregivers, Hsieh et al. (2017) note that many of the grandparents raising children today are survivors of the residential school system or similar experiences. Therefore, they are likely to continue to be affected by intergenerational effects of such trauma. They may have a conflictual or strained relationship with the mainstream health care and social systems and policies, especially those regarding child welfare, and they may be mistrustful of non-Indigenous caregivers.

The Indigenous grandparents raising grandchildren may also experience additional challenges including financial burden, inadequate housing, lack of access to formal support programs due to lack of knowledge of such services, lack of transportation or child care, and stigma associated with receiving support (Hsieh et al., 2017). Grandparents may need support for their own physical and mental health. It is critical that all health care providers understand the legacies of colonization, explore the needs and strengths of Indigenous grandparents who are caregivers, and link them to appropriate services where possible. It is equally important to recognize and support resilience and strengths inherent in individuals, families, and communities.

While the residential school system is no longer in existence, some would argue that in Canada it has been replaced by the child welfare system (Somos, 2021). In 2016, Indigenous children accounted for 7.7% of the child population but represented 52.2% of children in foster care (Government of Canada, 2021a). The Truth and Reconciliation Commission's (TRC) first call to action is on child welfare and calls upon the government to reduce the number of Indigenous children in care through actions such as monitoring neglect investigations, keeping children in culturally appropriate environments, keeping families together where it is safely possible, ensuring that social workers and other providers receive proper education and training to understand the impact of residential schools, and seeking out solutions for family healing in partnership with Indigenous families and communities (TRC, 2015). On January 1, 2020, the *Act Respecting First Nations, Inuit and Métis Children, Youth and Families* came into effect in Canada. "Co-developed with Indigenous, provincial and territorial partners, the act affirms the rights of First Nations, Inuit and Métis people to exercise jurisdiction over child and family services . . . [and] provides an opportunity for Indigenous people to choose their own solutions for their children and families" (Government of Canada, 2021a).

Cultural Competence in Action

First Build Trust, Then Understand the Story

Nathan, a 2-year-old child, had a follow-up appointment in the neurology clinic of an urban hospital. However, the family did not come for the appointment and did not notify the clinic in advance. The child is of Indigenous heritage and had been seen in the emergency department for seizures 2 days prior. The child was given medications and was discharged (rather than hospitalized) at the family's request, with a follow-up plan in the outpatient clinic. As the health care team reviewed the case, they noted that this was the third no-show appointment to the clinic in the past 3 months, although the family had been to the emergency department several times. Each time discharge from the emergency department indicated an agreed-upon plan for follow-up in the clinic. The clinic physician is concerned that the mother is unreliable and feels that the child may need to be taken from the family for care. The social worker reports that she has been calling the mother repeatedly but has been unable to reach the family.

- What factors might need to be considered in this situation to inform the next steps?
- Why might the family be so against hospitalization?

Consider the historical legacy of Indigenous families and the social determinants of health in your answer.

The team sought out assistance from Indigenous support services, and a social worker from that service (who was also Indigenous) was able to reach the family. They reported that the mother had no email and her cell phone had a limited service plan, which meant she had to be careful about usage. While not explicitly stated, it is also likely that she was avoiding the hospital calls, as the previous conversations that informed her of what was expected of her were somewhat accusatory in tone. The mother had also been ill and had been in and out of the hospital for care.

- With better understanding of the family story, how can the health care team proceed with a plan of care for this family?

Within the Indigenous population, there is a disproportionately higher number of grandparents—mostly grandmothers—who are caring for their grandchildren with no parent present. In this skip-generation family, the grandparent takes on the role of surrogate parent upon the request of either welfare workers or the adult parent themselves (Hsieh et al., 2017). The history of violence and abuse that the Indigenous population faced through attempted assimilations and forced separation of children from their culture and their displacement into residential schools have resulted in generational traumas and fractured families. Parents who experienced the trauma of the residential school system have had to deal with subsequent social issues, including loss of identity, lack of social skills, and chronic mental health issues related to violence and mistreatment (Hsieh et al., 2017). As a result, there is a disproportionately higher percentage of Indigenous children in foster care than for the non-Indigenous population. Consequently, more grandparents find themselves caring for their grandchildren when their adult children are unable to parent. In addition to the burden of parenting and anxiety over their adult children, Indigenous grandparents have to cope with social and health issues of poverty, housing insecurity, barriers to accessing care, mental health issues, and higher levels of disability (Hsieh et al., 2017).

Health care providers caring for the skip-generation Indigenous family need to provide care that is culturally sensitive and competent in addressing the impact of generational trauma. In some Indigenous cultures, no word exists for family. Family is defined in terms of relationships and kinship connections (Tam et al., 2017). This has strong implications for family assessments and care planning.

INTERGENERATIONAL TRAUMA

Intergenerational trauma can be defined as trauma that is transmitted across generations. It is often described as historical or collective trauma "in which the descendants of a person who has experienced a terrifying event show adverse emotional and behavioral reactions to the event that are similar to those of the person" (American Psychological Association, 2020). Intergenerational trauma has also been described as a collective trauma experienced by a group of people with shared identity or affiliation (Hudson et al., 2016). The trauma may be due to war, natural disasters, oppression and racism, forced displacement, cultural destruction (e.g., holocaust, residential schools), and other events that lead to significant sustained impact on individuals, families, and communities (Boulton, 2018; Isobel et al., 2021). The impact includes neurobiological changes in the brain, heightened sense of vulnerability to further harm and helplessness, low self-esteem, shame, grief, increased anxiety and guilt, depression, suicidality, substance abuse, difficulty with relationships and attachment to others, difficulty in regulating aggression, physical health concerns including obesity, and extreme reactivity to stress (Bennett & Woodman, 2019; Hackett et al., 2016; Isobel et al., 2021).

Intergenerational trauma has been described among survivors of the Holocaust; Indigenous people in Canada, Australia, New Zealand, and the United States, with similar histories of colonization and cultural destruction (O'Neill et al., 2016); refugee communities; and racial and ethnic minorities, particularly Black people in the United States with a legacy of slavery and ongoing police brutality (Bryant-Davis et al., 2017; Watson et al., 2020). Linkages between historical legacies of trauma, present-day inequities in society, along with health disparities have been noted in a variety of communities. While the specific manifestations of intergenerational trauma may vary across populations and individuals, consistent themes have emerged. The literature on intergenerational trauma highlights silencing, communication challenges, relationship challenges, and acknowledgement as areas that require understanding and support. There is also emerging dialogue on factors that promote resilience and healing from intergenerational trauma.

Silencing

A key finding in intergenerational trauma research is that of silencing or a conspiracy of silence around the traumatic experience(s) (O'Neill et al., 2016). While silencing is part of communication, it is often identified separately because of its frequent referencing (Hudson et al., 2016). The trauma often "remains a secret" within families as it is not acknowledged or expressed verbally. Individuals who directly experienced the trauma have difficulty expressing it—as a means of coping with the shame and distress, fear related to a history of punishment for speaking out, and a means of protecting family members (Hackett et al., 2016; Hudson et al., 2016; O'Neill et al., 2016). Thus silence can be both a protective and an avoidance tool. Although the next generation may not verbally access or acknowledge the trauma, they still experientially learn not to trust anyone and not to communicate their experiences (Hackett et al., 2016). In addition, the silence can lead to an exacerbation of the impact of trauma, resulting in negative impact on physical and mental health, social adjustment, and cognitive abilities (Hudson et al., 2016). It can also become a barrier in accessing opportunities for healing for individuals, families, and communities (Hudson et al., 2016). Parents do not bring up the trauma, to protect the children, and children do not ask because they do not want to further upset the parent(s) (O'Neill et al., 2016).

The silence of historical trauma occurs at multiple levels. Not only are individuals and families directly and indirectly affected by the trauma, society may also embrace the silence because of lack of knowledge, discomfort, or guilt. Such "social amnesia" (O'Neill et al., 2016) can exacerbate the trauma. While the Holocaust trauma has been widely acknowledged across many countries, the historical trauma of Indigenous people has only recently received broad recognition and acknowledgement within Canadian society with the work of the TRC and the government apology (O'Neill et al., 2016). For racialized and Black communities such dialogue is emerging in the context of multiple and widespread incidents of police injustices in the United States and Canada and the increasing support of the Black Lives Matter movement (Watson et al., 2020).

The social silence also extends to the health care sector. Research shows that health care providers may not bring up such topics because of pressures of time; a sense of inadequacy fuelled by feelings of discomfort, guilt, and fear of making things worse; and perceived lack of support within the system (Isobel et al., 2021; Watson et al., 2020). Recognizing the potential impact of intergenerational trauma is the first step. However, the awareness has to be accompanied by a willingness to listen and explore narratives of the individual and family to better understand the role of silence and the extent to which historical trauma is understood and acknowledged within the family.

Communication and Relationship

Intergenerational trauma can affect family communication and relationships between the generations in different ways. Children, including adult children, may not be aware of the trauma impact and thus unable to recognize it as a contributing factor to their parents' or their own health, well-being, and ability to integrate into society (O'Neill et al., 2016). Parents' feelings of anger, guilt, and shame may be transmitted to children. Children may experience guilt for parental suffering even though they had no role in the trauma, or they may try to somehow (over) compensate for parental losses (Hudson et al., 2016). In circumstances where there is frequent telling and re-telling of the traumatic events, children may be at risk for vicarious trauma or may take on a protective parental role (O'Neill et al., 2016). Thus health care providers must take note of the cultural communication within the family and the role of disclosure, nondisclosure, guilt, and anger and identify cultural barriers to health (Hudson et al., 2016), as well as strengths and opportunities for healing.

Though it may make memories more vivid, remembering and situating individual experiences in the context of community and historical experiences is important for healing. Taking the cues from the patient and family, it is important that health care providers demonstrate sensitivity and a willingness to listen and to acknowledge historical trauma and its potential impact on the current situation. Isobel et al. (2021) describe this as a theme of "looking back and forward," where both the past and future are considered to address issues in the present. Remembering can also be facilitated through use of art as a means of expression, exploring public places of remembrance (museums or exhibits), and connecting with others who have experienced similar trauma (Hudson et al., 2016). Understanding the link of the individual to the cultural and historical trauma is important to reduce the internalization of inadequacy that can accompany intergenerational trauma (O'Neill et al., 2016). Similarly, acknowledgement of the existence and impact of systemic racism and health inequities can support healing (Watson et al., 2020). More recently, the approach of restorative justice has gained recognition as a promising practice. **Restorative justice** is an approach that is used to repair harm and promote healing by providing an opportunity for connection between those who have been harmed and those who have contributed to the harm (Government of Canada, 2021b). Acknowledging the harm of systemic racism, colonization, and residential schools can support healing and reinforce commitment(s) to Black Lives Matter, Indigenous Lives Matter, and Every Child Matters.

It is important to support individuals and families by recognizing the strengths and resilience that is embedded within families and communities who have survived generations of injustice and violence. Cultural and social support from family, friends, and community has been noted as an important protective factor to support healing and resilience (Hsieh et al., 2017; Hudson et al., 2016). Hsieh et al. (2017) note that Indigenous grandparents raising grandchildren express pride, satisfaction, and happiness in knowing that they are able to provide for and share cultural values and cultural identity with their grandchildren. Traditional healing and cultural practices, faith and spirituality, and community networks and connections have been recognized as important approaches to strengthen resilience and promote healing in intergenerational trauma (Betancourt et al., 2015; Bryant-Davis et al., 2017; O'Neill et al., 2016).

Cultural Considerations in Care

The Impact of Race, Assumptions, and Labels

Curtis, a 14-year-old boy, came to the clinic, accompanied by his dad. Curtis was having difficulty in school and there were potential concerns regarding his cognitive abilities. Curtis was very quiet and withdrawn while his dad was quite agitated. The family was Black. When asked about the history, Curtis's dad was clearly upset. He spoke for several minutes describing Curtis's experiences of having difficulty and not getting the help that he needed. Curtis was having difficulty with comprehension and would get frustrated at not understanding and not getting help; however, his frustration was interpreted by others as aggression. In response, sometimes Curtis would just withdraw and become silent. However, this led to him being called "lazy" repeatedly. His dad, who was a teacher, was sad and frustrated, and stated that it made him "uncomfortable" that the system that should be helping his son was failing him.

The doctor and team caring for this family recognized the potential impact of racism and unconscious bias on Black families and the harm that can come from labels. They also felt "uncomfortable" with the racism experienced by this family and others. They demonstrated the importance of building trust and conveying respect by listening to the dad's story and validating the family's feelings of frustration and sadness. This initial trust-building was significant in the family's response to future follow-up, as subsequent investigation identified neurocognitive issues that required treatment. Acknowledgement of being "uncomfortable" with the racism that health care providers witness or hear about is an important factor in the team being able to support each other and the patients and families they serve.

Role of Families in Health and Illness

Families play a significant role in maintaining and restoring health. Health promotion behaviours (including diet, exercise, and other activities associated with specific healing traditions) are primarily learned within the family. Families can play a significant role in when and where to seek help for health needs, and they take on caretaking behaviour(s) when family members are ill or injured (Kaakinen, 2018a).

Wright et al. (1996) believe that, in the same way that the illness of an individual affects the whole family, the family, in turn, will affect the illness. They propose that the effect lies more in the beliefs about the illness than with the illness itself. Such beliefs might be about the diagnosis, etiology, healing and treatment, control, prognosis, and religion and spirituality, as well as the role of the illness in life. Rather than constraining family beliefs, which could cause suffering, health care providers are in a position to work with the family to come up with options that take their beliefs into account.

All health decisions, behaviours, and practices are influenced by and take place within the context of families (Kaakinen, 2018a). As discussed earlier, families are interdependent in their roles, thus illness within a family may be viewed as a family event in which illness in one member impacts all others to some extent. Families influence health maintenance and help-seeking behaviours and can play a significant role in all aspects of health and illness management.

HEALTH MAINTENANCE AND HOME TREATMENTS

Many cultural behaviours and rituals can have a direct or indirect effect on health maintenance. Members of the Seventh-Day Adventist Church, for example, view their bodies as the temple of God and will avoid using substances that are harmful to it, such as alcohol, tobacco, caffeine, and drugs. This behaviour, even though practised for religious rather than health reasons, will still have a direct (positive) effect on health maintenance (Giger & Haddad, 2021).

When patients experience symptoms, they interpret them within the context of their cultural outlook and explanatory models. Patients may believe that their symptoms are due to germs, a curse or magic, or a yin/yang (passive/active) imbalance. They could also view symptoms as being allowed by God as punishment for sin. The explanations that patients accept will determine the action they take to maintain health or seek treatments. Patients usually share their interpretation of symptoms with their families. The family, as a source of support and security, will then influence the decisions regarding health maintenance or looking for help. Some patients may be encouraged to seek home remedies, instead of, or in addition to, being steered toward health care providers.

Patients and their families may seek help from traditional healers or use home remedies because these therapies are viewed as more effective or more acceptable in certain circumstances. Knowing what the patient is using for treatment, and why, is important for health care providers because although many treatments (e.g., cupping and coin rubbing) are not harmful to the patient, others (e.g., some herbal remedies) may have a direct physiological effect or may interact with prescribed treatments (see Chapter 8 for discussion of healing traditions and complementary and alternative therapy).

Cultural Competence in Action

Sensitivity to Stigma Helps Reframe Problem

A 22-year-old Lebanese woman presented to the family physician with a several-week history of vise-like headaches, insomnia, weight loss, and weakness. Physical assessment and diagnostic testing revealed no physiological reason for the symptoms.

The patient and her husband became visibly upset when the physician suggested a psychological cause for the symptoms. The couple, upon the recommendation of the husband's mother, sought the second opinion of a Lebanese family doctor. The Lebanese physician, being more culturally sensitive to the stigma associated with psychiatric symptoms within the Lebanese culture, was able to work with the couple to identify sources of stress on the wife.

Apparently, the couple had been married less than a year and the wife had left her family in Lebanon and moved to Canada only recently. The husband worked all day while she stayed at home. Even though she spoke English, she had not yet made any friends within the community. The psychological label of depression was reframed as loneliness and acculturation stress. The couple agreed to continue to follow up with the physician until the symptoms were resolved.

ILLNESS MANAGEMENT

Family rules and roles influence the illness behaviour of family members, such as whether individuals take an active or passive role in their illness experiences and deciding whether they are exempt from the obligations of their roles within the family. Research shows that families can play a significant role in illness management and can both facilitate and impede recovery (Aldersey & Whitley, 2015). Family support can be moral support, concrete tangible support, or both (Aldersey & Whitley, 2015; Whitehead et al., 2018). Moral support may take the form of ensuring the patient does not feel isolated or alone; serving as advocates, consultants, and supporters in navigating the illness and health system; providing advice and validation for action; and maintaining normalcy by focusing on non–illness-related matters and activities (Aldersey & Whitley, 2015; Whitehead et al., 2018). Practical support may take the form of financial aid, providing transportation to and from health appointments, providing reminders for health actions, and caregiving of other family members (including pets) while the individual is unable to care for them in the same way (Aldersey & Whitley, 2015). Thus family roles are adjusted and realigned based on circumstances, to ensure family obligations and harmony are maintained. Readjustments and realignments may be needed as circumstances change, and while some families may be able to evolve with changing circumstances, others may find such tasks more challenging.

Although families can have a significant positive role in illness management, they can also be a source of stress in some circumstances. For some illnesses (e.g., mental illness), families may react out of fear based on stigma and prejudice rather than informed understanding, thereby becoming an additional barrier to recovery (Aldersey & Whitley, 2015). In chronic illness management, families often struggle with the balance between encouraging autonomy and self-management and "caring for" others out of a sense of duty or desire (Aldersey & Whitley, 2015; Whitehead et al., 2018). In families with collectivist worldviews and strong kinship ties, family members are more likely to assume the caregiver role of the sick or older person. Caregivers provide valuable work at a personal, physical, and emotional cost (Ng et al., 2016). The care is usually motivated by a personal sense of fulfillment and value because of a deep sense of love, loyalty, or faith; a sense of obligation or filial responsibility; or social pressure; or it is motivated by practical need when there is no one else available or willing to take on the caregiver role. Caregiver burdens include an interpersonal relationship cost with either the patient or other family members, pent-up emotions that are compounded by cultural values of discretion, and the difficulties of balancing other roles and activities around the caregiving responsibilities (Ng et al., 2016).

Significant caregiver burden has also been noted in families caring for family members with mental illness. Happell et al. (2017) note that the Mental Health Council of Australia and the Carers Association of Australia estimated that, in 2000, an individual caring for someone with a mental illness in Australia spent an average of 104 hours per week providing care. In addition, carers have been noted to have "significantly higher levels of depression and stress, and lower levels of subjective wellbeing, self-efficacy and physical health than those without carer responsibilities" (Happell et al., 2017, p. 128). Health care providers can provide support and encourage reflection and dialogue to negotiate a balance that contributes positively to the health and well-being of all family members. It is also important for health care providers to assess the caregiving burden and assist families in supporting the patient and in maintaining their own health and wellness.

IMPLICATIONS FOR HEALTH CARE PROVIDERS

Use of health care services is influenced by availability of, as well as trust and confidence in, the services. Factors that impact access to health care by immigrant and visible minority populations include the following (Debs-Ivall, 2016):

- Linguistic barriers

- Sociocultural barriers, especially in relation to how health is viewed as more than physical and rather as an interaction between the social, mental, and environmental dimensions
- Geographic barriers
- Socioeconomic barriers
- Lack of provider cultural competence
- Experiences of disrespect, discrimination, and racism
- A complex health care system with gatekeeping practices that complicate access

In 2016, immigrants to Canada comprised 21.9% of the population (Statistics Canada, 2019c) and are projected to represent close to 30% of the population by 2036 (Morency et al., 2017). As the diversity of the Canadian population increases there is a need for health care providers, in developing partnerships with families, to recognize that family members usually provide caring on an ongoing basis while the health care providers are regarded as invited, and sometimes uninvited, guests into their lives. Therefore, health care providers need to find ways to become part of the family system and provide care that fits with the cultural values and beliefs of their patients. However, this needs to be done in partnership with the patient and not based on assumptions that families are willing and able to take on caregiving roles. Health care providers also need to consider the burden that the caregivers are carrying and propose options and interventions to support them.

Some Western approaches to care might not fit with the cultural understanding of health and illness and could have a negative impact on the patient and on the relationship with the family. As such, health care providers need to engage the family in the care planning and decision making to ensure cultural relevance and safety of treatments and interventions. Research evidence shows that when family members are informed and supported, they are better able to support their family member (Aldersey & Whitley, 2015). Health care providers also need to consider a more expanded definition of health, beyond physical well-being, to include the emotional, social, and spiritual dimensions (Debs-Ivall, 2016). This will inform the family assessment, care planning, decision making, and evaluation of interventions. Access to health care remains an issue for diverse families. In addition to addressing the barriers noted earlier, health care providers need to advocate for change within the health care system for policies and processes that would facilitate access and address the discrimination and cultural incompetence that families experience.

Cultural Considerations in Care

A Simple Solution to Patient Passivity

Patient autonomy and independence are highly valued within the Western health care system. Often, patient education focuses on self-care practices to help patients gain back their pre-hospitalization independent status. However, in many non-Western cultures, the patient is expected to assume a passive "sick role" while the family members provide the care.

An enterostomal nurse specialist felt frustrated when she encountered such passive behaviour in Mr. Luciano, whom she was trying to teach how to care for his new colostomy stoma. The patient kept insisting his wife needed to learn, not him.

As the health care provider gained some understanding of the illness behaviour of the patient, she was able to negotiate an acceptable solution. When she reframed colostomy care as a normal part of everyday personal care, such as shaving and going to the washroom, the patient consented to learn the skill. As long as the patient viewed the colostomy care as part of his illness, he insisted that his family would take care of it. By reframing colostomy care as part of daily routines, he was able to take ownership for the colostomy routine.

PROVIDER ATTITUDES TOWARD FAMILIES

It is critical that health care providers reflect on their views and assumptions about family roles and family engagement in illness. While it is important to recognize cultural influences on potential family engagement, this must always be assessed and discussed, not imposed.

Ahmann and Lawrence (1999) challenge us to consider how we communicate not only with, but also about, families—even to other health care providers. Commonly used negative adjectives about families (e.g., "difficult," "demanding," "resistant," "indifferent," "nonreceptive") can be detrimental to the family–health care provider relationship, and to the family itself. Ahmann and Lawrence (1999) advocate that the negative words, which may in turn generate negative emotions within the health care provider, be replaced with words and beliefs that value and respect families. It is important for health care providers to recognize and name the family's strengths. A policy to consider is to use the same terminology in the family's absence as one would in the family's presence. See Table 7.2 for examples of this more positive approach.

Family Assessment and Approach to Care

Gathering information about the family should be done as part of the overall assessment of the patient. However, the type of family assessment will vary with the setting and role of the health care providers. It is important for health care providers to reflect on whether their role, focus, and opportunity is to care for the patient with family in the background as context or support or to provide care to the family as patient. Even when family is seen as supporting patient recovery, addressing the needs of the family caregivers is important for optimal engagement and support.

There are a variety of cultural assessment models that can be used for family assessment, each highlighting a different aspect of family diversity. The preferred tool will be based on the health care provider's discipline, area of practice, and preference. We provide below a brief description of one model from nursing as an example. To do a thorough family assessment appropriate to their clinical context, health care providers will likely use a combination of tools, in conjunction with a holistic assessment of the patient. An intentional focus on family that creates time and space for therapeutic interaction(s) is the foundation for an effective assessment and approach to care.

THE CALGARY FAMILY ASSESSMENT MODEL

The Calgary Family Assessment Model (CFAM) has received wide recognition since it was first introduced by Lorraine Wright and Maureen Leahey in 1984. It consists of three major categories of family assessments: structural, developmental, and functional. Each domain has additional sub-categories for added depth (Shajani & Snell, 2019) (Fig. 7.3). The model was

TABLE 7.2 ■ **Better Language to Describe Families**

Instead of This (Negative Language)	Use This (Positive Language)
Demanding	Strong advocate
Controlling	Actively involved, aware of own needs
Angry	Concerned, worried
Passive, indifferent, non-participatory	May need more time
Non-compliant	Has different priorities

From Ahmann, E., & J. Lawrence, J. (1999). Exploring language about families. *Pediatric Nursing, 25*(2), 221–224. Reprinted with permission.

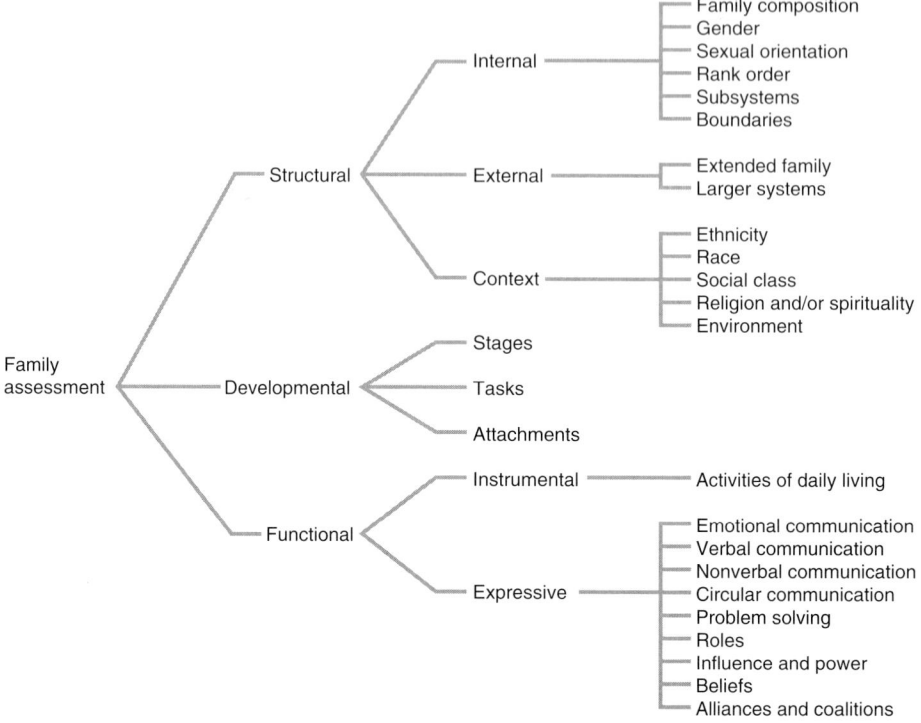

Fig. 7.3 Branching Diagram of the Calgary Family Assessment Model. (From Shajani, Z., & Snell, D. (2019). *Wright & Leahey's nurses and families: A guide to family assessment and intervention*. F. A. Davis Company, with permission.)

developed from clinical practice and has continued to be used widely within Canada and internationally (Leahey & Wright, 2016). The authors have developed assessment questions and interventions to accompany the model (see Shajani & Snell, 2019). It is important to note that not all aspects of the assessment need to be done at the same time, or at all. Health care providers need to establish which categories are relevant and appropriate to each family at any given time.

RELATIONAL APPROACH TO CARE

As discussed throughout the chapter, families and their approach to health and illness are embedded in larger sociocultural structures and processes. A **relational practice** approach recognizes the contextual relationships and complexities and "is oriented toward enhancing the capacity and power of people/families to live a life that is meaningful from their own perspective" (Kaakinen, 2018b). The approach consists of two components: a relational consciousness and inquiry as a form of action (Younas, 2020). Intentional focus on diverse factors that affect a situation allows the health care provider to identify and work with these intrapersonal, interpersonal, and sociocultural factors influencing the health–illness experience. The relational inquiry approach is guided by purpose, and practice develops in partnership with the patient and family. How the story evolves is influenced by how the family experiences the health care system and how the health care providers understand and respond to the family.

A culturally sensitive and relational approach to care recognizes that the health care provider's beliefs and approach will also influence the experience. It is therefore important for health care providers to understand their own views and assumptions about family roles and obligations as well as about family-centred care. It is also important not to judge, compare, or assume the best action for a family; rather, health care providers need to take their cue from families. Health care providers need to understand both the medical story and the illness story. "The medical story is about the patient who has the disease or health problem and includes signs and symptoms, medications, treatment regimen, and prognosis or trajectory of illness. The family illness story is how the family and each member live through the experience of the illness or health event" (Kaakinen, 2018b, p. 115).

Eliciting and understanding the family illness story can take many forms. It may begin with observation of family members' interactions with various parts of the health care system and each other, and progress to focused assessment and questions. Table 7.3 provides questions that can be used to elicit the family story. This is a beginning guide to initiate dialogue in the absence of a formal, structured tool.

Family desire and ability to collaboratively engage with health care providers is influenced by critical factors such as health literacy and the degree of trust (or mistrust) with health care providers based on past experiences. **Health literacy** refers to the ability to access, understand, appraise, and apply health information to make decisions about health and health care. This includes the ability to understand health care terminology, follow directions and instructions, and appreciate the consequences when such directions are not followed (Kaakinen, 2018b). It is important for health care providers to remember that sometimes a lack of follow-through on instructions is related not to understanding but rather to the ability to do so based on other factors. As well, families may have their own illness beliefs and preferred treatment, and it is important that such views be uncovered and discussed as part of the plan of care.

TABLE 7.3 ■ **Eliciting the Family Story**

I. Structure
  a. Who is in the immediate family?
  b. Are extended family members available or involved in family support?
  c. How is the family connected to the broader community?

II. Roles
  a. How are the various family members impacted by the illness?
  b. What are different family members most concerned or worried about?
  c. What strengths or supports can different family members provide?
  d. Who else should be involved in the patient's care (e.g., traditional Elder or healer, another family member)?

III. Engagement
  a. What is the desired level of family involvement?
  b. What factors facilitate or impede engagement (e.g., language, health, transportation, work, finances)?
  c. Who should the health care provider(s) communicate with on a regular basis?
  d. Who is involved in decision making?
  e. Past experience with illness managed in the home or within a health care setting?

IV. Beliefs
  a. What do you think has caused the problem?
  b. What do you fear most about the illness and treatment?
  c. What other actions could be taken to support your family member's care?
  d. Are there cultural, religious, or spiritual practices that are important in this situation?
  e. What are the most important results you hope are achieved?

In recent years the discourse and evidence of systemic racism within society and the health care system have shown that many people do not feel safe or receive safe, quality care. In particular, people who identify as Black, Indigenous, or People of Colour (BIPOC) are at increased risk for adverse outcomes (Roeder, 2019; Turpel-Lafond, 2020). The risk is not inherent in the racial or ethnic identity; rather it is embedded in factors such as unconscious bias and systemic racism. Although health care providers may recognize this reality, it is a difficult area to acknowledge and assess through direct inquiry until a therapeutic relationship and trust have been established. However, patient and family mistrust in the system may also be evident in emotions and behaviour such as detached silence, frustration, or anger. It is imperative that health care providers refrain from judgement and assumptions and instead intentionally engage with patients and family members to understand the reasons behind the silence, anger, or frustration.

Finally, it will be helpful to develop a family plan of care, with the family, that outlines the key elements of family goals, strengths, communication, and decision making, along with supports needed and desired (e.g., information, social supports, referrals, etc.). A critical role for health care providers is to help families see and discover their strengths as well as potential areas of conflict within the family. Families interact with the health care system in times of illness and injury when they are already experiencing greater stress and vulnerability. Curiosity, support, encouragement, and guidance are important ways in which health care providers can engage with patients in a partnership that optimizes health care experiences and outcomes.

Summary

Families play a pivotal role in maintaining health and seeking health care. Families are often regarded as the most basic unit in society. However, family demographics in society are changing. Families are diverse, consist of individuals who may or may not be legally related, and are dynamic in that both the composition and roles may change over time and context. Family-centred care is defined by core concepts of dignity and respect, information sharing, collaboration, and partnerships. This chapter discusses how culture influences our understanding of and ability to effectively convey respect to, collaborate with, and engage in mutual information sharing and goal setting with families as they encounter and navigate the health care system.

When caring for diverse families, areas that require particular consideration include characteristics such as race, ethnicity, and religion, but also worldviews, migration and acculturation, generational differences, socioeconomic status, and family structure. Recognizing, acknowledging, and addressing the impact of colonization and intergenerational trauma on Indigenous families is an imperative for health care providers. Individuals and families are more than their chief complaint and risk factors, and it is critical that health care providers understand both the medical and the family illness story, along with the social processes that contribute to ongoing health inequities. When working with patients from culturally diverse backgrounds, health care providers must recognize the role families play in all aspects of health and illness management. Health care providers also have opportunities to support families by acknowledging the impact of social factors, recognizing strengths, and mutually determining goals and supports needed for the patient and for family members to support the patient and maintain their own wellness.

Effective family assessment begins with the health care provider's ability to critically reflect on their own views and assumptions about families. It also requires a relational inquiry approach that recognizes the complexities of the family's experience in society as well the strength, expertise, and challenges that may exist within the family. A complete family story includes information about structure and roles as well as experiences, desired engagement, beliefs, and hope for the future.

 http://evolve.elsevier.com/Srivastava/culturalcompetence/.

Questions for Review and Discussion

1. Discuss how decision making differs between collectivistic and individualistic cultures.
2. Discuss how children in immigrant families might contribute to the settlement efforts of their families.
3. Define health literacy and discuss how it might have an impact on the health of individuals and families.

Group Activity

1. In a small group discuss the similarities and differences that you have observed or experienced between generations. How many generations live in your home? What are the factors that influence the similarities and differences across generations? Is importance placed on individual expression or family unity? Are children expected to grow away from or grow within the family? How do language, technology, migration, and economic situation impact generational differences?

References

Ahmann, E., & Lawrence, J. (1999). Exploring language about families. *Pediatric Nursing*, *25*(2), 221–224.

Albertini, M., Mantovani, D., & Gasperoni, G. (2019). Intergenerational relations among immigrants in Europe: The role of ethnic difference, migration and acculturation. *Journal of Ethnic and Migration Studies*, *45*(10), 1693–1706. https://doi.org/10.1080/1369183X.2018.1485202.

Alden, D. L., Friend, J., Lee, P. Y., et al. (2018). Who decides: Me or we? Family involvement in medical decision making in Eastern and Western countries. *Medical Decision Making: An International Journal of the Society for Medical Decision Making*, *38*(1), 14–25. https://doi.org/10.1177/0272989X17715628.

Aldersey, H. M., & Whitley, R. (2015). Family influence in recovery from severe mental illness. *Community Mental Health Journal*, *51*(4), 467–476. https://doi.org/10.1007/s10597-014-9783-y.

Al-Motlaq, M. A., & Shields, L. (2017). Family-centered care as a Western-centric model in developing countries: Luxury versus necessity. *Holistic Nursing Practice*, *31*(5), 343–347. https://doi.org/10.1097/HNP.0000000000000228.

American Psychological Association (APA). (2020). *Intergenerational trauma*. https://dictionary.apa.org/intergenerational-trauma

Australian Bureau of Statistics. (2016). *Family*. https://www.abs.gov.au/ausstats/abs@.nsf/Lookup/2901.0Chapter32102016

Banwait, K. (2019, January 23). An apology to our daughters-in-law: Patriarchal family dynamics in South Asian households. *Brown Girl Magazine*. https://browngirlmagazine.com/2019/01/apology-to-our-daughters-in-law-patriarchal-family-dynamics/

Battams, N. (2018). *A snapshot of family diversity in Canada*. The Vanier Institute of the Family. https://vanier-institute.ca/a-snapshot-of-family-diversity-in-canada-february-2018/

Bauer, E. (2016). Practicing kinship care: Children as language brokers in migrant families. *Childhood (Copenhagen, Denmark)*, *23*(1), 22–36. https://doi.org/10.1177/0907568215574917.

Beaujot, R., Liu, J., & Ravanera, Z. (2017). Gender inequality in the family setting. *Canadian Studies in Population*, *44*(1–2), 1–13.

Bennett, B., & Woodman, E. (2019). The potential of equine-assisted psychotherapy for treating trauma in Australian Indigenous people. *The British Journal of Social Work*, *49*(4), 1041–1058. https://doi.org/10.1093/bjsw/bcz053.

Bergnehr, D. (2018). Children's influence on wellbeing and acculturative stress in refugee families. *International Journal of Qualitative Studies on Health and Wellbeing*, *13*, 1–9. https://doi.org/10.1080/17482631.2018.1564517.

Berry, J. W., & Hou, F. (2016). Immigrant acculturation and wellbeing in Canada. *Canadian Psychology/Psychologie Canadienne*, *57*(4), 254–264. https://doi.org/10.1037/cap0000064.

Betancourt, T. S., Abdi, S., & Ito, B. S., et al. (2015). We left one war and came to another: Resource loss, acculturative stress, and caregiver-child relationships in Somali refugee families. *Cultural Diversity & Ethnic Minority Psychology*, *21*(1), 114–125. https://doi.org/10.1037/a0037538.

Boulton, J. (2018). History branded on the mind: Trans-generational trauma in Indigenous Australia. *Health and History*, *20*(2), 100–105. https://doi.org/10.5401/healthhist.20.2.0100.

Bryant-Davis, T., Adams, T., Alejandre, A., et al. (2017). The trauma lens of police violence against racial and ethnic minorities. *Journal of Social Issues*, *73*(4), 852–871. https://doi.org/10.1111/josi.12251.

Canadian Women's Foundation. (2019). *The facts about the gender pay gap in Canada*. https://canadianwomen.org/the-facts/the-gender-pay-gap/

Chan, S., & Lee, E. (2004). Families with Asian roots. In E. W. Lynch & M. J. Hanson (Eds.), *Developing cross cultural competence: A guide for working with children and their families* (3rd ed.). Paul Brookes Publishing Co.

Coehlo, D. P., Henderson, T. L., & Lester, C. (2018). The intersection of family policies, health disparities, and health care policies. In J. R. Kaakinen & D. P. Coehlo (Eds.), *Family health care nursing, 6e: Theory, practice, and research* (pp. 83–112). F. A. Davis Company.

Collins, C., Landivar, L. C., Ruppanner, L., et al. (2021). COVID-19 and the gender gap in work hours. *Gender, Work, and Organization*, *28*(SI), 101–112. https://doi.org/10.1111/gwao.12506.

Da, W., & Welch, A. (2016). *Educative and child-rearing practices among recent Chinese migrants in Australia: Continuity, change, hybridity*. Education in the Asia-Pacific Region: Issues, Concerns and Prospects book series (EDAP, Vol. 31). https://link.springer.com/chapter/10.1007/978-981-10-0330-1_17

Das, S. S. (2018). 'This is our culture!' or is it? Second generation Asian Indian individuals' perceptions of parents' socialization messages. *Journal of Family Studies*, *24*(2), 146–169. https://doi.org/10.1080/13229400.2016.1141110.

Debs-Ivall, S. (2016). *The lived experiences of immigrant Canadian women with the healthcare system*. Walden University. Unpublished doctoral dissertation.

Delgado, V. (2020). "They think I'm a lawyer": Undocumented college students as legal brokers for their undocumented parents. *Law and Policy*, *42*(3), 261–283. https://doi.org/10.1111/lapo.12152.

Erdem, G., & Safi, O. A. (2018). The cultural lens approach to Bowen family systems theory: Contributions of family change theory. *Journal of Family Theory & Review*, *10*(2), 469–483. https://doi.org/10.1111/jftr.12258.

Fuller-Thomson, E. (2005). *Grandparents raising grandchildren in Canada: A profile of skipped generation families*. https://socialsciences.mcmaster.ca/sedap/p/sedap132.pdf

Garcia-Sanchez. I. M. (2018). Children as interactional brokers of care. *Annual Review of Anthropology*, *47*, 167–184. https://doi.org/10.1146/annurev-anthro-102317-050050.

Giger, J. N., & Haddad, L. G. (2021). *Transcultural nursing: Assessment and intervention* (8th ed.). Elsevier.

Government of Canada. (2021a). *Reducing the number of Indigenous children in care*. https://www.sac-isc.gc.ca/eng/1541187352297/1541187392851

Government of Canada. (2021b). *Restorative justice*. https://www.justice.gc.ca/eng/cj-jp/rj-jr/index.html

Grammond, S., & Guay, C. (2016). Issues in research on Indigenous children and families. *Enfances Familles Générations*. https://journals.openedition.org/efg/1227

Guo, M., Xu, L., Liu, J., et al. (2015). Parent-child relationship among older Chinese immigrants: The influence of co-residence, frequent contact, intergenerational support and sense of children's deference. *Ageing and Society*, *36*(7), 1459–1482. https://doi.org/10.1017/S0144686X15000446.

Hackett, C., Feeny, D., & Tompa, E. (2016). Canada's residential school system: Measuring the intergenerational impact of familial attendance on health and mental health outcomes. *Journal of Epidemiology and Community Health*, *70*(11), 1096–1105. https://doi.org/10.1136/jech-2016-207380.

Hanna, A. M. V., & Ortega, D. M. (2016). Salir adelante (perseverance): Lessons from the Mexican immigrant experience. *Journal of Social Work*, *16*(1), 47–65. https://doi.org/10.1177/1468017314560301.

Happell, B., Wilson, K., Platania-Phung, C., et al. (2017). Physical health and mental illness: Listening to the voice of carers. *Journal of Mental Health*, *26*(2), 127–133. https://doi.org/10.3109/09638237.2016.1167854.

Hofstede, G. (2011). Dimensionalizing cultures: The Hofstede model in context. *Online Readings in Psychology and Culture, Unit 2*. http://scholarworks.gvsu.edu/orpc/vol2/iss1/8

Houle, R. (2019). *Results from the 2016 census: Earnings of immigrants and children of immigrants in official language minority populations. Insights on Canadian Society*. Statistics Canada. https://www150.statcan.gc.ca/n1/pub/75-006-x/2019001/article/00007-eng.htm

Hsieh, J. Y., Mercer, K. J., & Costa, S. A. (2017). Parenting a second time around: The strengths and challenges of Indigenous grandparent caregivers. *GrandFamilies: The Contemporary Journal of Research, Practice and Policy*, *4*(1), 76–123. https://scholarworks.wmich.edu/grandfamilies/vol4/iss1/8

Hudson, C. C., Adams, S., & Lauderdale, J. (2016). Cultural expressions of intergenerational trauma and mental health nursing implications for U.S. health care delivery following refugee resettlement: An integrative review of the literature. *Journal of Transcultural Nursing*, *27*(3), 286–301. https://doi.org/10.1177/1043659615587591.

Isobel, S., McCloughen, A., Goodyear, M., et al. (2021). Intergenerational trauma and its relationship to mental health care: A qualitative inquiry. *Community Mental Health Journal*, *57*(4), 631–643. https://doi.org/10.1007/s10597-020-00698-1.

Joyce, L., & Liamputtong, P. (2017). Acculturation stress and social support for young refugees in regional areas. *Children and Youth Services Review* (vol. 77[C], pp. 18–26). Elsevier.

Kaakinen, J. (2018a). Family health care nursing: An introduction. In J. R. Kaakinen, D. P. Coehlo, R. Steele, et al. (Eds.), *Family health care nursing: Theory, practice, & research* (6th ed., pp. 3–26). F.A. Davis.

Kaakinen, J. (2018b). Family nursing assessment and intervention. In J. R. Kaakinen, D. P. Coehlo, R. Steele, et al. (Eds.), *Family health care nursing: Theory, practice, & research* (6th ed., pp. 113–146). F.A. Davis.

Kim, S. C., Park, Y. S., Ho, B., et al. (2017). Family conflict, Asian cultural values, perceived parental control, and affectionate care among Asian American college students. *Journal of Asia Pacific Counseling*, *7*(2), 123–140. https://doi.org/10.18401/2017.7.2.2.

King, G., Desmarais, C., Lindsay, S., et al. (2015). The roles of effective communication and client engagement in delivering culturally sensitive care to immigrant parents of children with disabilities. *Disability and Rehabilitation*, *37*(15), 1372–1381. https://doi.org/10.3109/09638288.2014.972580.

Leahey, M., & Wright, L. M. (2016). Application of the Calgary Family Assessment and Intervention Models: Reflections on the reciprocity between the personal and the professional. *Journal of Family Nursing*, *22*(4), 450–459. https://doi.org/10.1177/1074840716667972.

Mao, W., Xu, L., Guo, M., et al. (2018). Intergenerational support and functional limitations among older Chinese immigrants: Does acculturation moderate their relationship? *Journal of Ethics and Cultural Diversity in Social Work*, *27*(4), 294–309. https://doi.org/10.1080/15313204.2018.1520170.

McFarland, M. R., & Wehbe-Alamah, H. B. (2015). *Leininger's cultural care diversity and universality: A worldwide nursing theory*. Jones & Bartlett Learning.

Menzies, C. R. (n.d.). *Canada First Nations families*. https://family.jrank.org/pages/199/Canada-First-Nations-Families.html

Mirabelli, A. (2018). *What's in a name? Defining family in a diverse society*. https://vanierinstitute.ca/whats-in-a-name-defining-family-in-a-diverse-society/

Morency, J.D., Malenfant, E. C., & MacIsaac, S. (2017). *Immigration and diversity: Population projections for Canada and its regions, 2011 to 2036* (Catalogue no. 91-551-X). Statistics Canada. https://www150.statcan.gc.ca/n1/en/pub/91-551-x/91-551-x2017001-eng.pdf?st=_MqbqQJl

Mostoway, K. (2020). The effects of immigration on families. *Canadian Journal of Family and Youth*, *12*(2), 60–68. http://ejournals.library.ualberta.ca/index/php/cjfy

Ng, H. Y., Griva, K., Lim, H. A., et al. (2016). The burden of filial piety: A qualitative study on caregiving motivations among family caregivers of patients with cancer in Singapore. *Psychology and Health*, *31*(11), 1293–1310. https://doi:10.1080/08870446.2016.1204450.

Nieuwenhuis, R., & Maldonado, L. (2018). *The triple bind of single-parent families: Resources, employment, and policies to improve wellbeing*. Policy Press.

Office for National Statistics. (2021). *Families and households statistics explained*. https://www.ons.gov.uk/peoplepopulationandcommunity/birthsdeathsandmarriages/families/articles/familiesandhouseholdsstatisticsexplained/2021-03-02

O'Neill, L., Fraser, T., Kitchenham, A., et al. (2016). Hidden burdens: A review of intergenerational, historical and complex trauma, implications for Indigenous families. *Journal of Child and Adolescent Trauma*, *11*(2), 173–186. https://doi.org/10.1007/s40653-016-0117-9.

Park, M., Giap, T. T., & Lee, M., et al. Patient- and family-centered care interventions for improving the quality of health care: A review of systematic reviews. *International Journal of Nursing Studies*, *87*, 69–93. https://doi.org/10.1016/j.ijnurstu.2018.07.006.

Phan, M. B., Banerjee, R., Deacon, L.et al. (2015). Family dynamics and the integration of professional immigrants in Canada. *Journal of Ethnic and Migration Studies*, *41*(13), 2061–2080. https://doi.org/10.1080/1369183X.2015.1045461.

Qian, Y., & Fuller, S. (2020). COVID-19 and the gender employment gap among parents of young children. *Canadian Public Policy*, *46*(S2), S89–S101.

Roeder, A. (2019). *America is failing its Black mothers.* Harvard Public Health. https://www.hsph.harvard.edu/magazine/magazine_article/america-is-failing-its-black-mothers/

Rothbaum, F., Morelli, G., Pott, M., et al. (2000). Immigrant-Chinese and Euro-American parents' physical closeness with young children: Themes of family relatedness. *Journal of Family Psychology, 14*(3), 334–348.

Shajani, Z., & Snell, D. (2019). *Wright & Leahey's nurses and families: A guide to family assessment and intervention.* F. A. Davis.

Smetana, J. G. (2017). Current research on parenting styles, dimensions, and beliefs. *Current Opinion in Psychology, 15*, 19–25. https://doi.org/10.1016/j.copsyc.2017.02.012.

Somos, C. (2021). Foster care replaced residential schools for Indigenous children, advocates say. *CTV News,* June 7. https://www.ctvnews.ca/canada/foster-care-replaced-residential-schools-for-indigenous-children-advocates-say-1.5459374

Stanhope, M., & Lancaster, J. (2018). *Foundations for population health in community/public health nursing* (5th ed.). Elsevier.

Statistics Canada. (2017a). *Children with an immigrant background: Bridging cultures. Census in Brief.* https://www12.statcan.gc.ca/census-recensement/2016/as-sa/98-200-x/2016015/98-200-x2016015-eng.cfm

Statistics Canada. (2017b). *Diverse family characteristics of Indigenous children aged 0 to 4.* https://www12.statcan.gc.ca/census-recensement/2016/as-sa/98-200-x/2016020/98-200-x2016020-eng.pdf

Statistics Canada. (2017c). *Families, households and marital status: Key results from the 2016 census: The Daily.* https://www150.statcan.gc.ca/n1/en/daily-quotidien/170802/dq170802a-eng.pdf?st=gWycKAjH

Statistics Canada. (2017d). *Infographic: Portrait of households and families in Canada.* https://www150.statcan.gc.ca/n1/pub/11-627-m/11-627-m2017024-eng.htm

Statistics Canada. (2017e). *Linguistic integration of immigrants and official language populations in Canada.* https://www150.statcan.gc.ca/n1/en/catalogue/98-200-X2016017

Statistics Canada. (2017f). *Same sex couples in Canada in 2016.* https://www12.statcan.gc.ca/census-recensement/2016/as-sa/98-200-x/2016007/98-200-x2016007-eng.pdf

Statistics Canada. (2019a). *Family matters: Adults living with their parents.* https://www150.statcan.gc.ca/n1/daily-quotidien/190215/dq190215a-eng.htm

Statistics Canada. (2019b). *Family matters: Grandparents in Canada.* https://www150.statcan.gc.ca/n1/en/daily-quotidien/190207/dq190207a-eng.pdf?st=LNzAsWq1

Statistics Canada. (2019c). *Immigration and ethnocultural diversity highlight tables, 2016 census.* https://www12.statcan.gc.ca/census-recensement/2016/dp-pd/hlt-fst/imm/index-eng.cfm

Statistics Canada. (2021). *Census family.* https://www23.statcan.gc.ca/imdb/p3Var.pl?Function=Unit&Id=32746

Stewart, M., Dennis, C. L., Kariwo, M., et al. (2015). Challenges faced by refugee new parents from Africa in Canada. *Journal of Immigrant and Minority Health / Center for Minority Public Health, 17*(4), 1146–1156. https://doi.org/10.1007/s10903-014-0062-3.

Tam, B. Y., Findlay, L. C., & Kohen, D. E. (2017). Indigenous families: Who do you call family? *Journal of Family Studies, 23*(3), 243–259. https://doi.org/10.1080/13229400.2015.1093536.

Triandis, H. (1995). *Individualism and collectivism.* Westview Press.

Triandis, H. (2018). *Individualism and collectivism: New directions in social psychology.* Routledge.

Truth and Reconciliation Commission of Canada (TRC). (2015). *Truth & reconciliation: Calls to action.* https://www2.gov.bc.ca/assets/gov/british-columbians-our-governments/indigenous-people/Indigenous-people-documents/calls_to_action_english2.pdf

Turcotte, M. (2019). *Results from the 2016 census: Education and labour market successes and challenges for children of immigrant parents. Insights on Canadian society.* Statistics Canada. https://www150.statcan.gc.ca/n1/pub/75-006-x/2019001/article/00016-eng.htm

Turpel-Lafond, M. E. (2020). *In plain sight: Addressing Indigenous-specific racism and discrimination in B.C. health care.* Government of British Columbia. https://engage.gov.bc.ca/app/uploads/sites/613/2020/11/In-Plain-Sight-Full-Report.pdf

Turner, A. (2016). *Insights on Canadian society: Living arrangements of Indigenous children aged 14 and under.* Statistics Canada. https://www150.statcan.gc.ca/n1/en/pub/75-006-x/2016001/article/14547-eng.pdf?st=5lizovj1

US Department of Health and Human Services. (2017). *Definition of family.* https://www.hrsa.gov/get-health-care/affordable/hill-burton/family.html

Valenzuela, A. (1999). Gender roles and settlement activities among children and their immigrant families. *American Behavioral Scientist*, *41*(4), 720–742.

Vanier Institute of the Family. (2021). *Definition of family*. https://vanierinstitute.ca/definition-of-family/

Watson, M. F., Turner, W. L., & Moore Hines, P. (2020). Black lives matter: We are in the same storm but we are not in the same boat. *Family Process*, *59*(4), 1362–1373. https://doi.org/10.1111/famp.12613.

Whitehead, L., Jacob, E., Towell, A., et al. (2018). The role of the family in supporting the self-management of chronic conditions: A qualitative systematic review. *Journal of Clinical Nursing*, *27*(1–2), 22–30. https://doi.org/10.1111/jocn.13775.

Wilk, P., Maltby, A., & Cooke, M. (2017). Residential schools and the effects on Indigenous health and well-being in Canada—A scoping review. *Public Health Reviews*, *38*(8). https://doi.org/10.1186/s40985-017-0055-6.

Wilson, K. (2018). *Pulling together: A guide for Indigenization of post-secondary institutions. A professional learning series*. BC campus. https://opentextbc.ca/indigenizationfoundations/

Wright, L. M., & Leahey, M. (2009). *Nurses and families: A guide to family assessment and intervention* (5th ed.). F. A. Davis.

Wright, L. M., Watson, W. L., & Bell, J. M. (1996). *Beliefs: The heart of healing in families and illness*. Basic Books.

Younas, A. (2020). Relational inquiry approach for developing deeper awareness of patient suffering. *Nursing Ethics*, *27*(4), 935–945. https://doi.org/10.1177/0969733020912523.

CHAPTER 8

Healing Systems and Traditions

Nikita Gupta, Linda Purushuttam, and Rani H. Srivastava

LEARNING OBJECTIVES

At the end of this chapter, the learner will be able to:
- Understand the experience of health and illness in the context of culture
- Explain the potential impact of religion on religious practices on health and well-being
- Develop a working familiarity with the major healing traditions of Ayurveda, Indigenous medicine, and traditional Chinese medicine
- Explore similarities and differences among the major healing traditions
- Differentiate between complementary, alternative, and integrative medicine
- Recognize the role and importance of complementary and alternative therapies in health and wellness

KEY TERMS

Acupuncture	Elder	Traditional Chinese medicine (TCM)
Allopathic medicine	Indigenous medicine	Traditional healing
Alternative medicine	Integrative care	Traditional medicine
Ayurveda	Intercessory prayer	Two-eyed seeing
Biomedicine	Naturopathic medicine	
Chiropractic medicine	Qi	
Complementary and alternative medicine (CAM)	Smudging	
Dosha	Sweat lodge	

Defined as the totality of beliefs, culture encompasses attitudes, behaviours, customs, and traditions. It is a "non-written link from the past to the present day, bridging the individuals in a society" (Değer, 2018, p. 40). As discussed in previous chapters, culture is multilayered and includes worldviews, traditions, history, politics, and power differentials, all of which have an impact on beliefs and behaviours. Culture influences individuals' perception and approach toward their health, illness, and treatment, as well as their ability to access and navigate the health care system. The Canadian health care system is primarily based on Western medicine and a biomedical approach to health. There are, however, other healing traditions that have been practised for centuries in many parts of the world. While historically colonization introduced biomedicine to many parts of the world, current globalization and immigration patterns are contributing to the spread of other healing traditions across the world.

The impact of colonization on the health inequities of Indigenous people across the globe is well documented. Loss of land, language, and culture, including access to Indigenous ways of maintaining and restoring health, are factors that are seen to perpetuate inequities (see Chapter 9).

The Truth and Reconciliation Commission (TRC) calls to action highlight the value of Indigenous healers and healing practices for the health and well-being of Indigenous communities (TRC, 2015). Recommendation 22 specifically "call(s) upon those who can effect change within the Canadian health-care system to recognize the value of Indigenous healing practices and use them in the treatment of Indigenous patients in collaboration with Indigenous healers and Elders were requested by Indigenous patients"[1] (TRC, 2015, p. 163). It is critical that health care providers recognize the impact of social determinants of health on Indigenous people and develop understanding of Indigenous health values, beliefs, and practices.

As societies become more global and diverse, there is increasing recognition of healing traditions from other parts of the world. Since biomedicine is the dominant system of care in North America, Europe, and Australia, it is the most familiar. Traditions that are different from biomedicine or allopathy may be viewed as alternative and, therefore, somehow seen by some as "less than" biomedicine (Cassidy, 2019). It is important for all health care providers to recognize that many of these healing traditions reflect centuries of knowledge and experience. These healing traditions are organized around inter-related concepts surrounding health and illness and are based on traditional ways of being, knowing, and approaches to care and cure. Such knowledge may be transmitted across generations in writing or through oral history.

Even when health care providers have respect for other traditions, lack of knowledge and familiarity may prevent them from understanding and engaging respectfully with patients and families who use these healing traditions for their health and well-being. This chapter presents a brief overview of select healing traditions from around the world. The aim is to familiarize health care providers with key concepts and frameworks so that they can engage in knowledgeable and respectful ways to provide culturally safe and responsive care. It is neither expected, nor possible, for health care providers to become experts in all of these traditions. Rather, our intent is to encourage health care providers to view and understand medicine through a different lens than the dominant, Western system of biomedicine. Indigenous tradition calls this **two-eyed seeing** and describes it as a "way of bridging two distinct and equally valuable ways of knowing, or worldviews" (Fijal & Beagan, 2019, p. 221). Neither the list of traditions nor the discussion should be considered exhaustive.

The chapter begins with a brief discussion on the potential impact of cultural diversity on health- and illness-related practices. Culture, religion, and health are inextricably linked. Thus it is important to consider the influence of religion on health maintenance, the meaning of illness, and healing. The discussion on healing traditions includes allopathic (biomedicine) medicine, Ayurveda, Indigenous medicine, and traditional Chinese medicine (TCM). These traditions have been chosen as they reflect the worldviews of cultures that are growing in numbers in Western countries, including Canada, the United States, Australia, and the United Kingdom (Migration Policy Institute, n.d.; The Migration Observatory, 2020). The chapter ends with a discussion of complementary therapies, including naturopathy, chiropractic medicine, and integrative care.

Religion, Health, and Healing

As current demographic trends indicate rapidly rising diversity among Canadians, there is a heightened need for understanding the importance of culture and its influences within health care. According to the 2016 census, Asia (including the Middle East) remains the primary location of emigration to Canada, with the majority of individuals who arrived in Canada between 2011 and 2016 being born in Asia (Statistics Canada, 2017b). A more diversified Canada also means increased religious diversity within the population. Population projections indicate that the number of people affiliated with non-Christian religions is expected to increase to 13–16% of

---

[1] We recognize that "Indigenous" is an older term; it is used here as it reflects the language of the TRC report.

the population as compared to 9% in 2011. People of South Asian origin, often reflecting Hindu, Sikh, and Muslim faiths, are over-represented among recent immigrants and these numbers are expected to grow (Statistics Canada, 2017a, 2017b).

Culture, religion, and spirituality are closely linked to health and well-being. Religious perspectives also influence the explanatory models of illness. For example, Hindus believe that illness and disease may be a direct result of one's *karma* or actions, while Muslims view it as a test and trial through which sins are removed (Attum et al., 2020). Both religions share a belief that recovery from illness lies directly in the hands of God, and patients may turn to traditional healing methods such as Ayurveda or to Muslim religious leaders called "Imams" to manage illness and disease.

Religious faiths across the globe often motivate and encourage people to be mindful of service to the human spirit or soul (Koenig, 2012). Upholding the idea that there is a higher power can also provide a framework for understanding oneself and the world and navigating life circumstances. Individuals with strong religious beliefs have been shown to demonstrate a stronger ability to embrace uncertainty and withstand adversities while keeping a positive attitude surrounding the matter. An adjusting and co-operative nature increases one's tolerance of uncertainty, enhanced coping, resourcefulness, and optimism (Koenig, 2012). Thus religion and the associated power of faith, ceremonies, and prayer can provide a deep sense of hope, purpose, discipline, and structure in one's life.

Prayer and spiritual healing have significance for many cultures. In the context of illness and disease, encouraging people to think positively and do their best, drawing on spirituality, religion, and faith, has consistently been shown to be an extremely positive coping mechanism (Hamilton et al., 2020; Koenig, 2012; Rao, 2015). Prayer may be used to support one's own health or the health of others. Praying on behalf of others is known as **intercessory prayer**. Prayer, intercessory prayer, and other activities undertaken with an "intention to heal" have been associated with positive outcomes on health and well-being (Hamilton et al., 2020; Roe et al., 2015).

Health care providers need to determine their own views regarding the value of prayer and recognize its importance for patients and families. Often health care providers may feel uncomfortable praying with patients, particularly if the religious traditions are different from their own. However, acknowledging the importance of prayer, encouraging patients and families to engage in prayer, and supporting patients through connecting them with multifaith or same-faith spiritual leaders are ways of demonstrating respect and cultural competence in care (Hamilton et al., 2020).

It is important for health care providers to understand the meaning of particular religious and spiritual practices from the perspective of the patient. For example, fasting is a regular practice in many cultures. Patients of Arab and Muslim origin may practise strict fasting regimens during the sacred month of Ramadan, when no food or water is ingested between sunrise and sundown, irrespective of one's health condition (Attum et al., 2020). Similarly, patients of Hindu faith are likely to partake in fasting or *upwas* during different festivals to restore good fortune, peace, and harmony. Some people who practise the Christian faith may give up particular foods or fast during the period of Lent, and Yom Kippur is a period of fasting for some who practise Judaism (Cultural Awareness International, 2015). Generally, religious fasts are undertaken as an expression of spiritual commitment or connection with God. However, fasting may also be associated with food insecurity (Yellow Bird, 2020). More recently, intermittent fasting has become popular in Western society as a means of weight control and better health management (Yellow Bird, 2020). We use the example of fasting here to illustrate that (1) many religions have similar beliefs but they may look different in how they are expressed in behaviour, and (2) similar actions (e.g., fasting) can have different meanings for individuals (spiritual or biological health). As well, even for people for whom fasts are a big part of their religion, there is considerable diversity within the culture with respect to how the fasting practice is conducted and under what circumstances it may be abandoned, even temporarily. It is therefore important for health care providers to ascertain the meaning related to the desired actions and consult with cultural and religious leaders for support and guidance to support desired health outcomes.

Cultural Considerations in Care

The Positive Impact of Faith and Community

Jean is a 55-year-old Filipino–Canadian who has two children: a 16-year-old daughter who has been diagnosed with cystic fibrosis, and an 8-year-old son. Jean works part-time at a jewellery store to support her two children and her 80-year-old mother, Gemma, who lives with her. Jean is a follower of Christianity and attends church regularly on a weekly basis. Recently, her divorce from her husband has led to an increase in roles and responsibilities surrounding the household. Adding to this, Jean just learned of her stage I breast cancer. Despite the recent challenges surrounding her, Jean maintains a positive attitude and is eager to battle cancer. She remains in good spirits to start chemotherapy soon and continues to attend church weekly. In addition, she has received overwhelming support from her church community, who have organized a volunteer system to help with household responsibilities.

Reflect on this case scenario and discuss findings with your colleagues. Consider how Jean's Filipino culture and faith may affect the burden of illness and individual coping.

Healing Traditions

The World Health Organization (WHO) defines **traditional medicine** as the "sum total of the knowledge, skill, and practices based on the theories, beliefs, and experiences indigenous to different cultures, whether explicable or not, used in the maintenance of health as well as in the prevention, diagnosis, improvement or treatment of physical and mental illness" (WHO, 2021). **Complementary and alternative medicine** (**CAM**) is defined as a "set of health care practices that are not part of that country's own tradition or conventional medicine and are not fully integrated into the dominant health-care system" (WHO, 2021). This definition recognizes that the "norm" in one culture may be considered as "alternative" in another cultural context. Over the last few decades, Western societies have been shifting toward an integrative and holistic approach to health. CAM such as chiropractic, naturopathic, and herbal therapies are sought after and readily available in most cities. In Canada, when such treatments are sought in addition to the biomedical approach, they are considered complementary; however, when they are chosen instead of biomedicine they are referred to as **alternative medicine** (Cassidy, 2019). Many traditional approaches to health and illness have a more holistic approach than biomedicine and focus on healing rather than cure and include the spiritual domain. France and Rodriguez (2019) distinguish between cure and healing by describing cure as a remedial strategy that fixes a problem, and healing as transformative approach that influences thoughts, feelings, energy levels, and how one lives life.

CONCEPT OF THE BODY (PHYSICAL, PSYCHOSOCIAL, SPIRITUAL, AND ENERGETIC)

Understanding healing traditions requires an exploration of how the concept of the body is understood across different systems and traditions. Cassidy (2019) describes the body–person as four intersecting circles: physical, psychosocial, spiritual, and energetic (Fig. 8.1). The intersecting nature of the four circles recognizes that what happens in one circle affects others to some extent; however, differences may exist in how this relationship is conceptualized.

The biomedical model focuses on the physical body and views it as the entry point for illness and the focus of treatment. However, there is a recognition of some indirect influence on the psychosocial since "a person who is functioning better may also *feel* better and be glad of it" (Cassidy, 2019, p. 459).

Other healing traditions and systems may begin with energy, mind, or spirituality as the initial focus or where illness begins, and the impact on physical aspects of the multidimensional body

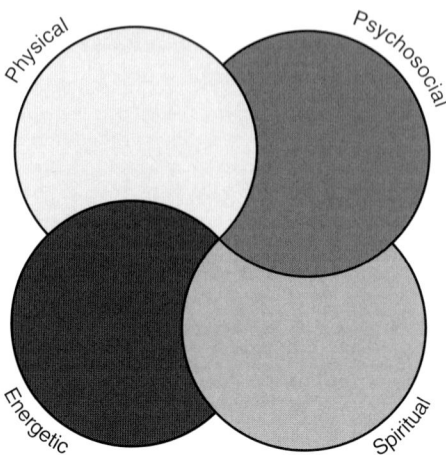

Fig. 8.1 The Four Bodies. (Adapted from Cassidy, C. M. [2019]. Social and cultural factors in medicine. In M. S. Micozzi [Ed.], *Fundamentals of complementary, alternative, and integrative medicine* [6th ed., pp. 451–474]. Elsevier.)

appear in the later stages. In other words, the problem may lie in the energy field or spiritual domain and the symptoms are evident in the body. Thus the treatment approach begins with a nonphysical dimension (e.g., *qi* that flows through the meridians in TCM) and the impact is subsequently evident in the physical, mental, and spiritual dimensions. Psychotherapy is similar in that it begins with a focus on the mind with subsequent impact on functioning and other somatic symptoms. If spiritual forces are seen as the primary source of illness, treatment or healing is often sought from spiritual or shamanic healers (Adu-Gyamfi & Anderson, 2019; Cassidy, 2019).

ALLOPATHIC MEDICINE (AKA BIOMEDICINE)

Biomedical or Western medicine is also known across the world as allopathy or allopathic medicine. The word *allopathic* comes from the Greek word for "other than disease" (More, 2016). Biomedicine has its roots in ancient Greek medicine (Cassidy, 2019; Osborn, 2021) and humoral theory originally proposed by Hippocrates. Humoral theory described the body as being comprised of four humors (fluids) that needed to be in balance in order for the individual to experience health; imbalance in humors led to disease (Breimeier, 2018). The four humors included phlegm, blood, black bile, and yellow bile. Each was associated with elements of water, air, earth, and fire. The humors were associated with seasons and with states of coldness, hotness, wetness, and dryness, and were influenced by factors such as planetary alignment, geography, and personal factors including age, sex, diet, and occupation. Diagnosis included examination of the fluids with a goal of removing impediments to restore the natural balance of the body. Since the humors were linked with personality types or temperaments, treatment was unique to the individual (as opposed to the disease) and included lifestyle and dietary changes (Breimeier, 2018).

The ideology and practices of humoral theory were prominent and commonly accepted until the nineteenth century. The shift from humoral theory to a more materialistic, scientific approach occurred in the nineteenth and twentieth centuries, and **biomedicine** became the predominant healing tradition in Europe and North America. **Allopathic medicine** views health as *the absence of illness* with a primary focus on cure (More, 2016). Based on the approach of hypothesis, experimentation, and outcome of experimentation, characteristics of allopathic medicine include a focus on symptoms and disease with minimal attention to the characteristics of the person with respect to age, body size, and, until more recently, gender (Cassidy, 2019). The concept of disease is also said to be associated with a framework in which the body is passive, at risk of "invasion" from the environment (pathogens), and each body responds similarly to the particular invader. Since each invader creates a different disease, the healer's job is to determine the invader (diagnose) and determine the approach to cure the patient by getting rid of the invader through removal, destruction, or immobility. In other words, the body's response and the treatment are based on the disease, not the person (Cassidy, 2019; More, 2016).

However, not all illnesses fit this paradigm and response to treatment is also influenced by individual factors. In particular, conditions that are chronic, degenerative, or influenced by stress do not fit nicely into the invasion paradigm (Cassidy, 2019). Thus for some people, biomedicine is seen as useful in urgent and emerging situations, but the stance of fighting is regarded as a "rigid medical approach" with associated concerns of adverse effects related to the treatment, particularly drug therapy (More, 2016). Over time, the biomedical approach has expanded to consider that (1) the body is not totally passive but plays some role in the origin of the disease; (2) disease is influenced by a range of environmental and psychosocial factors; and (3) the role of the healer or practitioner is not just to prescribe but also to educate (Cassidy, 2019). In addition, there is increasing recognition of a holistic approach to health and well-being.

AYURVEDA

Ayurveda originated in India over 5 000 years ago and is viewed as a holistic health care system. The word **Ayurveda** means the knowledge of living or the science of life, and is translated from the Sanskrit words *ayu* (life) and *veda* (knowing) (Shea, 2018). The key concepts in Ayurveda are balance and following a natural cycle; however, the balance between mind, body, and spirit also extends to connecting to oneself and a higher consciousness.

Ayurvedic medicine (AM) reflects a belief that health and health care are part of spirituality and spiritual practices. The knowledge source behind AM is considered to be divine revelation, which was subsequently transmitted orally and eventually transcribed into books. These books contain extensive knowledge of medicine, surgery, and pharmacology and are believed to date back to 400–200 BCE. Two major books are the *Charak Samhita* and the *Susrut Samhita*. The *Charak Samhita* describes the interconnections of mind, body, and spirit; identifies the causes of illness to include loss of faith in the divine, as well as external causes such as diet, lifestyle, exposure to chemicals, physical and biological agents; and identifies over 200 diseases and 150 pathological conditions and congenital defects based primarily on body organ systems and physiological functioning (Mishra et al., 2001). The *Susrut Samhita* is focused on surgery and provides detailed description of human anatomy, including fetal development, bones, nerves, and the circulatory system, along with descriptions of many surgical procedures. Other texts also exist and contain extensive descriptions of pharmacological properties of medicinal plants.

In AM the body is seen as a combination of **doshas** (mind and body elements), *dhatus* (tissues), and *malas* (wastes). Health is maintained by using the knowledge and understanding of the doshas to create a state of balance by addressing the root cause(s) of the imbalance. There are two types of doshas: (1) *sharirik doshas* are the biological elements, and (2) *mansik doshas* are the psychological elements or constitution of the mind. Ayurveda indicates that all human beings are composed of the five elements: air, earth, fire, water, and space. These elements form the doshas when combined in the human body, and these doshas are the life energies and control how the body functions.

Each *sharirik dosha* is a combination of two elements (Fig. 8.2; Table 8.1).

- **Vatha dosha** is made up of space and air, prevents movement and energy, and makes up the nervous system.

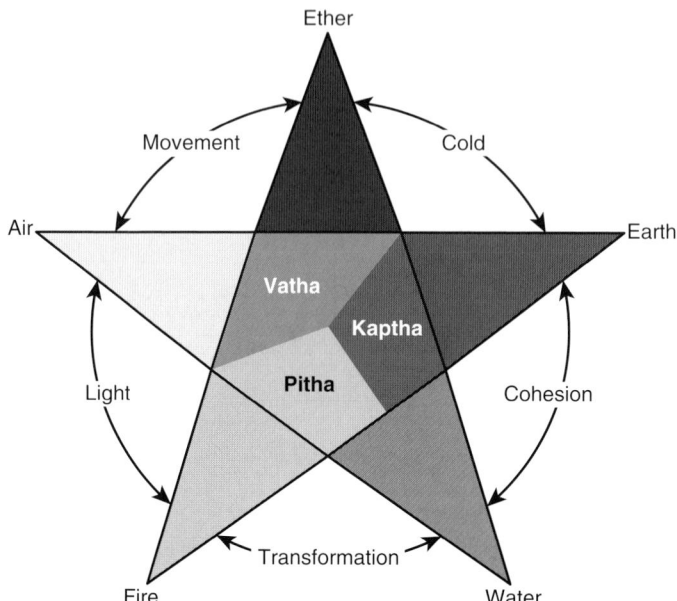

Fig. 8.2 Relationship of Doshas and Elements in Ayurveda. (Based on Gupta, S. [2015]. *10 Ayurvedic principles you should follow*. https://www.india.com/health/10-ayurvedic-principles-you-should-follow-281293/.)

TABLE 8.1 ■ A Description of the Three Doshas

Characteristic	Vatha Dosha	Pitha Dosha	Kaptha Dosha
Build	Lean or delicate, dry skin, fine hair	Medium build Muscular	Solid frame and thick bones
Expressiveness	Vibrant and energetic expression	Warm friends and fierce opponents	Calm, slow to act and react
Personality	Light of heart and quick to speak Highly creative and very changeable in mood, flexible in decision making and behaviour	Strong willed and passionate leaders Tend to be direct and take charge	Easy personality, loving and caring Move slowly and purposefully Are usually conservative

From Travis, F. T., & Wallace, R. K. (2015). Dosha brain-types: A neural model of individual differences. *Journal of Ayurveda Integrative Medicine, 6*, 280–285.

- **Pitha dosha** is composed of water and fire and controls light, heat, and transformation, and includes the metabolic and digestive systems.
- **Kaptha dosha** comprises earth and water and controls matter, cohesion, and preservation, including the bodily tissues.

There are three *mansik doshas*: (1) *sattva* is the positive quality and reflects characteristics such as compassion, knowledge, insight, and proper conduct; (2) *rajas* represents movement and activities that occur in the body; overactivity in this domain can lead to overfunctioning of emotions and sensations such as pain, desire, anger, aggressiveness, and severe anxiety; and (3) *tamas* leads to a tendency for evil conduct, lack of knowledge and insight, and physical and mental inertia (Mishra et al., 2001).

In addition to the doshas, the body also contains three *malas* (waste), which are feces, urine, and sweat, and seven *dhatus* (tissues), which are (1) *rasa*, fluids of digestion; (2) *rakta*, blood; (3) *mamsa*, muscle; (4) *meda*, fat; (5) *asthi*, bone; (6) *maija*, marrow; and (7) *shuka*, semen or reproductive fluids. The doshas regulate all physiological and psychological processes. Balance is necessary for health; either excess or deficiency presents as a symptom of illness (Shea, 2018).

An Ayurvedic clinical examination includes three diagnostic methods (*trividha pariksha*): inspection, interrogation, and palpation. Inspection involves observation of the body parts, for example, skin, hair, eyes, and tongue. Comprehensive understanding of medical history, symptoms, and psychological and physiological characteristics are covered during the interrogation. Palpation includes pulse and palpation of body parts (abdominal palpation, skin, etc.). The pulse diagnosis is significant and requires the practitioner to place the tips of three fingers on the radial pulse, and each finger assesses the characteristic of a particular *sharirik dosha* (index finger—Vatha, middle finger—Pitha, and ring finger—Kaptha) (Walia & Singh, 2010).

Treatment Approaches

In Ayurveda, treatment is holistic and addresses the interconnected factors that lead to imbalance. Imbalance occurs because of poor or inappropriate use of intellect or wisdom, over- or under-stimulation of senses, or seasonal variation. Ayurvedic practitioners utilize yoga, massage, and different rejuvenation and purification therapies. Some of the naturopathic products include combinations of diet, herbs, and oil therapy. The practitioner aims to preserve health and provides treatment of spirit, body, and mind, with a focus on self-healing. Overall good health is also related to good conduct; thus virtuous living is seen as essential for long life and well-being. Ayurveda recognizes air, food, water, sun, exercise, fasting, thoughts, and sleep as "natural doctors" that prevent or ameliorate disease (Dutta, n.d.). Treatment must be aligned with context, including the seasons, stage of life, the body constitution, and daily conduct.

INDIGENOUS MEDICINE

Indigenous people have used traditional healing methods for thousands of years. The Indigenous view of health is one of balance between the physical, mental, emotional, and spiritual components. As the individual is believed to be closely connected to family, community, and environment, approaches to health and well-being extend beyond the individual to the community, culture, and land (Fijal & Beagan, 2019; McArthur & Jakubec, 2018). The sense of inter-relatedness also means that disconnections from community, land, and culture are factors that can lead to imbalance and illness. For example, physical symptoms of illness may continue to appear until one accepts the relationship between the illness and the laws of nature.

A key component of Indigenous healing is the medicine wheel. The medicine wheel represents the culmination of life, health, and the values of the individual and their community. The medicine wheel has many teachings, interpretations, dimensions, and variations across different Indigenous groups. There are common understandings centred around the concepts of balance, with each side or perspective having equal weight or value and understanding life as a circular journey. The wheel is divided into four quadrants and represents the four aspects of health (physical, mental, spiritual, and emotional); four sacred medicines (sage, sweetgrass, tobacco, cedar); the four directions (west, north, east, south); four stages of life (adult-protection, elder-wisdom, child-innocence, youth-learning); and four seasons (fall, winter, spring, summer) (Charbonneau-Dahlen, 2019; Verwoord et al., 2011). See Fig. 8.3.

Indigenous medicine views illness or disease as resulting from a lack of attention to sacred, natural laws and imbalances amidst the fundamental constituents of the wheel. Indigenous medicine reinforces a notion centred around the belief of connections that an individual maintains to the land and environment. There is a fundamental value and significance placed on the earth as

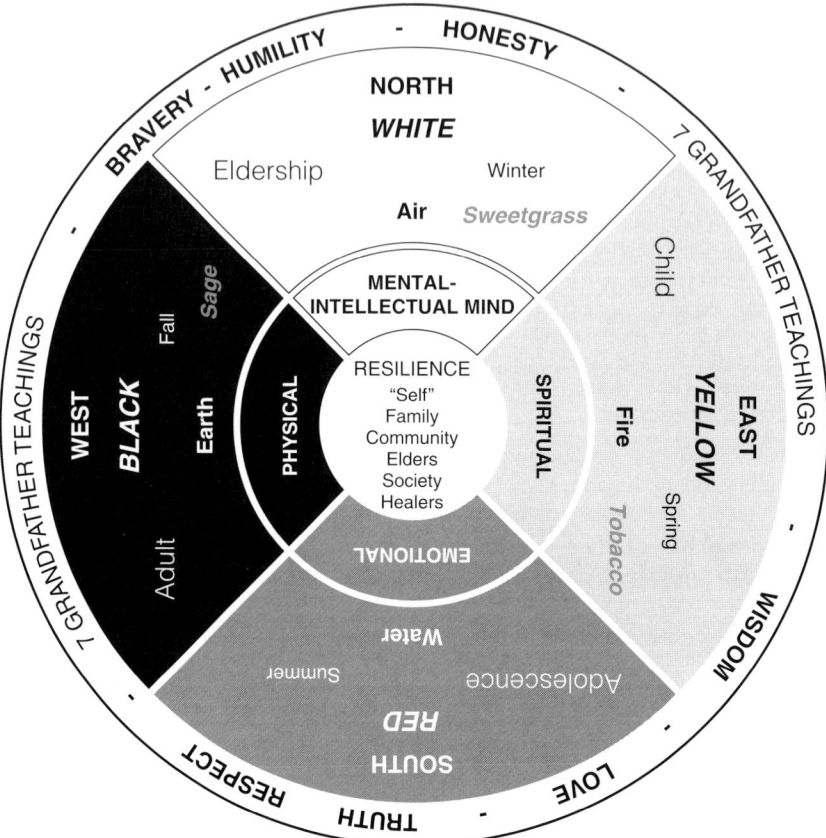

Fig. 8.3 Medicine Wheel Interconnections. (Adapted from Marsh, T. N., Young, N. L., Cote-Meek, S., et al. [2016]. Impact of Indigenous healing and seeking safety on intergenerational trauma and substance use in an Indigenous sample. *Journal of Addiction Research and Therapy*, 7, 3.)

a source of life rather than a resource and is often expressed through maintenance of authentic and intricate relationships to the land (Yu et al., 2020). Healing spaces need to be connected to the land and community in some way. There is a deep respect for all forms of life, and this sense of "universal kinship" extends to health and well-being of people within a family, community, and nation (Waterfall et al., 2017). Healing is seen as a journey, and spiritual, emotional, and physical healing are interconnected.

Treatment Approaches

Indigenous medicine supports a holistic approach to health. Maintaining or restoring balance, when it is disrupted by an illness, is an essential feature of Indigenous medicine. Various therapies involving herbs, sound, and sacred rituals (such as smudging and the sweat lodge) are used in an attempt to restore the balance of elements and energy within the medicine wheel. The four sacred herbs or medicines that are the main components of Indigenous medicine are paramount to Indigenous cultures and traditional healing practices. As noted earlier, there is considerable diversity across various Indigenous nations and the specific healing approaches may vary.

Elders have an important role in supporting the health of individuals and communities. An **Elder** is someone within the community who is considered to be wise and knowledgeable and who carries that knowledge in both the physical and spiritual realities (Marsh et al., 2015; Viscogliosi et al., 2017). Such knowledge may be acquired through visions, dreams, intuition, or ancestors and is believed to originate in the spirit and ancestral world (Marsh et al., 2015). In a scoping review of traditional Indigenous medicine in North America, Redvers and Blondin (2020) noted that "**traditional healing**" is more than "traditional medicine"; the former involves achieving spiritual connectedness and harmony with nature through fasting, prayer, mediation, ceremony, or use of traditional medicines.

Ceremonies are an important part of traditional healing for Indigenous people. These include smudging; sweat lodge ceremonies; traditional tobacco ceremonies; ceremonies associated with life events such as birth and puberty; and ceremony as a way of healing from trauma or passing of a loved one (Marsh et al., 2016; Redvers & Blondin, 2020). The **sweat lodge** ceremony is a central part of healing across various Indigenous groups and consists of both physical and spiritual purification. The lodge itself is constructed with great care and reverence for the ceremony as well as for the environment and the materials used. Rocks are heated in a sacred fire, and as water is poured on the glowing rocks, steam is created. The heating, bringing in of the rocks, and tending to the fire are sacred and important parts of the ceremony (Marsht et al., 2018). Sacred herbs are also added to further aid in cleansing. The Elder conducting the ceremony guides the participants through teaching, in lodge etiquette, and with care for the participants by encouraging them to drink water and attend to their comfort and discomfort. Participants who may be unable to participate by being in the lodge may also have the option to sit outside and still receive some benefits of the ceremony (Marsh et al., 2018).

Other less elaborate ceremonies include the sharing circle and smudging. **Smudging** is a sacred act that is part of many ceremonies and rituals. It involves burning a small amount of traditional medicine, such as sweetgrass, sage, tobacco, or cedar, and the smoke is used to cleanse and purify people and places. The smoke is spread over the body by a feather, a hand-held fan, or hand and is believed to bring calm, peace, and the opportunity for persons to connect inwardly, thereby allowing them to speak the truth (Government of Manitoba, 2019; Marsh et al., 2015; Waterfall et al., 2017).

Indigenous ways often convey spirituality through actions that involve "the sense of sight, sound, smell and touch" (Government of Alberta, n.d.). As such, dancing is viewed as praying and connection of mind, body, and emotions to the spiritual world. "The pow wow dance is an expression of strong deep-seeded heritage connecting Indigenous people to Mother Earth and all our relatives in Creation" (Absolon, 2021, p. 70). The ceremony is particularly significant, as it was outlawed under colonial rule and "these gatherings are now active acts of reclaiming and recreating Indigenous knowledge and traditions" (p. 70). The ceremony includes singing, dancing, and drumming. Drums are recognized as sacred objects and the drumbeat represents the "heartbeat of the nation" or "pulse of the universe" (Marsh et al., 2015, p. 8). Similarly, singing also fulfills a spiritual purpose; different songs exist and are tailored to the type of ceremony being held. Songs are seen as honouring the Creator and have a significant impact on healing. Lastly, there is a strong belief in healing circles; groups of people gather in a circle with the sole reason to impart healing. A talking stick, feather, or another object may be passed around the circle, giving each person an opportunity to speak and others to listen; this allows people to share their thoughts, feelings, and experiences as well as receive support and healing (Marsh et al., 2015; Redvers & Blondin, 2020).

Indigenous healers, Elders, and Indigenous healing traditions are being increasingly recognized to promote cultural safety and wellness, as a way of restoring the spiritual and land connection, and healing from the legacy and trauma of colonization.

TRADITIONAL CHINESE MEDICINE

With an extensive history of over 5 000 years, **traditional Chinese medicine (TCM)** focuses on balance and adopts a holistic approach to health that addresses both the symptoms and the cause (Shea, 2018). Similar to Ayurveda, TCM is said to originate through divine sources. Three divine beings are said to be responsible for the three major aspects of TCM. FuXi "is responsible for the *yin/yang* theory, Shen Nong is credited with the development of herbalism, and Huang Di is thought to have established **acupuncture** and diagnostic techniques" (Shea, 2018, p. 18).

"The philosophy of Chinese medicine begins with *yin* and *yang*. These two terms can be used to express the broadest philosophical concepts as well as the most focused perceptions of the natural world" (Ergil, 2019, p. 483). TCM philosophy notes that the universe consists of five elements (wood, fire, earth, metal, and water) and all phenomena can be categorized into two: *yin* and *yang*. The elements are associated with different body organs and the constitution of a person. Each individual has all five elements, albeit with different proportions. The constitution type also leads to inherent vulnerabilities that can lead to illness (Shea, 2018).

Yin and *yang* are complementary opposites that are interdependent and always exist in each other (Shea, 2018). There is a strong emphasis on maintaining a balance of *yin–yang*, referring to "dark–bright"—the notion that everything in nature is composed of two polarizing energies. The relationship between the two showcases the importance of having everything connected and complementary to one another. In terms of the body, *yin* refers to the lower body and cold; *yang* refers to the upper body and heat. An imbalance of *yin–yang* is seen from either an excess or deficiency of *yin* or an excess or deficiency of *yang*. However, the balance between the two yields health. Fig. 8.4 shows the relationship of *yin–yang* to the five elements.

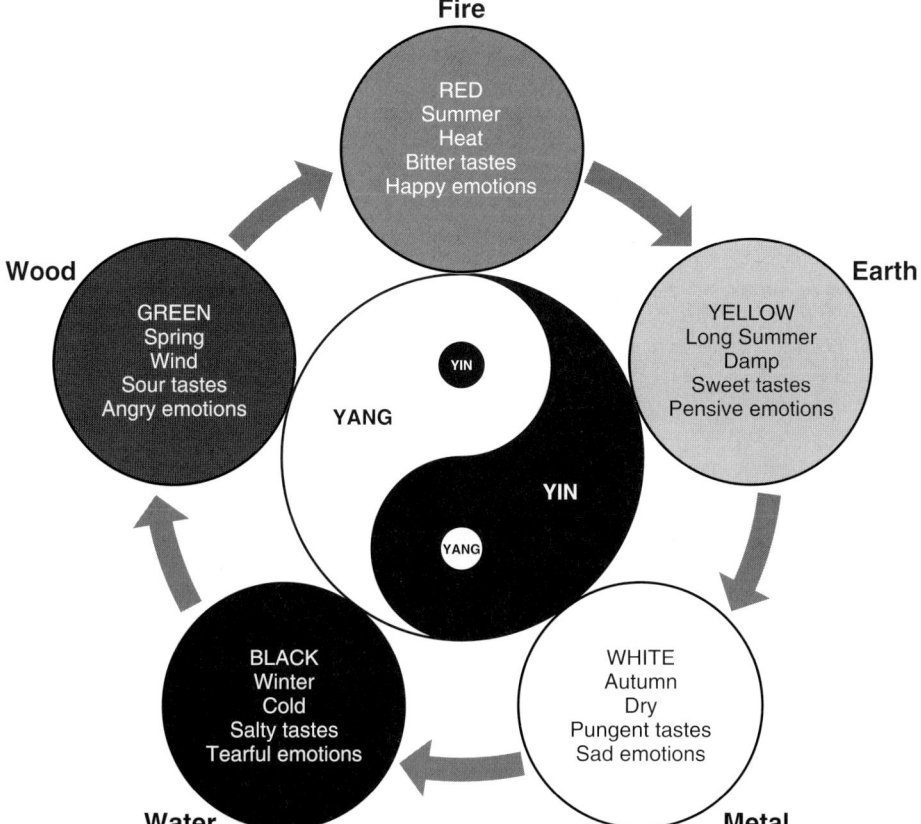

Fig. 8.4 Yin–Yang Theory. (Adapted from Ageless Herbs. *Yin yang theory*. https://agelessherbs. com/yin-yang-theory/.)

In addition to the elements and *yin* and *yang*, TCM also encompasses the concept of **qi** (pronounced "chee"), which is viewed as life energy that flows along different pathways (*jing luo* or meridians) within the body. While the presence of a free flow of *qi* directly correlates to health, its blockage or stagnation along these meridians yields illness or disease (HealthLinkBC, 2019). *Qi* might be imbalanced due to:

- External forces—related to environmental factors such as wind, cold, or heat
- Internal forces—related to emotional experiences such as joy, anger, or grief
- Lifestyle forces—related to any action or lifestyle choice an individual takes in relation to their health (e.g., poor diet, inadequate sleep, use of excessive alcohol, smoking) (HealthLinkBC, 2019)

Treatment Approaches

In TCM, imbalance is assessed through looking, listening, smelling, asking, and touching (Ergil, 2019). Pulse diagnosis along with examination of face, tongue, urine, and stool are used to determine balance between *yin–yang*, hot–cold, the five elements, and deficiency–excess (Shea, 2018). Through the examination a pattern is determined, and the treatment is targeted toward addressing the condition with opposing measures. The primary goal in TCM is to ensure and restore the body's balance and harmony between *qi* and the naturally occurring forces of *yin* and *yang*. Treatment also addresses the root cause of the illness and eliminates negative or evil influences (Ergil, 2019).

TCM emphasizes the importance of holistic healing, striving to yield restoration and balance between the body, mind, and spirit. This is primarily achieved through treatments that stimulate energy flow through needling, massage, herbal medicines, moxibustion, and movement therapies (Table 8.2).

TABLE 8.2 ■ Common Treatment Approaches in Traditional Chinese Medicine

Acupuncture	Key component of traditional Chinese medicine (TCM), it consists of inserting thin, solid, metal needles to introduce electrical stimulation. By doing so, it is believed the flow of *qi* can be improved, thereby yielding better health. Most commonly, acupuncture is used as a means of managing pain and discomfort associated with other diseases. These include headaches, menstrual cramps, fibromyalgia, and myofascial pain (Hopkins Medicine, n.d.; Mayo Clinic, 2020).
Acupressure	Similar to acupuncture, acupressure focuses on stimulating *qi* through deep massage and application of firm pressure to key meridian points within the body (UCLA Medicine, n.d.).
Cupping	The use of glass, plastic, or bamboo cups as suction devices, which are placed onto the skin. By doing so, it is believed that stagnated and congested blood will be broken to yield better flow of *qi*, thereby promoting health. Contrary to acupuncture and acupressure, it involves applying pressure to muscles through a gentle upward pull (NCCIH, 2018; Rushall, 2020).
Moxibustion	Heat therapy whereby dried plant materials called "moxa" are burned near the skin as a way to restore flow of *qi* and eliminate any pathogens. Moxa is generally made through use of a Chinese herb called mugwort but can be made of other substances too. It is commonly used to treat pain due to injury or arthritis, digestive problems, irregular elimination, and obstetrical conditions such as breech presentation in late pregnancy (Hafner, 2016).
Movement Therapy Qi Gong & Tai Chi	Ancient practices which focus on cultivating *qi* through a combination of movement, breathing, and meditation. It is believed that through movement and meditation, *qi* will become rejuvenated to further properly energize one's organs, systems, and the whole body (Wang et al., 2014). Drawing its attention on mental concentration and physical balance, tai chi and qi gong are viewed as a preventive strategy for various medical and psychological conditions.
Herbalism	Highly refined and classified according to their thermal properties, taste, the channel through which they enter the body, and primary mode of action. The medicines can be taken in the form of tea or powders that can be combined with food in different ways. Chinese medicinal products can also be used topically (Shea, 2018).

Cultural Considerations in Care

Blending Holistic Care and Complementary Therapies

Anjie is a young professional in her late 20s who, like many of her generation, embraces a "natural" way of life to the extent possible. She is a Hindu and religion is an important part of her life. Angie and her partner want to start a family; however, Anjie has been diagnosed with cancer, and she decides to undergo the toxic chemotherapy. Once her chemotherapy treatments are completed, Anjie turns her focus and attention to having a family and seeks out a traditional Chinese medicine practitioner to help her conceive. Following a pulse diagnosis, she is given a powdered blend of herbs and advised to exercise great care in choosing personal care products to ensure she avoids further toxicity. Fortunately, she is able to access an app that allows her to screen common products like shampoo, soap, detergent, and so on. She also draws strength and comfort from her Hindu religion and engages in a number of ceremonies and prayers to achieve her goal. Anjie follows the prescribed regimen for 6 months and, to her delight, is able to conceive and have a healthy pregnancy. In conversation she reflects that she felt she had to go with biomedicine for the cancer treatment, but she was very concerned about the toxic effects of the medications and therefore sought other therapies to restore her natural balance.

Anjie's story illustrates the opportunities that exist in a diverse culture with access to different healing traditions. The trend toward holistic care and increased use of complementary therapy is expected to continue. Thus it is important for all health providers to have an informed approach to the different ways of healing and promoting health.

Complementary Therapy and Integrative Care

CAM encompasses a wide range of treatment approaches that are not part of the conventional medical approach to care (Truant et al., 2015). If a practice is used *together with* conventional medical treatment, it is considered complementary; however, if a practice is used instead of conventional medical treatment, it is considered alternative. Integrative medicine or integrative health brings together conventional and complementary or traditional medicine in a coordinated manner (NCCIH, 2018).

Complementary medicine can be grouped under five main categories:

1. Whole medical systems or healing traditions such as TCM or Ayurveda
2. Mind–body medicine such as yoga, meditation, tai chi, and relaxation therapies, including guided imagery
3. Natural products or biological therapies, including herbs, vitamins, and minerals
4. Manipulative therapies such as massage and spinal, chiropractic, and osteopathic manipulation
5. Energy therapies such as reiki, acupuncture, and therapeutic touch

CAM continues to be widely adopted by Canadians to treat and manage chronic conditions. According to a report by the Fraser Institute (2016), complementary or alternative therapy utilization has continued to increase, with 79% of the survey respondents reporting use sometimes in their lives in 2016 as compared to 74% in 2006 and 73% in 1997. The most commonly used therapy was massage (44%), followed by chiropractic care (42%), yoga (27%), relaxation techniques (25%), and acupuncture (22%). The overall findings also show increasing generational acceptance, with "GenXers" reporting higher use than "young boomers" (those born in the early 1960s), and recent generations utilize CAM therapies not just for illness but also for health promotion and maintaining wellness (Canizares et al., 2017; Fraser Institute, 2016). The increased use can be attributed to a variety of factors, including a desire for holistic health as well as concerns over adverse effects of pharmaceuticals and other conventional treatments. In addition, many physicians and other health care providers are more engaged with CAM practices and therapies than in previous generations, leading to a wider range of options for the public. The increased use is occurring despite limited treatment coverage from publicly funded health systems.

The increased use and availability of CAM therapies has raised issues that require careful exploration. Additional cost of therapies can lead to uneven access, although for some patients the cost of CAM products may be less than the cost of pharmaceuticals. As health care in Canada falls under provincial jurisdiction, access to qualified and regulated CAM practitioners and therapies varies across the country. Although regulation is generally regarded as a positive step and a recognition of "legitimacy" within the Canadian context, there is also concern that regulation may negatively affect scopes of practice as well as the distinct worldviews that are reflected in CAM therapies, as traditional therapies are assessed and regulated within a biomedical paradigm (Ijaz et al., 2015).

A major concern with the increased use of CAM therapies is that of disclosure and communication. Patients may not disclose use of such therapies for a variety of reasons that range from not recognizing the use of a natural product as "therapy" to fear of judgement from the provider. It is critical that all health care providers initiate the conversation and include use of CAM therapies as part of their assessment to ensure negative interactions between products are avoided and any overlaps in care are beneficial. Regardless of their own views and values regarding particular therapies, all health care providers need to support patient choice and informed decision making. Acceptance of patient choice conveys respect and does not mean endorsement of a particular approach.

NATUROPATHY

Naturopathy evolved as a formal system of medicine in North America in the twentieth century. **Naturopathic medicine** is based on the philosophical approach of *vis medicatrix naturae* (the healing power of nature) (Broderick, 2019), where disease presents because of departure from natural ways of living.

Categorized as a "whole medical system," naturopathy contains "[other] complete systems of theory and practice that have evolved independently over time in different cultures" (Baars & Hamre, 2017) separate from Western or conventional medicine. The philosophy and foundation of principles of practicing naturopathy are consistent with that of "Eastern whole medical systems such as traditional Chinese medicine or Ayurveda" and homeopathy (Broderick, 2019, p. 3). In fact, naturopathy adopts its key tools and treatments from other healing traditions through use of TCM, Ayurveda, acupuncture, and homeopathy. It also strongly upholds the idea of lifestyle changes through eating healthy, staying fit, exercising regularly, and using personal empowerment.

Naturopathic medicine is defined by a set of principles rather than a specific therapeutic approach (Table 8.3). These principles are applied in the "context of a healing environment" and focus on educating, empowering, and motivating individuals to achieve optimal well-being (Broderick, 2019).

Logan et al. (2018) propose an additional principle, "Scientia Criticata." *Scientia* refers to "acquaintance with knowledge (vs. opinion)," and *criticus* is the Latin root of critical, as in decisive judgement, and refers to *kritos* meaning to separate or choose. Scientia Criticata is described as the "ability to critically analyze accumulated knowledge including scientific facts, knowledge about the self (critical consciousness) and values of the patient" (Logan et al., 2018, p. 367). It includes the need for critical self-reflection of clinician privilege and understanding of power dynamics that lead to health inequalities.

Treatment Approaches

The goal of naturopathic treatment is to restore optimal health through removing the cause of disease or illness and optimizing factors within the internal and external environment. Naturopathic medicine utilizes a blend of modern scientific knowledge and traditional forms of medicine to prevent disease, promote health, and treat illness (Canadian Association of Naturopathic Doctors, n.d.). Naturopathic treatment includes guidance on nutrition and herbal medicine, behaviour, and lifestyle changes, as well as tactile therapy such as massage, chiropractic treatment, and

TABLE 8.3 ■ Six Principles of Naturopathic Medicine

Vis Medicatrix Naturae (The Healing Power of Nature)	Recognizes the innate ability of organisms (plants, animals, people) to maintain and restore health. Optimal internal and external environmental conditions are necessary to support the natural healing ability.
Primum Non Nocere (First, Do No Harm)	Harm is minimized through the use of substances with minimal harmful effects; an approach of least possible force or intervention; avoiding symptom suppression; and respecting the self-healing process.
Docere (Doctor as Teacher)	Naturopathic doctors focus on education and emphasize self-responsibility. The patient–provider relationship is critical.
Tolle Causam (Treat the Cause)	Focus on the cause versus symptoms. When the cause is addressed, the symptoms go away.
Tolle Totum (Treat the Whole Person)	It is important to identify the cause of illness, which can be a result of factors within the physical, the mental, the emotional, genetic, environmental, social or spiritual domains.
Preventare (Prevention)	Recognize the importance of health, not just absence of disease. Health is achieved through assessment of risk factors and disease susceptibility and taking action to modify internal and external environment.

From Broderick. (2019). Naturopathic philosophy. In L. Hechtman (Ed.), *Clinical naturopathic medicine* (2nd ed., pp. 1–16). Elsevier; Logan, A. C., Goldenberg, J. Z., Guiltinan, J., et al. (2018). North American naturopathic medicine in the 21st century: Time for a seventh guiding principle - Scientia Critica. *Explore, 14*(5), 367–372.

acupuncture. Pharmacological drugs and surgery are beyond the scope of a naturopathic doctor (ND); however, the need for such treatment is recognized and addressed through referrals.

Naturopathic medicine is often regarded as a complementary or integrative therapy or approach to care that coexists alongside conventional medicine. This has led to the establishment of the naturopathic professional body (Canadian Association of Naturopathic Doctors, n.d.).

Over the years, NDs have gained much popularity, with increasing demands for their services. While conventional medicine may overlook the importance of holistic healing, many Canadians continue to seek NDs for ongoing support and care as both an alternative *and* as a complement to conventional medicine. The increased demand for NDs further led to creation of their regulation in six Canadian provinces, with Nova Scotia granting title protection in 2008. Being recognized as a separate entity from primary health care and upholding a distinct model from conventional medicine, naturopathy continues to expand. Consequently, many insurance companies recognize and cover the cost of certain visitations to NDs. Its transition from "alternative" medicine to "mainstream" medicine showcases the importance of upholding a holistic approach to treatments and healing. More importantly, its increasing popularity highlights societal change in perception of health and an adoption of values focusing on disease prevention and health promotion.

CHIROPRACTIC MEDICINE

The word *chiropractic* originated from the Greek words "kheir" (hand) and "praktikos" (do) and translates to mean "to do with the hand" (Kiroclinique.ca, n.d.). In 1895, the self-educated scientist Daniel David Palmer from the United States developed **chiropractic medicine** by proposing that the nervous system serves as the human body's control mechanism and any slight misalignment of the spine could significantly impact a person's health. Palmer viewed the human body as a machine, and the chiropractic practitioner "looks the human machine over, finds what parts are out of place, why the blood does not circulate freely to all parts, why the nerves cry out with pain" (Rosner, 2016, p. 35). Disease occurs when the body part arrangement is misaligned; the goal is to put them back in their proper place. Displacement of bones, muscles, or ligaments can result in pinched or strained nerves, leading to diseases of the nerves. Thus the chiropractic healing approach focuses on spinal manipulation therapy as the main treatment to correct spinal misalignment (Kirkley & Hall, 2019). This approach has evolved to include a focus on the spine, muscle, and nervous system as a complement to medical treatment and now plays a crucial role in managing conditions and injuries related to the musculoskeletal system.

Gliedt et al. (2017) argue that chiropractic practice is grounded in a biopsychosocial approach in that it recognizes the interdependence between mental/emotional, biochemical/nutritional, and structural influences on health. In addition, chiropractic practitioners recognize the importance of the provider–patient relationship, value kindness and patience, and are sensitive to the influence of psychosocial factors such as depression, anxiety, and unsupportive interpersonal relationships on pain and disability. Thus while the approach to care is more mechanistic, chiropractic practice itself can be viewed as more holistic.

With the advancement of the profession, chiropractors diagnose and treat various causes of pain. They use a noninvasive, drug-free, hands-on approach to correct low joint motion and restore proper body movement. Chiropractors have vast knowledge regarding the assessment, diagnosis, and conservative management of musculoskeletal conditions and are not limited to the back and neck. However, back pain, neck pain, and headaches are the primary neuromusculoskeletal conditions that bring patients to the chiropractor. They also treat strains, sprains, and arthritic pain (Ontario Chiropractic Association, 2022). The biomedical approach to the treatment of conditions such as muscle and joint pain includes the use of pain relievers and anti-inflammatory medications, which might temporarily alleviate symptoms but might not address the underlying causes. Chiropractic care goes beyond symptom management and can also be used to

- Improve flexibility, mobility, and posture
- Improve athletic performance
- Reduce the risk of any injury, for example, workplace and sports-related injuries, and so on

As a result, many people may choose chiropractic treatment to minimize the use of medications, improve functioning, and enhance quality of life. In this regard, chiropractic care can be regarded as complementary, alternative, or an integrative approach to care. While the acceptance and availability of chiropractic care have significantly increased over the years, access is limited by cost, as it is not covered by the provincial health plans and extended health benefits may have significant limitations in coverage.

As with other health care providers, chiropractors also recognize that culture matters in chiropractic practice and that it has a critical impact on patient experience. Chiropractors look for ways to adapt or modify their approach to care, as illustrated in the example below.

Cultural Considerations in Care

Respecting Modesty

Salma was a practicing Muslim, and her religion did not allow any of her skin to be exposed, especially in the presence of a man who was not her husband. The male chiropractor took extra time to explain what the treatment would entail and encouraged the option of having her male partner present during the assessment to make them both feel more comfortable. During the examination, the chiropractor did not expose any skin and did the palpation and orthopedic testing through Salma's clothes. After the initial assessment was completed, the findings and treatment options were discussed with the couple. During the treatment, the chiropractor took an extra step to make the patient feel more comfortable by asking his female kinesiologist to be present in the room and perform the setup of the therapeutic modalities. He left the room when direct intervention was not needed and returned once treatment was completed, and the patient was covered again. The practitioner recognized the importance of conveying respect and earning trust. He noted that "without trust, the patient will not let you do what is required to get better. Once that trust is earned, there is now a new level of comfort between the doctor and the patient, and this is the ultimate goal that all healthcare providers strive for with their patients."

From Dr. James Masellis, personal communication, December 29, 2020.

Integrative Care

Integrative care is the blend of conventional and traditional treatments offered in a coordinated manner. Although highly sought after, it is rarely seen in clinical practice and often lacks harmony in the way it is delivered. While Western medicine and providers may offer and recognize CAM therapies (e.g., yoga, mindfulness-based stress reduction exercises, therapeutic touch, music, art therapy, etc.), these are usually offered in a complementary approach. A strong emphasis is actively maintained toward conventional medicine as CAM therapies. Moreover, CAM therapies are utilized without formal collaboration and communication with conventional therapy providers, there is a risk of disintegrated care delivery, and additional burden is placed on patients in "connecting the dots" across various therapies (Truant et al., 2015).

Despite the true integration at a systems level, the trend is toward more utilization of CAM and traditional healing modalities. With the call to action from the TRC (2015) to provide access to Indigenous treatments and providers, many hospitals are integrating Indigenous healing into the care and services offered—both as an alternative and in a blended way (for example, see www.camh.ca/en/driving-change/shkaabe-makwa/resources). There are many examples of Indigenous-led or supported partnerships that are increasing access to culturally safe and effective care for Indigenous people (Allen et al., 2020; Marsh et al., 2015).

Integrative care is also increasingly evident for issues related to mental health, palliative care, and pain management, to name a few. Shafto et al. (2018) note that "knowledge of other healing systems, such as traditional Chinese medicine, Ayurveda, naturopathy, chiropractic and homeopathy, allows integrative medicine providers from an allopathic background to appreciate the role these fields play in healing, and appropriately counsel patients seeking care" (p. 75). They further note that combinations of mind–body techniques, such as acupuncture or acupressure, relaxation and stress-physiology regulation techniques, essential oils, botanicals and supplements and reiki, and pharmacological interventions, can be very effective in reducing distressing symptoms such as pain, nausea, and dyspnea. Examples of increasingly collaborative and integrative care approaches clearly highlight that the diversity of healing traditions and approaches adds to patient choice and providers' abilities to provide safe effective care through a broader range of alternatives.

However, different healing traditions and providing care with a two-eyed seeing approach is not always easy. Lucana and Elfers (2020) undertook a study to identify healing practices that would be appropriate for Western practitioners working with immigrant populations from Central and South America. Their findings illustrate the importance of and difficulties in navigating diagnostic categories and approaches between traditions, as illustrated below.

Cultural Competence in Action

Navigating Healing Traditions

Liz provided therapy for adolescent parents presenting with post-traumatic stress disorder (PTSD) and had many patients with Indigenous backgrounds in her practice. As she recognized that her approach did not always resonate with her patients, she began to shift her approach to work with patients' cultural practices as strengths by inviting them to talk about their dreams, ancestors, rituals, and other aspects of culture. She noticed that this change had a significant positive impact on reducing patient anxiety and sense of feeling overwhelmed. However, she also recognized that experiences of visions and dreams might be labelled and treated as psychotic episodes by many of her peers.

- How can Liz work with her patients in a culturally safe and responsive way while ensuring that she does not ignore symptoms that require attention?
- What supports can she seek out for herself as a practitioner as well as for her patients?

Adapted from Lucana, S., & Elfers, J. (2020). Sacred medicine: Indigenous healing and mental health. *The Qualitative Report*, 25(12), 4491.

Integrative care will continue to have increasing prominence due to the potential impact it has on the lives of individuals. By placing an emphasis on a "whole systems" approach, it reinforces the unique needs of a person seeking care first and aims to design individualized treatment plans based on the individual's assessment. As we move forward, Canadian health care providers must recognize ways to incorporate integrative care and participate in evolving research, promoting the use of different healing therapies.

Summary

This chapter explores the impact of culture, specifically religion and spirituality, on health and well-being. We provide an overview of major healing traditions that are encountered in Canadian society. These include allopathic medicine, Ayurveda, Indigenous medicine, and TCM. In addition, complementary medical approaches such as naturopathy and chiropractic medicine were also discussed. Through the discussion it is evident that there are many similarities between the various healing traditions. These include a holistic approach to health that recognizes the inter-relatedness of the physical, psychological, spiritual, and energetic body; the concept of balance both within the person and in terms of persons within their natural geographical environment; the idea of body type or constitution that requires an understanding of the person as well as an understanding of the illness or disease to determine an individualized approach to treatment; and treatments that draw on natural elements, the spiritual world, and activities of daily living.

Given the positive impact on health and well-being, the trends toward increasing diversification of society as well as healing traditions and therapies are expected to continue. Integrative care is the future, and while there are many challenges for true integration at the system level, it is critical that health care providers strengthen their own knowledge and skill to work with individuals across cultures and healing traditions. To do this effectively, providers will need to see culture as strength, view context of care as critical, be prepared to work with and learn from traditional healers, and adopt an expanded understanding of holistic care—one that extends to the spiritual, intergenerational, and natural world.

 http://evolve.elsevier.com/Srivastava/culturalcompetence/.

Questions for Review and Discussion

1. Briefly explain how religion and culture influence a person's decision making in the context of health and illness. List three examples.
2. What are some similarities in and differences between major healing traditions? Are there major concepts that can be utilized to initiate conversations with patients and families regardless of the specific tradition they may prefer?
3. Identify three to five different ways in which complementary, alternative, and integrative medicine have impacted the Canadian health care system.
4. Reflect on your own experience(s) with non-Western healing traditions. What factors support or challenge patients' and families' abilities to access their preferred tradition(s)? What concerns emerge with integrative approaches to health and healing, and how can they be addressed?

Group Experiential/Reflection Activity

In pairs or small groups, discuss the difference between cure and healing. Reflect on settings where you have practised in the past. Was there an emphasis on cure, healing, or both? From that experience, can you identify changes that are needed, at an individual and system level, to support patients?

References

Absolon, K. (2021). Four generations for generations: A pow wow story to transform academic evaluation criteria. *Engaged Scholar Journal: Community-Engaged Research, Teaching, and Learning, 7*(1), 66–85. https://doi.org/10.15402/esj.v7i1.70054.

Adu-Gyamfi, S., & Anderson, E. (2019). Indigenous medicine and traditional healing in Africa: A systematic synthesis of the literature. *Philosophy, Social and Human Disciplines, 1*, 69–100.

Allen, L., Hatala, A., Ijaz, S., et al. (2020). Indigenous-led health care partnerships in Canada. *Canadian Medical Association Journal, 192*, E208–216. https://doi.org/10.1503/cmaj.190728.

Attum, B., Hafiz, S., Malik, A., et al. (2020). Cultural competence in the care of Muslim patients and their families: *StatPearls*. StatPearls Publishing.

Baars, E. W., & Hamre, H. J. (2017). Whole medical systems versus the system of conventional biomedicine: A critical, narrative review of similarities, differences, and factors that promote the integration process. *Evidence-Based Complementary and Alternative Medicine, 2017*, 4904930. https://doi.org/10.1155/2017/4904930.

Breimeier, C. (2018). *The emergence of modern humoralism*. https://frontiersmag.wustl.edu/2018/04/28/the-emergence-of-modern-humoralism/

Broderick, K. (2019). Naturopathic philosophy. In L. Hechtman (Ed.), *Clinical naturopathic medicine* (2nd ed, pp. 1–16). Elsevier.

Canadian Association of Naturopathic Doctors. (n.d.). *About naturopathic medicine.* https://www.cand.ca/naturopathic-medicine-today/

Canizares, M., Hogg-Johnson, S., Gignac, M., et al. (2017). Changes in the use practitioner-based complementary and alternative medicine over time in Canada: Cohort and period effects. *PLoS ONE, 12*(5), e0177307.

Cassidy, C. M. (2019). Social and cultural factors in medicine. In M. S. Micozzi (Ed.), *Fundamentals of complementary, alternative, and integrative medicine* (6th ed., pp. 451–474). Elsevier.

Charbonneau-Dahlen, B. (2019). Symbiotic allegory as innovative Indigenous research methodology. *Advances in Nursing Science, 43*(1), E25–E35.

Cultural Awareness International. (2015). *Fasting around the world*. https://culturalawareness.com/fasting-around-the-world/

Değer, V. B. (2018). *Transcultural nursing*. IntechOpen. https://doi.org/10.5772/intechopen.74990.

Dutta, N. K. (n.d.). Ayurveda—natural way of healthy living. http://ayurvediccure.co/ayurveda.html

Ergil, K. (2019). Social and cultural factors in medicine. In M. S. Micozzi (Ed.), *Fundamentals of complementary, alternative, and integrative medicine* (6th ed., pp. 483–501). Elsevier.

Fijal, D., & Beagan, B. (2019). Indigenous perspectives on health: Integration with a Canadian model of practice. *Canadian Journal of Occupational Therapy, 86*(3), 220–231.

France, H., & Rodriguez, C. (2019). Traditional Chinese medicine in Canada: An Indigenous perspective. *Chinese Medicine and Culture, 2*(1), 1–5.

Fraser Institute. (2016). *Complementary and alternative medicine: Use and public attitudes 1997, 2006, and 2016*. https://www.fraserinstitute.org/sites/default/files/complementary-and-alternative-medicine-2017.pdf

Gliedt, J. A., Schneider, M. J., Evans, M. W., et al. (2017). The biopsychosocial model and chiropractic: A commentary with recommendations for the chiropractic profession. *Chiropractic & Manual Therapies, 25*, 16.

Government of Alberta. (n.d.). *Symbolism and traditions: Ceremonies.* https://www.learnalberta.ca/content/aswt/symbolism_and_traditions/documents/ceremonies.pdf?fbclid=IwAR3gMJuu-MRM0o_lb0uoyQXLoVpc2AZrvnFsa8S-eRfKeLBg0J7uHeNsl1Y

Government of Manitoba. (2019). *Smudging protocol and guidelines for school divisions*. https://www.edu.gov.mb.ca/iid/publications/pdf/smudging_guidelines.pdf

Gupta, S. (2015). *10 Ayurvedic principles you should follow*. https://www.india.com/health/10-ayurvedic-principles-you-should-follow-281293/

Hafner, C. (2016). *Moxibustion.* https://www.takingcharge.csh.umn.edu/explore-healing-practices/moxibustion#:~:text=Moxibustion%20is%20a%20form%20of,and%20dispel%20certain%20pathogenic%20influences

Hamilton, J., Kweon, L., Brock, L-U., et al. (2020). The use of prayer during life-threatening illness: A connectedness to God, inner-self, and others. *Journal of Religion and Health, 59*, 1687–1701. https://doi:10.1007/s10943-019-00809-7.

HealthLinkBC. (2019). *Traditional Chinese medicine.* https://www.healthlinkbc.ca/health-topics/aa140227spec

Hopkins Medicine. (n.d.). *Acupuncture.* https://www.hopkinsmedicine.org/health/wellness-and-prevention/acupuncture

Ijaz, N., Boon, H., Welsh, S., et al. (2015). Supportive but "worried": Perceptions of naturopaths, homeopaths, and Chinese medicine practitioners through a regulatory transition in Ontario, Canada. *BMC Complementary and Alternative Medicine, 15*, 312.

Kirkley, S., & Hall, B. (2019). The first chiropractor was a Canadian who claimed he received a message from a ghost. *National Post.* https://nationalpost.com/health/the-first-chiropractor-was-a-canadian-who-claimed-he-received-a-message-from-a-ghost

Kiroclinique.ca. (n.d.) *What is chiropractic?* https://kiroclinique.ca/en/chiropratic/what-is-chiropractic

Koenig, H. G. (2012). Religion, spirituality, and health: The research and clinical implications. *ISRN Psychiatry*, 278730. https://doi.org/10.5402/2012/278730.

Logan, A. C., Goldenberg, J. Z., Guiltinan, J., et al. (2018). North American naturopathic medicine in the 21st century: Time for a seventh guiding principle—Scientia Critica. *Explore (New York, N.Y.), 14*(5), 367–372.

Lucana, S., & Elfers, J. (2020). Sacred medicine: Indigenous healing and mental health. *The Qualitative Report, 25*(12), 4482–4495.

Marsh, T. N., Cote-Meek, S., Toulouse, P., et al. (2015). The application of two-eyed seeing decolonizing methodology in qualitative and quantitative research for the treatment of intergenerational trauma and substance use disorders. *International Journal of Qualitative Methods*, 1–13. https://doi.org/10.1177/1609406915618046.

Marsh, T. N., Marsh, D., Ozawagosh, J., et al. (2018). The sweat lodge ceremony: A healing intervention for intergenerational trauma and substance use. *International Indigenous Policy Journal, 9*(2). https://doi.org/10.18584/iipj.2018.9.2.2.

Marsh, T. N., Young, N. L., Cote-Meek, S., et al. (2016). Impact of Indigenous healing and seeking safety on intergenerational trauma and substance use in an Indigenous sample. *Journal of Addiction Research and Therapy, 7*, 3. https://doi.org/10.4172/2155-6105.1000284.

Mayo Clinic. (2020). *Acupuncture.* https://www.mayoclinic.org/tests-procedures/acupuncture/about/pac-20392763

McArthur, G., & Jakubec, S. (2018). Cultural considerations for psychiatric mental health nursing. In C. Pollard, S. Jakubec, & M. Halter (Eds.), *Varcarolis's Canadian psychiatric mental health nursing* (2nd Canadian ed., pp. 115–133). Saunders.

Migration Policy Institute. (n.d.). *The top sending countries of immigrants in Australia, Canada, and the United States.* https://www.migrationpolicy.org/programs/data-hub/top-sending-countries-immigrants-australia-canada-and-united-states

Mishra, L., Singh, B. B., & Dagenais, S. (2001). Ayurveda: A historical perspective and principles of the traditional healthcare system in India. *Alternative Therapies in Health and Medicine, 7*(2), 36–42.

More, B. (2016). Overview of medicine—its importance and impact. *DJ International Journal of Medical Research, 1*(1), 1–8. https://doi.org/10.18831/djmed.org/2016011001.

National Center for Complimentary and Integrative Health (NCCIH). (2018). *Cupping.* https://www.nccih.nih.gov/health/cupping

Ontario Chiropractic Association. (2022). *What is chiropractic care?* https://chiropractic.on.ca/chiropractic-care/about-chiropractic-care/what-is-chiropractic-care/

Osborn, D. K. (2021). *The four humors.* http://www.greekmedicine.net/b_p/Four_Humors.html

Rao, A., Sibbritt, D., Phillips, J., et al. (2015). Prayer or spiritual healing as adjuncts to conventional care: A cross sectional analysis of prevalence and characteristics of use among women. *BMJ Open, 5*(e007345). http://doi.org/10.1136/bmjopen-2014-007345.

Redvers, N., & Blondin, B. (2020). Traditional Indigenous medicine in North America: A scoping review. *PLoS ONE, 15*(8), e0237531. https://doi.org/10.1371/journal.pone.0237531.

Roe, C., Sonnex, C., & Roxburgh, E. (2015). Two meta-analyses of noncontact healing studies. *Explore, 11*(1), 11–23. http://dx.doi.org/10.1016/j.explore.2014.10.00.

Rosner, A. (2016). Chiropractic identity: A neurological, professional, and political assessment. *Journal of Chiropractic Humanities, 22*(1), 36–45.

Rushall, K. (2020). *The many benefits of Chinese cupping.* https://www.pacificcollege.edu/news/blog/2014/09/20/many-benefits-chinese-cupping-1

Shafto, K., Gouda, S., Catrine, K., et al. (2018). Integrative approaches in pediatric palliative care. *Children*, *5*, 75. https://doi.org/10.3390/children5060075.

Shea, B. (2018). *Handbook of Chinese medicine and Ayurveda*. Healing Arts Press.

Statistics Canada. (2017a). *Immigration and diversity: Population projections for Canada and its regions, 2011 to 2036*. Statistics Canada Catalogue no. 91-551-X. https://www150.statcan.gc.ca/n1/pub/91-551-x/91-551-x2017001-eng.htm

Statistics Canada. (2017b). *Immigration and ethnocultural diversity: Key results from the 2016 census*. Statistics Canada Catalogue no. 11-001-X. https://www150.statcan.gc.ca/n1/daily-quotidien/171025/dq171025b-eng.htm

The Migration Observatory. (2020). *Migrants in the UK: An overview*. https://migrationobservatory.ox.ac.uk/resources/briefings/migrants-in-the-uk-an-overview/

Travis, F. T., & Wallace, R. K. (2015). Dosha brain-types: A neural model of individual differences. *Journal of Ayurveda and Integrative Medicine*, *6*, 280–285.

Truant, T. L., Balneaves, L. G., & Fitch, M. I. (2015). Integrating complementary and alternative medicine into cancer care: Canadian oncology nurses' perspectives. *Asia-Pacific Journal of Oncology Nursing*, *2*, 205–214.

Truth and Reconciliation Commission of Canada (TRC). (2015). *Honouring the truth: Reconciling for the Future*. Author.

UCLA Medicine. (n.d.). *Acupressure for beginners*. https://exploreim.ucla.edu/self-care/acupressure-and-common-acupressure-points/

Verwoord, R., Mitchell, A., & Machado, J. (2011). Supporting Indigenous students through a culturally relevant assessment model based on the medicine wheel. *Canadian Journal of Native Education*, *34*(1), 49–66.

Viscogliosi, C., Asselin, H., Basile, S., et al. (2017). A scoping review protocol on social participation of Indigenous elders, intergenerational solidarity and their influence on individual and community wellness. *BMJ Open*, *7*, e015931. https://doi.org/10.1136/bmjopen-2017-015931.

Walia, R., & Singh, M. (2010). *Pulse based diagnosis system using the concept of Ayurveda*. https://www.research-gate.net/publication/321624488_Pulse_Based_Diagnosis_System_Using_the_Concept_of_Ayurveda

Wang, F., Lee, E. K., Wu, T., et al. (2014). The effects of tai chi on depression, anxiety, and psychological well-being: A systematic review and meta-analysis. *International Journal of Behavioral Medicine*, *21*(4), 605–617.

Waterfall, B., Smoke, D., & Smoke, M. L. (2017). Reclaiming grassroots traditional Indigenous healing ways and practices within urban Indigenous community contexts. In S. L. Stewart, R. Moodley, & A. Hyatt (Eds.), *Indigenous cultures and mental health counselling: Four directions for integration with counselling psychology*. ProQuest Ebook Central (pp. 34–45).

World Health Organization (WHO). (2021). *Traditional, complementary and integrative medicine*. https://www.who.int/health-topics/traditional-complementary-and-integrative-medicine#tab=tab_1

Yellow Bird, M. (2020). Decolonizing fasting to improve indigenous wellness. *Cultural Survival Quarterly Magazine*, June. https://www.culturalsurvival.org/publications/cultural-survival-quarterly/decolonizing-fasting-improve-indigenous-wellness

Yu, Z., Steenbeek, A., Biderman, M., et al. (2020). *Characteristics of Indigenous healing strategies in Canada: A scoping review*. https://www.researchgate.net/publication/343822574

CHAPTER 9

Cultural Safety for Indigenous Health Equity

R. Lisa Bourque Bearskin, Andrea Kennedy, and
Sonya L. Jakubec

LEARNING OBJECTIVES

At the end of this chapter, the learner will be able to:
- Understand how to create respectful relationships with Indigenous people
- Describe the historical and sociopolitical experiences of colonialism
- Explain the consequences of colonization and historical trauma for Indigenous people
- Define concepts associated with constructivist and anti-colonial knowledge
- Discuss the role of racism, discrimination, and oppression related to the determinants of Indigenous health
- Describe interpersonal and systems-level influences for Indigenous health equity
- Identify key relational practices that support cultural safety including the processes of cultural humility, cultural competency, and structural competency

KEY TERMS

Anti-colonial knowledge
Anti-oppressive practice
Colonialism
Constructivist knowledge
Cultural competence
Cultural humility
Cultural safety
Decolonization
Ethical space
Genocide

Indigenous health equity
Indigenous Knowledges
Intersectionality
Oppression
Racism
Relational practice
Residential school
 system
Self-determination
Sixties Scoop

Strengths-based
 approaches
Structural competency
Systemic racism
Structural violence
Terra nullius
Trauma-informed care
Treaties
White supremacy

The focus of this chapter is to explore how health care providers may develop knowledge and skills for cultural safety with Indigenous people. Through anti-oppressive practices, practitioners can advocate, individually and within systems, to take action for health equity with Indigenous people. This chapter provides an overview of Indigenous people health in Canada, focusing on core knowledge and skills for culturally safe practice. This chapter addresses key concepts of constructivist, anti-colonial knowledge and relationality with Indigenous people. These are a foundation to understanding the historical and sociopolitical impact of colonialism, counteracted through relational practices and trauma-informed care. Through practical vignettes, examples, and relevant research highlights, a rights-based approach forms the starting place for cultural safety with Indigenous people. The Cultural Considerations in Care box reflecting on culturally safe care with Peter highlights the process of cultural humility.

Cultural Considerations In Care

Reflecting on Culturally Safe Care With Peter

Peter is a Cree-Métis mooshum (Grandfather) with bright green eyes and short dark hair. You are meeting Peter for the first time for follow-up diabetes care. In the chart, you see that Peter is a residential school survivor who is raising three school-aged grandchildren while their daughter works up North. They enjoy spending time hunting in the bush and working in their extended family's large vegetable garden. The community looks up to Peter for guidance as a traditional knowledge holder for medicines. Peter greets you with "tansi" (Cree expression of "hello" and "how are you"?) and a warm smile.

Rather than slipping into "automatic pilot" assumptions, you remember the importance of cultural humility. While engaging with respect and curiosity about Peter's lived experience, you return the smile, take a deep breath, and reflect on the following reflective questions:

What are my beliefs, values, assumptions, and understanding of Indigenous people?

What are my biases around race, gender, and social hierarchies?

How does Peter's knowledge of traditional medicines help to inform his diabetes care?

How do I appreciate strengths when I tend to focus on deficits?

How do I need to respectfully communicate with Peter to ensure cultural safety?

After Peter leaves the clinic, you reflect on this interaction and think about how to expand institutional policies and societal views of Indigenous people.

Land Acknowledgement and Authors' Positionality

It is important to begin this chapter with a land acknowledgement as part of reconciliation to honour the traditional lands, Indigenous Knowledges, and relationships cultivated by Indigenous people for thousands of years. In this way, we humbly and respectfully acknowledge the ancestors, knowledge holders, and lands where we live and work.

In respect for tradition of one's self in place and community, we introduce ourselves, so the reader knows our positionalities and locations (Bourque Bearskin et al., 2020). The authors are Canadian Indigenous and non-Indigenous (Settler) nursing scholars. Bourque Bearskin is a *nêhiyaw-iskwêw* (Cree woman) from Beaver Lake Cree Nation, raised in Métis culture, dedicating her life to nursing with First Nations, Inuit, and Métis communities. As Canadian Institutes of Health Research (CIHR) Indigenous Health Research Chair in Nursing in British Columbia and past president of the Canadian Indigenous Nurses Association, her work stems from the re-member-ing of original healers and helpers to support Indigenous health nursing and the application of Indigenous nursing knowledge to inform renewed Indigenous health governance systems for community wellness. Kennedy is of European Settler and Métis ancestry with traditionally adoptive families from Tsuut'ina Nation and Hawai'i who have supported her cultural reconnection. She is originally from Robinson-Huron Treaty territory and is now a guest on Treaty 7 traditional lands and faculty at Mount Royal University. Her work is focused on advancing equity and reconciliation in nursing, health care, and higher education. Jakubec is of European Settler ancestry, now a visitor in Treaty 7 traditional lands; she is originally from the unceded territory of the Syilx/Okanagan Nation where learning and respect for the land was baked in with the Okanagan sun. She has also lived and learned as a nurse in Treaty 6, in unceded Witsuwit'en territory and alongside Indigenous people in Aotearoa/New Zealand, West Africa, and South India.

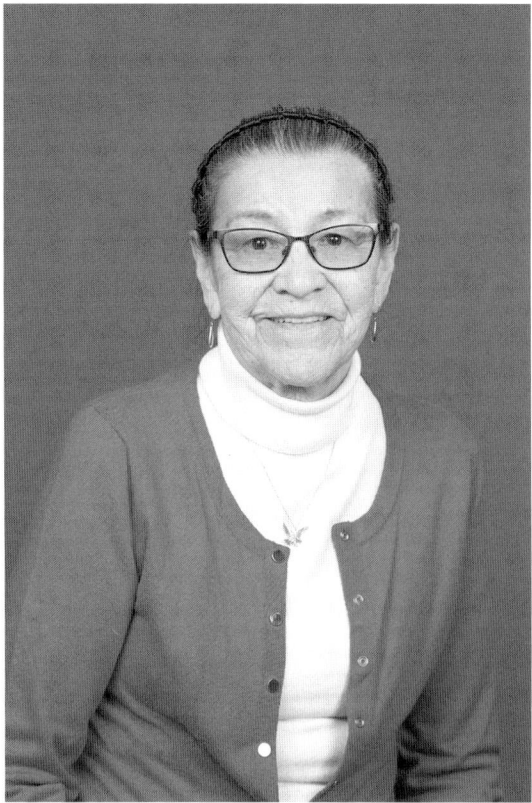

Fig. 9.1 Grandmother Doreen Spence, Saddle Lake Cree Nation. (Courtesy of Doreen Spence.)

We come together with humility and respect for health equity with Indigenous people from across the globe.

This chapter was supported and guided by two highly respected Indigenous Elders. Grandmother Doreen Spence (Saddle Lake Cree Nation) is a traditional healer, retired nurse, member of the Order of Canada, and global human rights advocate (Fig. 9.1). Kupuna Francine Dudoit Tagupa (Hawai'i) is Director of Native Hawaiian Healing at Waikiki Health, traditional healer, nurse, and political activist; she is also the *hanai* (traditionally adoptive) mother to Kennedy (Fig. 9.2). Both Elders have generously offered support to the author team by imparting wisdom from their respective traditions; their teachings are shared throughout this chapter.

As nursing scholars, we have been deeply impacted by dominant Westernized approaches to health care, policies, and evidence-informed practice. Our interdisciplinary experiences have informed this chapter for health care providers. While this discussion is from a critical perspective respecting Indigenous ways, we struggle with Westernized terms such as *knowledge* and *health* to describe related Indigenous concepts. Therefore we offer the following discussion with respect, humility, and ideas in flux as part of our ongoing decolonizing process. We encourage learners to similarly engage in a self-implicated critique: an examination that stresses we all have a position within colonization and responsibility for consciousness and action, to advance decolonization and reconciliation (Andreotti et al., 2015; McGibbon et al., 2013).

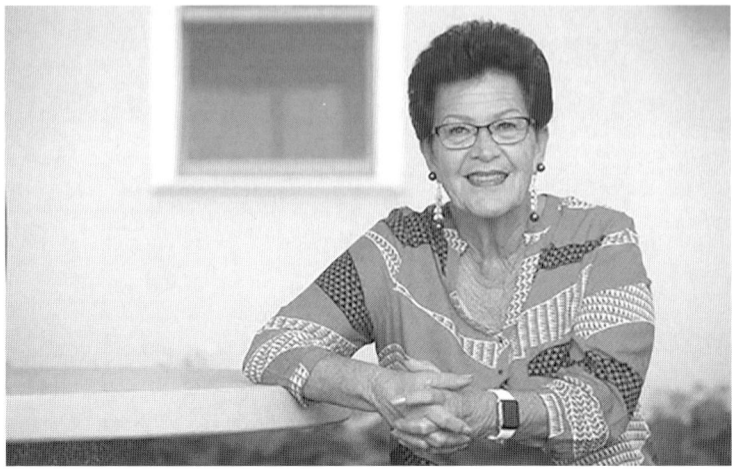

Fig. 9.2 Kupuna Francine Dudoit Tagupa, Hawai'i. (Photo courtesy of Kapuna Francine Dudoit Tagupa.)

We make particular use of several important terms that frame this chapter:

- While we use the term *Indigenous*, we resist a pan-Indigenous approach and respect the diversity of Indigenous people and knowledge systems.
- *Indigenous people* is capitalized for respect and pluralized to acknowledge diversity.
- In Canada, Indigenous people are constitutionally recognized as First Nations, Inuit, and Métis.
- Racialized identities are capitalized for respect and distinction, including "White," "Indigenous," and "Settler."
- The term *Indigenous* is not preferred given links to colonialism and destruction of Indigenous identities, land ownership, language loss, and other oppressive acts.
- The term *Indigenous* is used in keeping with human rights movements, and refers to the original inhabitants across the world, regardless of borders, constitutional, or legal definitions.
- The preferred way of acknowledging Indigenous people is connected to their original communities, such as Tk'emlups te Secwepemc (First Nations), Pangnirtung (Inuit), or Red River Settlement (Métis).
- The term **Indigenous Knowledges** is pluralized to respectfully acknowledge diversity in the knowledge systems of First Nations, Inuit, and Métis people in Canada.

Knowledge, History, and Rights-Based Foundations for Cultural Safety

I have lived through the darkest of times and never thought I would see the day when the rights of Indigenous people were recognized. And in my lifetime, I am beginning to see this change. I have been part of this change for many years. We need to remember that we share this responsibility.

—Grandmother Doreen

This is a critical time in history to recognize that "race" is a colonial Settler concept intended for social division and domination; **racism** results from discrimination of race-related traits, such as physical attributes and culture. While health care providers often focus on the discriminatory interactions of interpersonal racism, we must look more broadly at **systemic racism** "enacted through societal systems, structures, and institutions in the form of requirements, conditions, practices, policies, or processes that maintain and reproduce avoidable and unfair inequalities across ethnic/racial groups" (Paradies et al., 2008, cited by First Nations Health Authority [FNHA], 2018, p. 9). This is important to ensure the health care practice outcome of **cultural safety** "based on respectful engagement that recognizes and strives to address power imbalances inherent in the health care system. It results in an environment free of racism and discrimination, where people feel safe when receiving health care" (FNHA, 2018, p. 5). Recognizing that health is a human right, a rights-based approach prohibits racial discrimination and affords everyone equal protection under the *Charter of Rights and Freedoms* (Government of Canada, 2020). Constructivist and anti-colonial ways of knowing, along with understanding colonial history and Indigenous rights, are foundational to supporting cultural safety and **Indigenous health equity** so that Indigenous people can achieve their full potential: "Globally, health disparities between Indigenous and non-Indigenous populations are ubiquitous and pervasive and are recognized as being unfair, avoidable, and remediable. These inequities exist because of a breach of rights including the right to health. We reaffirm the sovereignty and rights of Indigenous people worldwide, including the right to health" (Jones et al., 2019, p. 512).

CONSTRUCTIVIST KNOWLEDGE

Health care providers are well positioned to engage in a rights-based caring practice. Questioning what practitioners can offer to the growth of healthy people and communities is critical to transforming our collective consciousness. Informed by a constructivist perspective (Lincoln & Guba, 2016), knowledge is constructed through interactions from multiple realities within the context of culture. **Constructivist knowledge** is based on philosophies stemming from social and educational theories of how people learn, act, and relate, based on their own realities (Brandon & All, 2010; Phillips, 2018). Knowledge is historically situated and embedded in cultural values and practices (Lincoln & Guba, 2016). The individual mind is replaced by a concern for relational processes as the foundation for claims of knowledge, truth, objectivity, rationality, and morality (Gergen, 2001, 2007). Health care providers are active agents in constructing, deconstructing, and co-constructing knowledge, which depends on the practitioner's level of community participation and negotiation. From this perspective, practitioners must commit to organizing and questioning information through critical reflective practices including constructive, collaborative, and active inquiry (Antonio, 2019).

Cultural Considerations In Care

Understanding Knowledge and Relationship to Self and Others

My Hawaiian name Makaonaona means "many eyes that see the truth". My grandmother's cultural teachings guide me. I take care of Native people and non-Native people with traditional healing. I also can walk in two worlds and bring in my nursing skills and knowledge of Western medicine. I am a fully integrated practitioner, but I am first and foremost a Native Hawaiian practitioner.

—Kupuna Francine

Reflective practice: Consider how knowledge that may seem very separate or incompatible can come together. Reflect on how contradictions in your own life coexist. How do you experience discord and harmony? How do you integrate or bring together different ways of knowing and different knowledge?

Health care providers are encouraged to respectfully draw from diverse knowledge systems based on how people understand their own lived experiences. Constructivist knowledge generated between people can transform ideas to productive opportunities for social action (Iverson et al., 2005). This practice is vital for understanding people truth within their cultural contexts. When practitioners recognize people as diverse cultural beings, this transforms dialogues where assumptions are explicitly considered and contextualized. This view situates practice in the patient's culture while considering how the determinants of health intersect with the health care system and societal institutional structures (Peters, 2000; Reading, 2015). Consider how revealing a person's cultural identity within the historical context opens reality. Going beyond preconceived notions, this constructivist learning approach strongly positions health care providers to critically examine culture in terms of sociopolitical history and exposes different views of identity (Bourque Bearskin, 2011).

ANTI-COLONIAL KNOWLEDGE

While colonialism seeks to maintain power over Indigenous people, **anti-colonial knowledge** helps health care providers to address the oppression of imposed and unjust colonial rule by challenging assumptions that normalize and privilege them (Van Herk et al., 2011). Application of anti-colonial knowledge reorients understanding of health care systems with respect for Indigenous people as collaborative partners with equal opportunities and rights. Anti-colonialism "recognizes the importance of locally produced knowledge emanating from cultural history and daily human experience and social interactions" (Dei & Asgharzadeh, 2001, p. 300). Power and privilege sanctioned by the state are critically examined along with the perpetuation of inequalities. This dominant discourse often goes unchecked in health care.

Anti-colonial knowledge guides health care providers in an ongoing **decolonization** process to undo the impact of colonialism and dominance over Indigenous people (Canadian Association of Schools of Nursing, 2020). Racism is unjust, maintaining Westernized Eurocentric Whiteness as superior over people who are not White (FNHA, 2018; Waite & Nardi, 2019). Imagine the possibilities for health equity by challenging the denial of colonialism, while opening possibilities for health care providers to decolonize their respective disciplines and practices. This presents an era of reawakening our social consciousness for truth and justice. It is no longer acceptable to provide care based on the dominant and colonial views of society (Griffiths et al., 2016). Growing voices of health care providers and Indigenous people are publicly decrying racism and resisting oppression based on racial differences. The vignette describing the tragic death of Joyce Echaquan in a Quebec hospital while health care providers insulted her and minimized her needs is one example of too common racist abuse. Now is our time to act.

Cultural Considerations In Care

How Do We Learn From Tragedy?

Joyce Echaquan (Manawan First Nation) courageously spoke out, yet tragically died while seeking care amidst an unsafe and racist health care environment at the Joliette Hospital in Quebec. Over centuries, similar events have occurred as described by Grandmother Doreen and the National Inquiry into Missing and Murdered Indigenous Women and Girls (MMIWG, 2019). There is a growing body of evidence related to systemic racism and the adverse impact on Indigenous people health care. Health care providers are called to learn from the tragic story of Brian Sinclair, who was "ignored to death" in a Winnipeg hospital (Brian Sinclair Working Group, 2017) and the dangers of complicity with Indigenous-specific racism "in plain sight" in health care (Turpel-Lafond, 2020).

Reflective practice: What did we learn from these tragedies? What can practitioners do differently to create positive change?

Defining and describing anti-colonial approaches with respect for Indigenous people in Canada is our shared challenge and priority. Positive change will remain hidden in the longstanding denial of colonialism in Canada unless we examine how historic sociopolitical contexts shape health care and society (Decolonial Futures, n.d.). Colonialism is a determinant of health that is embedded in historical trauma (Czyzewski, 2011). Critical self-reflexive analysis is required to disrupt the role of health care providers as colonial agents in reconciliation (Symenuk et al., 2020). This next section highlights the importance of applying *constructivist* and *anti-colonial knowledge* in practice informed by Canadian colonial history. Moving toward a dynamic constructive change, anti-colonialism offers opportunities for practitioners to critique colonial structures and processes.

COLONIALISM AND HISTORICAL KNOWLEDGE

Yes, I am responsible for myself, but my actions are all about being a member of my family and community. Each and every one of us belongs to each other. The land takes care of us all, so we need to take care of the land. You can use anything I have, but it is not yours to take—we share with respect.

—Kupuna Francine

The sociopolitical history of colonialism is deeply rooted in the confederation of Canada when it became an official country in 1867 (Government of Canada, n.d.). Learning chronology and sociopolitical history is essential to understanding the longitudinal impacts on Indigenous people health. The Auditor General's Report on Access to Health Services of First Nations People (2015) outlines injustices of the continued burden of ill health of Indigenous people as compared with the general population. This is manifested by misaligned systems and structures of care and geographic diversity of rural and remote areas where there are increased rates of injury and chronic illness, and access to appropriate health care is grossly insufficient (Nurses and Nurse Practitioners of BC [NNPBC], 2018). Overall, the pervasive influence of colonialism on Indigenous health equity is intertwined with geography, identity, power, displacement, and devolution of **self-determination** to political governance without interference by colonial structures (Cox & Taua, 2017; McKillop et al., 2013). Therefore, health care providers are called to understand colonialism and reflect on how this is misaligned with human rights and professional ethics.

Colonialism is the historical and contemporary use of imposed and unwanted power over the removal of rights to land, culture, and community resources resulting in multigenerational dispossession and dependency on the state by Indigenous people (Alfred, 2009). Important terms to understand include the doctrine of **terra nullius**, which refers to the "principle of 'empty lands' asserting that North America was not populated by humans before the arrival of Europeans" (p. 45). Based on this inaccurate description, the British Crown and Canadian government developed policies to force assimilation and dispossession of Indigenous people through residential schools, Indian hospitals (Lux, 2016), and the *Indian Act* of 1876. This resulted in marginalization of Indigenous people culture, language, and governing laws for education, justice, and health (Borrows, 2016; Goodman et al., 2017).

Treaties

My ancestor Jane Howse was highly respected in our community. She wrote some books in Cree, spoke several languages, and was a translator for the Treaties. However, since she was an Indigenous woman, I am not sure if the White male officials listened to her.

—Grandmother Doreen

Indian and Northern Affairs Canada's long history of treaty-making in Canada is in the foreground of current relationships between Indigenous people and Settlers. Decolonizing, trauma-informed, and culturally safe practices rely on awareness of this history. Early European Settler colonists were supported by imperialist countries to take over the "New World," yet needed support by Indigenous people for survival, to advance the booming fur trade industry, and for military protection of growing colonies. Realization of this critical relationship led to the first **Treaties** as formal agreements initiated by the Crown with Indigenous people.

The Royal Proclamation of 1763 defined the western boundary of the colonies as "Indian Territories"; there could be no settlement or trade without approval from the British Crown's military administration of the Indian Department. This proclamation was the first time the Crown recognized Indigenous people rights to title and lands. Previously, the Indian Department was concerned with the commercial and military assistance that Indigenous people provided to Settler colonists. The Crown's view shifted as more Settlers arrived, and the Indian Department began trying to assimilate "Indians" (Indigenous people). Subsequently, the Robinson–Huron and Robinson–Superior Treaties of 1850 were designed to relinquish lands and rights to the Crown; in return the Anishinaabe Nations (as "Ojibewa Indians") were promised reserves, annuities, and sustained rights to hunt and fish on unoccupied Crown land. These Treaties became the model for the "Numbered Treaties" signed after confederation.

The Dominion of Canada was created in 1867 and the *British North America Act* outlined the Canadian federal government's responsibility for "Indian and Lands reserved for Indians." This was another critical change in the relationship between Indigenous people and Settlers. Subsequently, the Department of Indian Affairs developed the *Indian Act*, which denied Indigenous people basic freedoms by taking control over Indigenous governance, lands, and resources while attempting to strip away language, culture, and identity. In 1896, the Hudson's Bay Company sold the "Rupert's Land Charter" to Canada, which then gained control of most of western Canada. Indigenous people were not consulted, and Indigenous rights to title and lands were now ignored. This provoked the Red River Rebellion led by Louis Riel, which was resolved in 1870 by creating the province of Manitoba. From 1871 to 1921, 11 "Numbered Treaties" were signed in prairies because of epidemics and famine, caused by diminishment of buffalo herds (Indian and Northern Affairs Canada, 2010).

Before European settlement, Indigenous groups were sovereign nations that governed their respective territories (McNeil, 2007). Rights to resources and lands still exist because of precontact sovereignty. With the 1876 *Indian Act*, Canada replaced well-established Indigenous self-governance with a colonial Settler version of elected chief and council with limited power. Yet, traditional systems of Indigenous self-governance persisted and were often concealed from colonial authorities. This speaks to the resilience of Indigenous people throughout attempted assimilation and erasure by colonial Settlers.

From 1927 to 1951, an amendment to the *Indian Act* made it illegal for Indigenous people to hire lawyers for land claims (Henderson & Parrot, 2018). In 1960, status "Indians" were granted the right to vote in the federal election. In 1969, the federal government proposed the "White Paper" to assimilate Indigenous people and repeal the *Indian Act*. Indigenous people were against this proposal and rallied together, demanding that treaty and inherent "Indigenous" rights be respected.

Indigenous people lobbied during the creation of the 1982 *Constitution Act to* make sure Indigenous sovereign and human rights were protected. They were successful with the inclusion of Section 35(1) stating that "The existing Indigenous and treaty rights of the Indigenous people (First Nations, Inuit and Métis) of Canada are hereby recognized and affirmed" (McNeil, 2007). Recognition of First Nations Treaty rights was a major milestone that continues to shape dialogue and legal battles for Indigenous rights. Colonial frontier logic characterized Canada as uninhabited land (Donald, 2012). This signalled a symbolic narrative among Settlers to purchase large amounts of land in the name of progress, while literally relegating Indigenous people to ditches. These margins gave way to the "roadside allowance people," also known as Métis, who established their own settlements and distinct way of life (Campbell, 1995). Health care providers should consider how denying Indigenous people right to self-determination negatively impacts health outcomes (United Nations [UN], 2007).

Residential Schools

The babies—keiki—the children are most cherished because they are our future generation and how our culture is propagated and perpetuated. Our culture is done if we do not take care of them.

—Kupuna Francine

Residential schools will forever leave a stain on our collective existence. On May 27, 2021 (Tk'emlúps te Secwépemc, 2021), the Tk'emlups te Secwepemc Kukpi7 (Chief), Chief Rosanne Casimir, announced the discovery of 215 unmarked children's grave sites at the old Kamloops Indian Residential School in British Columbia. This news shook most Canadians to their core. This discovery has intensified the pain experienced by Indigenous people, while validating what had long been described by people impacted by the historical and contemporary trauma (Newton, 2021). The Truth and Reconciliation Commission of Canada's (TRC, 2015) final report regarding residential schools elevated critical social understanding of the government-mandated, church-run **residential school system** for Indigenous people who had no desire to be assimilated. Tragically, this colonial assimilation policy led to **genocide** as "coordinated actions aimed at the destruction of [Indigenous people]" (National Inquiry into Missing and Murdered Indigenous Women and Girls [MMIWG], 2019, p. 50). The first residential school opened in the 1820s. Starting at the tender age of 5 years, children were forcibly taken away from their families and homes to be schooled in a foreign language within Western colonial society. Residential schools were seen as a way to solve the "problem" of Indigenous independence and "savagery." Many children suffered the loss of identity, language, and cultural teachings from their parents, grandparents, and community. It was not until 1998 that the last residential school was closed.

In 2007, the Indian Residential Schools Settlement Agreement with residential school survivors was established in response to the largest class action suit in Canadian history. In 2008, Prime Minister Stephen Harper offered a full apology on behalf of Canadians for the Indian residential school system; yet at a G20 Summit meeting in 2009, this same prime minister denied colonialism in Canada (Wherry, 2009). Despite the material reality and discoveries of thousands of unmarked graves at residential schools across the country, systemic denial perpetuates harm by rendering colonialism invisible (and therefore untouchable).

Amidst this denial, strength prevails with collective healing among Indigenous people, who are speaking their truths as first- and second-generation children of residential school survivors. The devastating impacts of residential schools are countered by survivors who courageously share their residential school experiences and stories of intergenerational trauma, while noting how Indigenous traditional culture is a key intervention for healing (Methot, 2019).

Sixties Scoop

The **Sixties Scoop** describes cultural genocide in Canada that peaked in the 1960s when thousands of First Nations, Inuit, and Métis children were removed from birth families and placed in non-Indigenous environments (Sinclair, 2007). In 1951, a new section of the *Indian Act* granted the Canadian provinces and territories jurisdiction over child welfare, leading to the removal of Indigenous children from their homes and communities. This was experienced more on reserves given poor health and living conditions stemming from colonial policies (National Collaborating Centre for Indigenous Health, 2017). By the 1980s, Indigenous communities began developing their own child and family services for people living on and off reserve (National Collaborating Centre for Indigenous Health, 2017). While these agencies aimed to provide culturally appropriate and holistic services, they had limited impact because of colonial legislation and funding shortages (Blackstock, 2009). Health care providers need to acknowledge the truth of these historic events, address systemic racism, and resist blaming Indigenous people for poor health outcomes.

Present-Day Indigenous Child Apprehension

The TRC (2015) noted that despite the closure of residential schools, Indigenous children were still being removed from their families and communities—just through a different means. Based on the 2016 census, Indigenous children represent 7.7% of the population yet comprise 55.2% of children in the foster care system (Indigenous Services Canada, 2021). This over-representation of Indigenous child apprehension is related to intergenerational trauma from assimilation practices and policies such as residential schools and the Sixties Scoop. The current proportion of Indigenous children in child welfare has reached alarming record levels, exceeding those during the Sixties Scoop and the period of residential schools (Blackstock, 2003). Although numerous Indigenous communities now have jurisdiction over child and family social services, many communities are not able to meet the needs of Indigenous people or provide culturally relevant care (National Collaborating Centre for Indigenous Health, 2017). We need to respond to this crisis through social justice aims and critically examine how present-day child welfare policies are rooted in colonial assimilation.

WHITE SUPREMACY AND RACISM

We are all equal. No one is above or below anyone else.

—Grandmother Doreen

White supremacy is a colonial Settler racist ideology that people who are not White are inferior, providing justification for maintaining power, wealth, and status by White people. This racial contract (Mills, 1997) organizes social and political contexts for White dominance over Black people, Indigenous people, and People(s) of Colour (BIPOC) (Dumbrill & Ying Yee, 2019). Dominant Whiteness places Western culture and beliefs as the societal standard; this standard authorizes Whiteness as a superior racialized identity driving White privilege (Diangelo, 2018). Health care providers are faced with an important opportunity to check their own social position and privilege.

Rather than normalizing racism as an individual moral defect, systemic racism is understood through **intersectionality** of race with gender, abilities, age, and social identity that privileges Western ways of being, knowing, and doing (Van Herk et al., 2011). How we respond to racial differences is connected to the **structural violence** within systems, including health, education, economics, and legal, and the political intentions of society (Dei, 1996; Diangelo, 2018). Ongoing dominance of Whiteness is created through racial discourses to "legitimize racial inequalities, and to protect white advantage" (Diangelo, 2018, p. 17). For example, "dominionization" is a social process that privileges Western knowledge systems with entrenched ownership of expertise in mainstream academic institutions (McGowan et al., 2020). Realizing how White privilege is entrenched in systems structures helps us to understand why reports of longstanding oppression against Indigenous people often result in little action. Health care providers should consider the MMIWG (2019) Calls for Justice and the TRC (2015) Calls to Action to guide practice toward positive change for equity within insidious health systems (Downey, 2020; Jones et al., 2019).

Canadian compliance with White supremacy resulted in the genocide of Indigenous people (MMIWG, 2019; Starblanket, 2020). The continuance of policies such as legislated identities, the *Indian Act*, and Non-Insured Health Benefit Programs impact the delivery of Indigenous health care, education, judicial, and social services. If left unchallenged, this manifestation of racism will continue to widen the health inequities gap between Indigenous and non-Indigenous people (Starblanket, 2020). Ignoring the racist harms of White supremacy is contrary to the Canadian Nursing Association's (CNA, 2017) *Code of Ethics* to "uphold principles of justice by safeguarding human rights, equity and fairness and by promoting the public good" (p. 15). Rather than hide in denial, health care providers are encouraged to examine the implications of colonial White supremacy on Indigenous people.

OPPRESSION

We need to all be sitting at the same table together and have our voices heard as equals. Not just Indigenous to Indigenous, or non-Indigenous to non-Indigenous, but all of us who live and work together as free people. We need to do what we do best - love each other and our work. We are not being loving if we ignore when somebody is hurting somebody and making them small and not respecting their freedom - we have to be in the truth, speak up and act for the greater good.

—Kupuna Francine

Oppression refers to a pressing down, a burdening, and an overpowering (Chambers Dictionary of Etymology, 2006), indicating an unjust exercise of power (Merriam-Webster, 2020). We must understand the challenges associated with colonialism and racialization to appreciate how identity politics is embedded in Indigenous people colonial history and health outcomes (Griffiths et al., 2016). Critical analysis of oppression in anti-racist education highlights cultural differences justifying inequality of Indigenous people well beyond cross-cultural misunderstanding (St. Denis, 2007). There is a serious need to recognize the conditions and effects of colonial oppression. For example, the education of First Nations, Inuit, and Métis people is often described as a "value conflict" between European and other cultures; this inaccurately suggests that inequality is an inevitable effect of different orientations to work, education, and family. When adverse conditions and effects are attributed to a "conflict of values," and interventions such as cross-cultural training are employed, these strategies have little impact on systems transformation. Such individuated interventions ultimately dislocate and minimize the harm of oppression, rendering colonial Whiteness invisible, further entrenching the status quo of structural inequities. In short, systemic problems require systemic solutions.

In attempts to debunk the hegemony of institutional governance and Whiteness in health care, Van Herk et al. (2011) examined how race, gender, and class intersect with Indigenous women's well-being; findings revealed barriers to relational practice and identified how the structures of power, equity, and social injustice are maintained. This signals an important starting point for health care providers to attend to their own social location and position within the care relationship. Understanding assumptions in how oppression operates at the individual level through prejudices shows how biases (unconscious/conscious) inform our practice and provide a glimpse into systemic challenges.

To move from colonization to decolonization, anti-oppression must be named and identified at individual and societal levels. Hope may be realized by creating a safe space and honoured place in our history for the truthful stories of trauma experienced by Indigenous populations. The individual and collective response of health care providers who enact the Calls to Action (TRC, 2015) and Calls to Justice (MMIWG, 2019) offers meaningful steps toward equity with Indigenous people as outlined in the Government of Canada's (2020) *Charter of Rights and Freedoms* and the UN (2007) *Declaration on the Rights of Indigenous People* (UNDRIP).

RIGHTS AND JUSTICE

I spent decades working as an Elder with the United Nations to make sure the voices of Indigenous people were heard. Everyone from around the globe needs to pay attention to how the Declaration of Rights on Indigenous People protects our cultural identity. We do not have to justify our existence or apologize for speaking up if these rights are not respected.

—Grandmother Doreen

"Cultural rights are of particular relevance for Indigenous people given that indigenous people are culturally distinct from the majority societies in which they live. Cultural rights involve protection for traditional and religious practices, languages, sacred sites, cultural heritage, intellectual property, oral and traditional history, etc. And, economic, social, and cultural rights are deeply rooted in the lands, territories and resources as well as the lifeways of indigenous people." (UN, 2015, p. 1).

The UN (2007) Declaration on the Rights of Indigenous People emphasizes cultural rights as indispensable to the survival, dignity, and well-being of Indigenous people. A rights-based approach provides a framework ensuring Indigenous people remain distinct to pursue economic, social, education, and health priorities. Understanding Indigenous people human rights and leg-islated identities is key to culturally safe care. According to Statistics Canada (2016), Indigenous people represent 4.9% of the overall Canadian population as three distinct groups: First Nations (58.4%), Inuit (3.9%), and Métis (35.1%). An additional 2.7% represent different or multiple Indigenous origins. There are over 700 different First Nations communities and 70 languages. The Indigenous population is the youngest and fastest growing population in Canada.

The World Health Organization (WHO, 2017, 2020) constitution is built on the premise that health is a "basic human right" as a holistic "state of complete physical, mental, and social well-being and not merely the absence of disease or infirmity" (para 1). These two key features of "rights" and "wholism" are interpreted by complex factors known as the social determinants of health (Reading & Wien, 2009, 2013). Health care providers often readily see the "proxi-mal" determinants of health with political, social, and economic origins and need to further respect the impact of deeper "distal" determinants of Indigenous health, including self-gov-ernance, colonialism, globalization, poverty, and cultural continuity. "Distal" determinants are also known as "root causes" of deeply embedded inequities in the historical and current socio-political context. Key strategies in addressing distal determinants of health requires training addressing Indigenous-specific racism. In British Columbia, a government-sponsored health care study revealed that 80% of Indigenous people experienced racism, with clear links between "colonial attitudes and beliefs that underpin the healthcare system, and cause harm and suffer-ing to Indigenous people" (Turpel-Lafond, 2020, p. 53). Health care providers are encouraged to engaged in a rights-based approach to disrupt racism, which is often taken for granted and fuelled by longstanding patterns.

From this perspective of relationality, consider how colonial Settler ways of being, knowing, and doing perpetuate White supremacy, privilege, and racism. The following section offers an alternative to oppression through a rights-based approach that respects Indigenous Knowledges as a foundation of health among Indigenous people.

Indigenous Knowledges for Health and Wellness

This is about relationships – living our lives in a good way according to the values of Kisewatisiwin with loving gentle kindness of caring for each other, our nations, communities and all beings.

—Grandmother Doreen

In this section, we focus on Indigenous ways of being, knowing, and doing in relationship with Indigenous people. We are concerned that non-Indigenous health care providers are striving to adopt Indigenous Knowledges without establishing authentic relationships, which is core to nurs-ing practice. Practicing in the spirit of reconciliation, health care providers are called to develop anti-colonial approaches that support Indigenous people who are reclaiming Indigenous ways of knowing. Diverse place-based Indigenous Knowledges are the basis for Indigenous health, well-ness, and traditional healing; this connection is key to upholding human rights and advancing health equity with Indigenous people who thrived for thousands of years pre-contact. However, Settler colonization and Eurocentric ways of being, knowing, and doing often go unchecked, thus implicitly and explicitly marginalizing non-Westernized knowledge systems. Colonial diminishing of Indigenous Knowledges violates the rights of Indigenous people to engage in traditional ways of being, knowing, and doing to advance health, wellness, and healing. Rather than rejecting Western ways, we are advocating for mutual understanding and intercultural co-learning to respectfully uphold human rights and advance health equity with Indigenous people (Blignault et al., 2018; Sherwood et al., 2011).

While Indigenous rights are clearly defined in the Canadian Treaties and the UNDRIP (2007), Indigenous knowledge systems are often marginalized in mainstream health care. Colonial harms may be countered by a relational ethic (Bourque Bearskin, 2011) that recognizes how Indigenous knowledge systems and healing practices are key to achieving Indigenous health equity. Health care providers have a shared opportunity to advance health equity through "ethical space" (Ermine, 2007) at the intersection of Western and Indigenous ways of being, knowing, and doing. Hence, this section first emphasizes *how* we respectfully engage with Indigenous people, followed by a discussion on Indigenous Knowledges and traditional healing practices.

ETHICAL SPACE

All of humanity is one. No one is above or below another. But that does not mean we are the same. Indigenous people have a different way of understanding the world because of our connection to the land and all beings. And we need to have different ways of seeing things so that all of humanity can all help each other.

—Grandmother Doreen

Ethical space honours the equality of people with disparate knowledge systems. Western and Indigenous knowledge systems have different intentions and assumptions that influence the relationality of an "ethical space of engagement" (Ermine, 2007). This requires respectful acceptance of differences without defaulting to Westernized views as the sanctioned "truth." "Ethical space is generated when both parties acknowledge these differences, as a first step, and navigate ways to work together through humility, honesty and commitment. Ultimately, dialogue within an ethical space leads to an agreement to interact across the cultural divide" (Alberta Health Services, 2018, p. 10). **Ethical space** is a "neutral zone between entities or cultures" (Ermine, 2007, p. 202) which offers an opening for reconciliation through mutual respect: "no one is above or below another—we are equals" (personal communication, Grandmother Doreen Spence, 2020).

Considering Indigenous people rights (UN, 2007) and how health is a human right (WHO, 2017), we are called to an "ethical space of engagement" (Ermine, 2007) between Western and Indigenous Knowledges. Amidst cultural differences, an authentic relationship of equals is possible through mutually respectful relationships (Bourque Bearskin, 2011; Deloria, 1999; Ermine, 2007). Moreover, ethical space requires healthy boundaries that honour how Indigenous Knowledges cannot be acquired, extracted, or mastered in the Western sense. Rather, health care providers are called to critically examine the "undercurrent" (Ermine, 2007, p. 197) of historical and social factors that reinforce "unchecked" (p. 198) Westernized views. Self-implicated critique is important in order to consider beliefs, attitudes, and values that shape how we see "truth" as the basis for evidence-informed practice. Ethical space requires an anti-colonial approach recognizing the merit of Indigenous Knowledges, with an ongoing commitment to future generations of Indigenous people for wellness and self-determination.

An anti-colonial relational ethic also requires communication that is mutually clear and respectful, practices explored later in this chapter. "Rules of engagement" (Ermine, 2007, p. 200) in communication support cultural rights and are "informed and asserted through Indigenous knowledge" (p. 201). Mere inclusion of Indigenous content or consultation is not enough; ethical space calls for a greater "radical reform" (Andreotti et al., 2015, p. 25) with transformative change that respectfully engages with Indigenous people and knowledge systems. In contrast to Westernized education, Indigenous Knowledges are based on a grassroots stronghold in relationship with Elders and knowledge holders who preserve land and language for the wellness of Indigenous people (Deloria, 1999). Relationship is the starting place of Indigenous Knowledges, in the same way that land is the starting place of decolonization. Examining yourself and relationships through questions such as those in the following Cultural Consideration in Care box provides a place for self-awareness that establishes the possibility for respectful engagement with Indigenous Knowledges.

Cultural Considerations In Care

Self-awareness: Examining You and Your Relationships

Whatever your experience, it is important to pause and reflect on the challenges and strengths needed to develop respectful relationships with Indigenous people; then consider how to extend perspectives of developing different ways of knowing.

Reflective questions: Do you feel yourself leaning in with curiosity? Do you sense impatience to "just get to the point" as you seek to learn about Indigenous Knowledges?

INDIGENOUS KNOWLEDGES

What is Indigenous Knowledge? You know we don't talk like that, but you can talk like that if it helps to build a bridge. It's not about what we know, it's about what we do for the good of the land and the people. It's about propagating, protecting and perpetuating culture for those reasons. We are all connected and responsible for each other.

—Kupuna Francine

Indigenous Knowledges have been "systematically excluded" (Battiste, 2013, p. 115) from contemporary education and health care. Considering such exclusion, we need to resist defining, evaluating, and assimilating Indigenous Knowledges from a Westernized worldview and process. The following introduction to Indigenous Knowledges respects complex inter-relatedness with Indigenous people health; however, it is not the role of non-Indigenous health care providers to adopt Indigenous Knowledges as part of their practice. Rather, it is the responsibility of health care providers to create ethical space for Indigenous people to reclaim their knowledge systems and healing practices. "Indigenous knowledge as a distinct knowledge system … is the expression of the vibrant relationships between the people, their ecosystems and the other living beings and spirits that share their lands" (Battiste & Youngblood Henderson 2000, p. 39–42).

Knowing is dynamic and situated in direct experience, focusing on *how one knows* through direct experiences rather than *what one knows*. Indigenous Knowledges and "truths" are dynamic, subjective, contextual, relational and mutualistic in a "self-generating path …. [of vast] ecologies and their forces" (Battiste & Youngblood Henderson, 2000, p. 39). Thus Indigenous Knowledges do not fit into a reduced compartment of Westernized definitions. Rather, Indigenous Knowledges are developed through direct participation with the natural world as relational ecologies that are place-based, active, circular, intergenerational, community-derived, and holistic (Battiste, 2013; Ermine, 1995). "Indigenous knowledge is fundamentally relational, linked to the land, language, and the intergenerational transmission of songs, ceremonies, protocols, and ways of life" (Greenwood & Lindsay, 2019, p. 82).

Indigenous Knowledges are based on a worldview linked to the ecosystem, with reality structured by language and shared responsibility between generations to care for traditional knowledge (Battiste, 2013; Battiste & Youngblood Henderson, 2000). Indigenous worldview focuses on developing an introspective "inner space" that extends outward in relationship with the natural world; this is held in tension with Western knowledge for dominance that often fragments and conquers "outer space" (Ermine, 1995, p. 101).

Since Indigenous Knowledges are developed through relationships with local ecosystems and processes, learners need to engage with local Indigenous knowledge holders (Smylie ct al., 2009). Considering that Indigenous Knowledges are generated in the community, related learning displaced in the Western academy or health system may "fall short" (Smylie et al., 2014, p. 17). We recognize this as an opportunity to develop new intercultural co-learning relationships (Sherwood et al., 2011) which may include "building a contemporary evidence base on all aspects of healthcare including use of traditional healing" (Blignault et al., 2018, p. 1355). Innovation is needed for positive change to challenge the Western status quo through respectful engagement with Indigenous people and knowledge systems. The following reflective practice on cultural care offers a point of entry to respectful engagement with Indigenous people and knowledge systems for health.

Cultural Considerations In Care

Challenging Status Quo Western Dominance

Health care based on Westernized knowledge, practices, and policies is viewed as "mainstream" and integral for all people. Traditional healing based on Indigenous Knowledges is also integral for Indigenous people, yet marginalized as "complementary."

Reflective questions: Consider how you have come to know what health and well-being are and what best practices should be. What knowledge dominates and what is diminished? How may we engage in ethical space, challenge colonial status quo, and resist dominance and diminishing of what is known?

Indigenous Knowledges for Health, Wellness, and Healing

Cultural [traditional] medicine can be integrated with western medicine, and this needs trust and relationships between the practitioners for the good of the client. This is not about being stuck in one world. We need to work together and help the people with all of our gifts and talents. But know that we have different gifts and this needs to be respected. The western world can't take this away from us because it comes from the community and culture and the land.

—Kupuna Francine

Indigenous people view health as an ongoing action through individual agency and collective responsibility grounded in place-based Indigenous Knowledges (Battiste & Youngblood Henderson, 2000). "The old paradigm of ascribed wellness, atikowisi miýw-āyāwin, where health and wellness are granted by outside sources, has to be replaced by the new paradigm kaskitmasowin miýw-āyāwin-achieved wellness, where health and wellness are earned through individual autonomy and creative genius to the fullest extent possible" (Dion Stout, 2012, p. 13).

Holistic well-being of mind, body, emotions, and spirit (Boot & Lowell, 2019; Isaak & Marchessault, 2008) is dynamic given the interconnected relationships of inner and outer worlds (Ermine, 1995). Active participation in health is circular and collaborative in essence (wholeness) and direction (ongoing change); thus the whole person is engaged in co-learning through animating wellness practices. This is not about "getting it right," but rather about moving forward in a good way with evolving understanding and action.

Many Indigenous groups have teachings and images to represent dynamic holistic health, including the First Nations Perspective on Health and Wellness (FNHA, 2020) (Fig. 9.3).

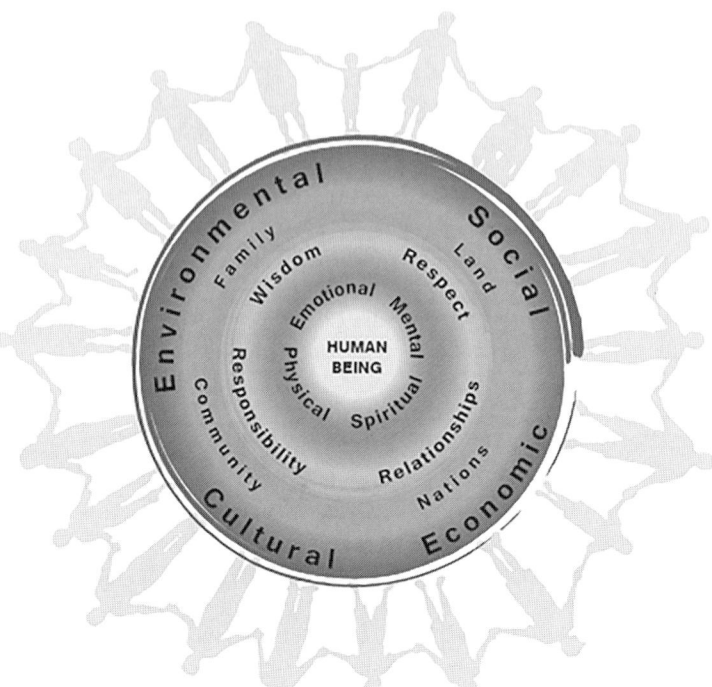

Fig. 9.3 First Nations Perspective on Health and Wellness. (From First Nations Health Authority. [2021]. https://www.fnha.ca/wellness/wellness-and-the-first-nations-health-authority/first-nations-perspective-on-wellness.)

This may be contrasted with a Westernized understanding of Indigenous health and wellness indicators of "demographics, health status and outcomes, determinants of health, and health system performance" (Government of Canada, 2018, para 1). Such contrasts are important "ethical space" reminders to respectfully acknowledge distinct Western and Indigenous Knowledges. At this intersection, intercultural co-learning is a necessary step toward Indigenous health equity. For example, Kílala Lelum is an Urban Indigenous Health and Healing Cooperative that works in partnership with Indigenous Elders and health care providers to provide holistic community care in Vancouver's Downtown Eastside. While the Cooperative has a complex model of care, their logo (https://kilala-lelum.ca/), designed by Coast Salish artist Chrystal Sparrow, reflects how people may transform—like the butterfly—on their healing paths. The symbol also represents the medicine wheel, the land and seasonality, and holistic (mental, physical, spiritual) aspects of health (Kilala Lelum, n.d.).

Land and language are the source of Indigenous Knowledges for health, wellness, and healing (Battiste & Youngblood Henderson, 2000; Lamouche, 2010; Robbins & Dewar, 2011). Reclaiming identity and knowledge systems is key to advancing health with Indigenous people and requires connecting Indigenous-informed evidence to guide Indigenous health promotion (Greenwood & Lindsay, 2019). Wellness is understood through local Indigenous Knowledge, which revitalizes empowerment and identity: "Indigenous community is the primary expression of a natural context and environment where exists the fundamental right of personhood to be what one is meant to be" (Ermine, 2007, p. 200). "Land, health, and knowledge are so closely intertwined for Indigenous people that it is impossible to consider any of them in isolation of the others. Indigenous knowledge and Indigenous health are both deeply rooted in the land—nurturing and protecting both requires nurturing and protecting the land" (Greenwood & Lindsay, 2019, p. 84).

Indigenous Knowledges for well-being are embedded in dependent relationships with ecosystems including land, waterways, persons, plants, and animals (Battiste & Youngblood Henderson, 2000). Indigenous health knowledge is rooted in the land and shared within families, communities, traditional ceremonies, and medicines that reflect relationships with local ecosystems (Smylie et al., 2014). Indigenous Knowledges extend current Western understanding of health by emphasizing individual agency and collective responsibility in direct relationship with the natural world. Indigenous-informed health literacy "is critical to decolonising health care … to access, appraise, and communicate health-related information, to navigate and engage with the healthcare system, and to advocate and maintain personal and community health and wellbeing" (Boot & Lowell, 2019, p. 2).

Indigenous Wellness and Healing Practices

I learned from my grannies who raised me in the bush. I retired from nursing, but you don't ever retire from traditional healing and supporting the community.

—Grandmother Doreen

You don't learn traditional healing from a book. You learn by working from healers recognized by the community. My grandmother was a healer and she raised me to do what she did for the people. This takes years and years. I had no choice. This is my kuleana [responsibility and privilege].

—Kupuna Francine

In this section, we will focus on Indigenous wellness and healing practices stemming from place-based Indigenous Knowledges. Indigenous traditional wellness is globally supported from a rights-based approach given in the UNDRIP: "Article 24. Indigenous people have the right to their traditional medicines and to maintain their health practices, including the conservation of their vital medicinal plants, animals and minerals. Indigenous individuals also have the right to access, without any discrimination, to all social and health services" (UN, 2007, p. 18).

As equals, we are called to respect Indigenous Knowledges and not relegate Indigenous traditional healing as "complementary," "integrative," or "folk medicine" in a downgraded comparison with Western approaches. Indigenous Knowledges are an "invaluable resource in addressing the global health crisis in low- and middle-income countries (Blignault et al., 2018, p. 1355). Holistic Indigenous Knowledge–based health practices are related to "preventative and long-lasting health benefits … [including] the potential to strengthen culturally safe practices and opportunities for self-determination, enhance health communication, and to foster relationships that are built on trust and mutual respect" (Boot & Lowell, 2019, p. 3). Furthermore, since health care providers are mainly educated in a Westernized system, it may be challenging—but necessary—to acknowledge the differences between Westernized institutional health spaces and Indigenous healing ecosystems (Robbins & Dewar, 2011). It is, however, not for non-Indigenous people to integrate *into* medical models. Rather, the respect, awareness, and freedoms for Indigenous people to learn and practice their own healing modalities will enable Indigenous Knowledge–based practices to, in turn, enable traditional health and well-being. "Traditional wellness is a term that encompasses traditional medicines, practices, approaches and knowledge. Traditional wellness is based on a holistic model of health and is often overlooked in the prevention and treatment of chronic conditions and in the promotion of health and wellness. Traditional medicines and practices are found worldwide in Indigenous communities. In many developing countries, it is the primary health option" (FNHA, 2014, p. 13).

Traditional wellness encompassing traditional medicine and healing practices is understood from a local context. There is a persistent barrier among health care providers who marginalize traditional healing practices. This barrier may be addressed through an ongoing process of "self-reflection to understand personal and systemic biases and to develop and maintain respectful processes and relationships based on mutual trust. **Cultural humility** involves humbly acknowledging oneself as a learner when it comes to understanding another's experience" (FNHA, 2018, p. 7). Such bridging is based on health care that "*respect* [patients] for who they are, that is *relevant* to their view of the world, that offers *reciprocity* in their relationships with others, and that helps them exercise *responsibility* over their own lives" (Kirkness & Barnhardt, 2001, p. 1). Practitioners need to resist Westernized inclusion of Indigenous Knowledges in health care as a "benevolent gift" (Stein & Andreotti, 2016, p. 373). Furthermore, equitable access to traditional medicine needs to be considered on the primary health care continuum by considering the power structures and knowledge ownership in health care systems (Redvers et al., 2019).

In a Canadian study by Zubek (1994) on family physicians' understanding and attitudes toward traditional healing, respondents lacked awareness of Indigenous healing methods and strongly disagreed "with their patients' use of traditional Native medicines in hospitals" (p. 1928). A more recent study surveyed arthritis health care providers' awareness of traditional healing practices including herbal, ceremonial/spiritual, and wellness counselling (Logan et al., 2020). Similarly, participants reported being "unclear or unaware of what Indigenous healing practices were" (p. e5), yet "expressed interest in the concept of creating space for Indigenous healing practices" (p. e5). While this shift may seem promising, findings revealed that inclusion of Indigenous healing practices is implemented "but with a colonial construct of medicine, demonstration of an evidence bias, and hierarchy of medicine" (p. e5). We need to move beyond mere inclusion of Indigenous Knowledges and traditional healing and respect that such ways of being, knowing, and doing are critical to the wellness of Indigenous people.

Ongoing collaboration among health care educators, professionals, service providers, policymakers, and community members are encouraged so that Indigenous people health needs are supported by traditional healing. In collaboration with community members and key stakeholders, the FNHA (2014) established directives to "protect, incorporate and promote First Nations knowledge, beliefs, values, practices, medicines and models of health and healing into all health programs and services that serve BC [British Columbia] First Nations" (p. 6). Traditional wellness is guided by four key values: respect, wisdom, responsibility, and relationships (FNHA, 2014, p. 25). A traditional wellness strategy framework was developed with five key objectives:

1. Support Building Understanding
2. Develop Knowledge Resources
3. Increase Knowledge Transfer
4. Promote Partnership
5. Advocate and Support Traditional Healers and Communities (FNHA, 2014, p. 29)

This framework exemplifies the ethical space of engagement that respects the integrity of Indigenous Knowledges at the intersection of Westernized health care. Health care providers are encouraged to consider how Indigenous and non-Indigenous practitioners have a shared role in promoting traditional healing, with an ethical space of engagement for Indigenous-led health care partnerships. Anti-colonial efforts to uphold such innovations may be supported by challenging Westernized assumptions and respectfully engaging with Indigenous Knowledges to restore and sustain wellness (Saskamoose et al., 2017; St. Denis & Walsh, 2017).

In concluding this section, we invite further reflection on the unique challenges faced by Indigenous health care providers in "accessing and applying Indigenous and Western Knowledges in their practice" (Rogers et al., 2019, p. 9). Consider the impact of Indigenous-specific racism in interpersonal encounters with patients and colleagues; this is further compounded by structural discrimination that is within institutional practices and policies (Allan & Smylie, 2015; Bond et al., 2019). Critical examination of our social and institutional processes is necessary to create positive change that protects Indigenous human rights to a safe space and place for Indigenous Knowledges and traditional healing for patients and providers alike.

Structural Competency and Strengths-Based Approaches

While interpersonal relational efforts are often emphasized, we must also consider how to advance Indigenous health at a systems level through key **structural competencies**:

1. Recognizing the structures that shape clinical interactions
2. Developing an extra-clinical language of structure
3. Rearticulating "cultural" formulations in structural terms
4. Observing and imagining structural interventions
5. Developing structural humility (Metzl & Hansen, 2014, p. 126)

From a structural competency lens, acknowledging the systemic impact on Indigenous people health from historical and social contexts enables movement toward health care framed by equity (Crowshoe et al., 2019). In this movement, we need to consider the strengths of Indigenous people, held in tension with the structural inequities imposed by society.

For example, in Canada it was illegal for Indigenous people to speak their language or practice traditional healing until the 1950s (Robbins & Dewar, 2011). Societal norms and structures perpetuate Indigenous-specific racism. An important anti-colonial challenge for health care providers is to focus on the inherent value of Indigenous people and Knowledges, while also attending to the structural inequities that perpetuate health disparities (Fogarty et al., 2018). Indigenous people face an unequal distribution of health resources and high illness burden amidst "power imbalances … and institutional discrimination" (Smylie et al., 2014, p. 18). To move past victim blaming, we need to try to locate the root of Indigenous health disparities within historical, societal and institutional structures. Widespread institutional support, strategic planning, policy, and intensive community engagement is imperative for this education and to result in culturally safe practice (Kurtz et al., 2018). This education and movement may also be supported by strengths-based approaches, such as resiliency to guide efforts in Indigenous health promotion, including trauma-informed care.

Cultural Considerations In Care

Choose to See Strengths

With a focus on Indigenous Knowledges and a goal of culturally safe practice, Indigenous perspectives must include strengths while not losing sight of health disparities.

To this end, search perspectives and accounts that uphold strengths. For example, review the First Nations Health Authority (2020) First Nations Perspective on Health and Wellness: https://www.fnha.ca/wellness/wellness-and-the-first-nations-health-authority/first-nations-perspective-on-wellness.

Reflective questions: Thinking of Indigenous Knowledges and health, what strengths do you recognize in this framework? How can strengths be highlighted and supported as individual, community, and system sites of practice?

RESILIENCE AND TRAUMA-INFORMED CARE

In Hawaiian, "imua" is about the encouragement and lesson to always move forward with strength. One of our greatest strengths is learning to love ourselves so that we can truly love others, be free, and do what we are meant to do.

—Kupuna Francine

In this section, we will focus on strengths-based approaches to equity and empowerment among Indigenous people through resilience and trauma-informed care. This may be achieved in partnership with Indigenous people through critical review of communication, programs, and policies that

1. Recognize positive experiences and attributes that facilitate wellness
2. Centre good relations with Indigenous people
3. Recentre power relationships and self-determination
4. Attend to structural determinants of health (Askew, 2020; Kennedy et al., 2020)

We may extend our capacity as health care providers by employing a strengths-based approach to address structural determinants of Indigenous health. These skills remain rooted in human rights and respectful engagement with Indigenous people and Knowledges as the basis for health.

Resilience

When I am having a tough time, I pray and ask for guidance from Creator. I give humble gratitude for my life and know that I am never alone. Remember to ask for help when you need it. We can all help each other, and we all need help from each other. This is another way that we are all equals. This is from a place of love.

—Grandmother Doreen

Strengths-based approaches refer to a variety of practices that focus on positive attributes of human flourishing to create and sustain health, while still acknowledging systemic health disparities (Fogarty et al., 2018). Since Indigenous Knowledges are local, strengths are understood within a place-based context. Health care providers are cautioned against imposing Westernized values that determine "strengths." It is important to understand how Indigenous people themselves describe their own strengths (Askew et al., 2020).

Indigenous resilience "is based on Indigenous people innate capacities and focuses on success rather than overcoming challenges" (McGuire, 2010, p. 121). The concept of resilience has been described within various Indigenous contexts (Hansen & Antsanen, 2016; Kirmayer et al., 2011; McGuire, 2010), reiterating how resilience is understood through local Indigenous Knowledges as direct experiences that support Indigenous identity and health.

Resilience is a place-based, holistic, and relational process "that can be acquired and developed" (Hansen & Antsanen, 2016, p. 1). A Canadian study with several diverse Indigenous communities on the "Roots of Resilience" (Kirmayer et al., 2011) resulted in a framework to guide local interpretation of four main Indigenous resilience processes:

1. Regulating emotion and supporting adaptation through relational, ecocentric, and cosmo-centric concepts of self and personhood
2. Revisioning collective history in ways that valorize collective identity
3. Revitalizing language and culture as resources for narrative self-fashioning, social positioning, and healing
4. Renewing individual and collective agency through political activism, empowerment, and reconciliation (Kirmayer et al., 2011, p. 84)

These processes are aligned with Indigenous Knowledges and understood within the dynamic nature of individuals' and communities' relationships with ecosystems that support health through "Indigenous agency and identity" (p. 84). Health care providers may support resilience by engaging with cultural humility and co-learning with Indigenous people who describe their own strengths and good relations with body, mind, emotions, and spirit. Consider how to refocus patient interactions that inspire discovery of the four main resilience processes (Kirmayer et al., 2011). Strength is often held in tension with struggle and magnified in trauma-informed care.

Trauma-Informed Care

My grandmother closed the shutters so no one would hear her speak Hawaiian with my aunties. I was not allowed to speak Hawaiian. It was a struggle to not be free to be myself. I know that

I am not alone. We have all fallen on hard times. We need to do what we do best and love each other through hard times. We live aloha. If not, we need to regroup and keep finding our way back.

—Kupuna Francine

Trauma-informed care is an approach that assumes patients and colleagues have experienced trauma, while shifting perspective from "what is wrong" to "what has happened" (Alberta Health Services, 2020). This approach is highly relevant given that over 75% of "Canadian adults report some form of trauma exposure in their lifetime" (BC Provincial Mental Health and Substance Use Planning Council, 2013, p. 9). Core principles of trauma-informed care include "trauma awareness; safety; trustworthiness; choice and collaboration; and building of strengths and skills" (BC Provincial Mental Health and Substance Use Planning Council, 2013, pp. 13–14).

All health care providers may learn trauma-informed care as a general approach, distinguished from specialized trauma-specific services. Key actions in trauma-informed care include the following:

- Realize the widespread impact of trauma and understand paths for recovery
- Recognize the signs and symptoms of trauma in patients, families, and staff
- Integrate knowledge about trauma into policies, procedures, and practices
- Actively avoid re-traumatization (Center for Health Care Strategies, 2019)

Trauma is understood as an event and response, with types of trauma including historical, intergenerational, cultural, domestic, developmental, interpersonal, vicarious, and system-oriented (Alberta Health Services, 2020). This section will focus on intergenerational trauma as an aspect of colonial historical trauma among Indigenous people. Historical trauma is transmitted psychologically, physiologically, and socially between generations, and repeatedly experienced at individual and collective levels over the lifespan (Alberta Health Services, 2020; Aguiar & Halseth, 2015).

Trauma responses are recognized across Indigenous generations with a holistic impact on physical, mental, emotional, cultural, economic, and spiritual health tragically marked by genocide (Aguiar & Halseth, 2015; Haskell & Randall, 2009; Wesley-Esquimaux & Smolewski, 2004). Historical trauma responses include "survivor guilt, depression, somatic (physical) symptoms, low self-esteem, intense fear, [and] vitality in [one's] own life seen as a betrayal to ancestors who suffered" (Brave Heart, 2017). This results in intergenerational trauma responses with "high rates of traumatic stress, grief, depression, substance abuse, domestic violence and suicide" (Alberta Health Services, 2020) and complex post-traumatic stress disorder (Haskell & Randall, 2009). Collective trauma impacts Indigenous people health within families, communities, and society.

Health care providers need to engage in a trauma-informed care guided by cultural humility with Indigenous people when considering "what happened to you" with respect to historical trauma rooted in societal colonialism. Furthermore, a strengths-based approach supports practitioners to respectfully engage with Indigenous people to describe resilience and challenges from their own context (Fogarty et al., 2018; Haskell & Randall, 2009).

We use rattles for healing with the good energy of the spirit. Even when I am protesting and the noise is all around, I am quiet in my heart and know my purpose to help bring change and healing through unconditional love.

—Grandmother Doreen

Local Indigenous Knowledges and traditional wellness practices are key supports for individual and collective healing (Brave Heart et al., 2011). Holistic healing of historical trauma, including disruption of intergenerational trauma, is best supported by a local cultural context that is inclusive and empowering for individuals, families, and communities (Aguiar & Halseth, 2015). Brave Heart et al. (2011) raised awareness of how to "alleviate psychological suffering and unresolved grief ... by developing culturally responsive interventions driven by the community" (p. 282). "Our aim is to restore and empower Indigenous people, to reclaim our traditional selves, our traditional knowledge, and our right to be who we are and should be as healthy, vital, and vibrant communities, unencumbered by ... traumatic responses. In essence, we strive to transcend our collective traumatic past" (Brave Heart et al., 2011, p. 288).

Historical trauma threatens Indigenous Knowledges and cultural continuity, yet healing is rooted in the strength of Indigenous ways of being, knowing, and doing. Thus collective resistance is required to challenge the status quo and enact positive change. Health care providers have a shared responsibility to advocate for Indigenous rights and health equity. In the following section, we examine how to advocate through rights-based, *anti-oppressive*, *relational practices* that incorporate *structural competency* and *cultural safety*.

Anti-Oppressive Practices for Cultural Safety

When the northern hospital was forcing sterilization on an Indigenous girl, I gave her breakfast so she couldn't go to the OR. This got me into a lot of trouble at every layer of that system, from the head nurse to the government. I asked Creator for help, and someone in administration got me on a plane out of there that very night. The power of the system was trying to erase our Indigenous lives; but there were some brave people who saw how this was fundamentally wrong. Every one of us has the choice to tap into our wisdom and either maintain or challenge the status quo for the sake of our common humanity.

—Grandmother Doreen

Through the bridges of the trauma-informed care and strengths-based approaches discussed earlier, how can health care providers practice in their daily work and within the institutions and organizations that have ties to oppression and harm? In this final section we explore anti-oppressive practices, actions and principles for relational practice and communication, and cultural humility in action, all leading toward culturally safe practice.

Anti-oppressive practice requires practitioners to consider history, trauma, power dynamics, and identity intersectionality while building on the strengths of individuals and communities without imposing their own biases (Van Herk et al., 2011). In this practice, health care providers need to be aware of their own traditions, values, beliefs, and biases toward healing and health care practices. This starting place of anti-oppressive practice cuts through "the rhetoric of caring" to acknowledge the history of discrimination, White privilege, scientific dominance, and oppression within the profession (Smith, 2020). For the purpose of this chapter, we understand that anti-racism fits within the broader approach of anti-oppressive practice.

Values of inclusivity, respect, celebrating differences, equity, and commitment support culturally safe care for individuals, families, groups, and communities (Jakubec & Bourque Bearskin, 2020). These values should be embedded in all processes, policies, and practices of health care providers and professional organizations (Registered Nurses' Association of Ontario [RNAO], 2007). Culturally safe care is provided not only to individuals of racial or ethnic groups but also to individuals belonging to groups based on factors such as age, religion, sexual orientation, and socioeconomic status. Practitioners must provide care that meets diverse people needs and reframes the profession to become a relevant and responsive ally. Culturally safe care begins with self-awareness—with specific practices discussed later in this chapter; however, it does not end there. Racism and oppression that shape unsafe care and environments are institutionalized, systemic, and organizational practices (Nzira & Williams, 2009).

A model of positive action for anti-oppressive practice at an organizational level incorporates activities that shape professions within the health care system (Jakubec & Bourque Bearskin, 2020). Dismantling the systematic language, practices, and activities that uphold oppression requires multiple levels of action—at interpersonal and relational levels, certainly, but right at the heart of the technologies and mechanisms of organizations. Organizational action can range from meeting minimal basic, foundational legal requirements for diversity and antidiscrimination, to specific positive action measures, equality schemes, and mainstreaming equal opportunities (Nzira & Williams, 2009). Organizations can choose to make position statements, reorient their work, and require Indigenous hiring in ways that enable Indigenous Knowledges to have an open and respected forum.

Moving beyond minimum legal requirements could involve taking proactive steps within the parameters of the law toward positive action that challenges discrimination within group dominance such as professional nursing or health organizations (Jakubec & Bourque Bearskin, 2020). Positive action means providing disadvantaged people and groups with special training and focused encouragement. Positive action does not put in place reverse discrimination quotas or preferential treatment, but rather applies an approach to diversifying a professional group in all roles to support better representation to counteract the effects of past discrimination and help eliminate sex and race stereotyping. Additional far-reaching equality schemes and mainstreaming of integrated organizational approaches (such as specific equality measures or new policies within an organization) can extend the reach of positive action to begin to shift institutionalized discrimination, inequity, and racism (Nzira & Williams, 2009). Mainstreaming positive action and anti-oppressive practices requires organizational policy and activities at multiple levels, including pre- and in-service training and education (Smith, 2020). Decolonizing practices focus on the unsettling of dominant approaches through Indigenous leadership and Knowledges. Health professions' education increasingly includes curricular and experiential engagement with awareness, allyship, and action for Indigenous health and equity. It is a moral responsibility to face the historic racism and discrimination from within and beyond health professions, and so individual and systemic practices are necessary at once.

RELATIONAL PRACTICE

All my Relations - We are One - Pohai O Kealoha

—Grandmother Doreen and Kupuna Francine

Dismantling oppressive practice and achieving cultural safety, as with inviting Indigenous Knowledges, is predicated on relationship and relational practice (Jakubec & Bourque Bearskin, 2020). **Relational practice** "is guided by conscious participation with patients using a number of relational skills including listening, questioning, empathy, mutuality, reciprocity, self-observation, reflection and a sensitivity to emotional contexts" (College of Nurses of Ontario, 2014, p. 13). It helps health care providers make better informed culturally competent decisions about the best care for diverse patients (e.g., patients of different gender identities, sexual orientation, abilities, spirituality, income, language, and geographic locations) (RNAO, 2006). Relational practice places care within the context of relationships (Bergum & Dossetor, 2005; Pollard, 2015). It asks practitioners to look beyond the restrictive labels of ethnicity, visible minority, age, and so on to see patients as individuals with their own history and identity (Hartrick Doane & Varcoe, 2020). Relational practice has been shown to improve health outcomes for patients and the job satisfaction of health care providers (Andersen & Havaei, 2015; Johannessen et al., 2013).

The hallmark of professional health care practice organized around relational practice is that care is safe, patient-focused care founded on trusting therapeutic relationships. There are many examples of how trusting therapeutic relationships have been severed in clinical practice. The earlier account of Joyce Echaquan, a 37-year-old Atikamekw woman who died on September 28, 2020 in hospital in Joliette, Quebec, is a particularly raw example, and yet there are many other experiences of broken relationships, and failed capacities to care. Cultural safety scholars have noted the prevalence of stereotyping, perceived discrimination, and derogatory comments by health care providers (Allan & Smylie, 2015; Martin & Kipling, 2006). In June 2020, British

Columbia's Minister of Health commissioned a review to investigate systemic Indigenous racism after claims surfaced about a "Price is Right" game allegedly being played in some BC hospital emergency departments, in which health care workers were guessing blood alcohol levels of Indigenous patients. The commission report found widespread Indigenous-specific racism in health services and care in the province. Recommendations for training in these practices for cultural safety at all levels (including pre-service and system-wide) as well as supporting processes and accountability for complaints of racist and oppressive practices were among the recommendations within "In Plain Sight" (Turpel-Lafond, 2020).

Hartrick Doane and Varcoe (2020) explain that relational practice builds on the strengths of individuals and recognizes the processes and practice that entrench power dynamics and systematic oppression involved in delivering health care services to patients. Relational practice helps health care providers work to address the power dynamic at the core of oppression in its many forms. Key concepts in relational practice are a heightened sense of self-awareness in relation to others, a holistic perspective of the context and culture, and capacity for relational practice. Self-awareness requires ongoing reflection and honesty. In anti-oppressive practice, such honesty means examining one's prejudices.

Cultural Considerations In Care

Examining Your Prejudices

1. Reflect on your own prejudices and biases to assess what has influenced some of your beliefs about race.
2. Take the test at the Implicit Project link https://implicit.harvard.edu/implicit/ (refer back to Chapters 1 and 3 for more discussion on values and biases).
   Reflective questions: Were you surprised at your results? What actions will you take to address your prejudices and biases?

Relational capacities are not just personal and reflective, but ways of being in a relationship; that is, being able and willing to understand others and express or share one's own personal meaning. Health care providers who engage in relational practice are fully present with people and demonstrate mindfulness, mutuality, intentionality, genuineness, warmth, respect, care, knowledge of boundaries, the ability to provide and receive constructive feedback, assertiveness, conflict-resolution skills, and a willingness to share information in meaningful ways (Hartrick Doane & Varcoe, 2020). In short, relational practice requires skilled communication that holds the relationship as the value over communication techniques. No amount of paraphrasing and parroting in conversation can get past oppression and abuse of power.

Communication

We need to learn to listen more than we talk. Creator gave us two ears and one mouth.

—Grandmother Doreen

We need to listen and speak with respect for ourselves and others.

—Kupuna Francine

Communication techniques are not the goal of communication, relationship is. Active listening skills, nonverbal communication skills, awareness, and compassion only serve to facilitate the health care provider's ability to develop effective therapeutic relationships with patients. They also provide practitioners with greater self-awareness and awareness of patients' cues that can reveal the root causes of pain, suffering, or challenging behaviours (Hartrick Doane & Varcoe, 2020). This expanded awareness of context and emancipatory action is necessary to motivate anti-oppressive action at multiple levels (e.g., individual, group, policy).

Cultural Humility

I ask permission before I visit Canada. I pray to Ke Akua (Creator) and ask the land, the ancestors, the Elders, and the people for permission for me to enter. I am humbled to be acknowledged when I visit and join in ceremony. I have great love and respect for the Elders from your traditional territories who welcome me like a sister.

—Kupuna Francine

The concept of cultural humility is relatively new for health care providers. It is a process that requires health care providers to continually engage in self-reflection and self-critique as life-long learners and reflective practitioners. Cultural humility also brings into check the power imbalances that exist in the dynamics of the health care setting (Tervalon & Murray-Garcia, 1998). Practitioners will be better prepared for culturally safe practice by learning cultural humility (Levi, 2009). Approaching health care with cultural humility goes beyond the concept of cultural safety to encourage individuals to identify and acknowledge their own biases. Cultural humility acknowledges that it is impossible to be adequately knowledgeable about cultures other than one's own and requires that we take responsibility for our interactions with others beyond acknowledging or being sensitive to our differences (Juarez et al., 2006). Elder Doreen Spence explains that having a sense of humility is being comfortable with a position of not knowing and not being the expert, approaching practice with the tenderness of the heart and strength of deep respect.

My life is an offering of humble gratitude for all the gifts and experiences Creator has given me. When I think about my days in nursing, I wonder what would have happened if we all had humble gratitude for the Native patients instead of it being up to me as the Native nurse. We need to understand that when we work together, we are healing each other. How can we say that nurses are "caring" when it does not show up in our actions? This needs to come straight from our hearts with humility and respect.

—Grandmother Doreen

Cultural humility is not an end in itself; rather, it is a commitment to a way of being and an active process of relating to one another (FNHA, 2020; Racher & Annis, 2007). Hoskins (1999) outlined five major processes that can help people work toward cultural humility: (1) acknowledging the pain of oppression, (2) engaging in acts of humility, (3) acting with reverence, (4) engaging in mutuality, and (5) maintaining a position of not knowing.

Personal trait development is emphasized in cultural humility at intra- and interpersonal levels. Traits include respect, empathy, and critical self-reflection with respect and openness to the patient's worldview, partnership building, and commitment to a lifelong process of cultural engagement (Chang et al., 2012). Combined with the relational and communication skills, cultural humility enables fundamental self-awareness skills for systemic actions; examples in the Cultural Considerations in Care box include position statements by professional and health service organizations. Institutions committed to system-level cultural humility ultimately influence individual and interpersonal levels, with flow and action throughout.

Cultural Considerations In Care

Cultural Humility in Action

Practical steps for system-level cultural humility:
1. Critical assessment of an institution's or organization's current practices and culture
2. Development or incorporation of cultural humility principles into the organization's mission and vision statements
3. Provision of training and resources for staff and employees
4. Continuous periodic evaluation of efforts and progress

Practical examples of organizations taking steps to promote system-level cultural humility:
1. The First Nations Health Authority (FNHA, 2018) developed and implemented a vision for a culturally safe Indigenous health system with staff training toward this goal.
2. The Canadian Association of Perinatal and Women's Health Nurses (CAPWHN, 2019) position statement on cultural safety and humility seeks to advance Indigenous health equity through righting relations.
3. The British Columbia College of Nurses and Midwives (BCCNM, 2022) practice standard for cultural safety, humility, and anti-racism.

Reframing Cultural Competency

In response to Canada's diverse cultural landscape, the demand has grown for health care providers to provide high-quality, effective, and safe care. Various definitions of cultural competence exist and many are contested for their essentialist views of culture. Essentialism suggests there is some natural and unchanging characteristics of people from cultural groups, making claims of defined categorization (Wesp et al., 2018). **Cultural competence**, in this way, is viewed as an ongoing process and "call to action" for health care providers and systems (TRC, 2015) to develop the capacity and skills to deliver culturally safe care with Indigenous people.

In the process and pursuit of competent care, Indigenous people cultures remain in the foreground with practice guided by cultural humility. In this way, health care providers are aware of their own cultural identity and views, constantly building awareness, reviewing their biases and limitations, and expanding their relational capacities. To address unique individuals in their specific contexts and environments, health care providers must move beyond essentialist cultural perspectives while abandoning a checklist of competency attributes (Gray & Thomas, 2006; Gregory et al., 2010).

The concern, then, is not a prescribed checklist, but a process of inquiry. This ongoing strengths-based process begins by acknowledging the fundamental variations in the ways people respond to health care challenges and wellness opportunities. Health care providers can begin by asking *all patients* about health inequities, policies, and practices regarding access to appropriate services (Rowan et al., 2013). At the same time, health care providers should seek to understand the patient's health promotion activities, social connections, ability to cope, spiritual practices, and culturally specific beliefs. We wish to emphasize the relational process and skills used toward culturally safe care.

Cultural Safety

There is no checklist or communication technique that constitutes cultural safety. Indigenous Knowledges, trauma-informed and strength-based practices, cultural humility, and relational practices come together in a process of relationship that acknowledges and addresses oppression. In this process, as explained by Hartrick Doane and Varcoe (2020), awareness of power is key to developing a culturally safe relationship and requires advanced critical reflection and humility. Cultural safety is recognized as an outcome of cultural humility by acknowledging barriers to clinical effectiveness from power imbalances between provider and patient (Curtis et al., 2019). A culturally safe practitioner–patient relationship requires that health care providers understand the following: Indigenous people access to traditional health care practices and ceremonies; engagement, dialogue, and consultations with health care administrators and providers; health administrators' and providers' respect for the rights of diverse knowledge; and the enactment of ethical commitments toward health equity, culturally safe practices, and collective thinking. These elements can lead to a holistic understanding of culture and a sense of humility to raise health care providers' consciousness of power and enactment of culturally safe practices.

Research by Browne et al. (2016) illuminates dimensions of equity-oriented Indigenous health care along with practical ways of operationalizing these approaches and strategies to promote health care equity. In their ethnographic study of two Indigenous health centres in Canada, Browne et al. (2016) interviewed over 100 participants (patients and staff) and conducted over 900 hours of field observations to explore strategies to enhance health care equity among Indigenous populations. They identified four key dimensions of equity-oriented health services foundational for supporting the health and well-being of Indigenous people: (1) inequity-responsive care, (2) culturally safe care, (3) trauma- and violence-informed care, and (4) contextually tailored care. To tailor these dimensions to local contexts, the researchers found that partnerships with Indigenous leaders, agencies, and communities were essential, as was the work of taking action at all levels, attending to local and global histories, and attending to the unintended and potentially harmful consequences of each of the 10 identified strategies to optimize effectiveness. These 10 strategies are as follows:

1. Explicitly committing to fostering health equity in partnership with Indigenous people in mission, vision, or other foundational policy statements
2. Developing organizational structures, policies, and processes to support the commitment to health equity
3. Optimizing use of place and space to create a welcoming milieu
4. Re-visioning the use of time
5. Continuously attending to power differentials
6. Tailoring care, programs, and services to local contexts, Indigenous cultures, and knowledge systems
7. Actively countering systemic and individual experiences of racism and intersecting forms of discrimination
8. Ensuring opportunities for meaningful engagement of patients and community leaders in strategic planning decisions
9. Tailoring care, programs, and services to address interrelated forms of violence
10. Tailoring care to address the social determinants of health for Indigenous people

These strategies provide a basis for organizational-level interventions to promote the provision of more equitable, responsive, and safe services for Indigenous people. They have been the foundation of an expanded learning program and other implementation strategies through EQUIP, a cross-disciplinary research program focused on growing organizational capacity to provide equity-oriented health care, particularly for those who experience significant health and social inequities (Browne et al., 2016). For more information on EQUIP see https://equiphealthcare.ca/.

In their review of the education of health sciences students in Australia, Canada, New Zealand, and the United States, Kurtz and colleagues found that cultural safety education and application to practice were linked to improved relationships, healthier outcomes, and increased number of Indigenous people entering health education programs and graduates interested in working in diverse communities (Kurtz et al., 2018). In their review of cultural safety practices in diabetes care in Canada, Australia, New Zealand, and the United States, Tremblay and colleagues also found that health outcomes improved through educating health providers, modifying clinical environments, and integrating Indigenous health providers in the workforce (Tremblay et al., 2020). Ultimately, culturally safe care is defined by people themselves, so safe practice means inquiring into what would be important for individuals and their community (Hughes, 2018). Cultural safety and achievement of safe practice can also be measured through the health equity and core

TABLE 9.1 ■ Core Principles of Cultural Safety

1. Be clearly focused on achieving health equity, with measurable progress toward this endpoint.
2. Be centred on clarified concepts of cultural safety and critical consciousness rather than narrow-based notions of cultural competency.
3. Be focused on the application of cultural safety within a health care systemic/organizational context in addition to the individual health provider–patient interface.
4. Focus on cultural safety activities that extend beyond acquiring knowledge about "other cultures" and developing appropriate skills and attitudes and move to interventions that acknowledge and address biases and stereotypes.
5. Promote the framing of cultural safety as requiring a focus on power relationships and inequities within health care interactions that reflect historical and social dynamics.
6. Do not limit curricula to formal education programs, rather extend across all training/practice environments, systems, structures, and policies.

From Curtis, E., Jones, R., Tipene-Leach, D., et al. (2019). Why cultural safety rather than cultural competency is required to achieve health equity: A literature review and recommended definition. *International Journal of Equity in Health, 18*, 174. https://doi.org/10.1186/s12939-019-1082-3.

principles seen in Table 9.1. The Indigenous Nurses Association of Canada website provides further information on its cultural safety initiative (see https://indigenousnurses.ca/).

Summary

This chapter raises awareness on how to bring rights-based, anti-colonial, trauma-informed, anti-oppressive relational practices for health care to Indigenous people. While health care providers need to be individually reflective and self-aware, we must also recognize how systems and structures deeply impact the determinants of health; this includes how historical and sociopolitical factors influence Indigenous people lived experiences and health outcomes. Through cultural humility, we create important opportunities to respectfully engage with Indigenous Knowledges as the basis for Indigenous people wellness and culturally safe care. Anti-oppressive practices serve as the counterbalance to the harms of racism. Together, we can advance health equity with Indigenous people and "transform healing paths" (Kílala Lelum, n.d.).

 evolve.elsevier.com/Srivastava/culturalcompetence/.

Questions for Review and Discussion

1. How can health care providers enact cultural safety to create respectful relationships with Indigenous people?
2. What is the impact of colonialism on health care experiences of Indigenous people?
3. How can health care providers make a difference in addressing Indigenous-specific racism?
4. What does Indigenous health equity mean to you?
5. How can health care providers engage in strengths-based care with Indigenous people?

Group Experiential/Reflection Activity

As a group, explore the following questions:
- What is Indigenous health equity?
- What does Indigenous health equity look like in your direct clinical care area (or a selected health care area)?
- What does Indigenous health equity look like in the broader health care system?

Then, brainstorm practical strategies based on the following questions:

- How can cultural safety, relational practice, and strengths-based and other approaches support Indigenous health equity at interpersonal and institutional levels of intervention in your health care work? What specific strategies can you envision in your care area and the wider health care system? How will you know if the strategies have been successful?

References

Aguiar, W., & Halseth, R. (2015). *Indigenous people and historic trauma: The processes of intergenerational transmission*. National Collaborating Centre for Indigenous Health.

Alberta Health Services. (2018). *Indigenous health transformational roadmap 2018-2020*. Population, Public and Indigenous Health: SCN Indigenous Health. https://albertahealthservices.ca/assets/about/scn/ahs-scn-ppih-ih-roadmap.pdf

Alberta Health Services. (2020). *Trauma informed care (TIC). Information for health professionals*. https://www.albertahealthservices.ca/info/Page15526.aspx

Alfred, G. T. (2009). Colonialism and state dependency. *Journal of Indigenous Health, 5*, 42–60.

Allan, B., & Smylie, J. (2015). *First people, second class treatment: The role of racism in the health and well-being of Indigenous people in Canada*. The Wellesley Institute.

Andersen, E., & Havaei, F. (2015). Measuring relational care in nursing homes: Psychometric evaluation of the relational care scale. *Journal of Nursing Measurement, 23*, 82–92.

Andreotti, V. D. O., Stein, S., Ahenakew, C., et al. (2015). Mapping interpretations of decolonization in the context of higher education. *Decolonization: Indigeneity, Education & Society, 4*(1), 21–40. https://jps.library.utoronto.ca/index.php/des/article/view/22168

Antonio, G. C. B. (2019). Constructivism: An approach in training nursing students in the clinical setting. *International Journal of Nursing, 5*(2). https://www.ijnonline.com/index.php/ijn/article/view/270

Askew, D. A., Brady, K., Mukandi, B., et al. (2020). Closing the gap between rhetoric and practice in strengths-based approaches to Indigenous public health: A qualitative study. *Australian and New Zealand Journal of Public Health, 44*(2), 102–105.

Battiste, M. (2013). *Decolonizing education*. Purich Publishing, Ltd.

Battiste, M., & Youngblood Henderson, J. (2000). *Protecting Indigenous knowledge and heritage challenge*. Purich Publishing, Ltd.

BC Provincial Mental Health and Substance Use Planning Council. (2013). *Trauma informed practice guide*. https://bccewh.bc.ca/wp-content/uploads/2012/05/2013_TIP-Guide.pdf

Bergum, V., & Dossetor, J. (2005). *Creating environment. Relational ethics: The full meaning of respect*. University Publishing Group.

Blackstock, C. (2003). First Nations child and family services: Restoring peace and harmony in First Nations communities. In K. Kufeldt & B. McKenzie (Eds.), *Child welfare: Connecting research policy and practice* (pp. 331–343). Wilfrid Laurier University Press.

Blackstock, C. (2009). The occasional evil of angels: Learning from the experiences of Indigenous people and social work. *First People Child & Family Review, 4*(1), 28–37.

Blignault, I., Hunter, J., & Mumford, J. (2018). Integration of Indigenous healing practices with Western biomedicine in Australia, Canada, New Zealand and the United States of America: A scoping review protocol. *JBI Database of Systematic Reviews and Implementation Reports, 16*(6), 1354–1360. https://doi.org/10.11124/JBISRIR-2017-003468.

Bond, C., Singh, D., & Kajlich, H. (2019). *Canada–Australia Indigenous health and wellness racism working group discussion paper and literature review, discussion paper series*. The Lowitja Institute.

Boot, G. R., & Lowell, A. (2019). Acknowledging and promoting Indigenous Knowledges, paradigms, and practices within health literacy-related policy and practice documents across Australia, Canada, and New Zealand. *International Indigenous Policy Journal, 10*(3), 1–28. https://doi.org/10.18584/iipj.2019.10.3.8133.

Borrows, J. (2016). Unextinguished: Rights and the Indian Act. *University of New Brunswick Law Journal, 67*, 3–35.

Bourque Bearskin, R. L. (2011). A critical lens on culture in nursing practice. *Nursing Ethics, 18*(4), 548–559. https://doi.org/10.1177/0969733011408048.

Bourque Bearskin, R. L., Kennedy, A., Bourque, D. H., et al. (2020). Nursing leadership in Indigenous health. In J. I. Waddell & N. A. Walton (Eds.), *Yoder-Wise's leading and managing in Canadian nursing* (2nd ed., pp. 54–89). Elsevier.

Brandon, A., & All, A. (2010). Constructivism theory analysis and application to curricula. *Nursing Education Perspectives*, *31*(2), 89–92.

Brave Heart, M. (2017). *The return to the sacred path: Reflections on the development of historical trauma healing*.   https://www.ihs.gov/sites/telebehavioral/themes/responsive2017/display_objects/documents/slides/historicaltrauma/htreturnsacredpath0513.pdf

Brave Heart, M. Y. H., Chase, J., Elkins, J., et al. (2011). Historical trauma among Indigenous people of the Americas: Concepts, research, and clinical considerations. *Journal of Psychoactive Drugs*, *43*(4), 282–290. https://doi.org/10.1080/02791072.2011.628913.

Brian Sinclair Working Group. (2017). *Out of sight: Interim report of the Sinclair Working Group*. http://ignored-todeathmanitoba.ca/index.php/2017/09/15/out-of-sight-interim-report-of-the-sinclair-working-group/

British Columbia College of Nurses and Midwives (BCCNM). (2022). *Indigenous cultural safety, cultural humility, and anti-racism*. https://www.bccnm.ca/Documents/cultural_safety_humility/All_PS_cultural_safety_humility.pdf

Browne, V., Varcoe, C., Lavoie, J., et al. (2016). Enhancing health care equity with Indigenous populations: Evidence-based strategies from an ethnographic study. *BMC Health Services Research*, *16*(1), 544. https://doi.org/10.1186/s12913-016-1707-9.

Campbell, M. (1995). *Stories of roadside allowance people*. Theytus Books.

Canadian Association of Perinatal and Women's Health Nurses (CAPWHN). (2019). *CAPWHN position statement on cultural safety/humility*. https://capwhn.ca/wp-content/uploads/2019/10/CAPWHN_Position_Statement_on_Cultural_Safety_Humility_Final.pdf

Canadian Association of Schools of Nursing (CASN). (2020). *Framework of strategies for nursing education to respond to the calls to action of Canada's Truth and Reconciliation Commission*. https://www.casn.ca/wp-content/uploads/2020/11/EN-TRC-RESPONSE-STRATEGIES-FOR-NURSING-EDUCATIONTRC-Discussion-Paper-Revised-date-Final.pdf

Canadian Nurses Association (CNA). (2017). *Code of ethics for registered nurses*. https://cna-aiic.ca/en/nursing-practice/nursing-ethics

Chang, E. S., Simon, M., & Dong, X. (2012). Integrating cultural humility into health care professional education and training. *Advances in Health Sciences Education: Theory and Practice*, *17*(2), 269–278. https://doi.org/10.1007/s10459-010-9264-1.

College of Nurses of Ontario. (2014). *Competencies for entry-level registered nurse practice*. Author.

Cox, L., & Taua, L. (2017). Understanding and applying cultural safety: Philosophy and practice of a social determinants approach. In J. Crisp, D. Waters, C. Douglas, et al. (Eds.), *Potter and Perry's fundamentals of nursing—Australian version* (5th ed.). Elsevier Australia.

Crowshoe, L., Henderson, R., Jacklin, K., et al. (2019). Educating for equity care framework. Addressing social barriers of Indigenous patients with type 2 diabetes. *Canadian Family Physician*, *65*, 25–33.

Curtis, E., Jones, R., Tipene-Leach, D., et al. (2019). Why cultural safety rather than cultural competency is required to achieve health equity: A literature review and recommended definition. *International Journal for Equity in Health*, *18*(1), 174. https://doi.org/10.1186/s12939-019-1082-3.

Czyzewski, K. (2011). Colonialism as a broader social determinant of health. *The International Indigenous Policy Journal*, *2*(1). http://ir.lib.uwo.ca/iipj/vol2/iss1/5

Decolonial Futures. (n.d.). *Denials*. https://decolonialfutures.net/4denials/

Dei, G. S. (1996). *Anti-racism: Theory and practice*. Fernwood.

Dei, G., & Asgharzadeh, A. (2001). The power of social theory: The anti-colonial discursive framework. *The Journal of Educational Thought*, *35*(3), 297.

Deloria, B., Foehner, K., & Scinta, S. (Eds.). (1999). *Spirit and reason: The Vine Deloria, Jr., reader*. Fulcrum Publishing.

DiAngelo, R. (2018). *White fragility: Why it's so hard for White people to talk about racism*. Beacon Press.

Dion Stout, M. (2012). Ascribed health and wellness, atikowisi miýw-āyāwin, to achieved health and wellness, kaskitamasowin miýw-āyāwin: Shifting the paradigm. *The Canadian Journal of Nursing Research*, *44*(2), 11–14.

Donald, D. (2012). Forts, colonial frontier logics, and Indigenous-Canadian relations: Imagining decolonizing educational philosophies in Canadian contexts. In A. Abdi (Ed.), *Decolonizing philosophies of education* (pp. 91–111). SensePublishers. https://doi.org/10.1007/978-94-6091-687-8_7.

Downey, B. (2020). Completing the circle: Towards the achievement of IND-equity – A culturally relevant health equity model by/for Indigenous populations. *Witness: The Canadian Journal of Critical Nursing Discourse*, 2(1), 97–110. https://doi.org/10.25071/2291-5796.59.

Dumbrill, G. C., & Ying Yee, J. (2019). *Anti-oppressive social work: Ways of knowing, talking and doing*. Oxford University Press.

Ermine, W. (1995). Indigenous epistemology. In M. Battiste & J. Barman (Eds.), *First Nation education in Canada: The circle unfolds* (pp. 101–111). UBC Press.

Ermine, W. (2007). The ethical space of engagement. *Indigenous Law Journal*, 6(1), 194–203.

First Nations Health Authority (FNHA). (2014). *Traditional wellness strategic framework*. https://www.fnha.ca/WellnessSite/WellnessDocuments/FNHA_TraditionalWellnessStrategicFramework.pdf

First Nations Health Authority (FNHA). (2018). *Creating a climate for change*. https://www.fnha.ca/Documents/FNHA-Creating-a-Climate-For-Change-Cultural-Humility-Resource-Booklet.pdf

First Nations Health Authority (FNHA). (2020). *First Nations perspective on health and wellness*. https://www.fnha.ca/wellness/wellness-and-the-first-nations-health-authority/first-nations-perspective-on-wellness

Fogarty, W., Lovell, M., Langenberg, J., et al. (2018). *Deficit discourse and strengths-based approaches: Changing the narrative of Indigenous and Torres Strait Islander health and wellbeing*. The Lowitja Institute.

Gergen, K. (2007). *An invitation to social construction*. SAGE.

Gergen, K. J. (2001). *Social construction in context*. SAGE Ltd.

Goodman, A., Fleming, K., Markwick, N., et al. (2017). "They treated me like crap and I know it was because I was native": The healthcare experiences of Indigenous people living in Vancouver's inner city. *Social Science & Medicine*, 178, 87–94. https://doi.org/10.1016/j.socscimed.2017.01.053.

Government of Canada. (2018). *First Nations and Inuit health and wellness indicators*. https://health-infobase.canada.ca/fnih/

Government of Canada. (2020). *Guide to the Canadian Charter of Rights and Freedoms*. https://www.canada.ca/en/canadian-heritage/services/how-rights-protected/guide-canadian-charter-rights-freedoms.html

Government of Canada. (n.d.). *Confederation. Our country, our parliament. An introduction to how Canada's parliament works*. https://lop.parl.ca/about/parliament/education/ourcountryourparliament/html_booklet/confederation-e.html

Gray, P. D., & Thomas, D. J. (2006). Critical reflections on culture in nursing. *Journal of Cultural Diversity*, 13(2), 76–82.

Greenwood, M., & Lindsay, N. (2019). A commentary on land, health, and Indigenous knowledge(s). *Global Health Promotion*, 26(3 suppl), 82–86. https://doi.org/10.1177/1757975919831262.

Gregory, D., Harrowing, J., Lee, B., et al. (2010). Pedagogy as influencing nursing students' essentialized understanding of culture. *International Journal of Nursing Education Scholarship*, 7(1), 1–17.

Griffiths, K., Coleman, C., Lee, V., et al. (2016). How colonisation determines social justice and Indigenous health—a review of the literature. *Journal of Population Research*, 33(1), 9–30. https://doi.org/10.1007/s12546-016-9164-1.

Hansen, J. G., & Antsanen, R. (2016). Elders' teachings about resilience and its implications for education in Dene and Cree communities. *The International Indigenous Policy Journal*, 7(1). https://doi.org/10.18584/iipj.2016.7.1.2.

Hartrick Doane, G., & Varcoe, C. (2020). *How to nurse: Relational inquiry in action* (2nd ed.). Walters Kluwer.

Haskell, L., & Randall, M. (2009). Disrupted attachments: A social context complex trauma framework and the lives of Indigenous people in Canada. *Journal of Indigenous Health*, 5(3), 48–99.

Henderson, W. B., & Parrot, Z. (2018). *Indian Act. The Canadian Encyclopedia*. https://www.thecanadianencyclopedia.ca/en/article/indian-act

Hoskins, M. L. (1999). Worlds apart and lives together: Developing cultural attunement. *Child and Youth Care Forum*, 28(2), 73–85.

Hughes, M. (2018). Cultural safety requires "cultural intelligence." *Nursing New Zealand*, 24(6), 24–25.

Indian and Northern Affairs Canada. (2010). *A history of treaty making in Canada*. https://www.rcaanc-cirnac.gc.ca/DAM/DAM-CIRNAC-RCAANC/DAM-TAG/STAGING/texte-text/ap_htmc_treatliv_1314921040169_eng.pdf

Indigenous Services Canada. (2021). *Reducing the number of Indigenous children in care*. https://www.sac-isc.gc.ca/eng/1541187352297/1541187392851

Isaak, C. A., & Marchessault, G. (2008). Meaning of health: The perspectives of Indigenous adults and youth in a northern Manitoba First Nations Community. *Canadian Journal of Diabetes, 32*(2), 114–122. https://doi.org/10.1016/S1499-2671(08)22008-3.

Iverson, R., Gergen, K., & Fairbanks, R. II. (2005). Assessment and social construction: Conflict or co-creation? *British Journal of Social Work, 35,* 689–708.

Jakubec, S. L., & Bourque Bearskin, L. (2020). Chapter 14: Decolonizing and anti-oppressive nursing practice: Awareness, allyship and action decolonizing. In L. McCleary & T. McPharland (Eds.), *Ross-Kerr and Wood's Canadian nursing issues & perspectives* (6th ed., pp. 243–268). Elsevier.

Johannessen, A-K., Werner, A., & Steihaug, S. (2013). Work in an intermediate unit: Balancing between relational, practical and moral care. *Journal of Clinical Nursing, 23,* 586–595. https://doi.org/10.1111/jocn.12213.

Jones, M., Crowshoe, L., Reid, P., et al. (2019). Educating for Indigenous health equity: An international consensus statement. *Academic Medicine, 94*(4), 512–519. https://doi.org/10.1097/ACM.0000000000002476.

Juarez, J. A., Marvel, K., Brezinski, K. L., et al. (2006). Bridging the gap: A curriculum to teach residents cultural humility. *Family Medicine, 38,* 97–102.

Kennedy, A., Szabo, J., McGowan, K., et al. (2020). *Strengths-based Indigenous health promotion.* Unpublished manuscript.

Kílala Lelum. (n.d). *Our logo.* https://kilalalelum.ca/clinics-programs/our-logo/

Kirkness, V. J., & Barnhardt, R. (2001). First Nations and higher education: The four R's: Respect, relevance, reciprocity, responsibility. In R. Hayoe & J. Pan (Eds.), *Knowledge across cultures: A contribution to dialogue among civilizations* (pp. 1–18). University of Hong Kong, Hong Kong Comparative Education Research Centre. http://www.afn.ca/uploads/files/education2/the4rs.pdf

Kirmayer, L. J., Dandeneau, S., Marshall, E., et al. (2011). Rethinking resilience from an Indigenous perspective. *Canadian Journal of Psychiatry, 56*(2), 84–91. https://doi.org/10.1177/070674371105600203.

Kurtz, D. L. M., Janke, R., Vinek, J., et al. (2018). Health sciences cultural safety education in Australia, Canada, New Zealand, and the United States: A literature review. *International Journal of Medical Education, 9,* 271–285. https://doi.org/10.5116/ijme.5bc7.21e2.

Lamouche, J. (2010, February). *Indigenous people health within the health sciences: A Métis, Inuit & First Nations specific health series.* In M. Anderson (Keynote Speaker), First Nations health session. McMaster University, Hamilton, Ontario.

Levi, A. (2009). The ethics of nursing student international clinical experiences. *Journal of Obstetric, Gynecologic, and Neonatal Nursing, 28*(1), 94–99. https://doi.org/10.1111/j.1552-6909.2008.00314.x.

Lincoln, Y. S., & Guba, E. G. (2016). *The constructivist credo.* Routledge. https://doi.org/10.4324/9781315418810.

Logan, L., McNairn, J., Wiart, S., et al. (2020). Creating space for Indigenous healing practices in patient care plans. *Canadian Medical Education Journal, 11*(1), e5–e15. https://journalhosting.ucalgary.ca/index.php/cmej/article/view/68647

Lux, M.K. (2016). *Separate beds: A history of Indian hospitals in Canada, 1920s-1980s.* University of Toronto Press.

Martin, D., & Kipling, A. (2006). Factors shaping Indigenous nursing students' experiences. *Nurse Education Today, 26*(8), 688–696.

McGibbon, E., Mulaudzi, F. M., Didham, P., et al. (2013). Toward decolonizing nursing: The colonization of nursing and strategies for increasing the counter-narrative. *Nursing Inquiry, 21*(3). https://doi.org/10.1111/nin.12042.

McGowan, K., Kennedy, A., El Hussein, M., et al. (2020). Decolonization, social innovation and rigidity in higher education. *Social Enterprise Journal, 16*(3), 299–316. https://doi.org/10.1108/SEJ-10-2019-0074.

McGuire, P. (2010). Exploring resilience and Indigenous ways of knowing. *Pimatisiwin: A Journal of Indigenous and Indigenous Community Health, 8*(2), 117–131.

McKillop, A., Sheridan, N., & Rowe, D. (2013). New light through old windows: Nurses, colonists and Indigenous survival. *Nursing Inquiry, 20*(3), 265–276. https://doi.org/10.1111/nin.12005.

McNeil, K. (2007). *A brief history of our right to self-governance pre-contact to present.* National Centre for First Nations Governance. http://www.fngovernance.org/publication_docs/Self-Governance_Right_CFNG.pdf

Merriam-Webster. (2020). *Oppression.* https://www.merriam-webster.com/dictionary/oppression

Methot, S. (2019). *Legacy: Trauma, story and Indigenous healing.* ECW Press.

Metzl, J. M., & Hansen, H. (2014). Structural competency: Theorizing a new medical engagement with stigma and inequality. *Social Science & Medicine, 103*, 126–133. https://doi.org/10.1016/j.socscimed.2013. 06.032.

Mills, C. (1997). *The racial contract*. Cornell University Press.

National Collaborating Centre for Indigenous Health. (2017). *Indigenous children and the child welfare system in Canada*. https://www.nccih.ca/495/Indigenous_Children_and_the_Child_Welfare_System_in_Canada. nccih?id=203

National Inquiry into Missing and Murdered Indigenous Women and Girls (MMIWG). (2019). *Reclaiming power and place. The final report of the National Inquiry into Missing and Murdered Indigenous Women and Girls.* https://www.mmiwg-ffada.ca/final-report/

Newton, P. (2021, June 1) '*Unthinkable' discovery in Canada as remains of 215 children found buried near residential school.* CNN. https://www.cnn.com/2021/05/28/world/children-remains-discovered-canada-kamloops-school/index.html

Nurses and Nurse Practitioners of British Columbia (NNPBC). (2018). *Enhancing rural and remote nursing practice for healthier BC* [Policy brief]. https://www.nnpbc.com/pdfs/policy-and-advocacy/rural-and-remote/Enhancing-Rural-&-Remote-Nursing-Practice-for-a-Healthier-BC.pdf

Nzira, V., & Williams, P. (2009). *Anti-oppressive practice in health and social care*. SAGE.

Office of the Auditor General of Canada (OAGC). (2015). *Access to health services for remote First Nations communities*. https://www.oag-bvg.gc.ca/internet/English/parl_oag_201504_04_e_40350.html

Paradies, Y., Harris, R., & Anderson, I. (Eds.). (2008). *The impact of racism on indigenous health in Australia and Aotearoa: Towards a research agenda*. Discussion paper no. 4. Cooperative Research Centre for Indigenous Health, Darwin. https://dro.deakin.edu.au/eserv/DU:30058493/paradies-impactofracism-2008.pdf

Peters, M. (2000). Does constructivist epistemology have a place in nurse education? *The Journal of Nursing Education, 39*(4), 166–172.

Phillips, B. (2018). Learning theories. In M. Oermann, J. Degane, & B. C. Phillips (Eds.), *Teaching in nursing and the role of the educator* (2nd ed., pp. 11–27). Springer Publishing Company.

Pollard, C. L. (2015). What is the right thing to do: Use of a relational ethic framework to guide clinical decision-making. *International Journal of Caring Sciences, 8*(2), 362–368.

Racher, F. E., & Annis, R. C. (2007). Respecting culture and honoring diversity in community practice. *Research and Theory for Nursing Practice, 21*(4), 255–270.

Reading, C. (2015). Structural determinants of Indigenous people health. In M. Greenwood, S. De Leeuw, N. M. Lindsay et al. (Eds.), *Determinants of Indigenous people health in Canada* (pp. 3–15). Canadian Scholars' Press.

Reading, C. L.et al.Wien, F. (2009, 2013). *Health inequities and social determinants of Indigenous people health*. National Collaborating Centre for Indigenous Health. https://www.ccnsa-nccah.ca/docs/determinants/ RPT-HealthInequalities-Reading-Wien-EN.pdf

Redvers, N., Marianayagam, J., & Blondin, B. (2019). Improving access to Indigenous medicine for patients in hospital-based settings: A challenge for health systems in northern Canada. *International Journal of Circumpolar Health, 78*(1), 1–5. https://doi.org/10.1080/22423982.2019.1577093.

Registered Nurses' Association of Ontario (RNAO). (2006). *Establishing therapeutic relationships—best practice guideline*. http://rnao.ca/bpg/guidelines/establishing-therapeutic-relationships

Registered Nurses' Association of Ontario (RNAO). (2007). *Embracing cultural diversity in health care: Developing cultural competence*. http://rnao.ca/bpg/guidelines/embracing-cultural-diversity-health-care-developing-cultural-competence

Robbins, J. A., & Dewar, J. (2011). Traditional Indigenous approaches to healing and the modern welfare of traditional knowledge, spirituality and lands: A critical reflection on practices and policies taken from the Canadian Indigenous example. *The International Indigenous Policy Journal, 2*(4), 1–17. https://doi. org/10.18584/iipj.2011.2.4.2.

Rogers, B. J., Swift, K., van der Woerd, K., et al. (2019). *At the interface: Indigenous health practitioners and evidence-based practice*. National Collaborating Centre for Indigenous Health. https://www.nccih.ca/docs/ context/RPT-At-the-Interface-Halseth-EN.pdf

Rowan, M. S., Rukholm, E., Bourque-Bearskin, R. L., et al. (2013). Cultural competence and cultural safety in Canadian schools of nursing: A mixed methods study. *International Journal of Nursing Education Scholarship, 10*(1), 1–10. https://doi.org/10.1515/ijnes-2012-0043.

Sasakamoose, J., Bellegarde, T., Sutherland, W., et al. (2017). Miỳo-pimātisiwin developing Indigenous cultural responsiveness theory (ICRT): Improving Indigenous health and well-being. *The International Indigenous Policy Journal, 8*(4). https://ir.lib.uwo.ca/iipj/vol8/iss4/1

Sherwood, J., Keech, S., Keenan, T., et al. (2011). Indigenous studies: Teaching and learning together. In N. Purdie, G. Milgate, & H. R. Bell (Eds.), *Two way teaching and learning. Toward culturally reflective and relevant education* (pp. 189–202). ACER Press.

Sinclair, R. (2007). Identity lost and found: Lessons from the Sixties Scoop. *First People Child & Family Review, 3*(1), 65-82. https://fpcfr.com/index.php/FPCFR/article/view/25

Smith, K. (2020). Facing history for the future of nursing. *Journal of Clinical Nursing, 29*(9–10), 1429–1431. https://doi.org/10.1111/jocn.15065.

Smylie, J., Kaplan-Myrth, N., & McShane, K. (2009). Indigenous knowledge translation: Baseline findings in a qualitative study of the pathways of health knowledge in three Indigenous communities in Canada. *Health Promotion Practice, 10*(3), 436–446. https://doi.org/10.1177/1524839907307993.

Smylie, J., Olding, M., & Ziegler, C. (2014). Sharing what we know about living a good life: Indigenous approaches to knowledge translation. *The Journal of the Canadian Health Libraries Association, 35*, 16–23. https://doi.org/10.5596/c14-009.

Starblanket, T. (2020). *Suffer the little children: Genocide, Indigenous nations and the Canadian state.* Clarity Press Inc.

Statistics Canada. (2016). *2016 census topic: Indigenous people.* https://www12.statcan.gc.ca/census-recensement/2016/rt-td/ap-pa-eng.cfm

St. Denis, V. (2007). Indigenous education and anti-racist education: Building alliances across cultural and racial identity. *Canadian Journal of Education, 30*(4), 1068–1092.

St. Denis, N., & Walsh, C. (2017). Traditional healing practices in an urban Indigenous setting: An autoethnography. *Journal of Indigenous Social Development, 6*(2), 50–64.

Stein, S., & Andreotti, V. D. O. (2016). Decolonization and higher education. In M. Peters (Ed.), *Encyclopedia of educational philosophy and theory* (pp. 370–375). Springer Science+Business Media.

Symenuk, P., Tisdale, D., Bourque Bearskin, D.H., et al. (2020). In search of the truth: Uncovering nursing's involvement in colonial harms and assimilative policies five years post Truth and Reconciliation Commission. *Witness: The Canadian Journal of Critical Nursing Discourse, 2*(1), 84–96. https://doi.org/10.25071/2291-5796.51.

Tervalon, M., & Murray-Garcia, J. (1998). Cultural humility versus cultural competence: A critical distinction in defining physician training outcomes in multicultural education. *Journal of Health Care for the Poor and Underserved, 9*(2), 117–125.

Tk'emlúps te Secwépemc. (2021). *Remains of Kamloops residential school discovered.* https://tkemlups.ca/wp-content/uploads/05-May-27-2021-TteS-MEDIA-RELEASE.pdf

Tremblay, M. -C., Graham, J., Porgo, T. V., et al. (2020). Improving cultural safety of diabetes care in Indigenous populations of Canada, Australia, New Zealand and the United States: A systematic rapid review. *Canadian Journal of Diabetes, 44*(7), 670–678. https://doi.org/10.1016/j.jcjd.2019.11.006.

Truth and Reconciliation Commission of Canada (TRC). (2015). *Honouring the truth, reconciling for the future. Summary of the Final Report of the Truth and Reconciliation Commission of Canada.* http://www.trc.ca/assets/pdf/Executive_Summary_English_Web.pdf

Turpel-Lafond (Aki-Kwe), M. E. (2020). *In plain sight: Addressing Indigenous-specific racism and discrimination in B.C. healthcare.* British Columbia Health Ministry. https://engage.gov.bc.ca/app/uploads/sites/613/2020/11/In-Plain-Sight-Full-Report.pdf

United Nations (UN). (2007). *United Nations Declaration on the Rights of Indigenous People.* https://www.un.org/development/desa/indigenouspeople/wp-content/uploads/sites/19/2018/11/UNDRIP_E_web.pdf

United Nations (UN). (2015). *Economic, social and cultural rights.* UN Permanent Forum on Indigenous Issues -14th Session: Concept note for discussion. https://www.un.org/esa/socdev/unpfii/documents/2015/concept-notes/escr.pdf

Van Herk, K. A., Smith, D., & Andrew, C. (2011). Examining our privileges and oppressions: Incorporating an intersectionality paradigm into nursing. *Nursing Inquiry, 18*(1). https://doi.org/10.1111/j.1440-1800.2011.00539.x.

Waite, R., & Nardi, D. (2019). Nursing colonialism in America: Implications for nursing leadership. *Journal of Professional Nursing, 35*(1), 18–25. https://doi.org/10.1016/j.profnurs.2017.12.013.

Wesley-Esquimaux, C.C., & Smolewski, M. (2004). *Historic trauma and Indigenous healing.* Indigenous Healing Foundation.

Wesp, M., Scheer, M., Ruiz, M., et al. (2018). An emancipatory approach to cultural competency: The application of critical race, postcolonial, and intersectionality theories. *Advances in Nursing Science, 41*(4), 316–326. https://doi.org/10.1097/ANS.0000000000000230.

Wherry, A. (October 1, 2009). What he was talking about when he talked about colonialism. *MacLean's.* https://www.macleans.ca/uncategorized/what-he-was-talking-about-when-he-talked-about-colonialism/

World Health Organization (WHO). (2017). *Health is a fundamental human right.* https://www.who.int/mediacentre/news/statements/fundamental-human-right/en/

World Health Organization (WHO). (2020). *Constitution.* https://apps.who.int/gb/bd/PDF/bd47/EN/constitution-en.pdf?ua=1

Zubek. E. M. (1994). Traditional Native healing. Alternative or adjunct to modern medicine? *Canadian Family Physician, 4,* 1923–1931.

CHAPTER 10

Sexual and Gender Diversity

Julie Leising, Oriana Shaw, Emma Hillier, Phillip Hau, Alexandra Marshall, Katie McCann, Michelle Anderson, and Julia Chronopoulos

LEARNING OBJECTIVES

At the end of this chapter, the learner will be able to:

- Be aware of common health disparities and health care needs of sexually and gender diverse people
- Understand historical and current factors in the health care system and broader society that underlie these health disparities
- Be able to discuss strategies to apply as a health care provider to be more inclusive of sexually and gender diverse patients

Authors' Note: With the aim of presenting these topics in a rounded way, this chapter was written by a group of authors who have a variety of different sexual orientations, gender identities, racial identities, cultural backgrounds, and levels of expertise in health care. That said, it is impossible to comprehensively represent the views of all people in any given community. This chapter is intended to provide a starting point to learning how to provide care informed by cultural competence and humility to sexually and gender diverse (SGD) people.

KEY TERMS

2SLGBTQ+	Homonormativity	Resiliency
Cisnormativity	Intersex/Person with	Sex assigned at birth
Gender binary	"differences of sexual	SGD people
Gender dysphoria	development" (DSD)	
Heteronormativity	Intersectionality	

Many countries, despite having high-quality health care, have records of countless health disparities among sexually and gender diverse (SGD) people that are due to ongoing marginalization and discrimination. SGD individuals have indicated that they delay or avoid seeking health care for fear of judgement, stigma, and discrimination related to their sexual orientation, gender, or substance use, and because services are not targeted to them (Edmonton Men's Health Collective, n.d.; Lorenzetti et al., 2015; McPhailet et al., 2016). SGD people are less likely to have a regular family physician than their heterosexual, cisgender counterparts (Scheim et al., 2017). When care is sought, it may be inadequate because of the minimal formal education health care providers receive about sexual and gender diversity. These factors all contribute to SGD people having more unmet health care needs (Transgender PULSE Canada Team, 2020).

The aim of this chapter is to familiarize readers with language, cultural context, and many actionable changes critical to making health care more inclusive of SGD patients. We begin by explaining common terms used in discussions surrounding sexual and gender diversity. We then explore historical perspectives on sexual and gender diversity and the resulting impacts on SGD people. Subsequently, we describe the concepts behind approaches to providing inclusive care and reducing health disparities faced by SGD people. The remainder of the chapter delves more deeply into *how* health care providers can improve experiences for SGD people in various health care settings and at particular stages of life. We conclude with several key principles that all health care providers can use to guide future interactions.

Terminology

When discussing sexual and gender diversity it is important to recognize that sexual orientation and gender identity are distinct. Everyone has a sexual orientation and everyone has a gender identity. Heterosexual and cisgender identities predominate current society. A **heterosexual** person is one who is attracted to people who are not the same sex or gender as them. A **cisgender** person is one whose internal conception of their gender identity matches their sex assigned at birth.

There are many terms used to discuss identities that are not heterosexual and cisgender. The most common term is some arrangement of letters, for example, **2SLGBTQ+**[1]. This stands for "2-Spirit, Lesbian, Gay, Bisexual, Transgender, and Queer" with a "+" at the end to signify other identities. In some cases, this has been extended to something like LGBTTQQPIANU+ (Lesbian, Gay, Bisexual, Transgender, Two-Spirit, Queer, Questioning, Pansexual, Intersex, Asexual, Non-Binary, Unlabelled, and +), or even longer iterations. Such a strategy has obvious failings. It is unwieldy language that is difficult to use naturally. As well, the words people use to describe and relate to their identity shift as we improve our cultural understanding of these topics and as words are created or applied in new ways. Thus, attempts to be more inclusive can paradoxically leave some individuals feeling even more excluded.

Occasionally the word *queer* is used as an umbrella term under which all other labels for SGD identities can reside. Some use this term because they do not want to limit themselves to a particular description. This can be a way to avoid stereotypes associated with certain labels. Others may use this term to avoid disclosing the details of their identity, allowing for a degree of privacy if desired. However, the word's pejorative history can make it a dubious choice for many people. Despite its use academically and modern efforts at reclamation, it should only be used to refer to someone if they have expressed it as a term with which they self-identify. The same guidance applies to all terms used to describe gender identity and sexual orientation; identity should always be defined by those who experience it, not imposed by others.

For the purposes of this chapter, when referring to the community of people who do not identify as heterosexual or cisgender, we will use the term **SGD people**. This term is also imperfect. Any umbrella term that is used to describe a group of people or a community (such as for race, ethnicity, religion, etc.) can make the diversity within the group invisible. However, this term expresses a breadth of identities without highlighting or singling out any in particular. They are also sufficiently succinct to be used conveniently.

---

[1]"LGBTQ2" is the official acronym recognized by the Government of Canada's LGBTQ2 Secretariat. For the most current information regarding federal policies, programs, and laws affecting the LGBTQ2 community, please refer to https://www.canada.ca/en/canadian-heritage/campaigns/free-to-be-me.html.

Whichever term(s) a patient chooses to use, health care providers must understand that there is a broad range of identities. Awareness of some common terms can help to develop shared understanding and to engage in meaningful conversations (Table 10.1). It is important to recognize that terminology is constantly evolving. Thus, while we provide broad definitions, it is important to remember that each individual has a unique identity, has unique needs, and may relate to terms differently. As we discuss later, it is always important to find out how patients prefer to have their identity described and what that means to them.

For a more rounded understanding of sexual and gender diversity, it is imperative to understand the concept of intersectionality. **Intersectionality** refers to overlapping and interacting forms of discrimination (see the Cultural Considerations in Care box below for more on how this concept was developed). People experience the world differently because of each aspect of their identity—race, gender, sexuality, and abilities—and because of the combination of these factors. Writer and activist Audre Lorde famously proclaimed that "there is no hierarchy of oppressions" (Lorde, 1983). One aspect of a person's identity cannot achieve justice if the other aspects still experience discrimination. The person as a whole must be afforded "freedom from intolerance," which includes all of the interacting aspects of their identity (Lorde, 1983). For instance,

---

TABLE 10.1 ■ **Examples of Terminology Describing Identity With Respect to Sexual Orientation and Gender**

Asexual: a person who experiences no, little or intermittent feelings of sexual attraction to others

Bisexual/Bi: a person who is sexually or romantically attracted to two or more sexes or genders

Cisgender: those whose gender identity matches the sex that they were assigned at birth

Gay: a person who is sexually or romantically attracted to people who are the same sex or gender as themselves

Heterosexual: an individual sexually attracted to people of the opposite sex or gender

Homosexual: an individual sexually attracted to people of the same sex gender

Intersex/Person with "differences of sexual development" (DSD): a person born with a body that is neither stereotypically male nor female due to ambiguous genitalia, hormonal differences, or chromosomal anomalies. For example, a person may have XY chromosomes, a vagina and breast development, and no uterus.

Lesbian: a person whose sex or gender is female who is sexually or romantically attracted to people of the same sex or gender

Non-binary: a person whose gender identity is not wholly encapsulated within the category of male or female. Examples of non-binary gender identities include genderfluid and agender.

Pansexual: a person whose attraction to others is not limited by sex or gender

Queer: an umbrella term encompassing all sexually and gender diverse identities

Questioning: a person who is in the process of discovering their sexual orientation or gender identity

Transgender/Trans: a person whose internal conception of their gender identity does not match their sex assigned at birth

Transfeminine: a person whose sex assigned at birth was male, who identifies with a feminine gender identity (not necessarily female)

Transgender man: a person whose sex assigned at birth was female, who identifies as a man.

Transmasculine: a person whose sex assigned at birth was female who identifies with a masculine gender identity (not necessarily male)

Transgender woman: a person whose sex assigned at birth was male who identifies as a woman

Two-spirit: umbrella term for some Indigenous people who identify as having both a female and male spirit within them or whose gender identity, gender expression, sexual orientation, or spiritual identity is not limited by the binary classification of gender as woman or man

Unlabelled: a person who does not wish to identify under a specific label with respect to sexuality or gender

> **Cultural Considerations in Care**
>
> *Origins of Intersectionality*
>
> The idea of intersectionality was developed by a series of Black and Indigenous feminist scholars such as Zitkala-Sa and Sarah Winnemucca (Hopkins, 2008; Zitkala-Ša, 1921; Zitkala-Ša et al., 1924). Feminist scholar bell hooks[1] (Jankowski, 2019) called for inclusion of those experiencing all forms of oppression who were most marginalized (hooks, 1984). The term *intersectionality* was coined by Kimberlé Crenshaw in her seminal paper, "Mapping the Margins" (Crenshaw, 1991). The Combahee River Collective, Angela Davis, and Audre Lorde created language for discussions on intersectionality (Lorde, 1983; Combahee River Collective, 1977; Winter, 2005).

it will not be possible to achieve equity for Black Canadians if the transgender community is discriminated against and therefore there are many Black transgender Canadians still experiencing discrimination.

Historical Perspectives

Canada has a history of colonization and continued colonial legacies that have infiltrated the systems and institutions of the modern-day country—health care included (MacDonald & Steenbeek, 2015). Similar issues are present in many parts of the world. Unique Indigenous nations, identities, systems of care, and norms existed before colonization (Voyageur & Calliou, 2001). Many Indigenous nations had a variety of non-cisheteronormative concepts incorporated in their views. The term *two-spirit* was created more recently to "reflect traditional [Indigenous] gender diversity, including the fluid nature of gender and sexuality" (Hunt, 2016, p. 7). While not all nations were equally accepting, the contrast with settlers' views of SGD people is stark. Settlers introduced strictly patriarchal and cisheteronormative systems (Giroux & Depelteau, 2015; Morgensen, 2011). **Cisnormativity** refers to the cultural or societal assumption of exclusively cisgender identities. **Heteronormativity** refers to a cultural or societal assumption of exclusively heterosexual expression of sexuality in a **gender binary** (classification of gender into two distinct categories of male and female) system. From 1850 onward, settlers imposed binaries for race, gender, and sexuality. This had a substantial impact on Indigenous people, for example, with the gendered implications of the *Indian Act*. In the *Indian Act*, "status" was the Canadian government's definition of who qualified as Indigenous. Until 1985, a status woman who married a man without status lost her status, and so did their children, yet a status man who married a non-status woman would retain his status, and the woman and their children would gain status. Residential schools, forced adoptions, and particular Christian teachings further solidified heteronormativity (Hunt, 2016; Ristock et al., 2019). The attempted ban on Indigenous language use restricted the application and propagation of traditional ideas of gender and sexuality. This shaped the current prevalence of heteronormativity, and of homonormativity in our society. **Homonormativity** is a belief that SGD people should conform to the societal norms and models of heterosexual relationships, apart from the gender of their sexual partner(s). For example, middle-class, monogamous, White, cisgender homosexuality is often the most accepted and represented form of sexual diversity. Our Canadian health care system

---

[1] bell hooks is the pen name for Gloria Jean Watkins, a contemporary *feminist theorist* who addressesd issues of race, gender, class, and sexual oppression. She chose to use lowercase letters for her name to shift the focus from name and ego to her work and ideas (Jankowski, 2019; see https://www.thoughtco.com/bell-hooks-biography-3530371).

was founded on colonial ideals that assume a male–female binary and pathologize concepts of gender and sexuality that are recognized and normalized within certain Indigenous cultures. Consistent and concerted efforts are needed to decolonize health care practices, going beyond recognizing institutional values to building practices in a way that includes culturally grounded Indigenous alternatives (Coulthard, 2014).

In the nineteenth century, societal views on SGD people maintained a moralistic lens—that SGD people were the result of immoral choices. Although this shifted progressively to more of a medical framework, remnants of the moralistic perspective remained. In fact, homosexuality was only decriminalized in Canada in 1969 (Kimmel & Robinson, 2014). The pathologization of SGD people was initially highly influenced by the work of Austro-German psychiatrist Richard von Krafft-Ebing. Krafft-Ebing's publication, *Psychopathia Sexualis*, used Bénédict Morel's 1857 theory of degeneracy to posit that homosexuality and cross-gender identification were sexual pathologies caused by degenerate heredity (Krafft-Ebing, 1886). This early framework led to the inclusion of homosexuality in the first edition of the *Diagnostic and Statistical Manual of Mental Disorders* (DSM-I) as a "sociopathic personality disturbance," clustered with other disorders such as "transvestism, pedophilia, fetishism, and sexual sadism." Though the conceptualization of this diagnosis changed as the DSM evolved, homosexuality was not completely removed until the publication of the DSM-5 in 2013. This course has been similar throughout editions of the *International Classification of Diseases* (ICD), which continues to include "egodystonic sexual orientation" in the ICD-10. Both the DSM-5 and ICD-10 continue to include "gender dysphoria" and "transsexualism," respectively (see the Cultural Considerations in Care box below for more on gender dysphoria) (Drescher, 2015). These imply that pathology is inherent to non-cisheteronormative identities leading to stigma, discrimination, and both conscious and unconscious bias.

The inclusion of homosexuality as a diagnosis allowed for practices such as conversion or aversion therapy, which aimed to change a person's sexual orientation or gender identity. Aversion therapy involved pairing homoerotic stimuli with an aversive one, such as electric shocks or other painful stimuli to the hands or genitals, or nausea-inducing drugs. This approach also involved masturbatory reconditioning and visualization (Haldeman, 2002). Conversion therapy has often combined aversion techniques with "talk therapy," sometimes based on religious ideology. All practices aimed at changing a person's gender identity or sexual orientation are not only ineffective, they also have harmful effects, including depression, low self-esteem, avoidance of intimacy or romantic relationships, and sexual dysfunction (Haldeman, 2002). In a position

---

Cultural Considerations in Care

The Gender Dysphoria Controversy

The diagnosis of gender dysphoria and its DSM-IV precursor gender identity disorder have long been shrouded in controversy. The diagnosis of gender identity disorder has been widely perceived as stigmatizing because it implies that diverse gender identities are pathological. In the DSM-5 this diagnosis was changed to gender dysphoria. The latter refers to the distress experienced by individuals whose **sex assigned at birth** or assigned gender based on their external genitalia does not match their gender identity as perceived by themselves. The DSM-5 (American Psychiatric Association, 2013) defines gender dysphoria as "a strong desire to be rid of one's primary and/or secondary sex characteristics because of a marked incongruence with one's experienced/expressed gender, … a strong desire for the primary and/ or secondary sex characteristics of the other gender, … a strong desire to be of the other gender, … [and] … a strong conviction that one has the typical feelings and reactions of the other gender" (p. 452). This must also be "associated with clinically significant impairment in social, occupational, or other important areas of functioning" (American Psychiatric Association, 2013, p. 453).

paper recommendation, the Canadian Psychiatric Association (CPA) states: "The CPA opposes the use of reparative or conversion therapy, given that such therapy assumes that LGBTQ identities indicate a mental disorder and (or) the assumption that the person could and should change their sexual orientation and (or) their gender identity and gender expression" (Veltman & Chaimowitz, 2014, p. 3).

Throughout this chapter we use the term **gender dysphoria** to refer to distress experienced by a person whose sex assigned at birth or gender as perceived by others does not match their gender identity, acknowledging that this distress can be felt by individuals and is often also influenced by social and cultural discrimination.

Where We Are Today

The long-term pattern of institutional discrimination, exclusion, and maltreatment both inside and outside of the health care setting has had consequences for the health of SGD people. SGD individuals are more likely to experience mental health issues including depression, anxiety, substance use, and increased risk of suicide. Transgender and bisexual individuals in particular report worse mental health than other SGD people, which can be linked to increased experiences of marginalization (Zeeman et al., 2019). With respect to health disparities, SGD people are also at a greater risk of developing chronic illnesses (including certain cancers, autoimmune conditions, arthritis, cardiovascular disease, asthma, and other respiratory diseases) and of contracting sexually transmitted and blood-borne infections (STBBIs), including syphilis and HIV, compared to cisgender, heterosexual Canadians (Blondeel et al., 2016; Hafeez et al., 2017; Hottes et al., 2016; House of Commons Standing Committee on Health, 2019; Livingston, 2017; Meyer, 2003; Plöderl & Tremblay, 2015; Steele et al., 2016; The Trevor Project, 2020; Transgender PULSE Canada Team, 2020; Veale et al., 2017; Zeeman et al., 2019). These health disparities are not inherent to SGD identities but are instead linked to increased stress, marginalization, and discrimination, which increase allostatic load and vulnerability to negative health outcomes. Health disparities are exacerbated by covert and overt harm from the lack of cultural competency in health care. This can be attributed to lack of knowledge, fear of the unknown, and unconscious bias (Goldberg et al., 2017) when working with SGD people in health care and has particularly significant impacts on transgender patients (Safer et al., 2016).

Our health care system has largely functioned with the assumption that gender exists in binary categories of "man" and "woman," and that these categories correspond with the sex assigned at birth, based on external genitalia (Iskander & Keenan, 2021; Stryker, 2006). Predictably, health care is no exception from prevailing transphobia and homophobia. There is a lack of data regarding SGD people's health, and many health care providers do not receive adequate education about SGD identities, existence, and health care needs (Mulé et al., 2020; Scheim et al., 2017).

Outside of the immediate health care setting, SGD people face discrimination in multiple settings impacting income and societal roles, such as securing and retaining employment. This contributes to higher rates of poverty, food insecurity, and homelessness, which in turn lead to increased health risks. SGD youth are also at increased risk of homelessness, largely due to a lack of familial acceptance of their sexual orientation or gender identity (House of Commons Standing Committee on Health, 2019). This problem is exacerbated by a lack of shelters that adequately and safely serve SGD people. SGD people experience increased rates of physical and sexual violence and social rejection (Blondeel et al., 2016; Colpitts & Gahagan, 2016b; Egale, 2020; House of Commons Standing Committee on Health, 2019; Jaffray, 2020; Meyer, 2003; Plöderl & Tremblay, 2015; Roberts et al., 2010; The Trevor Project, 2020; Transgender

PULSE Canada Team, 2020; Williams et al., 2017). None of these disparities are inherent aspects of sexual orientation or gender identity, rather they are a reflection of how SGD individuals have been viewed and treated within our society.

A More Inclusive Approach

Once SGD people access care, a major aspect of the health care provider's role is to build rapport. Taking time to develop a therapeutic relationship allows the health care provider to gain the patient's trust and determine what the patient needs to feel safer in the care environment. The aim of cultural safety and cultural competence in care for SGD people is to move away from pathologizing and labelling the community and take a person-centred approach that recognizes lived experiences (Collins & Arthur, 2010). Health care providers must avoid making assumptions about sexuality and gender identity. Instead, we should ask patients to explain or clarify information to ensure care can be complete and appropriate (Fung et al., 2020).

A common attempt at inclusivity in recent years has been the creation of safe spaces—physical or symbolic spaces intended to be free from oppression, judgement, and harm. The idea of a "safe space" has origins with psychologist Kurt Lewin, who identified the need for psychological safety in a space for change and honesty to occur (Lewin, 1947). "Safe spaces" were furthered by psychologist Carl Rogers and by SGD people to become what they are today (Kenney, 2001; Rogers, 1971). However, "safer spaces" may be a more appropriate aim. The idea of a safe space is well intentioned, but often cannot be guaranteed. In many circumstances, safe spaces are not in fact protected from violence, ignorance, and bigotry because of the very nature of the systems that these spaces operate within. Additionally, people have different requirements for feeling safe (Mental Health Commission of Canada, 2019). Guaranteeing a "safe space" when it is not possible to do so can lead to distrust. With "safer spaces," we acknowledge that nothing is certain in this imperfect system, but that considerable efforts have been made for all participants to feel safe, respected, and not judged (Thompson, 2017). In a health care setting, there are many factors outside the control of an individual health care provider. A health care provider can, however, be nonjudgemental, actively listen to patient experiences, and provide compassionate care in collaboration with patients. One way to achieve these outcomes is through the FIRST approach, which has its roots in Mi'kmaq culture (Table 10.2) (Latimer et al., 2020; Sylliboy & Hovey, 2020).

It is important to note that in providing "safer spaces" we are making attempts to normalize and understand differences among people. It can be uncomfortable for people to challenge their notions

---

TABLE 10.2 ■ **FIRST Approach**

- **F**amily (consider family: immediate, extended or chosen)
- **I**nformation (consider *how* information is shared, be respectful, ask questions and listen with the goal of understanding)
- **R**elationship building (create trust, take interest, give patients choice and ask permission)
- **S**afer Space (understand cultural safety, be intentional with language use, cultivate a safer space; more details are provided in this chapter)
- Treat **T**ogether (come up with a treatment and follow-up plan *with* the patient, incorporating concepts and interventions beyond Western medicine when that best suits the patient)

Adapted from Latimer, M., Sylliboy, J. R., Francis, J., et al. (2020). Co-creating better healthcare experiences for First Nations children and youth: The FIRST approach emerges from two-eyed seeing. *Paediatric and Neonatal Pain, 2*(4), 104–112. https://doi.org/10.1002/pne2.12024.

of discrimination, violence, harm, and power relations, but this discomfort does not mean that their safety is in jeopardy (Thompson, 2017). It is vital as health care providers that we allow ourselves to feel uncomfortable so that we will be susceptible to different ideas that our patients may expose us to. Discomfort can disrupt institutional norms and provide transformative possibilities for reimagining previously held assumptions and beliefs (Goldberg, 2015).

Health Care Environment

Creating an inclusive health care environment for SGD people spans the physical setting as well as the attitudes, policies, and values espoused by organizations. These considerations must be consistently implemented through every interaction that SGD patients have within the health care setting to address and mitigate systemic barriers to care. Health care's cisheteronormative foundations can otherwise lead to what has been described as the informational and institutional erasure of transgender (and other SGD) people (Bauer et al., 2009). In other words, it is important to recognize that the norm within our health care system is based on systems, structures, and processes that privilege, almost exclusively at times, the norm of heterosexual, cisgender people. The needs of SGD people remain invisible and often ignored.

As discussed in earlier chapters, cultural competence requires sensitivity, knowledge, skills, and resources on the part of the health care providers; however, several studies report health care providers receiving minimal education on the needs of SGD people (Beagan et al., 2015; Gahagan & Subirana-Malaret, 2020; Stewart & O'Reilley, 2017). Stewart and O'Reilley (2017) undertook an integrative review exploring the attitudes, knowledge, and beliefs of nurses and midwives regarding the health care needs of the 2SLGBTQ+ population. They noted attitudes ranging from affirmation and advocacy, to treating everybody the same, as well as intrusion and judgement from health care staff and providers. Similarly, Beagan et al. (2015) explored family physicians' perceptions of working with LGBTQ patients and noted the following themes: (1) sexual/gender identity does not matter as they treat everyone equally; (2) sexual /gender identity does matter in order to provide holistic care and address the impact of stigma and discrimination; and (3) sexual identity both matters and does not matter when physicians described the tension between understanding social group needs and individualized care. Such findings clearly identify the need for health care providers to understand the difference between equality and equity in order to reduce health disparities, as well as the need for ongoing education and support.

In a health care environment, patients often first make contact with a receptionist or health care administrative staff person before having disclosed their name, gender, or pronouns. Although using language such as "sir," "ma'am," "Ms.," or "Mr." may be intended as a means of communicating respect, it is important to note that this language involves an assumption about gender. These terms can easily be avoided. Once known, the language that a patient uses to describe themselves and their identity should be mirrored by all health care providers (see Cultural Competence in Action box).

Completing initial assessment or documentation forms can set the stage for patient–provider interactions, and thus deliberate care should be taken to avoid assuming patients' sexuality and gender. A patient's name and gender may be incongruent with the name on legal health care documentation (such as a health card or birth certificate) or with their sex assigned at birth. Although it may be necessary to collect this legal information, it is important to also ask patients their name and pronouns. Information about patients' gender and pronouns should be documented in a way that is easily accessible to all staff involved in their care. It is important to also note that such information is confidential health information and should be treated accordingly. Intake forms can help collect information about settings in which a patient is comfortable having their gender affirmed. Some patients may prefer the use of different words in confidential settings than in a waiting room, by phone, or in the presence of family. It is crucial for this information to be collected and documented clearly, as "outing" a patient may erode trust, create discomfort, or decrease physical and emotional safety.

Using gender-neutral language (such as "spouse," "partner," "parent," "sibling," and "child") is a way of promoting inclusivity of SGD individuals. Forms and documentation should not constrain identity and sexuality into discrete and fixed categories; rather, they should allow patients to use their own words. Identity terms are not fixed, as both language and experience shape an evolving understanding of identity. SGD patients may use different terms to describe their identity depending on the context and their experiences. The terms may be shaped by identity categories such as race, class, and gender, in addition to historical, social, and cultural understandings of desire and sexuality (Yep et al., 2003). Though the nuances of sexual orientation and gender identity are not easily captured on forms, the structure of forms can be used to signal a health care provider's openness to such discussions as they pertain to the patient's health.

It is important that SGD people see themselves represented in the physical setting. Visible symbols of support and indications of no tolerance of abuse are commonly used. It is imperative that these visible signs of support be accompanied by corresponding actions and care. However, this type of representation should go beyond rainbow flags and stickers. It should include magazines and educational materials displayed in waiting rooms and offices, and posters displaying sexual and gender diversity. Examples of this includes the "check it out guys" campaign promoting regular pap smears for transmasculine patients, the "clear the air" posters aimed at promoting smoking cessation in SGD communities, and resources from the Native Youth Sexual Health Network that are inclusive of Indigenous SGD identities (see www.rainbowhealthontario.ca and https://www.nativeyouthsexualhealth.com) (Native Youth Sexual Health Network—Resources, n.d.; Rainbow Health Ontario, 2009, 2012). Signs of inclusive care in the physical health care setting also involve access to gender-neutral washrooms, change tables, and menstrual products in all washrooms. Prior to accessing a health care setting, patients commonly review online materials, which should similarly be tailored to be deliberately inclusive and representative of SGD people.

Safer care for SGD people involves awareness and acknowledgement that current systems may not be designed to be inclusive. Electronic medical records may be designed to only include information present on government-issued health care documents, or may auto-populate forms, requisitions, or referrals with that information. Labs or pharmacies may only be able to process information concordant with legal health care information. Availability of non-cisheteronormative educational materials may be limited. In any of these circumstances, as health care providers we have a role in advocating for change based on the needs of our patients. Our role involves recognizing and acknowledging these shortcomings to SGD patients and explaining why we may not yet be able to be affirming in such circumstances. In addition to promoting inclusion by

---

Cultural Competence in Action

Mistakes Happen!

Francis is a 26-year-old non-binary person who recently moved to a new city. They reached out to other transgender people in the city through a social media group to ask for recommendations for a transgender-competent family medicine clinic. Though they were nervous when they first arrived in the clinic,

Continued

> they noted both a rainbow flag and a transgender pride flag behind the front desk, as well as posters in the clinic depicting queer and transgender people. They were greeted by a receptionist who gave them an intake form to fill out. Francis was pleased to see that this form asked for both their legal information and their name, gender, and pronouns. They were called in, and first met with a nurse who went over their medical history and measured their vital signs. The doctor then entered, saying "Hi, I'm Dr. Jones, my pronouns are she/her. You must be Francis?" Francis was pleasantly surprised that their doctor had shared her pronouns instead of only asking what Francis' were. When reviewing their vital signs with the nurse, Dr. Jones accidentally asked what "her" blood pressure was. Dr. Jones quickly realized her mistake, turned to Francis, and said "my apologies, what was their blood pressure?" This correction communicated to Francis that Dr. Jones's intention was to provide affirming care. It helped them feel comfortable later telling Dr. Jones that they preferred the use of the term "chest" instead of "breast" when discussing binding. Though Francis felt apprehensive that Dr. Jones might react poorly to this correction, they were reassured when Dr. Jones responded with "thank you for letting me know."
>
> This example demonstrates how creating a safer space for SGD people (through flags, posters, language selection on intake forms, and staff attitudes) can enable SGD patients to collaborate with their providers and reduce systemic barriers to care.
>
> Mistakes happen, and if you notice a mistake you have made, you can offer an apology to your patient and move on. It's important to remember that even if this evokes feelings of guilt, you need to focus on your patient's experience and not your own reactions. If a patient corrects a mistake you have made, a simple "thank you for the reminder" can address any rupture that may have resulted and reaffirm a desire to provide safe and inclusive care.

determining, documenting, and using the patient's name and gender identity in all interactions, health care providers can also advocate for change at the system level.

While the elements described thus far indicate an intention to provide inclusive and safer care for SGD people, the policies and values of an organization must also reflect this. Explicitly stating terms such as "sexual orientation," "gender identity," and "gender expression" in nondiscrimination policies is a good first step. Clear standards should be set for all patients and staff regarding affirming and nondiscriminatory behaviour, and education should be provided accordingly.

Primary Care

In Canada, health care is predominantly accessed through primary care. However, as discussed in previous chapters, not all populations have equitable access to care. The aim of primary care is to provide a patient-centred medical home, where the patient's full context can be taken into account while providing integrated and appropriate care. For this to happen effectively, it is imperative that a person feel safe and included in that health care environment. SGD people may be reluctant to disclose their sexual and gender identity because of past negative experiences in health care and a lack of confidence in the ability of the care provider to be sensitive to SGD people and issues (Beagan et al., 2015; Gahagan & Subirana-Malaret, 2020). Health care providers often make assumptions about the patient's pronouns, gender, sexuality, partners, the sexual acts they participate in, the body parts they have and those used for sex, and even whether the individual is sexual. Similarly, gender and sexuality are often mistakenly conflated. Knowing about the patient's gender does not provide information about their sexuality, and vice versa (Mizock & Hopwood, 2016; Poteat et al., 2016). Making assumptions about patients can lead to overlooking critical factors required for providing appropriate health care. For instance, bisexual people have been viewed by health care workers as straight when their partners were a different gender and viewed as gay or lesbian when they were with a same-sex dating partner (Legge et al., 2018). The dismissal of bisexual people's sexual identity can not only result in inappropriate care but also lead to feelings of invisibility and invalidation (Ross et al., 2010).

Additionally, the language used in regularly conversing with patients can be heavily gendered. Rather than discussing the fact that women should get a pap test done every 3 years, a provider can state that a "person with a uterus needs a pap every 3 years." Screening discussions should be based on anatomy and behaviour, as opposed to gender. Physical exams and some investigations are also times to be particularly attuned to possible distress. Examinations that involve disrobing or removing protective garments such as binders can be vulnerable experiences. Time should be taken to discuss with patients when and why these tests might contribute to their care and how the provider could work with them to decrease the distress of these encounters.

In a primary care setting, assumptions are made particularly frequently during a sexual health history. Before conducting a sexual health history, it is important to consider two factors. First and foremost, determine whether a sexual history is needed at that time. Simply asking patients why they are seeking care is an important step (Collins & Arthur, 2010). Is knowledge of the patient's sexual orientation or gender identity important to the concerns prompting them to seek care? Many SGD

Cultural Competence in Action

Let's Talk About Sex

Zenya, a 31-year-old female with a history of polycystic ovarian syndrome (PCOS), presented to a walk-in clinic because of feeling excessively tired over the past month and missing her most recent period. As part of the history, the doctor asked her, "Do you have sex with men, women, or both?" Zenya answered honestly with "one woman, my partner Sarah." She did not offer additional details about Sarah's gender or anatomy as the doctor's question had communicated a binary, cisgender framework. The doctor expressed that Zenya's fatigue and delayed period were most likely secondary to her PCOS, but gave her a laboratory requisition for some basic blood work to rule out iron deficiency anemia.

Zenya got her bloodwork done but didn't feel comfortable at the walk-in clinic, so she sought further care at the nearby Rainbow Health Clinic in Edmonton, Alberta. At this clinic, Dr. Ramesh started asking her general questions about her health to get a sense of why she came in. He asked Zenya if she would be *willing to speak about sexual health*, and if she had *ever been sexually active*. Both answers were yes. He asked, *"Do you have any current sexual partners?"* Given the open phrasing of these questions, Zenya felt more comfortable sharing personal information. He then asked, *"Which body parts do you use for sex? Which body parts do your partners use?"* She disclosed that she uses her vagina and her parner Sarah, a transgender woman who uses her penis. The disclosure allowed for further questioning eliciting that Zenya's β-hCG level should also be tested because of the risk of pregnancy. It turned out that Zenya was indeed pregnant, which was the reason for her fatigue being beyond her baseline.

Phrasing, as this situation demonstrates, can have a drastic impact on therapeutic alliance, differential diagnosis, and the ultimate quality of care.

Note: The word "partners" was used here, as opposed to "partner," as this presupposes that a person might have more than one partner and avoids assumption of monogamous norms.

---

patients find that the focus of health interviews can inappropriately hinge around their sexuality or gender, when that is not the reason for their presentation. This contributes to SGD patients' reluctance to seek health care. Histories should generally begin by talking about non-sexual health–related topics. Once those have been addressed, health care providers can explore whether further history is required about sexual health. Health care providers should refer to previously identified data, if available, regarding a patient's sex assigned at birth, and information regarding the patient's medical and surgical history with attention to which body parts they have and any body parts that have been added, removed, or modified. For example, a transmasculine individual with ovaries who is on testosterone may not menstruate but can still be at risk for pregnancy (Boudreau & Mukerjee, 2019; Obedin-Maliver & Makadon, 2016). Conversations about screening and health can then be targetted to an individual's anatomy.

Once the topic of sexual health has been approached appropriately (see Cultural Competence in Action box above), the line of questioning must continue in a respectful way that does not limit the patient's answers. If the patient indicates having current sexual partners, following up with *"would you like to talk about sexually transmitted infection prevention or testing?"* can invite patients to spend further time discussing this. Further questions can help the provider determine a patient's anatomy and applicable sexual practices. Asking *"which parts of your body do you use for sex?"* allows the provider to swab the appropriate body parts to assess for sexually transmitted infections (STIs), as suggested by current guidelines (Workowski et al., 2021). This rationale should be explained to the patient.

Asking *"which parts of the body do your partners use for sex?"* varies considerably from the commonplace "do you have sex with men, women, or both?". The latter may not provide useful information. If the patient says "men," they could mean transgender men, cisgender men, people with penises, or people who identify as masculine. It also avoids the assumption that a person's sexual orientation aligns with their sexual practices. People may be exploring their sexuality, or have partners who do not align with traditional conceptions of the term they use to describe their sexuality (Boudreau & Mukerjee, 2019; Eckstrand & Ehrenfeld, 2016; Light et al., 2017; Obedin-Maliver & Makadon, 2016). Adding a question about whether pregnancy is a possibility in any of their relationships can open a conversation about contraceptive needs that is inclusive of all gender identities.

Phrased appropriately, these questions create a respectful, inclusive space for sexual health conversation and the assessment of further health needs, including risk of pregnancy and STIs. This information helps, for example, determine whether a patient might be a candidate for pre-exposure prophylaxis (PrEP), a daily pill taken for prevention of human immunodeficiency virus (HIV) acquisition, or may benefit from further contraceptive discussions.

Whenever health care providers discuss sexual health, it is important to keep in mind that there are different circumstances under which people might engage in sex. It might be as part of a romantic relationship, anonymous encounters, sex work, as a result of sexual violence, or any other context. A sexual history should elucidate such information, enabling providers to understand additional risk factors. For instance, two people who each have a uterus and ovaries in a monogamous relationship have no risk of pregnancy, but if one of these people had a nonconsensual sexual encounter with someone who produces sperm, there may now be a risk of pregnancy. Such discussions may also open the door to talking about personal safety and may lead to referrals to other services. Support, sensitivity, and choice should always be offered during sexual health histories and examinations.

Obstetrics and Gynecology

Fertility, pregnancy, and reproductive health have traditionally been tied to gender within the health care system. Obstetrics and gynecology (OBGYN) has often been equated with "women's health" or "female reproduction." Understandably, for SGD individuals, accessing OBGYN care can feel vulnerable and alienating (Eckstrand & Ehrenfeld, 2016). OBGYN care may involve discussing sexual practices and reproductive organs and function, and undergoing intimate physical examinations, all of which may expose SGD people to discrimination or stigma (Eckstrand & Ehrenfeld, 2016). This leads many SGD people to postpone care, decline care, or withhold information from their providers, contributing to ongoing health disparities (Eckstrand & Ehrenfeld, 2016; Hoffkling et al., 2017). Consider a transmasculine person experiencing pelvic pain or irregular bleeding, a non-binary person with ovaries and a uterus wondering about their family history of ovarian cancer, or a transfeminine person with new hair growth in her neo-vagina. By framing obstetrics as a binary, cisgender "women's" issue, we risk excluding and marginalizing an entire portion of our population (Besse et al., 2020; Hoffkling et al., 2017). As health care providers, we have the opportunity and responsibility to broaden our definitions of reproductive care to welcome and affirm all people. In this section, we will highlight a few key areas where an understanding of SGD experiences may provide occasions for more holistic and person-centred care.

The physical examination is a particularly vulnerable aspect of any person's medical care. Within gynecology, a pelvic examination involves assessing the reproductive organs. Unfortunately, some gender diverse individuals have described medical providers asking questions or performing exams that were seemingly more for the curiosity of the provider than for medical necessity (Hoffkling et al., 2017). If an examination is required, it is often helpful to describe what will happen, why it is important, and reiterate that consent can be withdrawn at any time.

A study in 2020 found that the majority of transmasculine and non-binary patients surveyed had never had physicians ask which terms to use for their anatomy, yet the majority of respondents reported wishing their doctor would ask (Klein & Golub, 2020). Unsurprisingly, people had a range of preferred terms to use for their bodies, and so assumptions should not be made that what is affirming for one person will make the next person comfortable (Klein & Golub, 2020; Schwartz et al., 2019). Careful language and thoughtful discussion can help gain trust and reduce discomfort (Besse et al., 2020; Eckstrand & Ehrenfeld, 2016).

Preventing unintended pregnancies is an important aspect of reproductive health for all people. Many people who were assigned female at birth and who identify as SGD face barriers to contraception access and have equal, if not higher, risks of unintended pregnancy compared to cisgender heterosexual women (Blunt-Vinti et al., 2018; Everett et al., 2017; Higgins et al., 2019; Stoffel et al., 2017). Consequently, contraception and abortion care providers must be aware that people of all genders and sexual orientations may seek their services and deserve inclusive, comprehensive care.

The decision to become pregnant and give birth is individual. We cannot assume that all people wish to, or are able to, have biological children. Alternative routes to create a family should also be valued (Eckstrand & Ehrenfeld, 2016). Any person with a uterus may choose to pursue pregnancy; this includes transmasculine and non-binary individuals. Even in medically uncomplicated pregnancies, SGD people can face unique challenges. Among transgender individuals who carry a pregnancy, a range of experiences is found. Some people find pregnancy dysphoria inducing and emotionally challenging, especially as it involves stopping hormone therapy. Others find the experience of pregnancy empowering as they connect to a part of their body that has never felt right (Hoffkling et al., 2017). Transgender people may face social stigma with pregnancy and may struggle to reconcile their gender identity and expression with the visible aspects of pregnancy (Besse et al., 2020; Hoffkling et al., 2017). Any of these factors may lead SGD individuals to need closer social support during pregnancy (Obedin-Maliver & Makadon, 2016).

The social navigation of pregnancy is layered onto navigating the health care system. Some transmasculine people have described feeling relieved to hear that they are not the only transgender patient that the provider has encountered. Others describe feeling positive when a provider without such experience takes the initiative to educate themselves in preparation for the next appointment (Hoffkling et al., 2017).

As in every clinical encounter, it is important to learn a patient's name(s) and pronouns. The names and pronouns of any partners should also be asked and documented—not assumed (Besse et al., 2020). The antenatal record provides an opportunity to communicate such information to the entire health care team.

Prenatal appointments also provide an opportunity for health care providers to collaborate with patients in developing a birth plan. Again, the values, priorities, and fears of each patient may vary. Some people desire elective Caesarean births, while others prefer an intimate home birth (Light et al., 2017). Some want to suppress lactation, and others hope to induce lactation for feeding their baby (Obedin-Maliver & Makadon, 2016). A hospital birth will be medically recommended for many patients, but a hospital may also include new providers, multiple internal examinations, and lack of control (Besse et al., 2020). For many people, a hospital environment can increase the possibility that their identity, or their relationship with their partner, will be invalidated.

Consider the culture in your institution. Are SGD people included in the ways outlined in the discussion on health care environment (earlier in chapter)? Are partners of all genders recognized in the delivery room? Is it okay if your patient does not want to assign a gender to their baby? Are there ways for your patient to communicate language they want used about their body? If not, consider avenues for change, education, and advocacy. Obstetric health has moved beyond binary, cisgender "women's health." Thoughtful, welcoming, culturally competent reproductive health care is critical for the care of all people, especially SGD individuals and families. (Also see Chapter 12.)

Children and Youth

Many children and youth have regular contact with health care providers through well-child visits spanning from the first days of life through the teenage years. In these visits, health care providers outline developmental milestones to parents or caretakers, often focusing on physical, language, motor, and social development. Although identity development is rarely discussed explicitly, this is an important domain in a person's health and wellness. As per the Canadian Paediatric Society, children are thought to start recognizing differences between "girls" and "boys" by 2 years of age. As children develop an understanding of these social identities, they may begin to identify themselves in a way that fluctuates with time or may not match their sex assigned at birth. By age 4 years, most children begin to have a more stable gender identity. Children typically express their gender in stereotyped ways before age 6. Stereotypical gender expression gradually reduces with age as children gain confidence that others recognize them in their gender. This may coincide with increased social anxiety for children whose gender identity does not correspond with their sex assigned at birth. Gender identity is further developed from age 8 onward. Pubertal changes may highlight a child's sense that their gender identity does not correspond with the sex assigned at birth (Canadian Paediatric Society [CPS], 2018). During this critical period, health care providers should encourage families to remain open-minded, accepting, and caring. Such attitudes contribute to an enduring stable pattern of attachment within interpersonal relationships for children, which predicts positive health and social outcomes (CPS, 2018; Sizemore et al., 2019).

Sexual identity has also been found to develop through childhood and teenage years. Awareness of same or different sex attraction is thought to begin at approximately 10 years old, and self-identification of sexual orientation around 16 to 17 years old (Boxer & Herdt, 1996). Although the developmental lens of sexual and gender identity suggests normative timelines, it does not account for ways that identities are explored and experienced throughout a person's life. Our understanding of ourselves is shaped by personal reflection, evolving experience, language, and sociocultural inputs. SGD youth themselves have shaped how their identities are described and understood by inventing new terminology for their experiences (Bragg et al., 2018; Cover, 2018). As media accounts of transgender youth expanded through the 2010s, so did the language used, including terms such as "gender nonconforming," "gender variant," "gender creative," "gender expansive," "gender independent," "non-binary," and "agender." Terminology used to describe sexual orientation has also expanded, including such concepts as "pansexual," "heteroflexible," and "asexual" (Iskander & Keenan, 2021). As terminology expands, so do the labels that individuals use to identify and understand themselves, further contributing to the fluidity that can naturally exist in gender and sexual identity.

As much as health care providers learn from listening to youth, providers also have an important role in educating youth and parents. Education settings also offer an opportunity to teach youth about these topics and promote health. However, standard sexual education may not cover topics important to SGD people. When these topics are covered, the focus is often on reducing homophobia and transphobia, with little attention to other identities. Inadequate sexuality and gender-affirming health education reinforces the structural marginalization of SGD young people and further exacerbates inequities (Grant & Nash, 2019).

Health care providers have a role in discussing and normalizing different gender identities and sexual orientations. With young children, it is important to discuss these topics in a developmentally appropriate manner. One method of facilitating this has been through the use of tools such as the Gender Unicorn or the Genderbread Person, which are simple graphics that describe the basics of sexual and gender identity concepts (Global Justice Collective, n.d.; Trans Student Educational Resources, n.d.). Although these graphics may represent accessible ways to introduce discussions of gender identity and sexual orientation, it is important to note that these concepts are individual, nuanced, and fluid.

It is important to take an intersectional approach with young people, recognizing that young adulthood is a critical time for identity development. Their racial, cultural, sexual, gender, and other evolving identities all impact their care needs and the care experience. In a discussion of inclusive care for Indigenous and Torres Strait Islander LGBTQ+ young people in Australia, Uink et al. (2020) note that young people may feel particularly isolated as they experience increased health risks due to homophobia, transphobia, racism, and discrimination and may lack knowledge and information of available services. Such isolation may be intensified in rural and remote settings. Individuals may also experience challenges in negotiating and reconciling their cultural or Indigenous identity with sexual and gender identity, leading to a further disconnect from family and community. Adopting an inclusive approach includes creating opportunities to provide information and feedback on needs and services (Uink et al., 2020). Other strategies include decreasing use of medicalized language to reduce power differentials, reinforcing the limits of confidentiality to create trust and safety, and integrating diverse ways of knowing and being. Ongoing reflection of health care providers on assumptions, approaches, and outcomes is also critical (Uink et al., 2020). As with adult patients, health care providers should endeavour to take an affirming approach to gender- and sexuality-related care with children and youth. If patients are experiencing gender dysphoria (distress related to gender assigned at birth, gender expression, or others' perceptions of one's gender) an affirming approach can involve medical interventions and strategies that focus on lessening a person's distress about their appearance or gendered perceptions of their body.

The ability of youth to access health care services or interventions without their parents or guardians providing consent differs across the world. It is important to know local guidelines and let youth know the limits of confidentiality. Wherever possible, health care providers can educate and advocate to increase familial and social supports for youth, as these variables are important predictors of SGD youths' mental health (Travers et al., 2012). Although it is ideal to optimize familial and social support, this is not always possible, and it is not prerequisite to care.

Transition and Gender-Affirming Care

Transition is the process by which gender diverse individuals take steps to align themselves more closely with their internal, self-conceptualized gender identity. It is a multifaceted process which can involve psychological, social, legal, medical, and surgical aspects (Thomas et al., 2017). Transitions do not have one defined end point. People have individual goals and may choose to undergo certain aspects of a transition but not others. This decision should be respected, and their gender identity is as valid as someone who undergoes additional steps.

Despite progress in certain parts of the world, such as legal changes expanding protections for gender diverse people (Parliament of Canada, 2017) and some funding provisions for surgical transition (Alberta Health Services, n.d.), there remain inherent institutional and systemic barriers that may be encountered at each possible stage of a person's transition (Reisner et al., 2016). These barriers can lead to significant mental and physical health disparities for transgender populations, particularly those facing intersecting facets of marginalization, such as transgender women of colour (Sevelius, 2013). In some cases these barriers prohibit people from achieving the transition they desire.

In countries that provide access to gender-affirming surgery, guidelines are similar as they are often informed by the World Professional Association for Transgender Health (WPATH) standards of care (Coleman et al., 2012); Alberta, Canada will be used here as an example. To access funding for gender-affirming surgery, a patient must be diagnosed with gender dysphoria by a psychiatrist and must have letters from two psychiatrists, or one psychiatrist and a specialized family physician, recommending gender-affirming surgery. Getting the required psychiatric appointments may entail lengthy waitlists. The patient must have "completed a minimum of 12 months of the appropriate hormone therapy," lived "at least one year of the 'real-life experience' (e.g., functioning in the desired gender, legal name changes)," have "an adequate support network, a stable lifestyle," and not have "current substance abuse problems (alcohol or drugs), antisocial or behavioural issues" (Government of Alberta, 2012). These are just a few of the many criteria required to access funding. Patients are unable to apply for funding directly; the application must be completed by a psychiatrist. Procedures not funded include "chest contouring, breast augmentation for those with breast growth, facial feminization, tracheal shave and voice pitch surgery." Phalloplasty, metoidioplasty, and vaginoplasty are eligible for funding but are only offered nearly 3 000 km away, in Montreal, Quebec. Even if a patient receives funding, they still must pay out of pocket for their accommodations while in Montreal and for all medications and equipment they take home with them during the postsurgical recovery process (Alberta Health Services, n.d.).

The WPATH model does recommend that psychological assessment be a part of transition care and supports many of the requirements for funding (Coleman et al., 2012). WPATH finds that these requirements give time to document consistent, lasting gender dysphoria and to process social adjustments before having irreversible surgery (Coleman et al., 2012). However, many patients perceive this process as gatekeeping, thus the "informed consent model" presents an alternative approach (Cavanaugh et al., 2016). The informed consent model views the onerous psychological consultation as a significant barrier to access that fails to respect the autonomy of the individual seeking gender-affirming care (Hale, 2007). It recognizes that some people pursuing surgical transition feel the need to access psychological or psychiatric care, but many do not. The model allows that patients themselves may be the ones best positioned to assess their transition- related needs (Cavanaugh et al., 2016). This model does not require external evaluation of the person seeking care; rather, it suggests that discussion with a health care provider of risks and benefits of the possible options can be sufficient. The informed consent approach is based on the principles of patient autonomy and informed consent that are applied for most other surgical procedures.

The majority of transgender people report moderate to high levels of transphobic treatment when seeking medical care (Cavanaugh et al., 2016). These experiences can lead transgender patients to seek affirming care outside of standard clinical practice, for example, procuring hormones without a prescription and without the advice and guidance of a medical provider (Bauer et al., 2015).

Given the many barriers and frequency of having their identity pathologized (see earlier section, Historical Perspectives), gender diverse people may be wary of the health care system. It is up to health care providers to ensure that they are compassionate with patients and to minimize barriers through reflection, advocacy, and making changes to their own practices.

Care of Older Persons

Accessing culturally responsive health care can be difficult for SGD people of all ages, but unique barriers are experienced by older SGD adults. They are likely to have grown up in a time when diversity was more stigmatized and pathologized than at present. Being open about their identity, or being outed without their consent, often meant decades of discrimination and harm (Fredriksen-Goldsen et al., 2015). As barriers to health care access and health disparities for SGD people were even greater in the past, this can also mean compounding effects of many years with insufficient care (Stinchcombe et al., 2018).

With age, people tend to experience more health concerns. If hospital-based care is required, there can be difficulties when no legally recognized marriage exists. For older SGD people, same-sex marriage was illegal for much or all of their young adulthood, thus legally recognized marriages are rare in this population. Life partners may not be permitted to be substitute decision makers. The default to next of kin as substitute decision makers may be inappropriate. Some SGD individuals, particularly older adults, may be supported by their chosen family rather than their biological family. This is also a barrier in health care settings where visits are restricted to partners by marriage and biological family (Stinchcombe et al., 2017).

Long-term care facilities or other supportive living situations create additional issues. They are often avoided by SGD individuals because of stereotypes, stigmatization, and fear of social isolation (Stinchcombe et al., 2017). There is the pressure to disclose sexual or gender identity to many new and unfamiliar people (Furlotte et al., 2016). Rooming of patients and staff support can be heavily focused on gender. People who may have been living as their authentic gender or sexual identity may feel pressure to conform and assume cisheteromonogamous norms in their senior years.

Irrespective of how a person presents themselves or the information they initially disclose, it is important to avoid assumptions. For instance, a person may have been in a heterosexual marriage or have been presenting themselves as cisgender for many decades and now be starting to explore another side to their sexuality or gender identity. It is very common for people to make assumptions about the gender, sexuality, and/or sexual practices of older persons. This leads to geriatric sexual health frequently being overlooked. Many older persons had scarce or nonexistent formal sexual education. When education was provided, it was in relation to cisheteronormative health care practices and systems (Stinchcombe et al., 2017).

It is often assumed that older people are not sexually active or physically intimate. Although some people may choose to avoid these activities, many do not and sexual health needs to be part of their care.

People currently in their senior years were young adults during a time when homosexuality was pathologized and criminalized in medical and social systems. In the early 1980s, when the HIV epidemic was in full force, many doctors refused to treat patients (predominantly men who had sex with men) with HIV (David, 2017). Many people who lived through these times have been left with a distrust of the health care system. Older SGD patients seek health care providers who are educated in SGD health, who are nondiscriminatory and compassionate, and who understand the potentially harmful history that they may have had in health care and beyond (Putney et al., 2018). As health care providers we must keep this important context in mind as we seek to provide inclusive care to older SGD adults. It is also important to remind ourselves and our patients that older SGD people can have a high quality of life, often associated with positive sexual identity, the development of resilience and crisis competence, and strong social relationships (Goldsen & de Vries, 2019).

Mental Health

Seeking health care is often a vulnerable experience, involving examination of both bodies and minds. This vulnerability can be emphasized in mental health care settings because of the sensitive nature of the material discussed, combined with longstanding stigma surrounding mental health. Finding mental health care providers with competence in working with SGD people can be particularly challenging (The Trevor Project, 2020; Transgender PULSE Canada Team, 2020).

SGD people experience a disproportionate burden of mental illness due to marginalization, pathologization, and discrimination. It is imperative that all health care providers be able to provide inclusive care with respect to mental health. Previous hostile, invasive, or pathologizing experiences experienced by SGD patients contribute to increased anxiety, decreased engagement, guardedness, or defensiveness when accessing care that is not inclusive or validating. The heightened anxiety experienced by SGD people may not represent a mental health disorder but may instead be rational fear given the increased violence faced by this population. Discussing patients' sexual orientation and gender identity may allow greater insight and opportunities to intervene regarding social determinants of mental health. Trauma-informed care and cultural competency and humility are crucial to decrease the health disparities experienced by SGD people.

Transgender and gender diverse people occupy a particularly precarious position with regard to mental health. As discussed earlier, current guidelines for gender-affirming surgery in Alberta, Canada require patients to meet DSM-5 criteria for gender dysphoria. The guidelines also state, "If significant medical or mental concerns are present, they must be reasonably well-controlled" (Coleman et al., 2012). Predictably, patients are left in a situation in which they may emphasize symptoms consistent with a gender dysphoria diagnosis or minimize other mental health concerns for fear of being denied care. For health care providers involved in mental health evaluations prior to providing access to gender-affirming care, it is important to note that patients have the best understanding of their own gender identity. Our role as health care providers is not to sleuth out a person's true gender identity; it is to support patients, including their ability to provide informed consent to care. This is best achieved in working collaboratively with patients and valuing their knowledge as well as professional expertise. Gender-affirming care can be profoundly beneficial to patients' mental health and often results in decreased anxiety or depression (Barranco, 2020). On the other hand, many patients describe the experience of hormone therapy as a "second puberty," which may also have emotional and temperamental impacts.

One approach that can be used to promote mental health is to include conversations around **resiliency**. Although resiliency is not uniformly defined, it evolves over time and circumstances and precedes or supports one's ability to cope with adversity (Colpitts & Gahagan, 2016a). It has been proposed that resiliency goes beyond personal attributes; it also encompasses the environmental factors that contribute to overcoming adversity (Ungar, 2011). This is particularly important for SGD people, whose mental health is often significantly impacted by social and environmental factors. Resiliency-oriented conversations place health outcomes in context and are strength-based in nature. It is important to differentiate resiliency from "positive thinking," which can involve a burdensome or excessive focus on happiness in the face of adversity (Andrade, 2019). Resiliency-based approaches can involve exploring supportive interpersonal, cultural, and institutional factors, such as having an affirming family or educational system, connection to SGD community, positive SGD role models, and positive media representation of SGD people. Resiliency-based approaches also stress personal qualities such as positive self-esteem, self-efficacy, cognitive ability to mediate stress, self-acceptance, proactive coping, self-care, shamelessness, and spirituality (Colpitts & Gahagan, 2016a). Resiliency-oriented conversations can foster hope and confidence (Short & Russell-Mayhew, 2009). This framework has been used to promote thriving in the face of adversity (Grace & Wells, 2015).

To be able to provide genuine, affirmative care as health care providers, we must take time to reflect on and address our own biases. An affirming health care provider simultaneously validates and acknowledges SGD people's experiences while embracing a view that celebrates diversity in all genders and sexualities (Glassgold, 2008; Hinrichs & Donaldson, 2017; Pepping et al., 2018).

Summary

Many health care providers shy away from SGD health because they feel intimidated, overwhelmed, and fearful of making mistakes. These feelings are understandable given how little education health care providers receive on SGD health. We hope that this chapter has demystified some of these topics. It is not more expensive nor more difficult to provide inclusive care, it just takes some knowledge, reflection, and intention. There are several key principles to remember.

Avoid assumptions. Many people do not fit into the cisheteronormative mould that our health care system was once set up for. Using language and lines of questioning that assume people fit into these limited categories directly harms the therapeutic alliance, reduces a patient's sense of safety in disclosing their sexual orientation or gender identity, and ultimately results in poor-quality or inappropriate care. Language and questions should be used in ways that remain open to many possibilities. Whenever possible, use open-ended questions. At the same time, ensure that questions are being asked for valid reasons and not simply to satisfy curiosity. Be transparent about why questions are being asked and how that information may be used to inform the patient's care.

Mistakes are allowed. If we catch our own mistake, a brief apology and correction are all that is needed. If a patient corrects us, we can thank them, then move forward.

Listen to understand. Often, SGD people have faced discrimination in greater society and in the health care system. This can lead to hesitancy to open up to a health care provider. When people do feel comfortable enough to open up to you, be compassionate and listen. Validate their experiences and take an affirming approach. Doing so not only helps relationship building, but can be a learning opportunity for us as health care providers.

Advocate, educate, and make change. More health care providers and trainees must be educated about the unique challenges faced by SGD patients and how to tackle these challenges. We must address our own biases as well as the stereotypes and negative attitudes that SGD people face when accessing health care (McPhail et al., 2016). Despite recent strides made toward improving education on these topics (Goez et al., 2020), education on sexual and gender diversity in health care is frequently insufficient. As health care providers we should not only advocate to improve formal education but also seek further opportunities to educate ourselves so we can do better by our patients and avoid perpetuating disparities. Reading this chapter is a good first step toward learning how to make changes within our own institutions and practices. The more we learn, the easier it becomes to recognize and pursue further avenues for change.

These concepts go beyond health care. Limiting, cisheteronrmative views remain in many systems, institutions, and minds. Openness to new information and ways of thinking as our societal understanding evolves will foster the health and wellness of SGD people and many other marginalized groups around the world.

 http://evolve.elsevier.com/Srivastava/culturalcompetence/.

Questions for Review and Discussion

1. You are a health care provider helping to set up a new clinic. Describe what you want patients to experience in the waiting room. What will the physical space look like? How will they be greeted? What will be on the forms for them to fill out? What name will be called when a room is ready for them?

2. You are talking to one of your family members and they say that SGD individuals tend to have worse health outcomes simply because of their identity. You have read this chapter so you know that is incorrect. You decide to explain the real underlying reasons for these health disparities. What will you say?

3. You are talking to Liza, a 12-year-old patient whose sex assigned at birth was female. This patient has just disclosed to you that they do not feel comfortable in their own skin, they don't "feel like a girl." How will you respond?

Group Experiential/Reflection Activity

ENGAGING A GUARDED PATIENT

Many SGD patients have faced discrimination and mistreatment within health care, leading some to be fearful of self-disclosing to their care providers. Previous upsetting or traumatic experiences in health care settings may lead SGD patients to be guarded, anxious, or minimally engaged in interactions (Burrow et al., 2018). Intersecting factors such as age, race, socioeconomic status, and overall privilege (or lack thereof) can accentuate such behaviour. These factors can all contribute to marginalization and discrimination, which have substantial impacts on mental health. In pairs or small groups discuss the following:

> How might you attempt to increase an SGD patient's engagement in order to provide care?
> How might these engagement strategies be different with a 14-year-old transgender patient or a 67-year-old gay male with a history of HIV?
> How might you frame a patient's experience and current concerns through a lens of resiliency instead of a deficit model?

References

Alberta Health Services. (n.d.). *Alberta's gender reaffirming program.* https://www.albertahealthservices.ca/info/Page15676.aspx

American Psychiatric Association. (2013). Gender dysphoria. In *Diagnostic and Statistical Manual of Mental Disorders* (5th ed.). https://doi.org/10.1176/appi.books.9780890425596.dsm14.

Andrade, G. (2019). The ethics of positive thinking in healthcare. *Journal of Medical Ethics and History of Medicine*, 12. https://doi.org/10.18502/jmehm.v12i18.2148.

Barranco, C. (2020). Gender-affirming therapy linked to mental health. *Nature Reviews Urology*, 17(10), 544. https://doi.org/10.1038/s41585-020-00377-6.

Bauer, G. R., Hammond, R., Travers, R., et al. (2009). "I don't think this is theoretical; this is our lives": How erasure impacts health care for transgender people. *The Journal of the Association of Nurses in AIDS Care: JANAC*, 20(5), 348–361. https://doi.org/10.1016/j.jana.2009.07.004.

Bauer, G. R., Zong, X., Scheim, A. I., et al. (2015). Factors impacting transgender patients' discomfort with their family physicians: A respondent-driven sampling survey. *PLOS ONE*, 10(12), e0145046. https://doi.org/10.1371/journal.pone.0145046.

Beagan, B., Fredericks, E., & Bryson, M. (2015). Family physician perceptions of working with LGBTQ patients: Physician training needs. *Canadian Medical Education Journal*, 6(1), e14–e22.

Besse, M., Lampe, N. M., & Mann, E. S. (2020). Experiences with achieving pregnancy and giving birth among transgender men: A narrative literatue review. *The Yale Journal of Biology and Medicine*, 93(4), 517–528.

Blondeel, K., Say, L., Chou, D., et al. (2016). Evidence and knowledge gaps on the disease burden in sexual and gender minorities: A review of systematic reviews. *International Journal for Equity in Health*, 15. https://doi.org/10.1186/s12939-016-0304-1.

Blunt-Vinti, H. D., Thompson, E. L., & Griner, S. B. (2018). Contraceptive use effectiveness and pregnancy prevention information preferences among heterosexual and sexual minority college women. *Women's Health Issues*, 28(4), 342–349. https://doi.org/10.1016/j.whi.2018.03.005.

Boudreau, D., & Mukerjee, R. (2019). Contraception care for transmasculine individuals on testosterone therapy. *Journal of Midwifery & Women's Health*, 64(4), 395–402. https://doi.org/10.1111/jmwh.12962.

Boxer, A., & Herdt, G. (1996). *Children of horizons: How gay and lesbian teens are leading a new way out of the closet.* Beacon Press.

Bragg, S., Renold, E., Ringrose, J., et al. (2018). 'More than boy, girl, male, female': Exploring young people's views on gender diversity within and beyond school contexts. *Sex Education*, 18(4), 420–434. https://doi.org/10.1080/14681811.2018.1439373.

Burrow, S., Goldberg, L., Searle, J., et al. (2018). Vulnerability, harm, and compromised ethics revealed by the experiences of queer birthing women in rural healthcare. *Journal of Bioethical Inquiry*, 15(4), 511–524. https://doi.org/10.1007/s11673-018-9882-5.

Canadian Paediatric Society (CPS). (2018). *Gender identity—Caring for Kids—Canadian Paediatric Society.* https://www.caringforkids.cps.ca/handouts/gender-identity.

Cavanaugh, T., Hopwood, R., & Lambert, C. (2016). Informed consent in the medical care of transgender and gender-nonconforming patients. *AMA Journal of Ethics, 18*(11), 1147–1155. https://doi.org/10.1001/journalofethics.2016.18.11.sect1-1611.

Coleman, E., Bockting, W., Botzer, M., et al. (2012). Standards of care for the health of transsexual, transgender, and gender-nonconforming people, Version 7. *International Journal of Transgenderism, 13*(4), 165–232. https://doi.org/10.1080/15532739.2011.700873.

Collins, S., & Arthur, N. (2010). Culture-infused counselling: A fresh look at a classic framework of multicultural counselling competencies. *Counselling Psychology Quarterly, 23*(2), 203–216. https://doi.org/10.1080/09515071003798204.

Colpitts, E., & Gahagan, J. (2016a). The utility of resilience as a conceptual framework for understanding and measuring LGBTQ health. *International Journal for Equity in Health, Article 60.* https://doi.org/10.1186/s12939-016-0349-1.

Colpitts, E., & Gahagan, J. (2016b). "I feel like I am surviving the health care system": Understanding LGBTQ health in Nova Scotia, Canada. *BMC Public Health, 16*(1), 1005. https://doi.org/10.1186/s12889-016-3675-8.

Combahee River Collective. (1977). *The Combahee River Collective statement.* https://www.loc.gov/item/lcwaN0028151/

Coulthard, G. S. (2014). Red skin, white masks: Rejecting the colonial politics of recognition. University of Minnesota Press.

Cover, R. (2018). *Emergent identities: New sexualities, genders and relationships in a digital era* (1st ed). Routledge. https://www.routledge.com/Emergent-Identities-New-Sexualities-Genders-and-Relationships-in-a-Digital/Cover/p/book/9781138098619

Crenshaw, K. (1991). Mapping the margins: Intersectionality, identity politics, and violence against women of color. *Stanford Law Review, 43*(6), 1241–1299. https://doi.org/10.2307/1229039.

David, R. (2017). The legacy of the HIV/AIDS fight in Canada. *Policy Options.* https://policyoptions.irpp.org/magazines/january-2017/the-legacy-of-the-hivaids-fight-in-canada/

Drescher, J. (2015). Queer diagnoses revisited: The past and future of homosexuality and gender diagnoses in DSM and ICD. *International Review of Psychiatry, 27*(5), 386–395. https://doi.org/10.3109/09540261.2015.1053847.

Eckstrand, K. L., & Ehrenfeld, J. M. (Eds.). (2016). *In lesbian, gay, bisexual, and transgender healthcare: A clinical guide to preventive, primary, and specialist care (Ch. 17).* Springer International Publishing. https://doi.org/10.1007/978-3-319-19752-4.

Edmonton Men's Health Collective (EMHC). (n.d.). *Edmonton LGBTQ2S+ substance use survey.* https://ourhealthyeg.ca/substance-use-survey

Egale. (2020). *National LGBTQI2S action plan.* https://egale.ca/awareness/nationalactionplan/

Everett, B. G., McCabe, K. F., & Hughes, T. L. (2017). Sexual orientation disparities in mistimed and unwanted pregnancy among adult women. *Perspectives on Sexual and Reproductive Health, 49*(3), 157–165. https://doi.org/10.1363/psrh.12032.

Fredriksen-Goldsen, K. I., Kim, H. -J., Shiu, C., et al. (2015). Successful aging among LGBT older adults: Physical and mental health-related quality of life by age group. *The Gerontologist, 55*(1), 154–168. https://doi.org/10.1093/geront/gnu081.

Fung, R., Gallibois, C., Coutin, A., et al. (2020). Learning by chance: Investigating gaps in transgender care education amongst family medicine, endocrinology, psychiatry and urology residents. *Canadian Medical Education Journal, 11*(4), e19–e28. https://doi.org/10.36834/cmej.53009.

Furlotte, C., Gladstone, J. W., Cosby, R. F., et al. (2016). "Could we hold hands?" Older lesbian and gay couples' perceptions of long-term care homes and home care. *Canadian Journal on Aging, 35*(4), 432–446. https://doi.org/10.1017/S0714980816000489.

Giroux, D., & Depelteau, J. (2015). LGBTQ issues as Indigenous politics: Two-Spirit mobilization in Canada. In *Queer mobilizations: Social movement activism and Canadian public policy* (pp. 64–81). UBC Press. https://www.academia.edu/12548593/LGBTQ_Issues_as_Indigenous_Politics_Two_Spirits_Mobilization

Glassgold, J. M. G. (2008). Bridging the divide. *Women & Therapy, 31*(1), 59–72. https://doi.org/10.1300/02703140802145227.

Goez, H., Lai, H., Rodger, J., et al. (2020). The DISCuSS model: Creating connections between community and curriculum – A new lens for curricular development in support of social accountability. *Medical Teacher*, *42*(9), 1058–1064. https://doi.org/10.1080/0142159X.2020.1779919.

Goldberg, L. (2015). Cultivating inclusivity with caring science in the area of LGBTQ education: The self-reflexive educator. *Faculty Focus, CULT*, *23*(3), 15–17. https://www.researchgate.net/publication/290434161_Cultivating_inclusivity_within_caring_science_in_the_area_of_LGBTQ_education_The_self-reflexive_educator

Goldberg, L., Rosenburg, N., & Watson, J. (2017). Rendering LGBTQ+ visible in nursing: Embodying the philosophy of caring science in nursing. *Journal of Holistic Nursing*, *36*(3), 262–271. https://doi.org/10.1177/0898010117715141.

Goldsen, K. F., & de Vries, B. (2019). Global aging with pride: International perspectives on LGBT aging. *International Journal of Aging & Human Development*, *88*(4), 315–324. https://doi.org/10.1177/0091415019837648.

Government of Alberta. (2012). *Alberta Health Care Insurance Plan Bulletin—Med 166A—Final stage gender reassignment surgery program*. Author.

Grace, A., & Wells, K. (2015). *Growing into resilience: Sexual and gender minority youth in Canada*. University of Toronto Press. https://www.chapters.indigo.ca/en-ca/books/growing-into-resilience-sexual-and/9781442629042-item.html

Grant, R., & Nash, M. (2019). Educating queer sexual citizens? A feminist exploration of bisexual and queer young women's sex education in Tasmania, Australia. *Sex Education*, *19*(3), 313–328. https://doi.org/10.1080/14681811.2018.1548348.

Hafeez, H., Zeshan, M., Tahir, M. A., et al. (2017). Health care disparities among lesbian, gay, bisexual, and transgender youth: A literature review. *Cureus*, *9*(4). https://doi.org/10.7759/cureus.1184.

Haldeman, D. C. (2002). Gay rights, patient rights: The implications of sexual orientation conversion therapy. *Professional Psychology: Research and Practice*, *33*(3), 260–264. https://doi.org/10.1037/0735-7028.33.3.260.

Hale, C. J. (2007). Ethical problems with the mental health evaluation standards of care for adult gender variant prospective patients. *Perspectives in Biology and Medicine*, *50*(4), 491–505. https://doi.org/10.1353/pbm.2007.0047.

Higgins, J. A., Carpenter, E., Everett, B. G., et al. (2019). Sexual minority women and contraceptive use: Complex pathways between sexual orientation and health outcomes. *American Journal of Public Health*, *109*(12), 1680–1686. https://doi.org/10.2105/AJPH.2019.305211.

Hinrichs, K., & Donaldson, W. (2017). Recommendations for use of affirmative psychotherapy with LGBT older adults. *Journal of Clinical Psychology*, 73. https://doi.org/10.1002/jclp.22505.

Hoffkling, A., Obedin-Maliver, J., & Sevelius, J. (2017). From erasure to opportunity: A qualitative study of the experiences of transgender men around pregnancy and recommendations for providers. *BMC Pregnancy and Childbirth*, *17*(Suppl 2), 332. https://doi.org/10.1186/s12884-017-1491-5.

hooks, b. (1984). *Feminist theory from margin to center* (1st ed.). South End Press.

Hopkins, S. W. (2008). *Life among the Piutes: Their wrongs and claims*. Dodo Press.

Hottes, T. S., Bogaert, L., Rhodes, A. E., et al. (2016). Lifetime prevalence of suicide attempts among sexual minority adults by study sampling strategies: A systematic review and meta-analysis. *American Journal of Public Health*, *106*(5), e1–e12. https://doi.org/10.2105/AJPH.2016.303088.

House of Commons Standing Committee on Health. (2019). *The health of LGBTQIA2 communities in Canada*. HESA Committee Report No. 28 – HESA (42-1) – House of Commons of Canada. https://www.ourcommons.ca/DocumentViewer/en/42-1/HESA/report-28/page-105

Hues Global Justice Collective. (n.d.). *Genderbread person v3.3*. https://www.genderbread.org/resource/genderbread-person-v3-3

Hunt, S. (2016). *An introduction to the health of two-spirit people: Historical, contemporary and emergent issues*. National Collaborating Centre for Indigenous Health. http://www.nccah-ccnsa.ca/en/

Iskander, L., & Keenan, H. B. (2021). Transgender identity. In J. N. Lester & M. O'Reilly (Eds.), *The Palgrave encyclopedia of critical perspectives on mental health*. Palgrave Macmillan.

Jaffray, B. (2020). *Experiences of violent victimization and unwanted sexual behaviours among gay, lesbian, bisexual and other sexual minority people, and the transgender population, in Canada, 2018*. Statistics Canada: Canadian Centre for Justice and Community Safety Statistics. https://www.150.statcan.gc.ca/n1/pub/85-002-x/2020001/article/00009-eng.htm

Jankowski, L. (2019). *Biography of bell hooks, feminist and anti-racist theorist and writer*. https://www.thoughtco.com/bell-hooks-biography-3530371

Kenney, M. (2001). *Mapping gay L.A.: The intersection of place and politics*. Temple University Press.

Kimmel, D., & Robinson, D. (2014). Sex, crime, pathology: Homosexuality and criminal code reform in Canada, 1949–1969. *Canadian Journal of Law and Society, 16*, 147–165. https://doi.org/10.1017/S082932010000661X.

Klein, A., & Golub, S. A. (2020). Enhancing gender-affirming provider communication to increase health care access and utilization among transgender men and trans-masculine non-binary individuals. *LGBT Health, 7*(6), 292–304. https://doi.org/10.1089/lgbt.2019.0294.

Krafft-Ebing, R. (1886). *Psychopathia sexualis*. Bell.

Latimer, M., Sylliboy, J. R., Francis, J., et al. (2020). Co-creating better healthcare experiences for First Nations children and youth: The FIRST approach emerges from two-eyed seeing. *Paediatric and Neonatal Pain, 2*(4), 104–112. https://doi.org/10.1002/pne2.12024.

Legge, M. M., Tarasoff, L., Flanders, C., et al. (2018). A critical examination of online news media representations of bisexual women who use cannabis. *Journal of Bisexuality, 18*(2), 206–229. https://doi.org/10.1080/15299716.2018.1460648.

Lewin, K. (1947). Frontiers in group dynamics: Concept, method and reality in social science; social equilibria and social change. *Human Relations, 1*, 5–41. https://doi.org/10.1177/001872674700100103.

Light, A. D., Zimbrunes, S. E., & Gomez-Lobo, V. (2017). Reproductive and obstetrical care for transgender patients. *Current Obstetrics and Gynecology Reports, 6*(2), 149–155. https://doi.org/10.1007/s13669-017-0212-4.

Livingston, N. A. (2017). Avenues for future minority stress and substance use research among sexual and gender minority populations. *Journal of LGBT Issues in Counseling, 11*(1), 52–62. https://doi.org/10.1080/15538605.2017.1273164.

Lorde, A. (1983). *There is no hierarchy of oppressions. Interracial Books for Children Bulletin: Homophobia and Education, 14*(3–4). https://digicoll.library.wisc.edu/cgi-bin/Literature/Literature-idx?type=article&did=Literature.CIBCBulletinv14n0304.i0006&id=Literature.CIBCBulletinv14n0304&isize=M&pview=hide

Lorenzetti, L., Wells, L., Callaghan, T., et al. (2015). *Domestic violence in Alberta's gender and sexually diverse communities: Towards a framework for prevention*. Shift: The project to end domestic violence, University of Calgary. https://doi.org/10.11575/PRISM/31393.

MacDonald, C., & Steenbeek, A. (2015). The impact of colonization and Western assimilation on health and wellbeing of Canadian Indigenous people. *International Journal of Regional and Local History, 10*(1), 32–46. https://doi.org/10.1179/2051453015Z.00000000023.

McPhail, D., Rountree-James, M., & Whetter, I. (2016). Addressing gaps in physician knowledge regarding transgender health and healthcare through medical education. *Canadian Medical Education Journal, 7*(2), e70–e78.

Mental Health Commission of Canada. (2019). *Safer space guidelines*. https://www.mentalhealthcommission.ca/wp-content/uploads/drupal/2019-03/safer_space_guidelines_mar_2019_eng.pdf

Meyer, I. H. (2003). Prejudice, social stress, and mental health in lesbian, gay, and bisexual populations: Conceptual issues and research evidence. *Psychological Bulletin, 129*(5), 674–697. https://doi.org/10.1037/0033-2909.129.5.674.

Mizock, L., & Hopwood, R. (2016). Conflation and interdependence in the intersection of gender and sexuality among transgender individuals. *Psychology of Sexual Orientation and Gender Diversity, 3*. 93–103. https://doi.org/10.1037/sgd0000157.

Morgensen. S. L. (2011). *Spaces between us: Queer settler colonialism and Indigenous decolonization*. University of Minnesota Press.

Mulé, N., Khan, M., & McKenzie, C. (2020) Queering Canadian Social Work Accreditation standards and procedures: A content analysis. *Social Work Education, 39*(3), 288-301. https://doi.org/10.1080/02615479.2019.1648408.

Native Youth Sexual Health Network. (n.d.). *Toolkits*. https://www.nativeyouthsexualhealth.com/toolkits

Obedin-Maliver, J., & Makadon, H. J. (2016). Transgender men and pregnancy. *Obstetric Medicine, 9*(1), 4–8. https://doi.org/10.1177/1753495X15612658.

Parliament of Canada. (2017). *Government Bill (House of Commons) C-16 (42-1)—Royal Assent—An Act to amend the Canadian Human Rights Act and the Criminal Code—First Session, Forty-second Parliament, 64-65-66 Elizabeth II, 2015-2016-2017*. https://www.parl.ca/DocumentViewer/en/42-1/bill/c-16/royal-assent

Pepping, C. A., Lyons, A., & Morris, E. M. J. (2018). Affirmative LGBT psychotherapy: Outcomes of a therapist training protocol. *Psychotherapy (Chicago, Ill.)*, *55*(1), 52–62. https://doi.org/10.1037/pst0000149.

Plöderl, M., & Tremblay, P. (2015). Mental health of sexual minorities. A systematic review. *International Review of Psychiatry*, *27*(5), 367–385. https://doi.org/10.3109/09540261.2015.1083949.

Poteat, T., German, D., & Flynn, C. (2016). The conflation of gender and sex: Gaps and opportunities in HIV data among transgender women and MSM. *Global Public Health*, *11*(7–8), 835–848. https://doi.org/10.10 80/17441692.2015.1134615.

Putney, J. M., Keary, S., Hebert, N., et al. (2018). "Fear runs deep:" The anticipated needs of LGBT older adults in long-term care. *Journal of Gerontological Social Work*, *61*(8), 887–907. https://doi.org/10.1080/0163437 2.2018.1508109.

Rainbow Health Ontario. (2009). *Pap campaigns—"Check it out" and "Check it out guys."* https://www.rainbow-healthontario.ca/pap-campaigns/

Rainbow Health Ontario. (2012). *Clear the air campaign.* https://www.rainbowhealthontario.ca/clear-the-air-campaign/

Reisner, S. L., Poteat, T., Keatley, J., et al. (2016). Global health burden and needs of transgender populations: A review. *The Lancet*, *388*(10042), 412–436. https://doi.org/10.1016/S0140-6736(16)00684-X.

Ristock, J., Zoccole, A., Passante, L., et al. (2019). Impacts of colonization on Indigenous two-spirit/LGBTQ Canadians' experiences of migration, mobility and relationship violence. *Sexualities*, *22*(5–6), 767–784. https://doi.org/10.1177/1363460716681474.

Roberts, A. L., Austin, S. B., Corliss, H. L., et al. (2010). Pervasive trauma exposure among US sexual orientation minority adults and risk of posttraumatic stress disorder. *American Journal of Public Health*, *100*(12), 2433–2441. https://doi.org/10.2105/AJPH.2009.168971.

Rogers, C. (1971). Carl Rogers describes his way of facilitating encounter groups. *AJN The American Journal of Nursing*, *71*(2), 275–279.

Ross, L. E., Dobinson, C., & Eady, A. (2010). Perceived determinants of mental health for bisexual people: A qualitative examination. *American Journal of Public Health*, *100*(3), 496–502. https://doi.org/10.2105/ AJPH.2008.156307.

Safer, J. D., Coleman, E., Feldman, J., et al. (2016). Barriers to health care for transgender individuals. *Current Opinion in Endocrinology, Diabetes, and Obesity*, *23*(2), 168–171. https://doi.org/10.1097/ MED.0000000000000227.

Scheim, A. I., Zong, X., Giblon, R., et al. (2017). Disparities in access to family physicians among transgender people in Ontario, Canada. *International Journal of Transgenderism*, *18*(3), 343–352. https://doi.org/10.10 80/15532739.2017.1323069.

Schwartz, A. R., Russell, K., & Gray, B. A. (2019). Approaches to vaginal bleeding and contraceptive counseling in transgender and gender nonbinary patients. *Obstetrics and Gynecology*, *134*(1), 81–90. https://doi. org/10.1097/AOG.0000000000003308.

Sevelius, J. M. (2013). Gender affirmation: A framework for conceptualizing risk behavior among transgender women of color. *Sex Roles*, *68*(11–12), 675–689. https://doi.org/10.1007/s11199-012-0216-5.

Short, J. L., & Russell-Mayhew, S. (2009). What counsellors need to know about resiliency in adolescents. *International Journal for the Advancement of Counselling*, *31*(4), 213. https://doi.org/10.1007/ s10447-009-9079-z.

Sizemore, K., Carter, J., Millar, B., et al. (2019). Attachment as a predictor of psychological and sexual wellbeing among transgender women in New York City. *Journal of Sex Research*, *56*(9), 1192–1202. https://doi.org /10.1080/00224499.2019.1644486.

Steele, L. S., Daley, A., Curling, D., et al. (2016). LGBT identity, untreated depression, and unmet need for mental health services by sexual minority women and trans-identified people. *Journal of Women's Health*, *26*(2), 116–127. https://doi.org/10.1089/jwh.2015.5677.

Stewart, K., & O'Reilly, P. (2017). Exploring the attitudes, knowledge and beliefs of nurses and midwives of the healthcare needs of the LGBTQ population: An integrative review. *Nurse Education Today*, *53*, 67–77. https://doi.org/10.1016/j.nedt.2017.04.008. Epub 2017 Apr 18. PMID: 28448883.

Stinchcombe, A., Smallbone, J., Wilson, K., et al. (2017). Healthcare and end-of-life needs of lesbian, gay, bisexual, and transgender (LGBT) older adults: A scoping review. *Geriatrics*, *2*(1). https://doi.org/10.3390/ geriatrics2010013.

Stinchcombe, A., Wilson, K., Kortes-Miller, K., et al. (2018). Physical and mental health inequalities among aging lesbian, gay, and bisexual Canadians: Cross-sectional results from the Canadian longitudinal study on aging (CLSA). *Canadian Journal of Public Health, 109*(5–6), 833–844. https://doi.org/10.17269/s41997-018-0100-3.

Stoffel, C., Carpenter, E., Everett, B., et al. (2017). Family planning for sexual minority women. *Seminars in Reproductive Medicine, 35*(5), 460–468. https://doi.org/10.1055/s-0037-1604456.

Stryker, S. (2006). (De)Subjugated knowledges: An introduction to transgender studies. In *The Transgender Studies Reader* (Vol. 1, pp. 17–34). Routledge. https://doi.org/10.4324/9780203955055-7.

Sylliboy, J., & Hovey, R. (2020). Humanizing Indigenous people engagement in health care. *Canadian Medical Association Journal, 192*, E70–E72. https://doi.org/10.1503/cmaj.190754.

The Trevor Project. (2020). *The Trevor project national survey 2020.* https://www.thetrevorproject.org/survey-2020/

Thomas, R., Pega, F., Khosla, R., et al. (2017). Ensuring an inclusive global health agenda for transgender people. *Bulletin of the World Health Organization, 95*(2), 154–156. https://doi.org/10.2471/BLT.16.183913.

Thompson, M. (2017). *The discomfort of safety.* https://www.societyandspace.org/articles/the-discomfort-of-safety

Transgender PULSE Canada Team. (2020). *Health and health care access for transgender and non-binary people in Canada.* https://transpulsecanada.ca/research-type/reports

Transgender Student Educational Resources (TSER). (n.d.). *Gender unicorn.* https://transstudent.org/gender/.

Travers, R., Bauer, G., Pyne, J., et al. (2012). *Impacts of strong parental support for transgender youth: A report prepared for Children's Aid Society of Toronto and Delisle Youth Services.* Transgender PULSE Project.

Uink, B., Liddelow-Hunt, S., Daglas, K., et al. (2020). The time for inclusive care for Indigenous and Torres Strait Islander LGBTQ+ young people is now. *The Medical Journal of Australia, 213*(5), 201–204. https://doi.org/10.5694/mja2.50718. e1.

Ungar, M. (2011). The social ecology of resilience: Addressing contextual and cultural ambiguity of a nascent construct. *The American Journal of Orthopsychiatry, 81*(1), 1–17. https://doi.org/10.1111/j.1939-0025.2010.01067.x.

Veale, J. F., Watson, R. J., Peter, T., et al. (2017). Mental health disparities among Canadian transgender youth. *The Journal of Adolescent Health, 60*(1), 44–49. https://doi.org/10.1016/j.jadohealth.2016.09.014.

Veltman, A., & Chaimowitz, G. (2014). Mental health care for people who identify as lesbian, gay, bisexual, transgender, and (or) queer. *Canadian Journal of Psychiatry, 59*(11), 1–8.

Voyageur, C., & Calliou, B. (2001). Various shades of red: Diversity within Canada's Indigenous community. *Undefined, 16*, 109–124.

Williams, C. C., Curling, D., Steele, L. S., et al. (2017). Depression and discrimination in the lives of women, transgender and gender liminal people in Ontario, Canada. *Health & Social Care in the Community, 25*(3), 1139–1150. https://doi.org/10.1111/hsc.12414.

Winter, A. (2005). Women, race and class. *Off Our Backs, 35*(1/2), 48–49.

Workowski, K. A., Bachmann, L. H., Chan, P. A., et al. (2021). Sexually transmitted infections treatment guidelines, 2021. *MMWR. Morbidity and Mortality Weekly Report, 70*(4), 1–187. https://doi.org/10.15585/mmwr.rr7004a1.

Yep, G., Lovaas, K., & Elia, J. (2003). Introduction: Queering communication: Starting the conversation. *Journal of Homosexuality, 45*, 1–10. https://doi.org/10.1300/J082v45n02_01.

Zeeman, L., Sherriff, N., Browne, K., et al. (2019). A review of lesbian, gay, bisexual, trans and intersex (LGBTI) health and healthcare inequalities. *European Journal of Public Health, 29*(5), 974–980. https://doi.org/10.1093/eurpub/cky226.

Zitkala-Ša. (1921). *American Indian stories.* Penguin Random House.

Zitkala-Ša, Fabens, C. H., & Sniffen, M. K. (1924). *Oklahoma's poor rich Indians: An orgy of graft and exploitation of the five civilized tribes, legalized robbery.* Office of the Indian Rights Association.

CHAPTER 11

Immigrant and Refugee Health

Branka Agic

> *An immigrant is a person who chooses to settle permanently in another country. Refugees are forced to flee their countries because of a well-founded fear of persecution. They are not able to return home.*
> Immigration, Refugees and Citizenship Canada (2019)

LEARNING OBJECTIVES

At the end of this chapter, the learner will be able to:
- Define the main immigrant and refugee categories
- Describe the healthy immigrant effect
- Explain social determinants of immigrant and refugee health
- Discuss ways of addressing the health needs of immigrants and refugees

KEY TERMS

Discrimination	Immigrants	Social exclusion
Health inequities	Refugees	Social inclusion
Healthy immigrant effect	Social determinants of health	Temporary residents

Many personal, social, economic, and environmental factors interact with each other to influence the health status of individuals and communities. This chapter discusses social determinants of immigrant and refugee health. It begins with an overview of different categories of immigrants and refugees to Canada. Next, it describes the healthy immigrant effect. Then, the social and economic factors shaping immigrant and refugee health are examined. Finally, the implications of findings for policymakers, health planners, and health care providers are discussed.

Overview: Immigrants and Refugees in Canada

Immigration has been an integral part of Canada's history. Millions of immigrants and refugees have resettled in Canada, contributing to the ethnic and cultural diversity of the population. According to 2016 census data, over one in five Canadians (21.9% of the Canadian population or about 7.5 million people) were foreign-born. Approximately 1.2 million people were recent

---

[1] *Recent immigrant* refers to a person who obtained a landed immigrant or permanent resident status up to 5 years prior to a given census year (Statistics Canada, 2017a).

immigrants (i.e., those who arrived between 2011 and 2016) (Statistics Canada, 2017a, b, c). In 2019, Canada accepted over 341,000 permanent residents, including 30,000 resettled refugees. In the same year, immigration accounted for 80% of Canada's population growth (Immigration, Refugees and Citizenship Canada [IRCC], 2021). Statistics Canada estimates that immigrants could represent 30.0% of Canada's population in 2036 (Morency et al., 2017).

Immigrants and refugees to Canada arrive from different parts of the world. The origins of Canada's immigrants have shifted dramatically since the 1960s, from largely European to largely non-European countries of origin (Statistics Canada, 2016). In 2016, over 250 ethnic origins were reported and 22.3% of Canadians identified as racialized (Statistics Canada, 2017c). In 2018, the top five source countries of new immigrants and refugees to Canada were India, the Philippines, China, Syria, and Nigeria (IRCC, 2019). According to the 2020 annual report to Parliament, permanent and non-permanent residents accounted for 80% of Canada's population growth in 2019 (IRCC, 2021).

Immigrants are not a homogeneous group; there is a great diversity between and within immigrant groups with respect to immigration category under which they entered Canada, length of stay in Canada, country of origin, race, ethnicity, age, socioeconomic status, education, and knowledge of English or French.

Since 2002, Canada's immigration programs have been based on the *Immigration and Refugee Protection Act* (IRPA) (Government of Canada, 2001). The IRPA sets out the core principles that govern Canada's immigration and refugee protection programs.

An **immigrant** is defined as a person who has been granted the right to live in Canada permanently (Statistics Canada 2019, 2021). Immigrants to Canada fall into four main categories:

1. Economic immigrants (includes immigrants selected for their ability to contribute to Canada's economy)
2. Immigrants sponsored by family (immigrants sponsored by a Canadian citizen or permanent resident)
3. Refugees (immigrants granted permanent resident status on the basis of a well-founded fear of returning to their home country due to persecution; includes people affected by war, armed conflict, or a massive violation of human rights)
4. Other immigrants (immigrants granted permanent resident status under a program that does not fall under any of the above categories) (Statistics Canada, 2019, 2021). In 2019, 58% of permanent residents were admitted under the economic category (IRCC, 2020a).

Refugees are different from immigrants in that they are forced to flee their country becasue of war, armed conflict, political violence, or a violation of human rights. A refugee is a person who cannot return to their home country becasue of "a well-founded fear of persecution for reasons of race, religion, nationality, membership in a particular social group, or political opinion, and are unable or, because of this fear, unwilling to seek protection from [their] country of origin" (Government of Canada, 2021; Immigration and Refugee Board of Canada, 2021). The Canadian refugee system has two main components:

1. The Refugee and Humanitarian Resettlement Program is for people who need protection from outside Canada. This includes government-assisted refugees (GARs), privately sponsored refugees (PSRs), and those in the blended visa office referred (BVOR) program; and
2. The In-Canada Asylum Program is for people making refugee protection claims at a port of entry or from within Canada because they have a well-founded fear of persecution or are at risk of torture or cruel or unusual punishment in their home countries. If their claim is determined to be eligible, refugee claimants go through a refugee determination process. Those who receive a positive decision on their refugee claim receive protected person status and access to a range of settlement and support services.

Individuals who receive a negative refugee decision may be able to appeal the decision. Once all appeal options are exhausted, the process to remove that individual from Canada is initiated (IRCC, 2019).

Temporary residents are foreign nationals authorized to stay in Canada temporarily. They include temporary foreign workers, international students, visitors, protected persons, refugee claimants (asylum seekers), and temporary resident permit holders. Temporary residents are a very diverse group of migrants and subject to various conditions including the length of their stay in Canada and restrictions on their ability to work, study, or use some public programs and services depending on the temporary resident category (IRCC, 2020b).

Some people residing in Canada have no official immigration status. They are often referred to as "non-status persons," "undocumented persons," or "irregular migrants." The exact number of

---

Cultural Competence In Action

Immigration Status and Potential Health Needs

For each of the persons described below, discuss the anticipated health needs for the individual and family and the kinds of supports needed.

M.S. is a 65-year-old Punjabi woman who came to Canada sponsored by her son. She doesn't speak English. As a Family Class immigrant, she is dependent on her son, who must support her financially for a period of 20 years. During the initial dependency period, she may not be eligible for social assistance.

F.A. is a 30-year-old computer engineer from Russia who immigrated to Canada with his wife, who is a civil engineer, and their two children. Both he and his wife speak English. They self-financed the immigration process and came to Canada as economic immigrants.

G.P. is a single mother who came to Canada as a Government Assisted Refugee (GAR) under the Canadian federal government's Resettlement Assistance Program (RAP).

When the Sudanese soldiers invaded her village, her husband was killed, but she managed to escape with their daughter and fled to Chad. Once she got to Chad, she was raped by a Chadian soldier outside of the camp. She suffered multiple physical injuries and psychological trauma.

---

people without official status in Canada is unknown but is estimated to be between 200 000 and 500 000 (Gushulak, et al., 2011; Magalhaes et al., 2010).

Immigration status influences health through various mechanisms, including differential access to resources, services, and opportunities. While undocumented persons and temporary residents face some unique health challenges, discussion of this group is beyond the scope of this chapter.

Healthy Immigrant Effect

The research literature has consistently shown a **healthy immigrant effect**, a phenomenon where new immigrants are generally healthier than the Canadian-born population with regard to mental health, chronic conditions, disability, and risk behaviours (Vang et al., 2015). Refugees applying for permanent residence are also required to complete a medical exam. Refugee claimants who make a refugee claim at a port of entry are required to get a medical exam within 30 days. Those who are expected to cause "excessive demand on the health care system" are denied immigration status. Furthermore, individuals who are healthy are more likely to immigrate (Government of Canada, 2022; Lu & Ng, 2019). The existence of the healthy immigrant effect has been documented among immigrants to other developed countries, including the United States, the Netherlands, and Australia (Dhadda & Greene, 2018; Hamilton, 2015; Lubbers & Gijsberts, 2019; Moniz et al., 2020).

The healthy immigrant effect varies across immigrant groups, across the life course, and for different health outcomes (Gushulak et al., 2011; Vang et al., 2015). The strongest health advantage is observed among economic-class principal applicants. The healthy immigrant effect is found to be stronger for family-class immigrants and much weaker among refugees (Lu & Ng, 2019). Still, even recent refugees, overall, have lower mortality rates than the Canadian-born population (Beiser, 2005).

However, the health advantage of new immigrants disappears with time and converges toward the health status of the Canadian-born population. Over time, immigrants report higher prevalence of some chronic conditions, including diabetes, heart disease, and arthritis (Long, 2010). The immigrant advantage disappears after spending over 10 years in Canada for some cancers, including colorectal and breast cancer. Furthermore, evidence shows a steady decline in cancer-specific survival over time (Shuldiner et al., 2018). Research evidence also demonstrates a deterioration of the healthy immigrant effect in self-reported mental health (SRMH). A recent Canadian study found differences in SRMH among immigrants by admission category, especially for refugees, length of time in Canada, and region of origin (Ng & Zhang, 2020). For example, South Asian immigrants, in particular South Asian immigrant women, have an increased risk of heart disease and hypertension with increasing length of stay in Canada (Tu et al., 2015).

Deterioration of health over time also varies across different immigrant groups. Evidence suggests that certain groups including refugees, low-income immigrants, and recent non-European immigrants are at risk for deteriorating health soon after arrival in Canada (Gushulak et al., 2011; Mental Health Commission of Canada [MHCC], 2016; Ng et al., 2005; Ontario Ministry of Long-Term Care [MOHLTC], 2014).

Research studies point to a number of factors associated with health decline among recent immigrants and refugees, including initial health status, age, gender, language skills, place or region of birth, experiences of discrimination, cultural differences, social environment, and health care system–related factors (Ahmed et al., 2015; Fuller-Thomson et al., 2011).

The healthy immigrant effect has important implications for Canada's economic growth as well as health care systems, particularly if the health advantage of new immigrants is to be preserved over time.

Determinants of Immigrant and Refugee Health

Determinants of health are factors and conditions that interact with each other to influence health of individuals and populations. They include socioeconomic environment, physical environment, individual behaviours, biology and genetic endowment, and health care services (Government of Canada, 2020; Ministry of Health, 2012).

Social determinants of health are "the conditions in which people are born, grow, work, live, and age, and the wider set of forces and systems shaping the conditions of daily life" (World Health Organization [WHO], 2011, 2020a). They include, but are not limited to, income; education; literacy; employment and working conditions; early childhood development; food security; housing; social inclusion, social support networks; health care services; gender; culture; race; ethnicity; age; and sexual orientation (MOHLTC, 2012; Office of Disease Prevention and Health Promotion, 2020; Raphael et al., 2020; WHO, 2017).

Overwhelming evidence shows that social determinants are more important in influencing health than the person's individual characteristics such as biology, genetics, and lifestyle choices as well as health care (Canadian Medical Association, 2013a, b; Raphael et al., 2020; WHO, 2020b). Reports from the Canadian Public Health Association (2020) and Canadian Medical Association (2013a) highlight the importance of the social determinants for the health of the Canadian population.

HOW SOCIAL DETERMINANTS INFLUENCE HEALTH

Social determinants impact health both directly and indirectly. They can act as protective or risk factors. People who are exposed to adverse social conditions including poverty, poor quality housing, food insecurity, inadequate working conditions, job insecurity, and various forms of discrimination based on race, gender, sexual orientations, and other individual characteristics over a longer period of time experience high levels of stress. Chronic stress created through these social conditions serves as an important pathway leading to various health problems. Research shows that chronic stress weakens the immune system and can lead to changes in neurohormonal systems, putting people at greater risk of illnesses such as high blood pressure, heart disease, and adult-onset diabetes and may contribute to anxiety and depression. Some people may try to relieve stress by smoking, using alcohol or other substances, or overeating. Adverse and stressful living conditions also make it very difficult to practise healthy habits (Brunner & Marmot, 2006; Raphael et al., 2020) (Fig. 11.1).

Social determinants of health are the root causes of health inequities, differences in health among population groups that are considered to be unfair, unjust, and avoidable (Whitehead, 1990; WHO, 2008). In Canada, population groups experiencing health inequities include those with lower socioeconomic status, Indigenous people, racialized populations, and recent immigrants and refugees (Public Health Agency of Canada [PHAC], 2018). **Health inequities** are systematic differences in the opportunities groups have to achieve optimal health, leading to unfair and avoidable differences in health outcomes (National Academies of Sciences, Engineering, and Medicine, 2017). (See Chapter 1.)

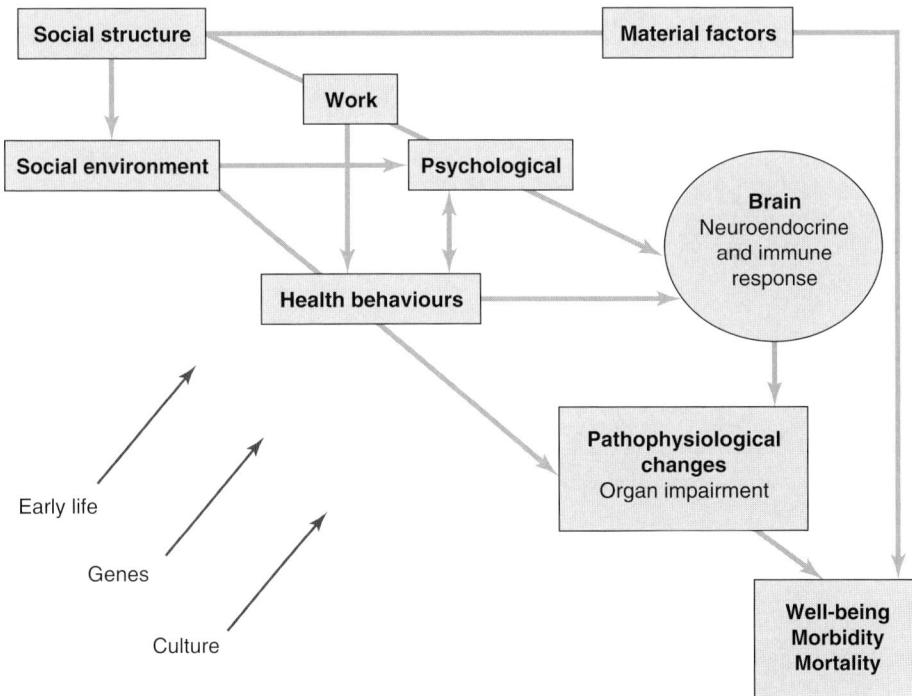

Fig. 11.1 Social Determinants of Health and the Pathways to Health and Illness. (From Brunner, E., & Marmot, M. G. [2006]. Social organization, stress, and health. In M. G. Marmot & R. G. Wilkinson [Eds.], *Social determinants of health*. Oxford University Press.)

Migration as a Social Determinant of Health

The health of immigrant populations is influenced by factors similar to those of Canadian-born people. However, there are additional factors that play an important role in shaping immigrant and refugee health. Migration is considered an additional layer to the factors listed above and is considered a social determinant of health. While migration itself is not a risk to health, circumstances surrounding migration can create risk for various health problems (Migration Data Portal, 2020).

Social determinants of immigrant and refugee health are usually viewed in terms of pre-migration, migration, and post-migration experiences (MOHLTC, 2016). Figure. 11.2 shows the pre-migration (Place of Origin), migration (Travel and Transit), and post-migration (Place of Destination) factors shaping immigrant and refugee health as well as other factors (Cross-cutting aspects) such as gender, age, and socioeconomic status that intersect with migration experiences. Migrants returning home often face additional challenges (Return), including social and economic integration. Pre-migration factors include income, socioeconomic status, and living conditions in the immigrant's country of origin such as epidemiological situation, availability and quality of health care services, and health beliefs and behaviours, as well as reasons for migration and experience of persecution, violence and injuries, and cumulative exposure to trauma (Davies et al., 2006; Hollander et al., 2012).

The migration factors include the living conditions and experiences during the transitional period, which may include living for a temporary period in another country or living in a refugee camp (Cooper-Jones, 2017). The ability to migrate through legal channels determines the impact of the migration journey on the health of migrants. Refugees who are forced to leave their countries because of war, armed conflicts, and human rights violations are at higher risk of adverse health outcomes. They are more likely to undergo dangerous journeys and be exposed to unsafe conditions, disease, exploitation, and discrimination and have a lack of access to health and support services (Davies et al., 2006). For example, Karen refugees resettled in Canada spent considerable time, up to 20 years, in a refugee camp in Thailand, stationed in a remote jungle area along the Thai–Burma border (Marchbank et al., 2014). Studies conducted on Syrian refugees in Lebanon, Jordan, Turkey, and Iraq indicated that noncommunicable diseases, pregnancy-related complications, mental health disorders, including post-traumatic stress disorder (PTSD) and depression, and some communicable diseases seem to be prevalent in refugee settings. They also found a gap in health care services provided to Syrian refugees in these countries (El Arnaout et al., 2019).

Post-migration factors, including immigration policies, working and living conditions in the host country, ability to speak the language of the host country, access to culturally and linguistically appropriate services, availability of family and social support, and, for refugee claimants, the refugee determination process, play a vital role in determining immigrant and refugee health (Gushulak et al., 2011). Certain subgroups of migrants are more vulnerable, including refugees, those with no legal status, socioeconomically disadvantaged people, women, older persons, and unaccompanied children.

The following section examines the key post-migration determinants of health for immigrants and refugees.

Income, Education, and Employment

Income. Income is perhaps the most important social determinant of health. Income determines the access to and quality of many other factors that affect health, including food security, housing, education, early child development, and other prerequisites of health. In Canada and in other developed countries, lower income is associated with shorter life expectancy and poorer overall health (Canadian Institute for Health Information [CIHI], 2016; Raphael et al., 2020).

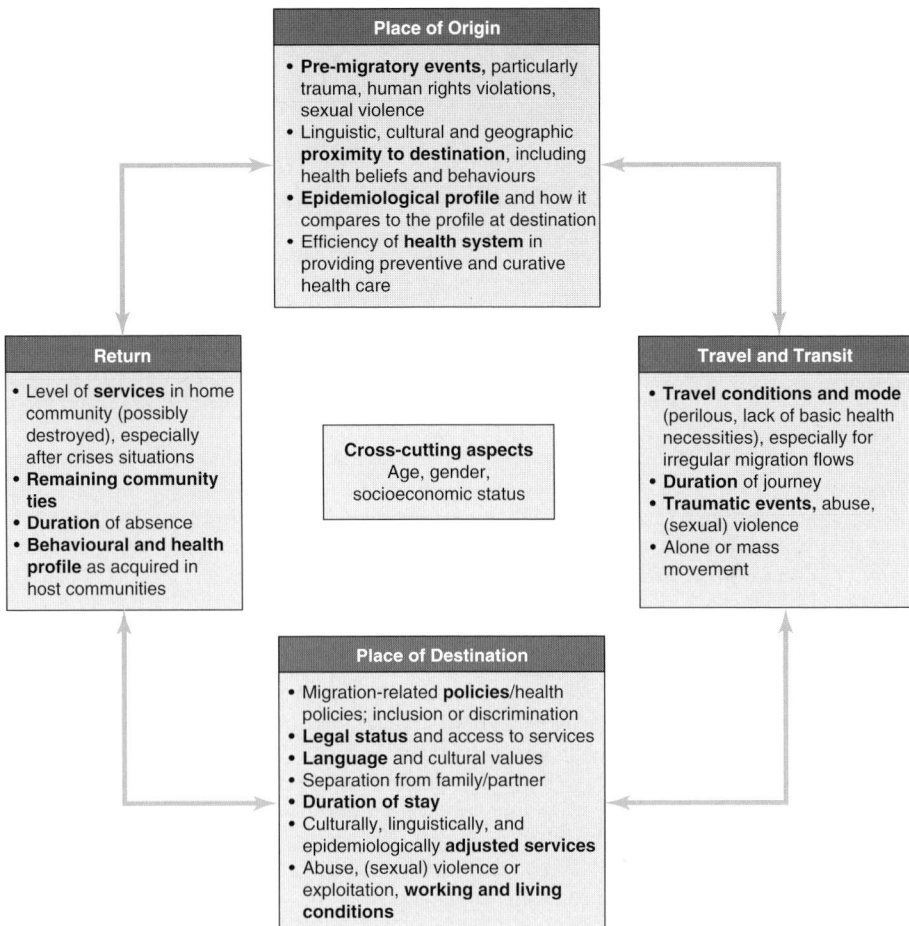

Place of Origin
- **Pre-migratory events,** particularly trauma, human rights violations, sexual violence
- Linguistic, cultural and geographic **proximity to destination**, including health beliefs and behaviours
- **Epidemiological profile** and how it compares to the profile at destination
- Efficiency of **health system** in providing preventive and curative health care

Return
- Level of **services** in home community (possibly destroyed), especially after crises situations
- **Remaining community ties**
- **Duration** of absence
- **Behavioural and health profile** as acquired in host communities

Cross-cutting aspects
Age, gender, socioeconomic status

Travel and Transit
- **Travel conditions and mode** (perilous, lack of basic health necessities), especially for irregular migration flows
- **Duration** of journey
- **Traumatic events,** abuse, (sexual) violence
- Alone or mass movement

Place of Destination
- Migration-related **policies**/health policies; inclusion or discrimination
- **Legal status** and access to services
- **Language** and cultural values
- Separation from family/partner
- **Duration of stay**
- Culturally, linguistically, and epidemiologically **adjusted services**
- Abuse, (sexual) violence or exploitation, **working and living conditions**

Fig. 11.2   The Migration Process and Health Outcomes. (From International Organization for Migration. [2020]. https://www.iom.int/social-determinants-migrant-health.)

In Canada, rates of low income among immigrants rose to historically high levels in the 1990s. Although the earnings of recent immigrants have increased over the past few years, immigrants continue to have higher rates of low income relative to the Canadian-born population (Picot & Lu, 2017). Recent immigrants experience the highest wage gap, earning 70% of what the general Canadian population earns (Ng & Gagnon, 2020). The 2016 census data show a significant income disparity between immigrants and Canadian-born people. Immigrants admitted to Canada in 2016 reported a median entry income of $25 900 compared to the Canadian population's median income of $36 100 (Statistics Canada, 2019b, 2021). Refugees admitted in 2015 had a median total income of $15 300 (Statistics Canada, 2016).

However, there are significant variations in low-income rates among different subgroups of immigrants. Racialized immigrants tend to earn less than White immigrants. Recent immigrants over the age of 65 are more likely to be represented within the low-income population. In 2016, approximately one-quarter of new immigrants aged 65 and over were low income (Kei et al., 2019). Immigrant women earn less than both immigrant men and Canadian-born women. Overall, immigrant women earn 13% less than immigrant men (Fitzsimmons et al., 2020). Immigrant racialized women in particular disproportionately experience the gender wage gap (Ontario Women's Health Network, 2017). Evidence shows that immigrants' economic outcomes improve with the number of years in Canada across all immigrant categories (Yssaad & Fields, 2018).

Compared to immigrants, refugees tend to fare worse in terms of economic integration, having lower incomes and employment rates than those for immigrants entering through other admission categories (Prokopenko, 2018; Yu et al., 2009).

Education. The association of education and health has been consistently observed in many studies. People with higher levels of education have longer life expectancy and overall better health compared to their less educated peers. Higher level of education is linked to better jobs and job security, higher income, retirement plans, and additional health benefits not covered by provincial health plans. Higher level of education is also associated with increased health literacy, which can contribute to healthier lifestyles, more use of preventive services, and better access to health care services (Bushnik et al., 2020; CPHA, 2020).

Immigrants to Canada are well educated. In general, immigrants are more likely to have post-secondary degrees than the Canadian-born population. According to the 2016 census, 40% of immigrants aged 25 to 64 had a bachelor's degree or higher, compared to 25% of the Canadian-born population (Statistics Canada, 2018a). Furthermore, over 50% of recent immigrants who arrived to Canada between 2011 and 2016 had a bachelor's degree or higher (Statistics Canada, 2018b).

However, new immigrants experience a range of challenges in Canada. They are more likely to be overeducated and underemployed compared to their Canadian-born counterparts. An estimated 29.6% of immigrants are overeducated for the jobs that they are working in, compared to 12% of Canadian-born workers (Hou et al., 2019). Again, there are differences among different groups of immigrants. Racialized immigrants from Asia, Africa, Latin America, and the Middle East fare worse than Canadian-born workers, while immigrants from Europe fare better than non-European immigrants. Non-recognition or devaluation of foreign credentials, limited official language skills, and lack of Canadian work experience continue to be barriers for immigrant labour–market integration (Ng & Gagnon, 2020).

Refugees to Canada are admitted for humanitarian rather than economic reasons. As a result, many refugees do not have postsecondary education or official language skills, and they face greater challenges in economic integration than other immigrants (Bevelander, 2016).

Employment. Employment and working conditions are the important contributors to health inequities. Employment provides income and a sense of financial security. It also provides a sense of purpose and identity and enhances person's social network (Government of Canada, 2013). The adequacy of a person's employment status also influences their health. Higher healthy life expectancy is strongly correlated with higher employment rates, particularly for men. On the other hand, underemployment is associated with higher rates of depression, anxiety, and suicide rates, as well as cardiovascular disease, hypertension, musculoskeletal disorders, and premature mortality (Pharr et al., 2011; Raphael et al., 2020).

Occupation and working conditions have powerful effects on health. Individuals working in higher status occupations have substantially better health and a lower risk of mortality than those working in lower status occupations (Burgard & Lin, 2013).

New immigrants have historically had lower employment rates than those for non-immigrants and long-term immigrants. Ng and Gagnon (2020) report that racialized immigrants from Asia (with the exception of immigrants from the Philippines), Latin America, and Africa have higher unemployment rates than those for the Canadian-born population. However, immigrants from Europe have lower unemployment rates than rates for the Canadian-born population. Recent immigrant women have the lowest employment rate (49.1%) (Ontario Women's Health Network, 2017).

In Canada, immigrants are overrepresented in lower-paying sectors such as accommodation and food services as well as in transportation, warehousing, and manufacturing. Recent racialized immigrants are overrepresented in low-paying industries such as hospitality, warehousing, and manufacturing. Yet many immigrants are also employed in sectors that pay relatively well, such as finance, insurance, and real estate, where they make up 34% of the workforce, and in professional, scientific, and technical services, where they account for 32% of the labour force (Ng & Gagnon, 2020).

Women immigrants are overrepresented in precarious, low-paying employment. Recent immigrant women are three times more likely to have part-time work and two-and-a-half times more likely to have temporary work than non-immigrant women (Hira-Friesen, 2017).

Relatively few studies of the economic outcomes of refugees have been conducted in Canada. A study looking over the labour market outcomes of refugees from 13 countries over the 1980–2009 period found that PSRs earned more in the first year in Canada compared to GARs. After 5 years in Canada, refugee men from 7 of the 13 countries had employment rates over 75%. However, refugees from Iran and Somalia had very low employment rates. Refugee women from Iraq, Afghanistan, Pakistan, and Somalia also had very low employment rates. The earnings of refugees from different countries varied significantly (Picot et al., 2019).

In addition to limited language skills, lack of Canadian work experience, and non-recognition of foreign credentials, factors specific to refugees include physical and mental health issues related to traumatic pre-migration experiences, a lack of legal documents, and long-term disruption of education and careers (Kaida et al., 2020).

Overall, refugees' economic outcomes during the initial settlement period were generally comparable to those of family-class immigrants, but were worse than those of economic immigrants. However, over their first 10 years in Canada, refugees' median annual earnings increased at a rate that was higher than that of all other immigrant entry groups. Yet, because refugees' initial disadvantage was so large, it would take them 12 to 18 years to reach the median earnings of all immigrants.

Social Inclusion, Social Exclusion, and Social Support

Social environment, social inclusion, and social support are important factors influencing health and well-being. **Social inclusion** refers to the ability to participate in and contribute to the social, political, cultural, and economic aspects of the society. Being socially connected, having access to different forms of social goods and resources, and being civically engaged are associated with positive physical and mental health (Mamatis et al., 2019).

Social Exclusion. By contrast, **social exclusion** refers to a lack of access to resources and opportunities to participate fully in society. Exclusion, including discrimination and racism, consists of interconnected processes driven by unequal power relationships interacting across four main dimensions: economic, political, social, and cultural. Exclusion occurs because certain population groups are systematically disadvantaged and discriminated against on the basis of their race, ethnicity, gender, sexual orientation, immigration status, and other forms of identity (Popay, 2010; Tilly, 2007). People who are socially excluded are more economically and socially vulnerable. In Canada, recent immigrants and refugees, in particular those from racialized groups, are one of the groups more likely to experience social exclusion (Raphael et al., 2020).

Compelling evidence shows that discrimination is harmful to health. **Discrimination** includes "any practice, judgment, and action that creates and reinforces oppressive relations or conditions that marginalize, exclude, and/or restrain the lives of those encountering discrimination" (Pollock et al., 2012). Discrimination may take many different forms—it may happen directly or indirectly; it may be overt, but is often subtle. Perceived discrimination has been linked to a range of physical and mental health problems, such as hypertension, self-reported poor health, cancer, depression, and anxiety. Research has shown that perceptions of discrimination could affect health

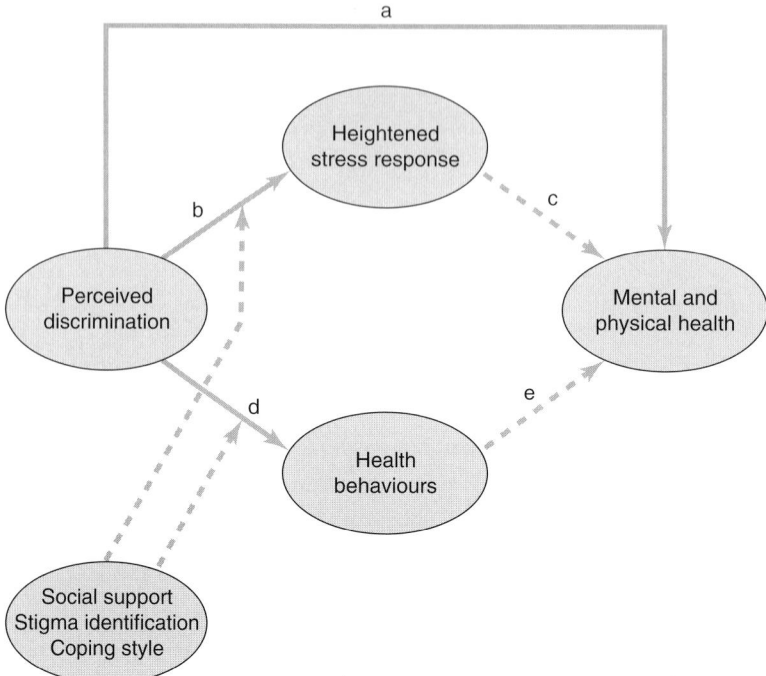

Fig. 11.3 Pathways by which perceived discrimination influences health outcomes. (From Pascoe, E. A., & Smart Richman, L. [2009]. Perceived discrimination and health: A meta-analytic review. *Psychological Bulletin, 135*[4], 531–554. https://doi.org/10.1037/a0016059. https://www.ncbi.nlm.nih.gov/pmc/articles/PMC2747726/.)

through the mechanisms of stress responses and health behaviours. Perceived discrimination has been associated with smoking, overeating, less sleep, and physical inactivity (Pascoe & Smart Richman, 2009; Sims et al., 2016). See Figure 11.3 for pathways by which perceived discrimination influences health outcomes. Perceived discrimination may affect mental and physical health directly (Path a) as well as through elevated stress responses (Path b). Chronic stress has been linked to various health problems including high blood pressure, heart disease, type II diabetes, and depression. Perceived discrimination may also contribute to health problems through allostatic load caused by chronic stressors (Path c). Allostatic load refers to the cost of chronic exposure to elevated or fluctuating endocrineor neural responses resulting from chronic stress or repeated challenges that are experienced as stressful (International Encyclopedia of the Social and Behavioural Sciences, 2001). Experiences of discrimination may affect health through participation in unhealthy or risky behaviours such smoking or use of other substances used to cope with chronic stress (Path d), which can have harmful effects on health. The solid lines in the figure indicate analyzed pathways; dashed line represent pathways hypothesized by past research (Pascoe & Smart Richman, 2009).

Racism is a prominent form of social exclusion and a key structural determinant of health (Hyman, 2009). The Ontario Human Rights Commission (OHRC, 2012) defines racism as "a belief that one group is superior to others. ... Racial discrimination is the illegal expression of racism. It includes any action, intentional or not, that has the effect of singling out persons based on their race, and imposing burdens on them and not on others, or withholding or limiting access to benefits available to other members of society ... ." Racism functions on multiple levels that often reinforce one another: individual, organizational, institutional, and systemic.

Systemic racism is embedded within society or an organization and supported by institutional policies. A substantial body of research indicates that racial discrimination is a significant risk factor for disease and is a contributor to racial disparities in health (Williams & Rucker, 2000; Williams et al., 2019). International research has found higher rates of infant mortality, high blood pressure, and diabetes among racialized group members compared to non-racialized group members (Levy et al., 2013).

More than 75% of immigrants who have arrived in Canada since 2001 are racialized. In 2016, the majority (61.8%) of newcomers were born in Asia, 13.4% were born in Africa (a four-fold increase from the 1971 census [3.2%]), while 27.7% of immigrants were born in Europe (Statistics Canada, 2017b). The healthy immigrant effect has been found to be stronger for non-European immigrants (including West Asian, South Asian, and Chinese individuals) than for European immigrants (Kim et al., 2013; Ng et al., 2005). De Maio and Kemp (2010) confirmed that racialized status was a statistically significant factor in the decline of immigrant health.

Perceived discrimination in health care settings is of particular concern because of its negative implications for health-seeking behaviour and health outcomes. Researchers have found that some health providers refuse to accept refugees as patients because of their complex health needs, linguistic barriers, and, in the case of refugee claimants, complicated insurance coverage delaying payment for services delivered. While discriminatory incidents are often isolated events, the stress of a single incident can lead to distrust of health care providers (Pollock et al., 2012).

Social Support. Evidence shows that support from families, friends, and communities is associated with better health. Individuals with greater levels of social support tend to have a lower incidence, prevalence, and severity of illness. Studies of mortality across industrialized nations show that individuals with the lowest level of involvement in social relationships are more likely to die earlier than those with greater involvement. There is compelling evidence linking a low quantity or quality of social ties with cardiovascular disease, high blood pressure, cancer and delayed cancer recovery, and slower wound healing (Umberson & Montez, 2010).

Recent immigrants and refugees must rebuild social networks in the new country to obtain needed social support. However, they often face social exclusion because of their race, language, religion, or immigrant status and have limited access to personal, social, and community resources (Hynie et al., 2011).

Social support plays an important role in immigrant settlement and has a positive impact on immigrant and refugee health. Support networks involving family and friends, as well as the host community, are important influences for immigrants to achieve life satisfaction. Research has found protective effects of social support networks against mental disorders such as anxiety, depression, and schizophrenia. Perceived family support is found to be the best protector of immigrant mental health. Interaction and social integration among and between immigrants and with the host community are among key elements for promoting immigrant health and well-being (Hombrados-Mendieta et al., 2019; Simich et al., 2005). Stewart (2014) suggests that "social support has the potential to decrease refugees' isolation and loneliness, enhance their sense of belonging and life fulfillment, mediate the stress of discrimination and facilitate integration into a new society."

Health Care Services

Both access to health care services and quality of care impact health outcomes. Despite Canada's universal health care system, new immigrants and refugees to Canada experience a number of barriers in access to and quality of health care. The most common barriers reported are language barriers, lack of information on accessing services, and cultural factors. Daily experiences of discrimination among racialized immigrants might lead to mistrust of health care systems. Other barriers include financial barriers, transportation barriers, and long wait times. These barriers to health care services lead to delays in receiving appropriate care, unmet health needs, inability to get preventive services, hospitalizations that could have been prevented, and overall poor health outcomes. Experiences related to barriers preventing access to health care may vary depending on the immigration category (Kalich et al., 2015).

While immigrants as well as GARs and PSRs are eligible for provincial health insurance, direct costs are still a significant obstacle for new immigrants seeking health care. In some provinces new immigrants must wait up to 3 months before they can get provincial health insurance. The Interim Federal Health Program (IFHP) provides temporary coverage of certain health care benefits to protected persons, including resettled refugees, refugee claimants, and certain other groups, during the period when they are not eligible for provincial or territorial health insurance (Government of Canada, 2017). New immigrants who need to access health care services during the waiting period for provincial health insurance might choose to delay seeking health care until the end of the waiting period because of financial barriers, which can lead to poor health outcomes (Goel et al., 2013).

Overall, recent immigrants use health care services less than the Canadian-born population, but there are significant differences within different groups of immigrants in terms of their patterns of utilization (Sarría-Santamera et al., 2016). A study conducted in British Columbia found the highest number of physician visits and hospitalization rates per person among refugees, followed by family class immigrants. Economic class immigrants utilized physicians the least and had lower hospitalization discharge rates (Long, 2010). The use of services increases with increasing length of residence in Canada.

Immigrant populations report higher rates of unmet health care needs compared to people born in Canada (Health Quality Ontario, 2016). Recent immigrants are less likely to have a primary care doctor than long-term immigrants and the Canadian-born population. Access to a primary care provider regularly offers opportunities for disease prevention and early intervention and is associated with better health outcomes regardless of a person's initial health status (Parlette, 2012; Vahabi et al., 2015).

Immigrants and refugees should be connected to primary health care as soon as possible after arrival. Research has found that newcomers are more likely to use health care services in an acute manner than for prevention However, immigrants without a primary care physician are also less likely to use the emergency department as a primary access point for care than Canadian-born respondents and, consequently, may receive different care than that provided non-immigrants (Ohle et al., 2018).

An Ontario study found that 84.6% of immigrants who have resided in Canada for less than a decade reported having a health care provider, compared to 94% of people born in Canada (Health Quality Ontario, 2016). A study exploring health care needs and service use among recent Syrian refugees in Canada found differences in the rates of unmet health care needs, based on sponsorship status and post-migration socioeconomic position. However, the reported rates of unmet health care needs both at baseline (48.2%) and at follow-up (42.6%) were much higher than rates for the general population in Canada (11.2%) (Tuck et al., 2019).

Canadian research has demonstrated that immigrants are under-screened for breast, cervical, and colorectal cancer. South Asian immigrant women have been found to have particularly low breast cancer screening rates. Research has also shown inequities in breast cancer diagnosis for immigrant women, in particular for immigrant women from Latin America, the Caribbean, and South Asia. Screening rates are significantly lower among recent immigrant women than for long-term immigrant women (Lofters et al., 2010; 2019).

In general, both immigrants and refugees are less likely than the Canadian-born population to use mental health care in primary care or specialty health care settings (Chen et al., 2009; Durbin et al., 2014, 2015; MHCC, 2016).

Culture

Culture is "a socially transmitted system of shared knowledge, beliefs and practices that varies across groups, and individuals within those groups" (Hernandez & Gibb, 2019). The influence of cultural norms, beliefs, and values on health is significant. Culture affects perceptions of health and illness, beliefs about causes of illnesses, how illnesses are experienced and expressed, how they can be cured or treated, and who should be involved in the process. Culture also affects acceptance of health promotion and prevention measures (Canadian Paediatric Society, 2020).

Immigrant and refugee groups bring their own perspectives, values, and behaviours to the health care system. Their health care beliefs and health practices may differ from those of the Canadian health system, which has been shaped by the dominant cultures. For example, some immigrants or refugees may prefer using alternative or traditional practices, medicines, or healers. Culture can also play a role in the level of family influence in patient care decisions (Canadian Medical Protective Agency [CMPA], 2014). Physician gender preferences, sharing hospital rooms, and stigma of certain illnesses such as mental illness or AIDS have also been identified as potential cultural barriers to health care (Ahmed et al., 2015; Ohle et al., 2018).

While culture is an important determinant of health, overemphasis on culture may lead to assumptions and stereotypes related to individuals from specific ethnic groups by equating individual beliefs with group beliefs. It is important to keep in mind that immigrant and refugee groups are not homogeneous—there is huge intragroup and intergroup diversity in terms of religion, language, education, rural and urban origin, and so on. Culture is also fluid and constantly changing. The immigration process requires adaptation to a new society. This process is complex and influenced by various socioeconomic factors. Therefore, perceptions of health and illness can vary widely within an immigrant group and over time (Kleinman & Benson, 2006; MHCC, 2016).

Both health care providers and patients are influenced by their respective cultures. Thus the culture of clinicians and the health care system need to be considered. Canada's health system has been shaped by the mainstream beliefs of historically dominant cultures. Cultural bias that introduces the dominant group's health values and behaviour as being the most highly valued can negatively affect access and quality of care for immigrants and refugees (Committee on Health Care for Underserved Women, 2018). Immigrants and refugees report experiences of insensitivity, cultural stereotyping, discrimination, and lack of knowledge about their religious and cultural practices. This includes instances of health care providers becoming frustrated when asked to respect specific religious or cultural beliefs and needs (Pollock et al., 2012; Reitmanova & Gustafson, 2008).

Providing culturally sensitive care improves treatment adherence, patient satisfaction, and health outcomes. Being aware of and respectful to cultural differences enables health care providers to ask about health beliefs or practices and to include that knowledge in treatment planning (Canadian Paediatric Society, 2020; Tucker et al., 2011).

Official-Language Proficiency

Language is a determinant of health for immigrants and refugees. Official-language proficiency determines participation in and integration into Canadian society, employment opportunities, and access to health care services. Limited official-language proficiency is significantly associated with poor self-reported health among both immigrant men and women (Bowen, 2015; Ng et al., 2011).

In 2016, almost four in five (78.5%) recent immigrants reported a language other than English or French as their mother tongue. Nine out of ten (89.6%) recent immigrants reported being able to conduct a conversation in English or French. However, 1 in 10 recent immigrants reported not being able to conduct a conversation in either English or French (Chavez, 2019). Less educated immigrant women, older women, and some immigration class groups such as spouse/dependents, family class, and refugees are more likely to have lower official-language proficiency on arrival (Adamuti-Trache et al., 2018).

Refugees in general tend to have limited skills in the official languages of Canada. However, there is a difference across different refugee groups. For example, according to the 2016 census, about 20% of GAR Syrian refugees knew English or French, compared to 67% of PSRs (Hou et al., 2019).

Evidence shows that language barriers have an adverse effect on initial access to health care services, including physician and hospital care, as well as health promotion and prevention programs. Language barriers result in poorer quality of care, lower patient and provider satisfaction, failure to obtain informed consent or protect patient confidentiality, and delayed treatment or misdiagnoses. Language barriers have been associated with increased risk of hospital admission and readmission, less adequate management of chronic diseases, and

---

Cultural Considerations In Care

Explanation and Understanding

A 45-year-old Hispanic immigrant, Mr. G., undergoes a job health screening and is told that his blood pressure is very high and he will not be allowed to continue work until his blood pressure is controlled. He goes to the local hospital and is given a prescription for a beta blocker and a diuretic. The doctor prescribes two medications known to be effective and simple for adherence because they each are supposed to be taken once a day.

Mr. G. presents to the emergency department 1 week later with dizziness. His blood pressure is very low, and Mr. G. says he has been taking the medicine just like it says to take it on the bottle. The puzzling case is discussed by multiple practitioners until one that speaks Spanish asks Mr. G. how many pills he took each day. "22," Mr. G. replies. The provider explains to his colleagues that "once" means "11" in Spanish.

When giving instructions to patients who require language support it is critical to support instructions with demonstration (where appropriate) and assess understanding by asking patients to do a return demonstration or explain their understanding in their own words (also see Chapter 6).

Scenario from Institute of Medicine (US) Committee on Health Literacy; Nielsen-Bohlman, L., Panzer, A. M., & Kindig, D. A. (Eds.). (2004). *Health literacy: A prescription to end confusion*. National Academies Press. https://www.ncbi.nlm.nih.gov/books/NBK216037/.

Cultural Competence In Action

Vital Role of Language Support

It's 2:00 A.M. when a man walks into an emergency department. The man, of Ethiopian background, is obviously distraught and his hands are covered in blood. He is speaking so fast in broken English and Amharic that no one can understand him. A physician treats the serious knife wounds to the man's hands. Seeing what he perceives to be the man's fear of whoever assaulted him, he decides to report the crime to the police.

If an interpreter had been called, the physician would have learned that the wounds were self-inflicted and arranged for the man to see a psychiatrist to help him through the crisis.

- What factors may have influenced the physician's decision not to seek interpretation services? How might this patient respond to police presence?
- What actions could have been taken to prevent the miscommunication and enhance health outcomes for this patient?

CAMH Immigrant and Refugee Mental Health Course, 2017.

higher number of adverse drug reactions (Al Shamsi et al., 2020; Bowen, 2015; de Moissac & Bowen, 2019).

The use of qualified professional interpreters in person or remotely by phone or videoconferencing improves equity in access and quality for those who are not fluent in English or French (Laher et al., 2018). Unfortunately, interpreter services are not mandated in the health care system.

Interpreter services also often pose challenges in terms of access to professional interpreters and the associated cost. In Canada, only some province and health regions provide interpretation services free of charge. As a result, health care providers may turn to ad hoc interpreters, including family and friends. While no interpreter is perfect, errors committed by ad hoc interpreters are more likely to have adverse consequences than those committed by qualified professional interpreters (Flores et al., 2012; Hansson et al., 2010; MHCC, 2016).

Family members or friends can be used as interpreters in an emergency. They may be prone to omissions, additions, substitutions, interpretations, and opinions. Furthermore, patients may not disclose sensitive personal information to family and friends. For example, if a refugee woman survivor of sexual violence is brought to the hospital by her family member who is then asked to interpret for her, the woman is not likely to reveal the history of sexual violence.

Children should never be used as interpreters. Asking children to interpret for their parents or other family members places children in inappropriate and potentially traumatic situations that can also negatively affect family dynamics (CAMH, 2017).

Refugee Determination Process

Individuals seeking refugee status from within Canada or at a port of entry must go through the refugee determination process. Not knowing whether they will be given refugee status can take a toll on refugee claimants. They may fear being turned down and deported back to their country of origin. This increases the risk of mental health problems including depression, anxiety, and PTSD (Agic et al., 2019).

Intersecting Identities

The social determinants of health approach recognizes that multiple identities such as race, class, ability, gender, sexual orientation, immigration status, and related structures of oppression and discrimination intersect and often reinforce each other to produce health inequities (Caiola et al., 2014; MOHLTC, 2012). Immigrants and refugees hold many intersecting identities (e.g., gender, education, race, ethnicity, religion, sexual orientation, ability). These intersections not only shape their vulnerability and resilience, but also their experiences and the health care system's responses to them.

Cultural Considerations In Care

The Intersectional Impact of Gender, Other Identities, and Discrimination

Racialized refugee women often experience discrimination in a different way than racialized men or even women as a gender. The effects of racism and gender discrimination often intersect, giving rise to compounded or double discrimination. When a woman's immigration status is factored into her experience, the triple burden of gender, immigration status, and racial discrimination overlap (Ontario Human Rights Commission, 2016).

Example: *Women with disabilities experience unique forms of discrimination. They may be singled out as targets for sexual harassment and sexual violence due to a perception that they are more vulnerable and unable to protect themselves. They may also experience discrimination related to their right to reproductive freedom. And they are more likely to be underemployed, unemployed, and live in poverty.*

Ontario Human Rights Commission (2016). *Intersecting grounds.* http://www.ohrc.on.ca/en/policy-ableism-and-discrimination-based-disability/4-intersecting-grounds.

Implications for Policymakers, Program Planners, and Health Care Providers

Canada depends on immigration for population and economic growth. Therefore, promoting and protecting the health and well-being of immigrants and refugees has powerful implications for the country's future success and prosperity. Addressing the health of immigrants and refugees "in an inclusive, comprehensive manner and as part of holistic efforts to respond to the health needs of the overall population" is also a human rights obligation of Canada (WHO, 2019). The WHO's Constitution states that "the enjoyment of the highest attainable standard of health is one of the fundamental rights to every human being without discrimination of race, religion, political belief, economic or social condition" (WHO, 1948). The right to health applies to every human being, "locals, refugees and migrants alike" (WHO, 2020a). The right to health is interrelated with other human rights, including social, economic, civil, political, and cultural rights. Therefore, the right to health extends to social determinants of health (Kuehlmeyer et al., 2019).

Reducing health inequities experienced by immigrants and refugees in Canada requires a comprehensive approach focusing on tackling living conditions fundamental to health and well-being, including income disparities, underemployment, and social exclusion, as well as inequities in access to health promotion, prevention, and treatment services.

Immigrants as well as refugees to Canada are a heterogeneous group. A blanket approach to policies, programs, and service models is not effective. Health status and risk factors differ across different groups of immigrants and refugees. The trend of declining health status over time is not universal to all immigrants. It has been well documented that certain groups are at higher risk of transitioning to poor health, including women, low-income immigrants, older persons, refugees, and recent immigrants from racialized groups. This finding suggests that program and policy responses should adopt an equity lens to better recognize and incorporate diversity between and within immigrant groups, and the complex interactions of the social, economic, political, and environmental circumstances of their lives (Gushulak, 2010; Simich & Jackson, 2010).

Research evidence further highlights the need for intersectoral collaboration; focusing on health promotion and illness prevention; involving members of immigrant and refugee communities in program and service planning; having a clear system of pathways to care and information on services available; increasing the diversity of programs and services; improving cultural sensitivity of health care provision; and ensuring access to professional interpreters (Agic et al., 2016; Gushulak et al., 2011; Hansson et al., 2010; Pollock et al., 2012).

HEALTH CARE PROVIDERS

Health care providers are in a key position to promote and protect the health of immigrants and refugees during the crucial post-migration period. Timely access to appropriate health care services and supports has a major impact on treatment outcomes. Some specific recommendations for health care service improvement include the following (British Medical Association, 2011; Marmot, 2017; Pottie et al., 2008):

- *Recognizing social determinants of immigrant and refugee health:* This means considering the patient as a person within the context of their pre-migration, migration, and post-migration circumstances, keeping in mind that the health needs of newly arriving immigrants and refugees often differ from those of Canadian-born population.
- *Providing linguistically appropriate services:* Health care providers need to use qualified, trained interpreters whenever possible and be aware of the potential consequences of using family and friends as interpreters, including confidentiality, privacy, accuracy, and neutrality issues; they should never use children as interpreters.

- *Demonstrating cultural awareness and sensitivity:* Health care providers need to avoid making generalizations and assumptions about immigrants or refugees and be aware of their own biases. They should respectfully asking about patients' health beliefs, norms, behaviours, and expectations and incorporate new knowledge into diagnosis and treatment planning.
- *Liaising with community-based organizations:* This involves identifying and addressing psychosocial needs and linking patients with local community-based organizations providing settlement services, language classes, employment counselling, or basic assistance such as housing or food programs.
- *Advocating for improved and equitable access to care and for immigrants and refugees at local, regional, national, and international levels.*

Summary

This chapter provided an overview of multiple interacting factors influencing the health and well-being of immigrants and refugees to Canada, in particular post-migration social determinants of health and their implications for policymakers, program planners, and health care providers. Immigrants and refugees to Canada are diverse groups with unique health care needs and challenges. The rates of health problems and disorders vary considerably between and within different groups, reflecting differences in exposure to and effects of social risk factors on specific subgroups. Upon arrival, new immigrants are healthier than the Canadian-born population, but this healthy immigrant effect disappears over time. Refugees, low-income immigrants, and recent immigrants from racialized groups are at increased risk of transitioning to poorer health soon after arrival. Promoting and protecting the health of immigrants and refugees is a human rights obligation of Canada that requires tackling social determinants of health and health inequities. Improving equity in access and quality of care for immigrants and refugees requires the provision of contextually tailored and culturally and linguistically appropriate health care services.

ⓔ http://evolve.elsevier.com/Srivastava/culturalcompetence/.

Questions for Review and Discussion

1. What is the healthy immigrant effect and how it differs across subgroups of immigrants?
2. Explain why migration is considered a social determinant of health.
3. Despite the universal health care system, new immigrants and refugees to Canada experience inequities in access to and quality of health care. Identify and discuss the most common barriers to health care services and how they impact immigrant and refugee health outcomes.
4. In what ways does "the triple burden of gender, immigration status, and racial discrimination overlap"? Explain what is meant by this statement.
5. Children should not be used as interpreters. What are the reasons for this?

Group Experiential/Reflection Activity

Working in small groups, research and discuss your findings on one of these topics:
Why do women refugees experience more discrimination and racism than other refugees?
Why are racialized women refugees with disabilities more at risk of mental health problems than other immigrant or refugee women?

References

Adamuti-Trache, M., Anisef, P., & Sweet, R. (2018). Differences in language proficiency and learning strategies among immigrant women to Canada. *Journal of Language, Identity & Education*, *17*, 1–18. https://doi.org/10.1080/15348458.2017.1390433.

Agic, B., Andermann, L., McKenzie, K., et al. (2019). Refugees in host countries: Psychosocial aspects and mental health. In T. Wenzel & B. Droždek (Eds.), *An uncertain safety*. Springer. https://doi.org/10.1007/978-3-319-72914-5_8.

Agic, B., McKenzie, K., Tuck, A., et al., on behalf of the Mental Health Commission of Canada. (2016). *Supporting the mental health of refugees to Canada*. https://ontario.cmha.ca/wp-content/files/2016/02/Refugee-Mental-Health-backgrounder.pdf

Ahmed, S., Shommu, N., Rumana, N., et al. (2015). Barriers to access of primary healthcare by immigrant populations in Canada: A literature review. *Journal of Immigrant and Minority Health*, *18*, 1522–1540. https://doi.org/10.1007/s10903-015-0276-z.

Al Shamsi, H., Almutairi, A. G., Al Mashrafi, S., et al. (2020). Implications of language barriers for healthcare: a systematic review. *Oman Medical Journal*, *35*(2), e122. https://doi.org/10.5001/omj.2020.40.

Beiser, M. (2005). The health of immigrants and refugees in Canada. *Canadian Journal of Public Health*, *96*(2), S30–S44.

Bevelander, P. (2016). Integrating refugees into labor markets. *IZA World of Labor*, *269*(2), 269. https://doi.org/10.15185/izawol.269.

Bowen, S. (2015). *The impact of language barriers on patient safety and quality of care*. Société Santé en Français.

Brunner, E., & Marmot, M. G. (2006). Social organization, stress, and health. In M. G. Marmot & R. G. Wilkinson (Eds.), *Social determinants of health*. Oxford University Press, Figure 2.2, p. 9.

Burgard, S. A., & Lin, K. Y. (2013). Bad jobs, bad health? How work and working conditions contribute to health disparities. *The American Behavioral Scientist*, *57*(8). https://doi.org/10.1177/0002764213487347.

Bushnik, T., Tjepkema, M., & Martel, L. (2020). Socioeconomic disparities in life and health expectancy among the household population in Canada. Statistics Canada Catalogue no. 82-003-X ISSN 1209-1367. *Health Reports*, *31*(1), 3–14. https://doi.org/10.25318/82-003-x202000100001-eng.

Caiola, C., Docherty, S. L., Relf, M., et al. (2014). Using an intersectional approach to study the impact of social determinants of health for African American mothers living with HIV. *ANS. Advances in Nursing Science*, *37*(4), 287–298. https://doi.org/10.1097/ANS.0000000000000046.

Canadian Institute for Health Information (CIHI). (2016). *Trends in income-related health inequalities in Canada. Technical report*. https://secure.cihi.ca/free_products/trends_in_income_related_inequalities_in_canada_2015_en.pdf?_ga=2.205007760.1662519056.1646018971-1423025675.1646018971

Canadian Medical Association. (2013a). *Health care in Canada: What makes us sick?: Canadian Medical Association Town Hall Report*. Author.

Canadian Medical Association. (2013b). *Health equity and the social determinants of health: A role for the medical profession*. https://policybase.cma.ca/media/PolicyPDF/PD13-03.pdf

Canadian Medical Protective Association (CMPA). (2014). *When medicine and culture intersect*. https://www.cmpa-acpm.ca/en/advice-publications/browse-articles/2014/when-medicine-and-culture-intersect

Canadian Paediatric Society. (2020). *How culture influences health. A guide for health professionals working with immigrant and refugee children and youth. Caring for kids new to Canada*. https://www.kidsnewtocanada.ca/culture/influence

Canadian Public Health Association. (2020). *What are the social determinants of health?* https://www.cpha.ca/what-are-social-determinants-health

Chavez, B. (2019). *Immigration and language in Canada, 2011 and 2016. Ethnicity, language and immigration thematic series*. Statistics Canada. https://www150.statcan.gc.ca/n1/en/pub/89-657-x/89-657-x2019001-eng.pdf?st=5B-S_Ot9

Committee on Health Care for Underserved Women. (2018). *Importance of social determinants of health and cultural awareness in the delivery of reproductive health care*. The American College of Obstetricians and Gynecologists, 729. https://www.acog.org/-/media/project/acog/acogorg/clinical/files/committee-opinion/articles/2018/01/importance-of-social-determinants-of-health-and-cultural-awareness-in-the-delivery-of-reproductive-health-care.pdf

Davies, A. A., Basten, A., & Frattini, C. (2006). *Migration: A social determinant of the health of migrants—Background paper*. IOM Migration Health Department. http://citeseerx.ist.psu.edu/viewdoc/download?doi=10.1.1.462.6286&rep=rep1&type=pdf

de Moissac, D., & Bowen, S. (2019). Impact of language barriers on quality of care and patient safety for official language minority francophones in Canada. *Journal of Patient Experience*, 6(1), 24–32. https://doi.org/10.1177/2374373518769008.

Dhadda, A., & Greene, G. (2018). The healthy migrant effect for mental health in England: Propensity-score matched analysis using the EMPIRIC survey. *Journal of Immigrant and Minority Health*, 20(4), 799–808. https://doi.org/10.1007/s10903-017-0570-z.

Durbin, A., Lin, E., Moineddin, R., et al. (2014). Mental health care use for non-psychotic conditions by immigrants in different admission classes and refugees in Ontario, Canada. *Open Medicine*, 8(4), e136–e146.

Durbin, A., Moineddin, R., Lin, E., et al. (2015). Examining the relationship between neighbourhood deprivation and mental health service use for immigrants in Ontario, Canada. *BMJ Open*, 5(3), e006690.

El Arnaout, N., Rutherford, S., Zreik, T., et al. (2019). Assessment of the health needs of Syrian refugees in Lebanon and Syria's neighboring countries. *Conflict and Health*, 13, 31. https://doi.org/10.1186/s13031-019-0211-3.

Fitzsimmons, S., Baggs, J., & Brannen, M. Y. (2020). The immigrant income gap. *Harvard Business Review*. https://hbr.org/2020/05/research-the-immigrant-income-gap

Flores, G., Abreu, M., Barone, C. P., et al. (2012). Errors of medical interpretation and their potential clinical consequences: A comparison of professional versus ad hoc versus no interpreters. *Annals of Emergency Medicine*, 60, 545–553. https://doi.org/10.1016/j.annemergmed.2012.01.025.

Fuller-Thomson, E., Noack, A. M., & George, U. (2011). Health decline among recent immigrants to Canada: Findings from a nationally-representative longitudinal survey. *Canadian Journal of Public Health*, 102(4), 273–280. https://doi.org/10.1007/BF03404048.

Goel, R., Bloch, G., & Caulford, P. (2013). Waiting for care: Effects of Ontario's 3-month waiting period for OHIP on landed immigrants. *Canadian Family Physician*, 59(6), e269–e275.

Government of Canada. (2001). *Immigration and Refugee Protection Act (IRPA)*. https://laws-lois.justice.gc.ca/PDF/I-2.5.pdf

Government of Canada. (2013). *What makes Canadians healthy or unhealthy?* https://www.canada.ca/en/public-health/services/health-promotion/population-health/what-determines-health/what-makes-canadians-healthy-unhealthy.html

Government of Canada. (2017). *Health care – Refugees*. https://www.canada.ca/en/immigration-refugees-citizenship/services/refugees/help-within-canada/health-care.html

Government of Canada. (2020). *Social determinants of health and health inequalities*. https://www.canada.ca/en/public-health/services/health-promotion/population-health/what-determines-health.html

Government of Canada. (2021). *Resettle in Canada as a refugee*. https://www.canada.ca/en/immigration-refugees-citizenship/services/refugees/help-outside-canada.html

Government of Canada. (2022). *Medical inadmissibility*. https://www.canada.ca/en/immigration-refugees-citizenship/services/immigrate-canada/inadmissibility/reasons/medical-inadmissibility.html#excessive-demand

Gushulak. B. (2010). *Canada's migration health – Legislation and policies: Over the centuries*. Health Canada.

Gushulak, B. D., Pottie, K., Hatcher Roberts, J., et al. (2011). Migration and health in Canada: Health in the global village. *CMAJ: Canadian Medical Association Journal*, 183(12), E952–E958. https://doi.org/10.1503/cmaj.090287.

Hamilton. T. G. (2015). The healthy immigrant (migrant) effect: In search of a better native-born comparison group. *Social Science Research*, 54, 353–365. https://doi.org/10.1016/j.ssresearch.2015.08.008.

Hansson, E., Tuck, A., Lurie, S., et al., for the Task Group of the Services Systems Advisory Committee. (2010). *Improving mental health services for immigrant, refugee, ethnocultural and racialized groups: Issues and options for service improvement*. Mental Health Commission of Canada.

Health Quality Ontario. (2016). *Measuring up 2016: A yearly report on how Ontario's health system is performing*. Queen's Printer for Ontario.

Hernandez, M., & Gibb, J. K. (2019). Culture, behavior and health. *Evolution, Medicine, and Public Health*, 2020(1), 12–13. https://doi.org/10.1093/emph/eoz036.

Hira-Friesen. P. (2017). The effect of labour market characteristics on Canadian immigrant employment in precarious work, 2006-2012. *Canadian Journal of Urban Research*, *26*(1), 1–15.

Hollander, A.-C., Bruce, D., Ekberg, I., et al. (2012). Longitudinal study of mortality among refugees in Sweden. *International Journal of Epidemiology*, *41*(4), 1153–1161. https://doi.org/10.1093/ije/dys072.

Hombrados-Mendieta, I., Millán-Franco, M., Gómez-Jacinto, L., et al. (2019). Positive influences of social support on sense of community, life satisfaction and the health of immigrants in Spain. *Frontiers in Psychology*, *10*, 2555. https://doi.org/10.3389/fpsyg.2019.02555.

Hou, F., Lu, Y., & Schimmele, C. (2019). *Recent trends in over-education by immigration status*. Statistics Canada Catalogue. no. 11F0019M—No. 436. https://www150.statcan.gc.ca/n1/en/pub/11f0019m/11f0019m2019024-eng.pdf?st=_ouZP24Z

Hyman, I. (2009). Racism as a determinant of immigrant health. https://citeseerx.ist.psu.edu/viewdoc/download?doi=10.1.1.516.7501&rep=rep1&type=pdf

Hynie, M., Crooks, V. A., & Barragan, J. (2011). Immigrant and refugee social networks: Determinants and consequences of social support among women newcomers to Canada. *CJNR*, *43*(4), 26–46.

Immigration and Refugee Board of Canada (IRB). (2021). *An introduction to Canada's refugee determination system*. https://irb.gc.ca/en/stay-connected/Pages/refugee-determination-transcript.aspx

Immigration, Refugees and Citizenship Canada (IRCC). (2019). *How Canada's refugee system works*. https://www.canada.ca/en/immigration-refugees-citizenship/services/refugees/canada-role.html

Immigration, Refugees and Citizenship Canada (IRCC). (2020a). *2019 annual report to Parliament on immigration*. https://www.canada.ca/content/dam/ircc/migration/ircc/english/pdf/pub/annual-report-2019.pdf

Immigration, Refugees and Citizenship Canada (IRCC). (2020b). *Temporary residents*. https://www.canada.ca/en/immigration-refugees-citizenship/corporate/publications-manuals/operational-bulletins-manuals/temporary-residents.html

Immigration, Refugees and Citizenship Canada (IRCC). (2021). *2020 annual report to Parliament on immigration*. https://www.canada.ca/content/dam/ircc/migration/ircc/english/pdf/pub/annual-report-2020-en.pdf

International Encyclopedia of the Social & Behavioral Sciences. (2001). *Allostatic load*. https://www.sciencedirect.com/topics/neuroscience/allostatic-load

Kaida, L., Hou, F., & Stick, M. (2020). *The long-term economic outcomes of refugee private sponsorship*. Statistics Canada Catalogue no. 11F0019M — No. 433. https://www150.statcan.gc.ca/n1/en/pub/11f0019m/11f0019m2019021-eng.pdf?st=rPA6m8Hh

Kalich, A., Heinemann, L., & Ghahari, S. (2015). A scoping review of immigrant experience of health care access barriers in Canada. *Journal of Immigrant and Minority Health*, *18*(3), 697–709. https://doi.org/10.1007/s10903-015-0237-6.

Kei, W., Seidel, M.-D. L., Ma, D., et al. (2019). *Results from the 2016 census: Examining the effect of public pension benefits on the low income of senior immigrants*. Statistics Canada Catalogue no. 75-006-X ISSN 2291-0840. https://www150.statcan.gc.ca/n1/en/pub/75-006-x/2019001/article/00017-eng.pdf?st=xQNwQV9V

Kim, I. -H., Carrasco, C., Muntaner, C., et al. (2013). Ethnicity and postmigration health trajectory in new immigrants to Canada. *American Journal of Public Health*, *103*(4), e96–e104.

Kleinman, A., & Benson, P. (2006). Anthropology in the clinic: The problem of cultural competency and how to fix it. *PLoS Med*, *3*, e294.

Kuehlmeyer, K., Klingler, C., & Huxtable, R. (Eds.) (2019). *Ethical, legal and social aspects of health care for migrants: Perspectives from the UK and Germany*. Routledge.

Laher, N., Sultana, A., Aery, A., et al. (2018). *Access to language interpretation services and its impact on clinical and patient outcomes: A scoping review*. Wellesley Institute. http://www.wellesleyinstitute.com/wp-content/uploads/2018/04/Language-Interpretation-Services-Scoping-Review.pdf

Levy, J., Ansara, D., & Stover, A. (2013). *Racialization and health inequities in Toronto*. Toronto Public Health. https://scholar.harvard.edu/files/davidrwilliams/files/racialization_health_toronto_2013.pdf

Lofters, A. K., Hwang, S. W., Moineddin, R., et al. (2010). Cervical cancer screening among urban immigrants by region of origin: A population-based cohort study. *Preventive Medicine*, *51*, 509–516.

Lofters, A. K., McBride, M. L., Li, D., et al. (2019). Disparities in breast cancer diagnosis for immigrant women in Ontario and BC: Results from the CanIMPACT study. *BMC Cancer*, *19*, 42. https://doi.org/10.1186/s12885-018-5201-0.

Long, M. (2010). Improving health care system responses to chronic disease among British Columbia's immigrant, refugee, and corrections population: A review of current findings and opportunities for change summary: Immigrant population. http://www.bccdc.ca/pop-public-health/Documents/RHILitReviewKeyFindingsImmigrants.pdf

Lu, C., & Ng, E. (2019). Healthy immigrant effect by immigrant category in Canada. *Health Reports*, *30*(4), 3–11. https://doi.org/10.25318/82-003-x201900400001-eng.

Lubbers, M., & Gijsberts, M. (2019). Changes in self-rated health right after immigration: A panel study of economic, social, cultural, and emotional explanations of self-rated health among immigrants in the Netherlands. *Frontiers in Sociology*, *4*, 45. https://doi.org/10.3389/fsoc.2019.00045.

Magalhaes, L., Carrasco, C., & Gastaldo, D. (2010). Undocumented migrants in Canada: A scope literature review on health, access to services, and working conditions. *Journal of Immigrant and Minority Health*, *12*(1), 132–151. https://doi.org/10.1007/s10903-009-9280-5.

Mamatis, D., Sanford, S., Ansara, D., et al. (2019). *Promoting health and well-being through social inclusion in Toronto: Synthesis of international and local evidence and implications for future action*. Toronto Public Health and Wellesley Institute. https://www.wellesleyinstitute.com/wp-content/uploads/2019/07/Social-Inclusion-Report.pdf

Marchbank, J. (July 2014). *Karen refugees after five years in Canada – Readying communities for refugee resettlement.* http://issbc.org/wp-content/uploads/2018/03/9_-_Karen_Refugees_After_Five_Years_in_Canada_CS.pdf

Mental Health Commission of Canada (MHCC). (2016). *The case for diversity: Building the case to improve mental health services for immigrant, refugee, ethno-cultural and racialized populations*. Author.

Migration Data Portal. (2020). *Migration and health*. https://migrationdataportal.org/themes/migration-and-health

Moniz, M., Abrantes, A., & Nunes, C. (2020). Healthy immigrant effect in non–European Union immigrants in Portugal: After a decade of (non-)integration! *Public Health*, *186*, 95–100. https://doi.org/10.1016/j.puhe.2020.07.006.

Morency, J. D., Malenfant, E. C., & MacIsaac, S. (2017). *Immigration and diversity: Population projections for Canada and its regions, 2011 to 2036*. Catalogue no. 91-551-X. Minister of Industry. https://www150.statcan.gc.ca/n1/en/pub/91-551-x/91-551-x2017001-eng.pdf?st=oGtYE2sU

National Academies of Sciences, Engineering, and Medicine. (2017). *The root causes of health inequity*. https://www.ncbi.nlm.nih.gov/books/NBK425845/

Ng, E. S., & Gagnon, S. (2020). *Employment gaps and underemployment for racialized groups and immigrants in Canada*. Diversity Institute. https://fsc-ccf.ca/wp-content/uploads/2020/01/EmploymentGaps-Immigrants-PPF-JAN2020-EN.pdf

Ng, E., Pottie, K., & Spitzer, D. (2011). Official language proficiency and self-reported health among immigrants to Canada. *Health Reports*, *22*(4), 15–23.

Ng, E., Wilkins, R., Gendron, F., et al. (2005). *Dynamics of immigrants' health in Canada: Evidence from the National Population Health Survey* (Catalogue no. 82-618-MWE2005002). http://www.statcan.gc.ca/pub/82-618-m/2005002/pdf/4193621-eng.pdf

Ng, E., & Zhang, H. (2020). The mental health of immigrants and refugees: Canadian evidence from a nationally linked database. Statistics Canada, Catalogue no. 82-003-X. *Health Reports*, *31*(8), 3–12. https://www150.statcan.gc.ca/n1/en/pub/82-003-x/2020008/article/00001-eng.pdf?st=OQZm8vVW

Office of Disease Prevention and Health Promotion. (2020). *Determinants of health*. https://www.healthy-people.gov/2020/about/foundation-health-measures/Determinants-of-Health#individual%20behavior

Ohle, R., Bleeker, H., Yadav, K., et al. (2018). The immigrant effect: Factors impacting use of primary and emergency department care – a Canadian population cross-sectional study. *CJEM*, *20*(2), 260–265. https://doi.org/10.1017/cem.2017.4.

Ontario Human Rights Commission (OHRC) (2012). *Racial discrimination*. https://www.ohrc.on.ca/en/racial-discrimination-brochure

Ontario Human Rights Commission. (OHRC). (2016). *Intersecting grounds*. http://www.ohrc.on.ca/en/policy-ableism-and-discrimination-based-disability/4-intersecting-grounds

Ontario Ministry of Health and Long-Term Care (MOHLTC). (2012). *Health Equity Impact Assessment (HEIA) workbook*. http://www.health.gov.on.ca/en/pro/programs/heia/docs/workbook.pdf

Ontario Ministry of Health and Long-Term Care (MOHLTC). (2014). *Health Equity Impact Assessment (HEIA). Immigrant populations supplement.* http://www.health.gov.on.ca/en/pro/programs/heia/docs/HEIA-Immigrant-Supplement.pdf

Ontario Women's Health Network. (2017). *Start from zero: Immigrant women's experiences of the wage gap.* Author.

Parlette, V. (2012). Social determinants of health and populations at risk. In A. S. Bierman (Ed.), *Project for an Ontario women's health evidence-based report* (Volume 2). https://www.ices.on.ca/Publications/Atlases-and-Reports/2012/POWER-Study

Pascoe, E. A., & Smart Richman, L. (2009). Perceived discrimination and health: A meta-analytic review. *Psychological Bulletin, 135*(4), 531–554. https://doi.org/10.1037/a0016059.

Pharr, J., Moonie, S., & Bungum, T. (2011). The impact of unemployment on mental and physical health, access to health care and health risk behaviors. *ISRN Public Health*, 2012. https://doi.org/10.5402/2012/483432.

Picot, G., & Lu, Y. (2017). *Chronic poverty among immigrants in Canada and its communities.* Analytical Studies Research Paper Series, Statistics Canada. Research Paper #397.

Picot, G., Zhang, Y., & Hou, F. (2019). *Labour market outcomes among refugees to Canada.* Statistics Canada Catalogue no. 11F0019M — No. 419. https://www150.statcan.gc.ca/n1/en/pub/11f0019m/11f0019m2019007-eng.pdf?st=gE2xLQQr

Pollock, G., Newbold, K. B., & Lafrenière, G., et al. (2012). Discrimination in the doctor's office: Immigrants and refugee experiences. *Critical Social Work, 13*(2), 60–79. https://ojs.uwindsor.ca/index.php/csw/article/view/5866/4843

Popay, J. (2010). Understanding and tackling social exclusion. *Journal of Research in Nursing, 15*, 295–297. https://doi.org/10.1177/1744987110370529.

Pottie, K., Ng, E., Spitzer, D., et al. (2008). Language proficiency, gender and self-reported health: An analysis of the first two waves of the longitudinal survey of immigrants to Canada. *Canadian Journal of Public Health, 99*(6), 505–510. https://doi.org/10.1007/BF03403786.

Prokopenko, E. (2018). Refugees and *Canadian post-secondary education: Characteristics and economic outcomes in comparison.* Statistics Canada Catalogue no. 89-657-X2018001.

Public Health Agency of Canada. (2018). *Key health inequalities in Canada. A national portrait.* https://www.canada.ca/content/dam/phac-aspc/documents/services/publications/science-research/key-health-inequalities-canada-national-portrait-executive-summary/key_health_inequalities_full_report-eng.pdf

Raphael, D., Bryant, T., Mikkonen, J., et al. (2020). *Social determinants of health: The Canadian facts.* Ontario Tech University Faculty of Health Sciences and York University School of Health Policy and Management.

Reitmanova, S., & Gustafson, D. (2008). They can't understand it: Maternity health and care needs of immigrant Muslim women in St. John's, Newfoundland. *Maternal and Child Health Journal, 12*, 101–111. https://doi.org/10.1007/s10995-007-0213-4.

Sarría-Santamera, A., Hijas-Gómez, A. I., & Carmona, R. (2016). A systematic review of the use of health services by immigrants and native populations *Public Health Reviews, 37*, 28. https://doi.org/10.1186/s40985-016-0042-3.

Shuldiner, J., Liu, Y., & Lofters, A. (2018). Incidence of breast and colorectal cancer among immigrants in Ontario, Canada: A retrospective cohort study from 2004-2014. *BMC Cancer, 18*(1), 537. https://doi.org/10.1186/s12885-018-4444-0.

Simich, L., Beiser, M., Stewart, M., et al. (2005). Providing social support for immigrants and refugees in Canada: Challenges and directions. *Journal of Immigrant and Minority Health, 7*, 259–268. https://doi.org/10.1007/s10903-005-5123-1.

Simich, L., & Jackson, B. (2010). *Social determinants of immigrant health in Canada: What makes some immigrants healthy and others not?* Migration and Health, Health Canada.

Sims, M., Diez-Roux, A. V., Gebreab, S. Y., et al. (2016). Perceived discrimination is associated with health behaviours among African-Americans in the Jackson Heart Study. *Journal of Epidemiology and Community Health, 70*(2), 187–194. https://doi.org/10.1136/jech-2015-206390.

Statistics Canada. (2016). *150 years of immigration in Canada.* Statistics Canada Catalogue no. 11-630-X. https://www150.statcan.gc.ca/n1/pub/11-630-x/11-630-x2016006-eng.htm

Statistics Canada. (2017a). *2016 census of population: Immigration and ethnocultural diversity, Canada.* Catalogue no. 98-501-X2016008. Minister of Industry. https://www12.statcan.gc.ca/census-recensement/2016/ref/98-501/98-501-x2016008-eng.pdf

Statistics Canada. (2017b). *Focus on geography series, 2016 census.* Statistics Canada Catalogue no. 98-404-X2016001 https://www12.statcan.gc.ca/census-recensement/2016/as-sa/fogs-spg/Index-eng.cfm

Statistics Canada. (2017c). *Immigration and ethnocultural diversity: Key results from the 2016 census.* https://www150.statcan.gc.ca/n1/en/daily-quotidien/171025/dq171025b-eng.pdf?st=pRq22mrs

Statistics Canada. (2018a). *Education in Canada: Key results from the 2016 census.* https://www150.statcan.gc.ca/n1/en/daily-quotidien/171129/dq171129a-eng.pdf?st=N9LnlN1z

Statistics Canada. (2018b). *Income and mobility of immigrants, 2016.* https://www150.statcan.gc.ca/n1/en/daily-quotidien/181210/dq181210a-eng.pdf?st=iOI3G2F0

Statistics Canada. (2019). *Definitions, data sources and methods. Classification of admission category of immigrant.* https://www23.statcan.gc.ca/imdb/p3VD.pl?Function=getVD&TVD=323293&CVD=323294&CLV=0&MLV=4&D=1

Statistics Canada. (2021). *Definitions, data sources and methods. Statistical units. Immigrant.* https://www23.statcan.gc.ca/imdb/p3Var.pl?Function=Unit&Id=85107

Stewart, M. J. (2014). Social support in refugee resettlement. In L. Simich & L. Andermann (Eds.), *Refuge and resilience: Promoting resilience and mental health among resettled refugees and forced migrants.* Springer Science + Business Media. (Vol. 7, pp. 91–107). https://doi.org/10.1007/978-94-007-7923-5_7.

Tilly, C. (2007). Poverty and the politics of exclusion. In D. Narayan & P. Petesch (Eds.), *Moving out of poverty: Cross-disciplinary perspectives on mobility.* World Bank. (Vol. 1, pp. 45–76).

Tu, J. V., Chu, A., Rezai, M. R., et al. (2015). The incidence of major cardiovascular events in immigrants to Ontario, Canada: The CANHEART Immigrant Study. *Circulation, 132*(16), 1549–1559. https://doi.org/10.1161/CIRCULATIONAHA.115.015345.

Tuck, A., Oda, A., Hynie, M., et al. (2019). Unmet health care needs for Syrian refugees in Canada: A follow-up study. *Journal of Immigrant and Minority Health, 21*(6), 1306–1312. https://doi.org/10.1007/s10903-019-00856-y.

Tucker, C. M., Marsiske, M., Rice, K. G., et al. (2011). Patient-centered culturally sensitive health care: Model testing and refinement. *Health Psychology, 30*(3), 342–350. https://doi.org/10.1037/a0022967.

Umberson, D., & Montez, J. K. (2010). Social relationships and health: A flashpoint for health policy. *Journal of Health and Social Behavior, 51*(Suppl), S54–S66. https://doi.org/10.1177/0022146510383501.

Vahabi, M., Lofters, A., Kumar, M., et al. (2015). Breast cancer screening disparities among urban immigrants: A population-based study in Ontario, Canada. *BMC Public Health, 15*, 679. https://doi.org/10.1186/s12889-015-2050-5.

Vang, Z., Sigouin, J., Flenon, A., et al. (2015). *The healthy immigrant effect in Canada: A systematic review.* Population Change and Lifecourse Strategic Knowledge Cluster Discussion Paper Series/Un Réseau stratégique de connaissances Changements de population et parcours de vie Document de travail: Vol. 3, Issue 1, Article 4. https://ir.lib.uwo.ca/pclc/vol3/iss1/4

Whitehead, M. (1990). *The concepts and principles of equity in health.* WHO Regional Office for Europe.

Williams, D. R., Lawrence, J. A., & Davis, B. A. (2019). Racism and health: Evidence and needed research. *Annual Review of Public Health, 40*(1), 105–125.

Williams, D. R., & Rucker, T. D. (2000). Understanding and addressing racial disparities in health care. *Health Care Financing Review, 21*(4), 75–90.

World Health Organization (WHO). (2008). *Closing the gap in a generation: Health equity through action on the social determinants of health.* Author.

World Health Organization (WHO). (2011). *Rio political declaration on social determinants of health.* https://www.who.int/sdhconference/declaration/Rio_political_declaration.pdf?ua=1

World Health Organization. (2017). *Determinants of health.* https://www.who.int/news-room/questions-and-answers/item/determinants-of-health

World Health Organization (WHO). (2019). *Promoting the health of refugees and migrants: Draft global action plan, 2019–2023.* Report by the Director-General. https://www.who.int/publications/i/item/promoting-the-health-of-refugees-and-migrants-draft-global-action-plan-2019-2023

World Health Organization (WHO). (2020a). *Refugee and migrant health. The right to health.* https://www.who.int/migrants/about/right-to-health/en/#:~:text=Health%20is%20a%20human%20right.&text=The%20principles%20of%20non%2Ddiscrimination,acceptable%20and%20of%20good%20quality

World Health Organization (WHO). (2020b). *Social determinants of health.* https://www.who.int/health-topics/social-determinants-of-health#tab=tab_1

Yssaad, L., & Fields, A. (2018). *The Canadian immigrant labour market: Recent trends from 2006 to 2017.* Statistics Canada Catalogue no. 71-606-X.

Yu, S., Ouellet, E., & Warmington, A. (2009). Refugee integration in Canada: A survey of empirical evidence and existing services. *Refuge, 24*(2), 17–34.

Specific Cultural Considerations

Rani H. Srivastava

Section Outline

In this section, which examines cultural considerations in specific populations, individual authors highlight how culture shapes the issues in the context of their practice. The discussion is not exhaustive and should be considered as a starting point toward achieving cultural competence in caring for specific clinical populations. The chapters also show a variety of ways that populations can be clinically grouped, reflecting the reality of our health care services. Sometimes health care services are organized by clinical specialty (for example, mental health); at other times by clinical issues (such as pain management) or developmental stage of life (for example, perinatal, end of life); and on occasion by areas of practice, such as community health.

This section reflects the author's experience that generally our work in health care is organized by such clinical specialties and shows that the specific cultural knowledge needed by health care providers depends on the nature of their practice and the population serve. Key concepts such as family, communication, and decision making are raised in several chapters, illustrating once again the need to bring an understanding of generic cultural knowledge to specific populations, such as families in the perinatal period, those experiencing end of life, and those in palliative care, and in navigating issues regarding pain management and mental health challenges. In bringing generic cultural knowledge to specific populations and issues, health care providers can focus on health promotion and community engagement.

Chapter 12 discusses the influence of cultural identity as families experience pregnancy and birth. It highlights the significant influence of unique and complex contexts of social and cultural determinants during all stages of the perinatal period for the pregnant person and their baby for effective and quality care. The chapter examines the need for health care providers addressing cultural issues, including racism and discrimination, to achieve cultural safety and equity in perinatal care. This is done through anti-racism education, compassionate care, respect for life, and understanding of cultural practices.

Chapter 13 discusses how culture shapes how people experience and respond to the end of a life. The chapter discusses how health care providers can work with people and their family as they approach the end of life. A brief discussion of medical assistance in dying (MAiD) within the Canadian context is presented. The chapter explores concepts such as a "good death," the meaning of suffering, and how critical life-and-death decisions are made. The chapter ends with a brief exploration of bereavement and the importance of rituals to support grief.

Chapter 14 discusses how culture influences views on mental health and mental illness. It identifies key issues within mental health care that are influenced by culture and presents specific and generic competencies that are necessary for health care providers. Cultural identity and cultural explanations are two important areas that require assessment before appropriate interventions can be determined. Power dynamics between health care providers and clients are highlighted through a discussion on the psychodynamics of this relationship and its potential impact on the therapeutic relationship. The chapter presents a care formulation exercise that illustrates how this tool can be used to incorporate the relevant clinical data into an overall assessment and plan of care.

Chapter 15 provides guidance on culturally sensitive pain management practice. The chapter discusses historical concepts of pain management among cultural groups, along with differences in how various cultural groups experience and express pain. Concepts of pain threshold, tolerance, catastrophizing, and stoicism, along with differences in affective response to pain are highlighted. Also explored are factors that affect access to pain care. Culturally sensitive, patient-centred approaches to the assessment and management of pain are discussed.

Chapter 16 explores social and structural determinants of health and health inequities. The chapter focuses on people of African descent living in Nova Scotia, for two reasons: 1) to make visible a distinct population in Canada and 2) to illustrate the impact of historical legacies of racism and discrimination and their ongoing impact on the health of individuals and communities. This understanding can be applied to other communities. The chapter begins with an exploration of the history and development of public health. It describes how public health evolved from a focus on individual health to population health with an emphasis on social and structural determinants of health using a social justice framework. The chapter provides examples of health promotion efforts to address health inequities at an individual, community, and societal level. It explores how COVID-19 has affected specific populations in Canada and exacerbated health inequities and highlights the need to improve racialized data collection and health indicators.

CHAPTER 12

Cultural Considerations at the Beginning of Life (The Perinatal Period)

Melba Sheila D'Souza and Paige Leslie

LEARNING OBJECTIVES

Upon completion of the chapter, the learner will be able to:

- Assess the sociocultural factors and social determinants of health of birthing people that influence pregnancy and child-bearing
- Examine the sociocultural influences and environmental-health factors that affect prenatal health and well-being of pregnant persons and their babies
- Describe culturally safe communication and the decision-making process between patients, families, and health care providers to enhance childbirth experiences
- Examine ways of knowing and ways of being that positively support the parent in the postpartum period based on individual needs and expectations
- Integrate cultural values and cultural practices to enable equitable access to health care and wellness for diverse ethnic and racial populations

KEY TERMS

Birth evacuation	Doula	LGBTQ2
Birth plan	Family-centred prenatal	Non-binary
Black, Indigenous, or	and newborn care	Pregnant person
People of Colour (BIPOC)	Female genital cutting	Transgender men
Clitoridectomy	Gender identity	
Cultural safety	Infibulation	

Pregnancy and childbirth are major life events for new parents, their families, and communities. Parenting and childbirth acquire a special significance for a person who is expecting a baby. A **pregnant person** (birthing person) experiences physiological, psychological, and social changes influenced by their emotional makeup and sociocultural background. During pregnancy, one can experience ambivalent feelings, introversion, acceptance, mood swings, and body image changes. These biological experiences also have interpersonal, spiritual, economic, and cultural meaning and implications for the entire family.

Equitable access to health care is crucial in this stage of life. Health care providers need to know these concepts and factors to provide respectful and safe care. Family-centred prenatal and newborn care aims for informed decision making by promoting awareness of culture's influence on unique needs and expectations during pregnancy. Interpretation of how the culture of health care is experienced must also be considered. Health care providers need to assess each situation individually to provide family-centred prenatal, intrapartum, and newborn care (Public Health Agency of Canada, 2020).

This chapter discusses the influence of cultural identity as families experience pregnancy and birth. It is recognized that health care providers reflect a range of disciplines, specialties, and collaboration for perinatal care that vary by province and within the practice context. This chapter is meant to serve as a guide, and a starting point, to understand sociocultural issues to improve patients' health and well-being and to enable discourse around concepts and outcomes of care during the perinatal period (the beginning of life). Traditionally, the childbirthing process was predominantly a feminine (women's) experience and a calling to motherhood, but we also acknowledge increasing supports for and recognition of gender diversity, sexual orientation, and the limitations of cisgender language. The terms *pregnant* and *birthing person* are meant to include women and persons who bear children but do not identify as women. This chapter provides gender-inclusive terminology and a focused discussion of sexual and gender diversity.

The aim of this chapter is to enhance cultural competency and safety of health care providers in caring for individuals and families experiencing pregnancy and childbirth. This chapter highlights ethical, cultural, and decision-making processes within a contextual approach to culturally responsive care. The chapter explores how social determinants of health, cultural traditions, ethnicity, race, sexual orientation, and gender identity impact the dynamic perinatal experience. We explore the three stages of the perinatal period: pregnancy (prenatal stage), childbirth (intranatal or labour), and the postpartum (postnatal) stages, and how each of these stages might be influenced by dynamic forces of culture. We acknowledge there are different definitions of the perinatal period; in this chapter, we adopt Garcia and Yim's (2017) definition of the perinatal period as pregnancy and the first year postpartum.

Changes in Population Demographic Trends

Parenthood and childbirth are empathetic experiences that impact family functioning, cultural identity, and cohesiveness, especially for people with diverse ethnic, racial, and cultural backgrounds. The way North American culture approaches child-bearing is undergoing a paradigm shift. From the 1800s to the mid-1900s, prenatal care in Canada typically took place in the local community, births occurred in the home with families, and midwives routinely provided care. The medicalization of childbirth in the later part of the twentieth century moved birth into hospitals and under the care of physicians. It viewed the birthing body as a machine. It created a risk- or fear-based approach to perinatal services rather than regarding childbirth as a normal physiological phenomenon (Vanier Institute of the Family, 2017).

The national Caesarean birth rate can serve as an example of the impact that medicalization of childbirth has on birthing Canadians. The World Health Organization (WHO) considers the ideal Caesarean birth rate to be 10–15% for all to be medically justifiable (WHO, 2015); however, in Canada, Caesarean births have increased from 17.6% in 1995–1996 to 29.4% in 2018 (Canadian Institute for Health Information [CIHI], 2020). Seeking further options for their birthing experience, Canadians are choosing to receive prenatal care through registered midwives and give birth at home rather than in the hospital. From 2016 to 2017, 10.8% of births in Canada were done by registered midwives. Registered midwives care for low-risk, healthy patients and work collaboratively with obstetricians and other health practitioners as needed. The midwifery profession was legalized in 1994 and has increasingly grown across Canada as a holistic approach to perinatal care, promoting the patient as the primary decision maker (Canadian Association of Midwives, 2021). Within Canada, growing recognition of midwives' role has corresponded with improved satisfaction with the pregnancy, birth, and post-birth stages (Ekström & Thorstensson, 2015; Okeke et al., 2016).

Interprofessional Collaborative Practice

In Canada, health care is generally an interprofessional collaborative practice. Care and special considerations during the perinatal period are no exception. Health care providers (regulated and licensed) who care for pregnant patients include family doctors, obstetricians, and registered midwives. Patients may also receive care from complementary and alternative care providers. While these health care providers may vary in competencies, standards, evidence-informed practice, and practice regulation, it is important to recognize the positive value they may have for patients. For example, chiropractors may provide services that include prenatal adjustments for back relief; naturopathic doctors may use traditional Chinese medicine, such as acupuncture, to assist with alternative forms of fertility treatment; registered dietitians can assist patients in achieving a healthy balanced diet; and registered massage therapists can provide hands-on relief for pregnancy discomfort (Curnow & Geraghty, 2019). Limited research on the effectiveness of some of these complementary and alternative care practices places responsibility on consumers to exercise extreme caution when utilizing these services and discuss the options with their primary health care provider.

Historically and across many cultures, birthing people's support network included a **doula**, a trained health care worker who provides continuous physical and emotional support to a patient before, during, and after birth. More recently, the doula profession has re-emerged as a part of the modern interdisciplinary perinatal team. In Canada, doulas serve as a source of information while providing labour and postpartum support. With the medicalization of childbirth, their role has expanded to include serving as an advocate for the patient within the health care system. One study shows that doulas improve patient satisfaction and decrease medical interventions, such as Caesarean births (Bohren et al., 2017).

These complementary perinatal health services provide additional physical support for patients, but access is often limited to those with higher socioeconomic status. Pregnant people may not seek out these services, as such care and advice were traditionally provided by family or community members, and the practitioner support may not be understood (Khanlou et al., 2017). Additionally, they might not access these services because of financial barriers. Knowing about local accessible complementary perinatal programs is imperative to family-centred care. This involves recognizing barriers that patients may face when accessing these services and creating a personalized plan for facilitating access. All health care providers can dismantle the medicalization of childbirth and promote culturally safe and family-centred prenatal and newborn care by acknowledging the barriers to care and respecting individual preferences their patients have for their child-bearing experience.

Sociocultural Diversity and Inclusive Practice

Cultural competence and cultural safety are important aspects for ensuring culturally appropriate care in a multicultural and multilingual society (for definitions and discussions see Chapter 1). The diversity of Canadian society is reflected in statistics that show more than one in five Canadians (21.9%) are foreign-born (Statistics Canada, 2016), and this may bring a desire for traditional healing practices. As well, according to the 2016 census, Indigenous people (including First Nations, Métis, and Inuk [Inuit]) accounted for 4.9% of Canadians (Statistics Canada, 2016). This population is relatively young compared to the non-Indigenous population (Statistics Canada, 2016), and many Indigenous people often seek culturally appropriate safe care as they reclaim their traditional practices. The traditional healing practices of newcomers and Indigenous people should be supported unless evaluated as harmful to the pregnancy or newborn outcome. Although practices may not directly contribute to physical health, they might be important factors for psychological and emotional well-being. Even when cultural practices are regarded as harmful, sensitivity and understanding are needed when discussing and providing care to patients who practise them. Understanding prenatal care from the birthing family's perspective is essential to understanding their social and health needs and expectations, to improve perinatal care, health care access, and quality of care.

When caring for immigrants, health care providers need to engage in a two-way dialogue and remain open to different ways of knowing and doing, communicating in a value-free and respectful tone, and tailoring care to the immigrant cultural context of the pregnant person and family (Merry et al., 2020). Immigrant status and rural residence are risk factors for poor pregnancy outcomes, and health care providers must be sensitive to patients' sociocultural context and needs (Khanlou et al., 2017). Birthing people may contrast their expectations and experiences between their country of origin and what they encounter in Canada. In an ethnographic study of North African birthing people in one Canadian city, differences in social support and the physical environment (both natural and built) between "back home" and "here" were commonly described in terms of opportunities to eat healthily, be physically active, and be emotionally well during their perinatal experience (Quintanilha et al., 2016). Overall, participants reported that, in Canada, they lacked the social and environmental factors perceived as critical enablers of healthy pregnancies and postpartum. It is essential to provide these patients with the sociocultural and environmental support they need in order to thrive during pregnancy and postpartum, especially while helping establish social and support networks "here" (Jessri et al., 2013; Joseph et al., 2019; Quintanilha et al., 2016). Health care providers play an important role in helping families understand and navigate the local health care system, while inquiring about and providing culturally appropriate care. Critical consciousness, listening, respecting preferences, recognizing differences, and supporting appropriate choices make health care providers accountable for nurturing, advocating, and caring for a person in the perinatal period.

According to 2016 census data, 22% of Canadians have a first language other than English, French, an Indigenous language, or American sign language (Brosseau & Dewing, 2018). In Canada, English is the predominant language of care (except in the province of Quebec). Individuals whose preferred language of care and communication is not English are likely to experience compromised communication with health providers, even if they have some English language proficiency. Key strategies to address this challenge include using printed or audiovisual translated materials, and using family members as interpreters. However, this can be problematic as translated materials are limited to a predetermined set of information, and interpreters may also be limited by their ability to convey the information precisely. Although partners and children in an immigrant family are often the first to acquire the local language, having them interpret in prenatal care is often inappropriate. Communication challenges and strategies for linguistically appropriate care are further discussed in Chapter 5.

History, Power, and Privilege

Many families face multiple barriers to optimal health and pregnancy outcomes related to social determinants of health, such as poverty, food insecurity, unsafe neighbourhoods, lack of access to education, and inadequate social support (Bethune et al., 2019). People who identify as **Black, Indigenous, or People of Colour (BIPOC)** are more susceptible to disadvantage based on social factors. Health care providers can identify the factors that are modifiable and encourage healthy public policy that provides an adequate social safety net. The term *BIPOC* gained popularity in 2019–2020 to acknowledge the violence and discrimination experienced by Black and Indigenous people in particular. While the term aspires to be inclusive, the reference to people of colour is controversial; it blends several groups into one and fails to recognize and name people and their experiences.

RACE, COLONIALISM, AND EQUITY-ORIENTED HEALTH CARE

Indigenous People

Key factors that affect Indigenous prenatal women include limited health care resources, health care services that do not consider socioeconomic and lifestyle barriers, and the impact of colonization on the relationship between health care providers and Indigenous women (Kolahdooz et al., 2016). Many Indigenous patients and those who are living in rural or remote areas of the country face unique challenges because of factors such as extended distances from medical facilities and specialized equipment; a limited number of practitioners and physicians available for on-call services; and fewer Caesarean birth and anaesthesia capabilities or services compared with services available in urban centres (Riddell et al., 2016; Winquist et al., 2016). Rural obstetrical care is provided by teams of family physicians, nurses, and registered midwives, and in some communities they are the only health care providing prenatal care. Given the limited availability of perinatal care providers and services in rural and remote regions, many pregnant people must travel to urban centres to give birth. However, several birthing centres have opened in Puvirnituq (Nunavik), Rankin Inlet (Nunavut), and Inukjuvak (Quebec) to fill the gap in health care service delivery in the Canadian North (National Indigenous Council of Midwives [NACM], 2014).

In British Columbia, the infant mortality rate for Indigenous babies is more than double that for non-Indigenous babies: 13.8 versus 6.1 deaths per 1 000 live births in rural areas, and 12.7 versus 6.1 deaths per 1 000 births in urban areas (Richmond & Cook, 2016). The lower health outcomes for Indigenous people can be attributed to colonial and postcolonial policies that have undermined Indigenous cultures, led to intergenerational trauma, and promoted Westernized medical approaches to health care and birthing (Anderson et al., 2016; Riddell et al., 2016). "In addition, these policies have compromised access to care due to geography, anti-Indigenous racism, as well as challenges associated with income, housing, and food insecurity" (Leason, 2018, p. 5). The colonization of birth and mandatory birth travel for Indigenous pregnant people (**birth evacuation**) is an "invisible" policy. The federal policy prioritizes privileged Western biomedicine in the obstetrical management of pregnant bodies. This policy serves to create a reliance on federal (off-reserve) obstetrical resources to ensure Indigenous pregnant people living on a reserve have access to intrapartum care, while devaluing traditional birthing practices and midwifery (Cidro et al., 2020). As a result, Indigenous pregnant people are forced to travel to urban areas to access intrapartum care, and they experience labour, delivery, and recovery (immediately postpartum) typically in isolation away from their families and communities. To address this, the Society of Obstetricians and Gynecologists of Canada (SOGC) policy statement affirms the belief that rural or remote low-risk Indigenous births should take place in their home communities (SOGC, 2010).

Health care inequities are ingrained in geographic distribution of and proximal access to birthing services and practitioners for Indigenous people (Smylie et al., 2021). Using data from a national population-based survey, Smylie et., al (2021) noted that mothers with Indigenous identity were more likely to travel 200 kilometres (124.3 miles) or more for birth than non-Indigenous mothers (9.8% vs. 2%), particularly in rural regions. This likelihood was independent of medical complications of pregnancy and birth complications (Smylie et al., 2021). Indigenous mothers were more likely to have experienced stressful events during pregnancy in rural areas than were non-Indigenous Canadian-born mothers (Smylie et al., 2016, 2021). For many Indigenous people, a positive experience from first entering the clinic or hospital is critical to feeling comfortable, welcomed, and safe. Therefore, taking time to build rapport and effective relationships with Indigenous families is an important aspect of providing culturally appropriate safe care. Birthing centres, midwifery, access to doulas, and full access to prenatal services are necessary for creating positive traditional birthing practices closer to home and in the hands of Indigenous midwives and birth helpers, which enhances Indigenous perinatal experiences. Indigenous midwifery integrates traditional knowledge, brings Indigenous birth back to the communities, and dismantles symbolic oppression (NACM, 2016). Indigenous midwives have been successful in lobbying for community-based health care (Vanier Institute of the Family, 2017).

Indigenous midwives are essential for culturally safe and relevant health care in any geographic area. They reduce birth evacuations from remote communities, keep families together during the birthing process, improve health outcomes, and increase patient agency and self-determination in health care (Vanier Institue of the Family, 2017). Indigenous midwives view their roles as caretakers of their patients. They recognize their traditional role in the community as both nation builders and "aunties" who take time to provide quality culturally grounded care, which includes relationship building and knowledge sharing. With this culturally relevant background, Indigenous midwives are able to better understand the diversity of traditional healing practices and individualistic preferences that exists between various Indigenous communities and can serve as an example to other health care providers on individualizing the experience between patients when working with Indigenous people (Tabobondung, 2014). Bringing birth back to Indigenous communities through trained Indigenous midwives knowledgeable in traditional birth customs can address the cultural and health gap elicited by forced birth evacuation and improve the access to health care services (WHO & UNICEF, 2020). Indigenous midwifery in remote and northern communities in Canada can provide better continuity of care, improve access to antenatal assessments, and promote traditional birth customs (NACM, 2016). In addition, the calls to action from the Truth and Reconciliation Commission (TRC, 2015) emphasize greater accessibility to health care services, integrating Indigenous healing practices and practitioners in models of care, and cultural birth practices in various health care settings (Amundsen & Kent-Wilkinson, 2020).

Cultural competence and cultural safety are essential concepts in the care of Indigenous people. Cultural safety is built on the understanding that "culture" is neither static nor superficial. Instead, it is fluid, dynamic, complex, and sociopolitical—culture is integral to social structuring, knowledge systems, and relationships. "**Cultural safety** is both a process and an outcome, and the only person who can define the care as culturally safe is the person receiving care" (Churchill et al., 2020, p. 4). It is essential to recognize that cultural safety may mean different things to different groups. Churchill et al. (2020) conducted a qualitative study on cultural safety in midwifery practice and noted that cultural safety is described both similarly and differently by patients who are Indigenous, Black, or of White European descent. They note that patients who reflected White European ethnicity conceptualized cultural safety in ways that were similar to core principles of the Ontario midwifery model of care (i.e., informed choice, continuity of care, and choice of birthplace, etc.). However, the concept of patient-centred care and getting to know the individual "may not foster cultural safety for Indigenous and racialized patients who understand relationships, knowledge, and space as interconnected manifestations of family, kinship-based societies" (Churchill et al., 2020, p. 10). Health care providers must understand their own view of cultural safety and also recognize what is essential for the patient. The unique needs of Indigenous women and considerations for emergency transport during prenatal care should be integrated where health services are delivered (Turpel-Lafond, 2020).

Cultural Considerations In Care

Cultural Safety in Indigenous Prenatal Care

In a recent study, Indigenous participants conceptualized cultural safety to highlight the survival and resurgence of Indigenous values, understandings, and approaches in cities like Toronto, and affirm the need for Indigenous midwives (Churchill et al., 2020). Three cultural safety domains emerged from the analysis: relationships and communication, sharing knowledge and practice, and culturally safe spaces. One participant noted: "We could smudge when I was in labour, and giving my daughter a cedar bath when she was born meant a lot to me. I am happy to be giving my children that because I understand it more, and I know a little more about my culture. They can pass it on" (First Nations participant, p. 7).

ACCESS TO HEALTH CARE AND TRADITIONAL PRACTICES

All people need to be empowered decision makers in their pregnancies. They need safe linguistic care (Bowen, 2015) and culturally appropriate care, along with support from their families, community members, and health care providers. COVID-19 has disproportionately impacted Indigenous communities along with other ethnic and racial minorities (Subedi et al., 2020). For many Indigenous people, the pandemic experience can retraumatize them because of their previous experiences that reflected racism and discrimination in the health care system, such as stereotyping, unacceptable interactions, and historically poor quality of care (Turpel-Lafond, 2020). Moreover, restrictions to prevent the transmission of COVID-19 have further limited Indigenous people's access to health services and cultural supports (Power et al., 2020). It is vital to identify ways to mitigate the pandemic's adverse impacts. These include healing centres like the sweat lodge, smudging, healing circles, support for sacred ceremonies, and family gatherings (Turpel-Lafond, 2020). The prenatal person needs support to be accompanied for medical visits during the COVID-19 pandemic. Such actions can help to create a culturally safe environment where Indigenous families feel respected and not discriminated against. It is critical for health care providers to support Indigenous families who are at risk of encountering racist behaviours, policies, and practices in prenatal care, and to ensure culturally safe care (Fig. 12.1).

RACE, INTERSECTIONALITY, AND SOCIAL JUSTICE

Black People

Mortality rates of birthing people can reveal disparities in perinatal care access, treatment, and outcomes when examined with a racial lens. Since Canada does not track data by race, we look to American research to learn about racism in the birthing experience that can be extended to the Canadian birthing experience. Racial and ethnic disparities in pregnancy-related mortality (PRM) were evident in 2007 and continued through 2016, with significantly higher PRM rates

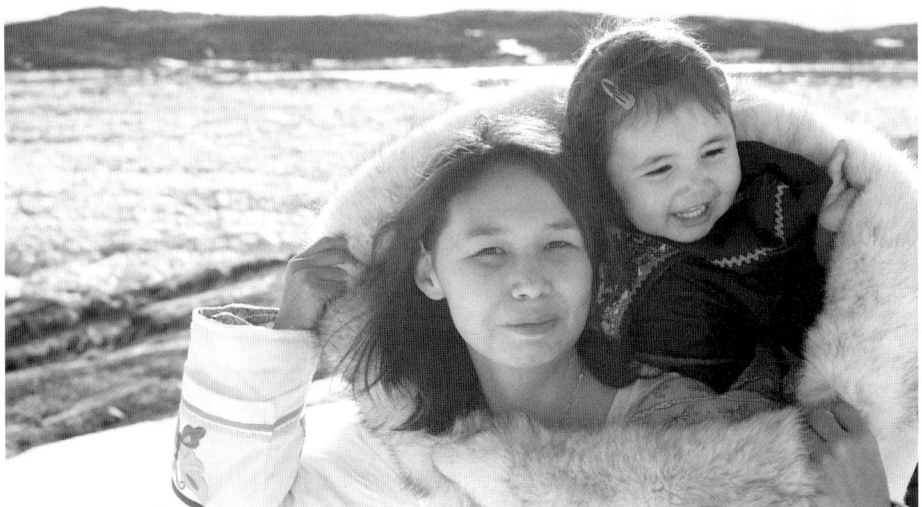

Fig. 12.1 An Inuit child being carried in the traditional way. (Courtesy iStock.com/RyersonClark.)

among Black and American Indian/Alaska Native women than among White, Asian, Pacific Islander, and Hispanic women (Petersen et al., 2019). In some studies, Black women have been shown to have more than five times the risk of dying in pregnancy or up to 6 weeks postpartum compared with White women (Knight, 2019; Petersen et al., 2019; Royal College of Obstetricians and Gynaecologists, 2020). The reasons for the disparity are varied and complex. Cardiomyopathy, thrombotic pulmonary embolism, and hypertensive disorders of pregnancy contributed to more PRM among Black women than among White women (Centers for Disease Control and Prevention [CDC], 2019). While poor access to care and other social determinants may be a contributing factor, a study in New York found that Black post-secondary–educated patients birthing at local hospitals were more likely to experience severe pregnancy or childbirth complications than White patients who never graduated from high school (Martin & Montagne, 2017). The data suggest that even social determinants of health such as education and income do not serve as protective factors for Black people (Johnson et al., 2015; Martin & Montagne, 2017).

Recently, stories of Black birthing people dying from preventable causes have come to the forefront of the media, highlighting health care racism (American Heart Association [AHA], 2019; National Partnership for Women and Families, 2018; Roeder, 2019). The stories reveal experiences of being marginalized. As the AHA (2019) reports, "Basically, Black women are undervalued. They are not monitored as carefully as White women are. When they do present with symptoms, they are often dismissed." This is highlighted by the postpartum experience of tennis star Serena Williams, who experienced a pulmonary embolism postpartum and had to advocate for herself over dismissive explanations of her symptoms. While Serena Williams had a positive outcome, others are not so fortunate, and the families are left with a devastating loss (Roeder, 2019). The common narrative in these stories is the differential treatment attributed to factors such as communication gaps, in which crucial details about a patient's medical history are not passed on or attended to; patient concerns being dismissed outright; superficial or delayed actions being taken by the health care provider(s) (AHA, 2019; Roeder, 2019); and women being discharged without adequate information on potential risks (Roeder, 2019). Stories from high-profile women such as tennis stars indicate that social advantage in access, income, and education is not sufficient to protect against the risk of PRM, leading to the conclusion that "racism is an undeniable thread running through the stories of Black mothers who die" (Roeder, 2019).

Cultural Competence In Action

Responding to Culturally Competent Care

Malika Selassie, a Black woman, was 36 years old when she had her hospital birth in Mississauga, Ontario. Malika and her family doctor knew her pregnancy was high risk. She was on prescribed medications for clotting disorders and had a history of high blood pressure. Malika was discharged after the Caesarean birth without any instructions on what symptoms to watch for, given her previous history. After she returned home, her health quickly deteriorated. For the next 4 weeks, she visited her primary care providers for a painful hematoma, draining abscess in her Caesarean incision, spiking blood pressure, continuous headaches, blurred vision, swelling legs, and rapid weight gain. Her husband took her to these appointments. Malika was assured that the symptoms were typical, and she just needed time to heal. In the fourth week, when Malika took her medications, she collapsed and died at home before reaching the emergency room.

The child-bearing experience of Black people is a teachable moment regarding racial bias and ethnic disparities. Consider factors that contributed to health care providers not recognizing the history and risk factors for Malika (clotting disorder and high blood pressure) and not taking Malika's concerns seriously enough to warrant immediate intervention for postpartum pre-eclampsia What would have changed the outcomes for Malika and her newborn baby, considering the barriers and facilitators for Black patients?

Black patients are also at increased risk of bias in pain assessment and management. A study by Hoffman et al. (2016) showed that false beliefs about biological differences between Black and White people (e.g., Black people have thicker skin than White people, or Black people feel less pain than White people) were endorsed by 50% of the White medical students and residents, and these views led to less accurate treatment recommendations. The researchers note that these false beliefs "dating back to slavery," continue to lead to "inadequate treatment recommendations for Black patients' pain" (p. 4300).

The preceding discussion shows that racism and discrimination have a strong influence on the health and wellness of the Black community. Child-bearing experience can be a vulnerable moment in prenatal care for all birthing persons. Recognizing and attending to the risk factors, including those associated with unconscious bias and systemic factors, are critical attributes of cultural competence and cultural safety—without this we continue to run the risk of inequities in care that lead to devastating outcomes for individuals and families. Informed and patient-centred decision making needs to be at the forefront of care to improve prenatal care satisfaction across cultures and ensure equitable outcomes.

Immigrants and Refugees

Immigrant pregnant people face challenges adapting to both Canada's cultural context and a new climate, which may influence pregnancy choices. Immigrant patients' experiences may also be linked to "transnational ties" through their connections with their home country. Through an integrative review of the literature from the United States, Canada, Australia, New Zealand, and Europe, Merry et al. (2020) noted transnational ties in two ways: "ways of being" and "ways of belonging" that influence the child-bearing and parenthood experiences in a new country. "Ways of being" refers to actions that maintain refugees' and immigrants' own cultural identity and relationships with the family and culture back home. Staying connected to family and friends back home may increase feelings of loneliness in a new place, but can also be a source of support. "Ways of belonging" refers to maintenance of aspects of cultural identity (e.g., religious, cultural/ethnic, linguistic, and political) in the new country. The findings show that although health care providers are aware of, acknowledge, and address "ways of belonging" in different ways, "important gaps remain" (Merry et al., 2020, p. 19). In addition, they found little evidence that "ways of being" were acknowledged and addressed by health care providers. It is important to recognize the potential role of family back home in terms of the supports and advice they can provide and how that can be integrated into care in the new country (Merry et al., 2020).

Immigrants and refugees also face barriers to accessing health care services, which then increases their risk for poor health outcomes throughout the perinatal period (Khanlou et al., 2017). Some of the social and health concerns are related to accessing health care, seeking health information, receiving care in their language from a female health care provider, absence of extended family support, and preference for home births. Immigrants and refugees who have migrated to Canada contend with cultural expectations both within the Canadian context and their country of origin. The family is often also adjusting to a new country and contending with discrimination and issues of resettlement (Khanlou et al., 2017). Immigrant and refugee families may be less aware of the health care system, have limited social networks, and have precarious health status or limited access to or eligibility for services. There is a complex interaction of cultural, environmental, and interpersonal factors contributing to challenges during pregnancy and childbirth for immigrants and refugees. The influence of cultural and language differences and lack of economic resources greatly diminishes the ability of low-income immigrant patients to negotiate and seek access to the best possible care and treatment (Khanlou et al., 2017).

Financial concerns can be significant for refugee and immigrant patients who might not yet have access to work benefits, health insurance, and social disability. For patients without insurance, efforts must include access to appropriate health care services and seeking out health care providers such as registered midwives. Ontario midwives have funding for anyone with a permanent residence in their catchment area, regardless of health insurance. There is also funding for consultations and laboratory testing, but hospital stays are still an out-of-pocket expense. Patients eligible for a home birth can utilize a midwife and therefore avoid the costs of a hospital stay (Association of Ontario Midwives, 2021); however, possible medical and hospital fees may occur and should be discussed ahead of time. Such discussion could include appropriate arrangements made with the hospital administration for patients who are required to pay for out-of-pocket services. In other provinces such as British Columbia, refugee patients may be covered by the interim federal health program, and they do not have to pay for midwifery services (Midwives Association of British Columbia, 2021).

Cultural Considerations In Care

Reducing Economic and Financial Costs

Sara Maria Henriques is a new immigrant who recently arrived in Hamilton, Ontario from Portugal. She is 36 weeks pregnant and attending her antenatal appointment. She learns that she will likely need a Caesarean birth for breech presentation with an obstetrician in the area, but she does not have health insurance. In addition to the obstetrical fees, procedure costs, and the $10 000 deposit the hospital requires, Sara Maria has become overwhelmed attempting to navigate the Canadian health care system just weeks before her baby is expected to be born. Sara Maria's obstetrician is aware of funded midwifery services in Ontario that are available to residents, regardless of health coverage. Midwifery care would be free, along with available funding for consultations, lab work, and ultrasound investigations, but the hospital fees would still be required. The obstetrician was able to connect Sara Maria with a midwife, even at this late stage. In the end, Sara Maria did not need a Caesarean birth as the baby's position had shifted, and she was therefore able to give birth at home and avoid the hospital expenditures. In this scenario, Sara Maria was able to avoid costs because of the availability of funding for midwifery care.

Immigrant patients may also experience racism and discrimination. Research has documented disrespectful care of immigrants during childbirth (Morton et al., 2018). The disrespectful behaviours include engaging in procedures without giving a woman time or the option to consider them; engaging in procedures explicitly against the patient's wishes; verbal abuse in the form of threats to the baby's life unless the woman agrees to a procedure; and failure to provide informed consent (Morton et al., 2018). The researchers noted that reporting the witnessed disrespectful care was infrequent; however, maternity support workers (doulas and nurses) who witnessed the disrespect were more likely to leave obstetrical support work within 3 years (Morton et al., 2018). Such findings are alarming and raise concerns for patients as well as affect the workforce. Perinatal care must be approached with greater sensitivity and support. Health care providers witnessing racism and abuse can and must directly impact care by taking on the role of ally or advocate (see Chapter 4). Identifying and overcoming institutional barriers to caring for this vulnerable population is vital. Health care providers need to ensure that pregnancy and postpartum care are adapted and culturally safe for migrants by using linguistically and culturally adapted materials; reflecting on their own culture, beliefs, and attitudes about "others"; and recognizing and avoiding stereotypes (Merry et al., 2020). Engaging patients from diverse backgrounds in various aspects of care, including in determining priorities, developing and delivering programs, and participating on institutional committees, such as a diversity and equity task force on quality of care, can support the provision of culturally appropriate care.

Family-Centred Prenatal and Newborn Care

Family-centred prenatal (maternal) and newborn (neonatal) care involves respect for cultural differences between individuals, families, and communities, while following the essential principles of care (Health Canada, 2000). Such care encourages increasing participation of the pregnant person and their families in the decision-making process concerning their pregnancy, birth, and early postpartum experiences, to promote optimal health and well-being for the pregnant person and child (Institute for Patient-and Family-Centered Care [IPFC], 2017). Pregnant people who receive early and regular prenatal and newborn care generally have better prenatal and health outcomes. However, not everyone in Canada has equal access to prenatal care or receives care consistent with their needs, preferences, and expectations. Access to health care and health outcomes can be compromised by social determinants of health including geography, cost, or lack of cultural appropriateness (Andermann, 2016).

Immigrant and BIPOC birthing people in Canada are generally given the opportunity for necessary health care services, but they can face many barriers in accessing and utilizing these services. For some women (for example, of Muslim faith), there may be discomfort in attending prenatal classes and participating in activities of a personal nature with men they don't know (Alzghoul et al., 2021). Personal and organizational barriers can also limit access to and adequacy and acceptability of health care for many immigrants (Higginbottom et al., 2016). Lack of understanding of the informed consent process, lack of respect for privacy and confidential information, short consultation times, immediate discharge from the hospital after birth, discrimination and stereotyping, cultural shock, and divergence in food choices and nutrition are some of the factors that lead to a negative perception of what should be quality prenatal care (Higginbottom et al., 2016).

INTERCULTURAL COMMUNICATION AND RELATIONSHIP

Good communication and trusting relationships are critical elements of quality health care. However, communication between health care providers and immigrant and refugee patients may be compromised by language, health literacy, and cultural differences (Mengesha et al., 2018). Canada's foreign-born population is projected to increase to 30% by 2036 (Statistics Canada, 2017) and linguistic diversity is also increasing (Statistics Canada, 2017). About one in five females have a first language other than English on their linguistic profile (Statistics Canada, 2017). Immigrant families with limited English proficiency struggle with the prenatal education topics' perceived relevance, as well as the health care provider's accent, terminology, jargon, and communication speed. Immigrant families do not feel comfortable asking questions because they feel intimidated and do not wish to challenge health care providers (Higginbottom et al., 2016). Health care providers need to ensure that they speak slowly, avoid using jargon, and verify if messages have been understood. While health care providers do not perceive themselves as having an accent, for many patients, the way of the provider's speaking, including the tone, terminology, and way of talking, may be new and unfamiliar and therefore difficult to understand. Health care providers may rely on written materials to support communication for informed decision making; however, such educational materials need to be in the patient's preferred language, if possible, and used to augment verbal communication—not replace it. Many patients may come from oral traditions and societies, and most families value interaction and an opportunity for engagement and clarification (Higginbottom et al., 2016).

As discussed earlier, BIPOC patients, and more specifically Black patients are more likely to experience racial injustices and health disparities when accessing care. The research of Vedam et al. (2019) explores the inequity and mistreatment of Black birthing people. Their findings highlight that Black patients are more likely to report mistreatment in obstetrics care than their White counterparts. In their study they found that effective communication improves the quality of care received by a Black patient. Such communication and informed choices can be achieved by listening to patient concerns, providing informed consent, and respecting patients' autonomy to make choices for their care, even if these decisions differ from those of the health care providers (Vedam et al., 2019).

Cultural Competence In Action

Compassionate Care and Having a Voice

Valerie Luther, a Black woman who was 5 months pregnant, was feeling uncomfortable and was at home when she started bleeding. She visited her doctor's clinic and waited a long time for her appointment in Thunder Bay, Northwestern Ontario. When the doctor checked Valerie, she said that the bleeding was normal and sent her home. At home, Valerie's buttocks started hurting. She took a warm bath and called her doctor. She was advised that it was constipation and was encouraged to have a bowel movement. Valerie experienced increased pain in her buttocks, and she could not sleep. She called the emergency unit and described her situation, but she did not receive immediate care. She visited the hospital early the next morning. Valerie had just enough energy to ask for painkillers and then lost consciousness. The baby was delivered via Caesarean birth but passed away. As Valerie and her husband were grappling with the loss of their baby, they had many questions about what happened, and wondered if anything could have been done earlier to save their baby. Sadly, they also received a comment as to why they did not recognize that she had been in labour and come in earlier. This blame, on top of the perceived mismanagement at the system level, led to feelings of anger, mistrust, and betrayal, at a time when they were struggling with profound grief at the loss of their child.

How would you support this family at this time of loss and grief? What factors potentially contributed to this outcome? What aspects of critical consciousness and compassionate care could have been taken earlier for a better and more positive care experience?

While we recognize that the comments of blame by a health care provider were inappropriate, unfortunately, such racism exists within the system. If you were to witness such a statement or sentiment, what would you do?

Implicit racial bias has been reported in the health care system and can affect patient–practitioner interactions, treatment decisions, adherence, and health outcomes (Hall et al., 2015). Important components of providing equitable health care include listening without being defensive, responding rapidly, empathizing, and collaborating with pregnant people after thoroughly understanding their concerns. Such actions can help to address racial disparities. Delivering culturally appropriate safe care requires knowledge of risk factors, along with enhanced communication and collaboration with the pregnant person and family as well as among health care providers throughout the perinatal period.

DIET AND NUTRITION

Diet is an essential aspect of monitoring the health and well-being of a pregnancy. A famous North American saying is that a pregnant person is "eating for two"; however, beliefs like this have led to excessive gestational weight gain, which carries an increased risk for Caesarean delivery, gestational hypertension, and gestational diabetes (Maxwell et al., 2019). Therefore, health care providers must appropriately address their patients' nutritional needs and discuss the importance of pregnancy diet for optimal outcomes. A cultural lens should also be considered, as many patients have beliefs and traditions regarding nutrition.

Across cultures, diet is adjusted in pregnancy to support positive and desired outcomes for the mother and baby (Higginbottom et al., 2018). For example, a sample of Chinese immigrant mothers described foods like eggs, soup, fish, nuts, and black sesame as associated with light-coloured flawless skin, brain development, and thick black hair—all desired attributes in the baby (Higginbottom et al., 2018). At the same time, women changed their diet to include milk and milk products based on the advice of their doctor (Higginbottom et al., 2018). Thus it is important to recognize that cultural considerations of food preferences are important, and it is also important to share recommendations based on practitioner knowledge.

Many cultures (e.g., Asian, Latin American, African) hold traditional beliefs about hot–cold properties of certain foods and conditions (Chakrabarti & Chakrabarti, 2019; Higginbottom et al., 2018; Lim & van Dam, 2020). Foods are considered either hot or cold on the basis of their humoral properties associated with traditional healing systems such as traditional Chinese medicine or Ayurvedic medicine, irrespective of the food's temperature. Pregnancy is often considered a "hot" condition; therefore, consumption of foods that are too "hot" are to be avoided prenatally but may be preferred after the birth of the baby. Other factors that influence dietary choices include social support and advice, as well as increased access to less nutritional convenience foods and lack of time for more traditional cooking (Higginbottom et al., 2018). A culturally safe approach to diet in pregnancy includes asking the patient to record a food journal and reviewing their diet to ensure pregnancy demands are met. Additionally, patients may benefit from referral to a registered dietictian, especially those who are experiencing food insecurity or are of a lower socioeconomic status. The diet of "traditional foods" or "special foods" should be encouraged among Indigenous and other populations. These foods have been shown to improve diet quality and are linked to Indigenous people's cultural identity (Health Canada, 2019).

PHYSICAL ACTIVITY AND EXERCISE

Pregnancy is often viewed in different ways in relation to physical activity. There may be a belief that pregnancy requires rest and that exercise and strenuous activity may damage the mother or baby (Greenhalgh et al., 2015). Other cultures may stress that too much rest is associated with laziness, creating labour problems (Watson et al., 2019). Pregnant people may receive advice from family, friends, and relatives that is trusted more than the advice from health care providers. Some patients may not be able to alter physical activity because of their work–life demands and individual needs. Health care providers should counsel patients on evidence-informed approaches to physical activity in the perinatal period while considering cultural differences. The SOGC recommends moderate-intensity exercise of 150 minutes a week for those without contraindications, to reduce rates of complications such as gestational diabetes, gestational hypertension, and Caesarean birth (Mottola et al., 2018).

EMOTIONAL AND MENTAL HEALTH

In a study of psychosocial stress, Robinson et al. (2016) found that participants who identified as ethnic minorities experienced more significant psychosocial stress than participants who identified as White. Ethnic identity was based on self-identification, and most pregnant people in this group were immigrants or first-generation Canadians. Those who identified as an ethnic minority were more likely to report inadequate social support, depressive symptoms, and poor emotional health and perceive their life as being more stressful. Other studies have also noted that migrant participants have a greater likelihood of prenatal depression, which may often be expressed as somatic symptoms (Khanlou et al., 2017). It is vital that culturally sensitive mental health screening and care be a component of prenatal care.

In some Asian cultures, the preference for a male child over a female may be significant and may influence how the baby is welcomed into the family, and whether the birthing person is supported or not (Mucina, 2018; Srinivasan, 2018). The complexity of the issue is beyond the scope of this chapter. (For further discussion, see Almond et al., 2013; Mucina, 2018; Qadir et al., 2011;

Srinivasan, 2018.) It is crucial that practitioners be sensitive to such dynamics, recognize how they may impact maternal mental and emotional health, and create a safe, nonjudgemental space for dialogue as needed.

A CULTURALLY SAFE AND SENSITIVE BIRTH PLAN

A **birth plan** outlines labour and birth preferences of a pregnant patient and their support people and is a good strategy to help prepare patients for birth. Recognizing that the birth experience can be unpredictable, it is crucial for health care providers to carefully walk through what the course of labour may look like for the patient, including routine practices and reasons for possible interventions. This also becomes an ideal opportunity to elicit cultural needs and traditions for the intra- and postpartum periods. Table 12.1 outlines some questions that aid in creating a culturally safe and responsive birth plan. An individual participatory approach to developing a culturally safe and sensitive birth plan provides an opportunity to have open dialogue. For example, for families who prefer female health care providers, it is crucial to have a respectful conversation regarding the possibility that this might not be possible during labour. The health care provider can ask if there are there ways in which it would be acceptable to have a male physician, together with a female nurse or midwife.

Lesbian, Gay, Bisexual, Transgender, Queer, Two-Spirit Communities

LGBTQ2 is the official acronym recognized by the Government of Canada's LGBTQ2 Secretariat and stands for Lesbian, Gay, Bisexual, Queer, and Two-Spirit (Government of Canada, 2020). Another acronym often used internationally is LGBTI (Lesbian, Gay, Bisexual, Transgender, Intersex) (Government of Canada, 2020). LGBTQ2 people can face discrimination, erasure, and stigma throughout the perinatal period (see Chapter 10). In countries such as Australia, Canada, New Zealand, the United States, and the United Kingdom, childbearing is typically a heteronormative and cisgender female experience. However, a growing number of individuals are embracing the fluidity and diversity of sexuality and **gender identity**, which is how an individual defines their gender. Many LGBTQ2 partners seek to have children and have faced numerous barriers to culturally competent care. Health care providers

---

TABLE 12.1 ■ Interview Guide for a Culturally Safe and Sensitive Birth Plan

1. Who will support and advise you during the prenatal, labour, and postpartum periods?
2. What religious or cultural traditions are essential for you during the birth and postpartum periods?
3. What is your gender preference for health care providers? If unable to achieve this, what can we do to create a positive and safe experience?
4. What terms or issues would you prefer your care team to use or avoid, such as disclosing the assigned sex of the fetus or baby's gender?
5. How would you like health care providers to refer to your labour pains?
6. What kind of specific pain relief options would you like to incorporate into your birth plan?
7. What safe birthing positions would you prefer while going into labour and delivery?
8. What personal preferences do you have for immediate contact with the baby?
9. Would you like access to your placenta for personal or cultural practices?
10. What are your priorities and your expectations from your health care providers regarding safety for you and for your baby?
11. What are your previous experiences with planned parenthood or the perinatal period (if any)?
12. What traditional health information or medicines are helpful for you at this time?

can validate LGBTQ2 families at various stages of the perinatal process. In this section on LGBTQ2 child-bearing families, pregnant non-binary people and transgender males will be highlighted, as they face a large amount of systemic inequity, erasure, and transphobia within the perinatal experience (Hoffkling et al., 2017). **Non-binary** refers to individuals whose gender identity does not fall under the binary of male or female (The Center, 2021). Transgender people's gender identity typically differs from the gender they were assigned at birth, based on their genitalia. For instance, **transgender men** were assigned female at birth and identify as male Identifying as transgender is not dependent on medical procedures or alterations to one's physical appearance (The Center, 2021). (Also see Chapter 10.)

Health care providers can cause discomfort by using binary terminology for anatomical features. Asking and documenting the patient's preferred name, pronouns, and language of anatomical structures is a way to affirm their gender identity and prevent administrative discrimination. Inclusive intake papers and clinic environments also serve to normalize the LGBTQ2 child-bearing experience. Transgender men often face social isolation, physical and emotional vulnerability, and fear of the medical system (Besse et al., 2020a). A trans-competent health care provider can help normalize their experience and plan with their patients in ways to best meet their needs to reduce discrimination in the health care system. Trans-competent care can also include discussing invasive procedures ahead of time. (Also see Chapter 10.) There are currently several avenues available for conception with assisted reproductive technology and fertility preservation mechanisms.

Trans-masculine and non-binary people face overt and systemic obstacles in the experience of child-bearing and in how they navigate a feminine-oriented system (Besse et al., 2020a, b; Hoffkling et al., 2017; Riggs et al., 2020). Fears of being misgendered when visibly pregnant and of inadequate health care provider education regarding LGBTQ2 issues can cause discomfort and dysphoric feelings (Besse et al., 2020a).

Cultural Consideration In Care

A Transgender Male's Child-bearing Experience

Matthew and his partner Neil are expecting their first child. They live in Steinbach, Manitoba. Matthew is worried about the care he will receive as a trans-male. At their first antenatal appointment, Matthew and Neil feel accepted as they enter the clinic when they see posters of lesbian, gay, bisexual, transgender, queer, and two-spirit (LGBTQ2) families. During the initial visit, their midwife asks them about their preferred pronouns and who is the gestational carrier. During Matthew's physical, his midwife asks his preferred terminology for his chest and pelvic body parts and how she can make examinations more comfortable for him. Matthew feels included in prenatal care by seeing LGBTQ2 representation in the clinical setting and how his midwife did not make assumptions regarding his gender identity.

Not making assumptions and increasing representation are important steps in promoting inclusive and culturally safe care for patients of various backgrounds and identities within the LGBTQ2 community. Each transgender and non-binary birthing experience will be unique. It is imperative that the care team create a care plan founded in respect and a willingness to learn the preferences of the patient, thus promoting quality and safe care. In one study, transmasculine people, non-binary people, and transgender men reported on emotional responses that were distressing after a pregnancy loss (Riggs et al., 2020). This study focused on the importance of asking about pronouns; advocating for system change ensuring that names, pronouns, and gender be correctly recorded; and ensuring that prenatal experiences following a pregnancy loss not add complexity to the potential grief experienced by men, transmasculine people, and non-binary people and their partners (Riggs et al., 2020).

Family-Centred Birthing

Canadians have the option to give birth in the hospital, at home, or in a birthing centre depending on where they live. The choices are affected by many factors, including controlling the birth experience and birth attendant(s). The influence of culture on the intrapartum period can be seen in the childbirth support person(s), birth position, pain management, and traditions that may accompany the birthing process. Patients desire support and attentive care during labour and birth. Caregivers can convey emotional support by offering their continued presence and words of encouragement.

In contemporary Western medicine and society, pregnancy and childbirth are seen as a "couple's" experience. The partner of the birthing patient is expected to be the primary support person. However, in some cultures, the norm is to have women present, such as the mother, mother-in-law, or sister by birth or choice. Health care providers can support a genuine intercultural experience. Consultation and facilitation of a shared approach to patient experiences and birth support persons are crucial indicators of better outcomes. For example, traditionally, South Asian patients may be used to and prefer having their mother or mother-figure for support during childbirth; however, lack of family and social support and acculturation into Western culture might mean their partner is instead present during labour. Caregivers who are sensitive to the potential cultural unfamiliarity in the role of birth support person for the partner can significantly impact the well-being of both partners. For example, a Muslim patient in Canada described her positive experience with her husband, noting that the help she received from her husband led to greater closeness (Alzghoul et al., 2021). It is also essential to be supportive and nonjudgemental of partners who choose to remain outside the birthing room.

Cultural Competence In Action

Informed Choices of Expectant Couples

Mariam Hussain is in early labour with her first child in a rural health centre and is in midwifery care. During her labour assessment in the maternal unit, the midwife informs Mariam and her husband, Mohammed, that she needs to consult with an obstetrician, as Mariam's blood pressure has become abnormally high. The midwife further explains that the obstetrician on call today is male, and after discussion, Mariam and Mohammed request the midwife to transfer Mariam to a hospital where there is a female obstetrician. As birth is not imminent, the midwife calls the hospitals in the surrounding area and plans to transfer Mariam to another hospital, which has a female obstetrician and is located 54 kilometers (33.6 miles) away from her home.

Are there risks to quality and safety in the chosen option? What if the nearest hospital was 150 km (93.3 miles) away and the intrapartum complications happened later in the labour period? How could the care have been improved with a culturally informed birth plan?

Health care providers should review preferences prenatally with the patient. Information gathered should include situations such as place of birth and gender identity of the care team. They should also discuss realistic expectations based on the patient's clinical picture, supports, and navigation of resources available to them in the area. Such discussions need to anticipate potential scenarios with how the birth may unfold so that plans and decisions can be made ahead of time.

BIRTHING POSITION AND LABOUR PAIN

With the medicalization of childbirth, patients often labour and birth while lying in bed. This practice likely evolved out of convenience for the health care provider as it may provide easier monitoring and assistance for delivery. The supine position is in sharp contrast to those used in other cultures, where childbirth occurs with Rebozo bands, or in upright and squatting positions (Fig. 12.2). There may be cultural beliefs about specific foods and drinks and applying particular substances like squash leaves on a labouring woman's abdomen to encourage labour. The extent to which these can be accommodated will depend on the individual situation. However, it is important to acknowledge such preferences, adjust where possible, and provide an honest explanation if these practices cannot be supported. It is important to inquire about preferred birth position as the patient may be unsure about their options and hesitant or unable to advocate for themselves in the midst of a labour experience.

Pain during labour is a universal experience; the intensity of pain and pain expression may vary across individuals and cultures. While expression of pain is the norm in Western culture, other cultures (e.g., Japanese, Chinese, Korean, East Indian, Nepal, Burmese, Malaysian) may view outward expressions of pain as culturally inappropriate and patients may remain quiet and be at risk for inadequate pain management (Ricci, 2020). It is therefore important to do frequent pain assessments and encourage honest communication of pain in a nonjudgemental way. In addition, pregnant people with chronic pain may have additional needs, and without intentional attention their right to adequate pain management may be compromised (Mellin, 2017). Increased knowledge of pain by the health care provider is related to a more positive attitude toward pregnant patients with chronic pain and is correlated with an increased intent to medicate pregnant people (Mellin, 2017). Health care providers are in an ideal position to provide child-bearing patients with balanced, concise information about effective nonpharmacological and pharmacological measures to relieve pain and ensure a safe birthing process. Other cultural traditions during the birthing experience may include, for Indigenous people, to smudging or having cedar, sage, or tobacco in the birth suite (Churchill et al., 2020). In addition, music for relaxation or spiritual support, and rituals of cord-cutting or disposing of the placenta can be incorporated into the birthing experience (Sharma et al., 2016). Culturally

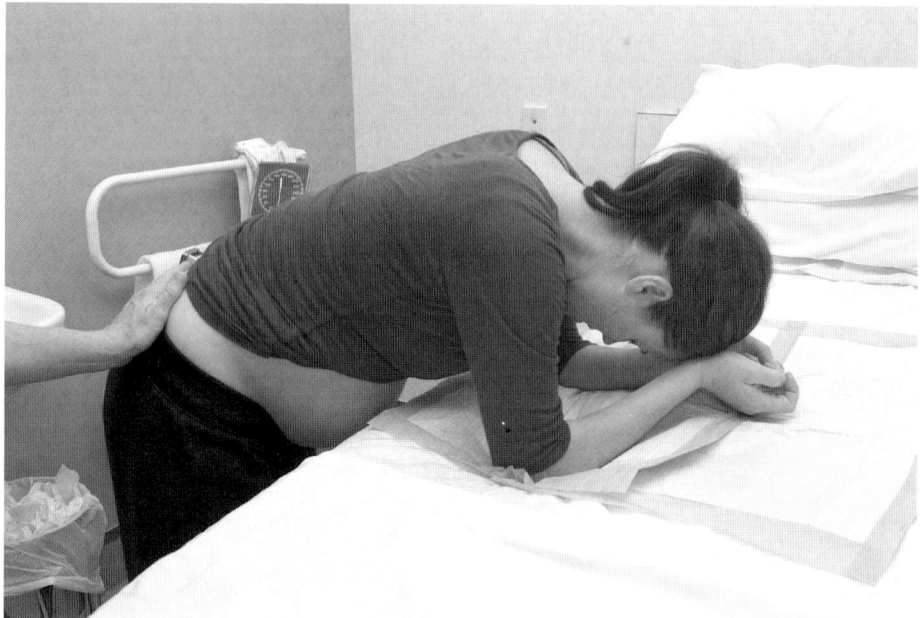

Fig. 12.2   Upright Birthing Position. (Courtesy iStock.com/chameleonseye.)

diverse child-bearing families in the labour and birth suites have the same needs and desires of as those of all families. It is essential to give them the same respect and sense of welcome, by integrating their needs, values, and preferences into care.

Cultural Competence in Action

A Culturally Safe Birth Plan

Ms. Oksana Rosa, a 23-year-old from the Philippines, is at 38 weeks with her second pregnancy and is in active labour. She labours quietly and speaks in Tagalog to her sister Juana from time to time. She was initially offered pain options such as epidural analgesia, Nitronox, or hydrotherapy; however, she refused. She seems to be coping fine with the support of her sister by her side. She says that she prefers to squat for a birthing position. The health care provider is more focused on monitoring the baby's well-being.

How would you describe the care being provided to Oksana? What factors might contribute to the health care provider's lack of engagement with Oksana? Consider assumptions about pain expression, the need for a practitioner since the patient has support from her sister, language barriers, and unfamiliarity with the preferred birth position. It is important for heath care providers to check their own biases and avoidance, and to ensure regular check-ins with labouring persons to provide comfort and pain relief.

Patients With Female Genital Cutting

Female genital circumcision, more recently known as **female genital cutting** (FGC), is a cultural practice occurring mainly in Africa and parts of the Middle East and Asia. The three types of FGC vary in severity. Type one involves **clitoridectomy**, the removal of the clitoris; type two, or excision, includes clitoridectomy and removal of the labia minora; and type three, also known as **infibulation**, consists of creating a narrow vaginal orifice by sealing the labia majora to the labia minora and potentially clitoridectomy (United Nations Children's Fund & Gupta, 2013). It is estimated that 200 million females currently have been affected by FGC worldwide. FGC is a nonmedical procedure performed on girls during puberty as a rite of passage. The procedures are often performed without aseptic technique and by lay medical personnel. It poses severe implications to reproductive and sexual health, such as a wound or urinary infection, death after the procedure, prolonged or obstructed labour, and increased risk of dying during birthing (United Nations Population Fund, 2018). Canadian health care providers must consider the legal implications of FGC as it is a criminal offence (Ontario Human Rights Commission, 2000).

Cultural Competence In Action

Reframing Cultural Practices and Identities

Fatima has recently immigrated to Canada from Sudan. She is 37 weeks pregnant and has presented to the birthing unit in active labour. Upon assessment, it is discovered that Fatima's perineum is infibulated. During her baby girl's birth, Fatima's pushing efforts are obstructed by the seal, requiring her obstetrician to cut the seal open to facilitate delivery of the baby's head. Her husband asks the obstetrician to repair her perineum and seal the urethra and vagina again, also known as re-infibulation. Fatima's obstetrician explains that they will repair the cut they made to arrest bleeding and promote optimal healing. However, they will not be able to reseal Fatima's infibulation as it carries risks to Fatima's pelvic health. The next morning after Fatima has been able to rest, the obstetrician returns to provide Fatima with more detailed reasoning, including the legal implications, as to why they did not perform the re-infibulation. Fatima did not realize the health risks of her cultural practice before meeting the obstetrician as it was performed on her as a young girl. Following this discussion, Fatima understands the reasoning for her obstetrician refuseding the request of re-infibulation.

Continued

> When met with a cultural practice that is not clinically recommended or has legal implications, health care providers should respectfully discuss the topic with their patients and respect their choices, while providing them with the clinical information as to why the provider cannot perform the service.

When providing care for patients affected by FGC, health care providers must have a nonjudgemental approach to this cultural practice, to help establish a relationship of trust and honesty. Terminology is also of the utmost importance, as referring to a patient's genitalia as "mutilated" may create an unsafe patient environment. The risks of FGC for reproductive and sexual health should be communicated to the patient, including the information that it is illegal for re-infibulation to be performed in Canada.

Culture Considerations In Care

Seeking Nonjudgemental Language and Empathy

Consider the following questions to pose to a patient who has undergone FGC: How would you like your perineal alteration to be referred to? What cultural significance does this practice have to you? What would you like your health care providers to do for your labour and birth to make you feel most comfortable?

Adequate, culturally competent, and culturally safe communication between health care providers and immigrants is essential in the access and delivery of health care. Health care providers must acquire a cultural understanding of the attitudes, behaviours, beliefs, and practices of minority subpopulations in order to improve timely access to prenatal care and improve newborn outcomes.

Family-Centred Postpartum Care

Many factors that affect health equity in prenatal care continue in the postpartum period, and some might be magnified during this period. If patients do not have a positive experience with the health care system and health care providers in the earlier part of their perinatal period, they are unlikely to trust and seek care post-delivery.

For many cultural communities, the postpartum period is defined by prescribed rituals to promote healing and bonding between the family and baby and by developing new roles as new parents or as parents with a new addition to the family. For collectivist cultures that are "we" oriented, this is a time to get support from others. People from these cultures have noted that perinatal care in Canada is more oriented toward the pre- and intrapartum periods with an expectation that couples will be actively engaged in and assume responsibility for caring for themselves and the new baby. Canadian parents are encouraged to get fresh air and stay active as ways to prevent postpartum mood disorders. However, in many cultures, there is a resting period of 40–50 days or more, when the new parent who gave birth is expected to rest, do minimal chores, and receive support, both emotional and tangible, in the form of special foods, assistance in care of the baby, and housework, from family and friends (Bolton et al., 2018; Evagorou et al., 2016; Higginbottom et al., 2016; Quintanilha et al., 2016; Sharma et al., 2016). Patients may fear potential postpartum pain and complications if they become active too soon. Many patients can have difficulty coping with the daily routine of looking after a baby in a country where they do not receive support from their extended family.

Another area of cultural difference between the Western culture and many other cultures is hygiene, specifically bathing. Many cultures have traditional customs that dictate avoiding baths and showers postpartum for a period of time ranging from 10 to 30 days. Bathing during these times is seen as a cause of ill health and rheumatism in old age. Sponge baths and steam baths can be used as alternatives. Some patients may object to having a shower immediately after giving birth and may find it easier to go through the motions than advocate or negotiate for their cultural traditions (Higginbottom et al., 2016), while others will reject this tradition while retaining others (Higginbottom et al., 2018; Joseph et al., 2019). Thus it is important to use such cultural knowledge to inquire into patients' needs and preferences and not make assumptions.

Health care providers may have views on what a new parent role looks like, concerning responsibility for care and infant bonding. This can lead to judgement and imposition of Western cultural norms as to what is best for parents and babies. If a baby is cared for by an extended family, it may be interpreted that the parent is not assuming responsibility and bonding between parent and infant is obstructed. Health care providers need to ensure that they share their expert clinical knowledge with the family and remain open to learning about cultural strengths from families.

POSTPARTUM DEPRESSION

In Canada, 23% of postnatal mothers reported feelings consistent with either postpartum depression or an anxiety disorder, ranging from 16% in Saskatchewan to 31% in Nova Scotia (Statistics Canada, 2019). Indigenous and immigrant women have been noted to have a higher risk of experiencing depressive symptoms in the postpartum period than non-Indigenous, Canadian-born pregnant people (Daoud et al., 2019). The increased risk for immigrants can be attributed to factors such as family discord, difficult external expectations of motherhood, poor nutrition and self-care practices, and economic dependence (Khanlou et al., 2017), as well as lack of social support, loneliness, and household burden (Jessri et al., 2013). It is important to recognize that some cultures have a tendency for somatization, where emotional distress presents as physical symptoms (Evagorou et al., 2016). Dietary patterns of the pregnant person have also been linked to postpartum mental health (Teo et al., 2018). Counselling, sunlight therapy, vitamin D supplements, seeking local support, and self-help can be helpful for ensuring support during postnatal care.

LACTATION AND INFANT FEEDING

The WHO recommends that infants receive breastfeeding (or chest feeding) exclusively for 6 months, and then alongside complementary foods for 2 years and beyond (WHO, 2018; WHO & UNICEF, 2020). Breastfeeding is the perfect nutrition for newborns as breast milk is dynamic in content and changes to match the infant's needs. Research has shown that breastfed infants have reduced rates of sudden infant death syndrome (SIDS), reduced likelihood of obesity, and decreased rates of ear and lung infections. It is also beneficial to the parent as it aids the mother–baby dyad and reduces risk of breast and ovarian cancer, diabetes, and heart disease (Government of Canada, 2020). In Canada, 90% of birthing parents initiate breastfeeding, but only 57% of those parents continue to breastfeed past 6 months. The main reasons for ceasing breastfeeding early are perceived to be low milk supply and difficulty with breastfeeding technique (Government of Canada, 2020). Across various cultures, breastfeeding is approached differently and is linked to beliefs about infant nutritional needs as well as religious and cultural beliefs (Jessri et al., 2013; Kanhadilok & McGrath, 2015). Breastfeeding is generally viewed positively across cultural groups. It is associated with cultural norms of being a good mother, maternal bonding, and doing what is best for the infant (Bolton et al., 2018; Gallegos et al., 2013; Kanhadilok & McGrath, 2015) (Fig. 12.3).

UNICEF recommends breastfeeding initiation within the first hour of postpartum (UNICEF, 2018; WHO & UNICEF, 2020). However, colostrum may be regarded as "dirty" or "old" milk by

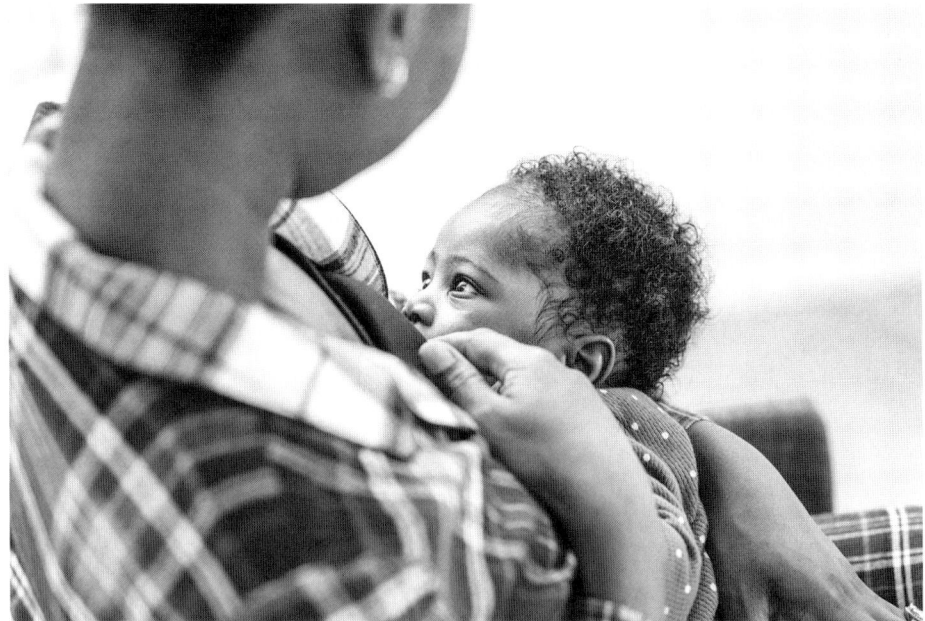

Fig. 12.3   A parent is breastfeeding their baby. (Courtesy iStock.com/kate_sept2004.)

some cultural groups (Legesse et al., 2015), and these mothers might delay breastfeeding until their mature milk comes in after a few days. Breastfeeding preferences should be discussed with the patient along with the evidence on the benefits of colostrum. Health care providers should work to meet the needs of their patients and, in this case, could recommend pumping colostrum to stimulate the patient's breasts during the days before mature milk begins. Cultures also vary in when other foods and drinks should be introduced to the infant—with many patients opting for traditional practices and advice from friends and family from the country of origin. Support from a partner, friends, and family is positively associated with breastfeeding success across cultures (Gallegos et al., 2013; Jessri et al., 2013; Kanhadilok & McGrath, 2015).

A body of research supports a multilevel approach to address the low level of breastfeeding among Black mothers (Hemingway et al., 2021; Johnson et al., 2015). Supportive breastfeeding initiatives must be combined through major institutions so that Black mothers may benefit from reliable breastfeeding education and care from health care providers and community lactation groups to attain heightened breastfeeding outcomes (Johnson et al., 2015).

Research across cultures has also identified several challenges to maintaining breastfeeding among groups such as Chinese, Middle Eastern, and African people. A frequently cited reason for not breastfeeding is public exposure. In many cultures, such as Middle Eastern cultures, modesty, particularly for women, is an important expectation, and lack of public spaces that support privacy can make it hard for mothers to continue breastfeeding. Similarly, adolescent mothers often feel embarrassed about exposure (Jessri et al., 2013). Many cultures report that, in general, they did not feel that Canadian and Australian societies support public breastfeeding (Mathews, 2019; Nesbitt et al., 2012). Another limiting factor is the need to return to work and not having adequate space and time to pump breast milk (Jiang et al., 2015). Other factors that make it harder for immigrant women to continue breastfeeding are lack of familiarity with services such as lactation consultants and breastfeeding hotlines, inability to access services due to linguistic barriers, and "conflicts of care" between Western and traditional cultural practices where women are expected to rest and focus on recovery for the first 30–40 days after birth. Immigrant mothers in Canada and Australia note that the culture in their new country is one of resuming physical activity quickly, feeding schedules, lack of support with household duties, and often an economic necessity to return to work (Gallegos et al., 2013; Jessri et al., 2013; Joseph et al., 2019). Dietary changes also affect perceptions of what is needed by women. Many cultures have "special foods" thought to stimulate breast milk production; however, if these foods are not available to women in their new country, they may turn to supplements such as solid foods, formula, and other liquids (Gallegos et al., 2013; Jessri et al., 2013; Joseph et al., 2019).

Racial disparities have been noted in both the initiation and continuation of breastfeeding in the United States. Hemingway et al. (2021) looked at breastfeeding practices in communities before and after their hospital's achievement of baby friendly hospital designation and noted that Black mothers were 2.4 times less likely to maintain breastfeeding than non-Black mothers. After baby friendly hospital initiative enactment, the racial gap in breastfeeding initiation decreased, but a significant difference persisted for continuous in-hospital breastfeeding (Hemingway et al., 2021). Factors that may be contributing to this disparity include "inherent presumptions that women of color will not breastfeed and so were given fewer lactation referrals, deprioritized in workflow, and received reduced attention and support. They also reported overt racist comments made by colleagues and increased referrals of Black mothers to social work and long-acting birth control" (Hemingway et al., 2021). Similar findings of negative perceptions of Black women, experiences of racism, and Black women receiving less advice or encouragement to breastfeed based on provider assumptions and being more likely to have formula offered to them have been consistently reported in the literature (DeVane-Johnson et al., 2017; Smith, 2018; Spencer & Grassley, 2013). Such findings have led to a call for understanding inequities in breastfeeding for Black mothers as an issue of social justice rather than just from a medical perspective (Hemingway et al., 2021).

Cultural Competence In Action

Breastfeeding Success and Early Communication

Sharon Avram is attending her 28-week antenatal appointment with her midwife. She is pregnant with her first child and is planning a hospital delivery. Today her midwife plans to discuss infant feeding and she asks how Sharon intends to feed her baby. Sharon says her friends and family have all formula-fed their babies, so she thinks she will do the same. Sharon further explains that in her predominantly Black community, breastfeeding is considered an old practice and not suitable for a working parent's lifestyle. What should be considered in order to provide a culturally safe discussion?

Sharon and her midwife spend some time reviewing the benefits of nursing for both the breastfeeding parent and the baby. After learning more about breastfeeding, she plans to breastfeed her baby with support and education. She signs up to receive further help with community resources. What additional supports would be helpful to support Sharon in her decision to breastfeed?

Summary

This chapter highlights the significant influence of unique and complex contexts of social and cultural determinants during all stages of the perinatal period for the pregnant person and their baby on effective and quality care. Changing demographics and evidence of inequities and challenges in the health care system experienced by birthing persons make cultural competency and cultural safety an urgent necessity. There is a need to create more critical consciousness and culturally safe spaces. Social determinants of prenatal health intersect with education and employment, race and gender, discrimination and inequalities, and cultural values and practices that influence family-centred prenatal and newborn care. Hence, this chapter has examined approaches to care to support families in the perinatal period by ensuring culturally safe communication, promoting access to appropriate care, and integrating cultural practices.

BIPOC individuals of diverse ethnic, racial, and cultural backgrounds may encounter challenges with birthing in Canada because of a lack of psychological and emotional support, competing social and work roles, socioeconomic distress, and stress. Challenges such as appropriate distribution of resources, power, freedom, and control will influence BIPOC patients' participation in perinatal care, and mitigation of these inequities can reduce their vulnerability to illness. Inequitable access to health care health care disparities, and adverse perinatal outcomes among Indigenous patients in Canada result from complex social determinants of health, including the legacy of residential schools and the intergenerational impacts of colonization. Health care providers need to recognize the roles of and relationships between Indigenous families, Indigenous midwives and traditional birth helpers, and cultural influences that impact Indigenous prenatal and newborn outcomes.

Parenthood and childbirth are essential developmental milestones influenced by cultural, psychosocial, emotional, mental-health, and behavioural factors. By integrating cultural competency in health care practices, the known risks and impact of unconscious bias and racism experienced by pregnant people of diverse cultures and Indigenous families can be reduced and the quality of care enhanced. Health care providers must address cultural issues including racism and discrimination to achieve cultural safety and equity in perinatal care through anti-racism education, compassionate care, respect for life, and understanding of cultural practices. This includes integrating Indigenous and other traditional healing practices in all health care interactions by creating safe spaces and services that provide a welcoming prenatal experience.

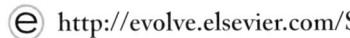 http://evolve.elsevier.com/Srivastava/culturalcompetence/.

Questions for Review and Discussion

1. "Health care is advancing because priorities and strategies change with care processes." Discuss some of the challenges and trends occurring in the health care system today with respect to perinatal care.
2. "Prenatal education is associated with positive outcomes." What factors facilitate the participation of pregnant persons and their support partners in prenatal classes?
3. What are some key cultural considerations that require further assessment when helping Indigenous patients develop a birth plan?
4. How can you integrate your knowledge of premature mortality risk for Black mothers into actions when caring for a Black family during the perinatal period?
5. What are some key cultural considerations for ensuring postpartum support for migrant families?

Group Experiential/Reflection Activity

SEEKING PRENATAL CARE IN A NEW COUNTRY

My-Duyen Choung is a young Vietnamese immigrant who is pregnant with her first child and speaks very little English. She lives in a large urban city in Canada and has come in for her first prenatal appointment. She listens quietly to the health care provider's questions, and although she appears confused, she asks no questions and becomes agitated. Thang Thao, her husband, nods and smiles frequently. He speaks more English than his wife but has difficulty responding to his wife's health questions.

1. What are some important considerations in providing culturally responsive, equitable care for this family?
2. Consider the following areas: patient/family engagement, prenatal education, and development of a birth plan.

References

Almond, D., Edlund, L., & Milligan, K. (2013). Son preference and the persistence of culture: Evidence from South and East Asian immigrants to Canada. *Population and Development Review*, *39*(1), 75–95.

Alzghoul, M. M., Møller, H., Wakewich, P., et al. (2021). Perinatal care experiences of Muslim women in Northwestern Ontario, Canada: A qualitative study. *Women and Birth*, *4*(2), e162–e169.

American Heart Association. (2019). *Why are black women at such high risk of dying from pregnancy complications?* https://www.heart.org/en/news/2019/02/20/why-are-black-women-at-such-high-risk-of-dying-from-pregnancy-complications

Amundsen, C., & Kent-Wilkinson, A. (2020). Prenatal evacuation: Addressing the birth customs and perinatal care needs of Indigenous women in Northern Canada. *International Journal of Nursing Student Scholarship*, *7*.

Andermann, A. (2016). Acting on the social determinants of health in clinical practice: A framework for health professionals. *CMAJ*, *188*(17–18), E474–E483.

Anderson, I., Robson, B., Connolly, M., et al. (2016). Indigenous and tribal people health (The Lancet–Lowitja Institute Global Collaboration): A population study. *The Lancet*, *388*(10040), 131–157.

Association of Ontario Midwives. (2021). *Uninsured clients*. https://www.ontariomidwives.ca/uninsured-clients

Besse, M., Lampe, N. M., & Mann, E. S. (2020a). Experiences with achieving pregnancy and giving birth among transgender men: A narrative literature review. *The Yale Journal of Biology and Medicine*, *93*(4), 517.

Besse, M., Lampe, N. M., & Mann, E. S. (2020b). Focus: Sex & reproduction: Experiences with achieving pregnancy and giving birth among transgender men: A narrative literature review. *The Yale Journal of Biology and Medicine*, *93*(4), 517.

Bethune, R., Absher, N., Obiagwu, M., et al. (2019). Social determinants of self-reported health for Canada's Indigenous people: A public health approach. *Public Health*, *176*, 172–180.

Bohren, M. A., Hofmeyr, G. J., Sakala, C., et al. (2017). Continuous support for women during childbirth. *Cochrane Database of Systematic Reviews, 7*(7), CD03766.

Bolton, K. A., Kremer, P., Hesketh, K. D., et al. (2018). Differences in infant feeding practices between Chinese-born and Australian-born mothers living in Australia: A cross-sectional study. *BMC Pediatrics*, *18*(1), 209. https://doi.org/10.1186/s12887-018-1157-0.

Bowen. S. (2015). *The impact of language barriers on patient safety and quality of care*. Société Santé en Français. https://www.reseausantene.ca/wp-content/uploads/2018/05/Impact-language-barrier-qualitysafety.pdf

Brosseau, L., & Dewing, M. (2018). *Canadian multiculturalism*. https://lop.parl.ca/sites/PublicWebsite/default/en_CA/ResearchPublications/200920E

Canadian Association of Midwives. (2021). *Midwives and midwifery-led births 2019*. https://canadianmidwives.org/2020/10/01/registered-midwives-midwifery-assisted-births-2019/

Canadian Institute for Health Information (CIHI). (2020). *QuickStats: Childbirth indicators by place of residence*. https://apps.cihi.ca/mstrapp/asp/Main.aspx?Server=apmstrextprd_i&project=Quick%20Stats&uid=pce_pub_en&pwd=&evt=2048001&visualizationMode=0&documentID=029DB170438205AEBCC75B8673CCE822

Centers for Disease Control and Prevention (CDC). (2019, September 5). *Racial and ethnic disparities continue in pregnancy-related deaths. Black, American Indian/Alaska Native women most affected* [Press release]. https://www.cdc.gov/media/releases/2019/p0905-racial-ethnic-disparities-pregnancy-deaths.html

Chakrabarti, S., & Chakrabarti, A. (2019). Food taboos in pregnancy and early lactation among women living in a rural area of West Bengal. *Journal of Family Medicine and Primary Care*, *8*(1), 86.

Churchill, M. E., Smylie, J. K., Wolfe, S. H., et al. (2020). Conceptualising cultural safety at an Indigenous-focused midwifery practice in Toronto, Canada: Qualitative interviews with Indigenous and non-Indigenous clients. *BMJ Open*, *10*(9), e038168. https://doi.org/10.1136/bmjopen-2020-038168.

Cidro, J., Bach, R., & Frohlick, S. (2020). Canada's forced birth travel: Towards feminist indigenous reproductive mobilities. *Mobilities*, *15*(2), 173–187.

Curnow, E., & Geraghty, S. (2019). Chiropractic care of the pregnant woman and neonate. *British Journal of Midwifery, 27*(5), 284–287.

Daoud, N., O'Brien, K., O'Campo, P., et al. (2019). Postpartum depression prevalence and risk factors among Indigenous, non-Indigenous and immigrant women in Canada. *Canadian Journal of Public Health, 110*(4), 440–452.

DeVane-Johnson, S., Woods-Giscombe, C., Thoyre, S., et al. (2017). Integrative literature review of factors related to breastfeeding in African American women: Evidence for a potential paradigm shift. *Journal of Human Lactation, 33*, 435–447.

Ekström, A. C., & Thorstensson, S. (2015). Nurses and midwives' professional support increases with improved attitudes-design and effects of a longitudinal randomized controlled process-oriented intervention. *BMC Pregnancy and Childbirth, 15*(1), 275.

Evagorou, O., Arvaniti, A., & Samakouri, M. (2016). Cross-cultural approach of postpartum depression: manifestation, practices applied, risk factors and therapeutic interventions. *Psychiatric Quarterly, 87*(1), 129–154.

Gallegos, D., Vicca, N., & Streiner, S. (2013). Breastfeeding beliefs and practices of African women living in Brisbane and Perth, Australia. *Maternal and Child Nutrition, 11*, 727–736.

Garcia, E. R., & Yim, I. S. (2017). A systematic review of concepts related to women's empowerment in the perinatal period and their associations with perinatal depressive symptoms and premature birth. *BMC Pregnancy and Childbirth, 17*(2), 1–13.

Government of Canada. (2020). *About the LGBTQ2 Secretariat*. https://www.canada.ca/en/canadian-heritage/campaigns/free-to-be-me/about-lgbtq2-secretariat.html

Greenhalgh, T., Clinch, M., Afsar, N., et al. (2015). Socio-cultural influences on the behaviour of South Asian women with diabetes in pregnancy: A qualitative study using a multi-level theoretical approach. *BMC Medicine, 13*(1), 1–15.

Hall, W. J., Chapman, M. V., Lee, K. M., et al. (2015). Implicit racial/ethnic bias among health care professionals and its influence on health care outcomes: A systematic review. *American Journal of Public Health, 105*(12), e60–e76.

Health Canada. (2000). *Family-centred maternity and newborn care: National guidelines*. https://www.canada.ca/en/public-health/services/maternity-newborn-care-guidelines.html

Health Canada. (2019). *Canada's dietary guidelines for health professionals and policy makers* (p. 55). https://food-guide.canada.ca/en/guidelines/

Hemingway, S., Forson-Dare, Z., Ebeling, M., et al. (2021). Racial disparities in sustaining breastfeeding in a baby-friendly designated Southeastern United States hospital: An opportunity to investigate systemic racism. *Breastfeeding Medicine, 16*(2), 150–155.

Higginbottom, G. M., Safipour, J., Yohani, S., et al. (2016). An ethnographic investigation of the prenatal healthcare experience of immigrants in rural and urban Alberta, Canada. *BMC Pregnancy and Childbirth, 16*(1), 1–15.

Higginbottom, G. M., Vallianatos, H., Shankar, J., et al. (2018). Immigrant women's food choices in pregnancy: Perspectives from women of Chinese origin in Canada. *Ethnicity & Health, 23*(5), 21–541. https://doi.org/10.1080/13557858.2017.1281384.

Hoffkling, A., Obedin-Maliver, J., & Sevelius, J. (2017). From erasure to opportunity: A qualitative study of the experiences of transgender men around pregnancy and recommendations for providers. *BMC Pregnancy and Childbirth, 17*(Suppl 2). https://doi.org/10.1186/s12884-017-1491-5.

Hoffman, K. M., Trawalter, S., Axt, J. R., et al. (2016). Racial bias in pain assessment and treatment recommendations, and false beliefs about biological differences between blacks and whites. *Proceedings of the National Academy of Sciences of the United States of America, 113*(16), 4296–4301.

Institute for Patient-and Family-Centered Care [IPFC]. (2017). *Advancing the practice of patient-and family-centered care in hospitals: How to get started*. http://www.ipfcc.org/resources/getting_started.pdf

Jessri, M., Farmer, A., & Olson, K. (2013). Exploring Middle-Eastern mothers' perceptions and experiences of breastfeeding in Canada: An ethnographic study. *Maternal and Child Nutrition (2013), 9*, 41–56. https://doi.org/10.1111/j.1740-8709.2012.00436.x.

Jiang, B., Hua, J., Wang, Y., et al. (2015). Evaluation of the impact of breast milk expression in early postpartum period on breastfeeding duration: A prospective cohort study. *BMC Pregnancy and Childbirth, 15*(1), 1–13.

Johnson, A., Kirk, R., Rosenblum, K. L., et al. (2015). Enhancing breastfeeding rates among African American women: A systematic review of current psychosocial interventions. *Breastfeeding. Medicine, 10*(1), 45–62.

Joseph, J., Liamputtong, P., & Brodribb, W. (2019). Postpartum breastfeeding experiences in the traditional biomedical crossroads: A qualitative study using drawing with Vietnamese and Myanmarese refugee women in Australia. *Journal of Advanced Nursing*, 75, 2855–2866. https://doi.org/10.1111/jan.14110.

Kanhadilok, S., & McGrath, J. (2015). An integrative review of factors influencing breastfeeding in adolescent mothers. *The Journal of Perinatal Education*, 24(2), 119–127. https://doi.org/10.1891/1058-1243.24.2.119.

Khanlou, N., Haque, N., Skinner, A., et al. (2017). Scoping review on prenatal health among immigrant and refugee women in Canada: Prenatal, intrapartum, and postnatal care. *Journal of Pregnancy*, 2017, 8783294.

Knight, M. (2019). The findings of the MBRRACE-UK confidential enquiry into maternal deaths and morbidity. *Obstetrics, Gynaecology & Reproductive Medicine*, 29(1), 21–23.

Kolahdooz, F., Launier, K., Nader, F., et al. (2016). Canadian Indigenous women's perspectives of maternal health and health care services: A systematic review. *Diversity and Equality in Health and Care*, 13(5), 334–348.

Leason, J. L. (2018). Exploring the complex context of Canadian Indigenous maternal child-health through maternity experiences: The role of social determinants of health. *Social Determinants of Health*, 4(2), 54–67.

Legesse, M., Demena, M., Mesfin, F., et al. (2015). Factors associated with colostrum avoidance among mothers of children aged less than 24 months in Raya Kobo district, North-eastern Ethiopia: Community-based cross-sectional study. *Journal of Tropical Pediatrics*, 61(5), 357–363. https://doi.org/10.1093/tropej/fmv039.

Lim, C. G., & van Dam, R. M. (2020). Attitudes and beliefs regarding food in a multi-ethnic Asian population and their association with socio-demographic variables and healthy eating intentions. *Appetite*, 144, 104461.

Martin, N., & Montagne, R. (2017). *Nothing protects Black women from dying in pregnancy and childbirth*. ProPublica.

Mathews, V. (2019). Reconfiguring the breastfeeding body in urban public spaces. *Social & Cultural Geography*, 20(9), 1266–1284.

Maxwell, C., Gaudet, L., Cassir, G., et al. (2019). Guideline no. 391—pregnancy and maternal obesity part 1: Pre-conception and prenatal care. *Journal of Obstetrics and Gynaecology Canada*, 41(11), 1623–1640. https://doi.org/10.1016/j.jogc.2019.03.026.

Mellin, P. S. (2017). *Adequately medicating pregnant women with pain: A survey of perinatal nurses*. The William Paterson University of New Jersey. [Unpublished doctoral dissertation].

Mengesha, Z. B., Perz, J., Dune, T., et al. (2018). Challenges in the provision of sexual and reproductive health care to refugee and migrant women: A methodological study of health professional perspectives. *Journal of Immigrant and Minority Health*, 20(2), 307–316.

Merry, L., Villadsen, S. F., Sicard, V., et al. (2020). Transnationalism and care of migrant families during pregnancy, postpartum and early-childhood: An integrative review. *BMC Health Services Research*, 20(1), 1–24.

Midwives Association of British Columbia. (2021). *Frequently asked questions*. https://www.bcmidwives.com/faq.html

Morton, C. H., Henley, M. M., Seacrist, M., et al. (2018). Bearing witness: The United States and Canadian maternity support workers' observations of disrespectful care in childbirth. *Birth*, 45(3), 263–274.

Mottola, M. F., Davenport, M. H., Ruchat, S. M., et al. (2018). No. 367-2019 Canadian guideline for physical activity throughout pregnancy. *Journal of Obstetrics and Gynaecology Canada*, 40(11), 1528–1537.

Mucina, M. K. (2018). Exploring the role of "honour" in son preference and daughter deficit within the Punjabi diaspora in Canada. *Canadian Journal of Development Studies/Revue Canadienne d'études du Développement*, 39(3), 426–442.

National Indigenous Council of Midwives (NACM). (2014). *Bringing birth back in Indigenous midwifery toolkit*. https://indigenousmidwifery.ca/wp-content/uploads/2018/10/Indigenous-Midwifery-Toolkit.pdf

National Indigenous Council of Midwives (NACM). (2016). *The landscape of midwifery care for Indigenous communities in Canada*. https://canadianmidwives.org/wp-content/uploads/2017/03/NACM_Landscape Report_2016_REV_July18_LOW.pdf

National Partnership for Women and Families. (2018). *Black women's maternal health: A multifaceted approach to addressing persistent and dire health disparities*. https://www.nationalpartnership.org/our-work/health/reports/black-womens-maternal-health.html

Nesbitt, S. A., Campbell, K. A., Jack, S. M., et al. (2012). Canadian adolescent mothers' perceptions of influences on breastfeeding decisions: A qualitative descriptive study. *BMC Pregnancy and Childbirth*, 12(1), 1–14.

Okeke, E., Glick, P., Chari, A., et al. (2016). The effect of increasing the supply of skilled health providers on pregnancy and birth outcomes: Evidence from the midwives' service scheme in Nigeria. *BMC Health Services Research*, 16(1), 425.

Ontario Human Rights Commission. (2000). *Policy on female genital mutilation (FGM)*. http://www.ohrc.on.ca/en/policy-female-genital-mutilation-fgm

Petersen, E. E., Davis, N. L., Goodman, D., et al. (2019). Racial/ethnic disparities in pregnancy-related deaths—United States, 2007–2016. *Morbidity and Mortality Weekly Report*, *68*(35), 762.

Power, T., Wilson, D., Best, O., et al. (2020). COVID-19 and Indigenous people: An imperative for action. *Journal of Clinical Nursing*, *29*(15–16), 2737–2741. https://doi.org/10.1111/jocn.15320.

Public Health Agency of Canada. (2020). *Family-centred maternity and newborn care: National guidelines*. https://www.canada.ca/en/public-health/services/maternity-newborn-care-guidelines.html

Qadir, F., Khan, M. M., Medhin, G., et al. (2011). Male gender preference, female gender disadvantage as risk factors for psychological morbidity in Pakistani women of childbearing age—a life course perspective. *BMC Public Health*, *11*(1), 1–13.

Quintanilha, M., Mayan, M. J., Thompson, J., et al. (2016). Contrasting "back home" and "here": How Northeast African migrant women perceive and experience health during pregnancy and postpartum in Canada. *International Journal for Equity in Health*, *15*, 80. https://doi.org/10.1186/s12939-016-0369-x.

Ricci, S. (2020). *Essentials of maternity, newborn, and women's health nursing* (5th ed.). Wolters Kluwer.

Richmond, C. A., & Cook, C. (2016). Creating conditions for Canadian Indigenous health equity: The promise of healthy public policy. *Public Health Reviews*, *37*(1), 2.

Riddell, C. A., Hutcheon, J. A., & Dahlgren, L. S. (2016). Differences in obstetric care among nulliparous First Nations and non–First Nations women in British Columbia, Canada. *CMAJ*, *188*(2), E36–E43.

Riggs, D. W., Pearce, R., Pfeffer, C. A., et al. (2020). Men, trans/masculine, and non-binary people's experiences of pregnancy loss: An international qualitative study. *BMC Pregnancy and Childbirth*, *20*(1), 1–9.

Robinson, A. M., Benzies, K. M., Cairns, S. L., et al. (2016). Who is distressed? A comparison of psychosocial stress in pregnancy across seven ethnicities. *BMC Pregnancy and Childbirth*, *16*(1), 1–11.

Roeder, A. (2019). America is failing its black mothers. *Harvard Public Health*. https://www.hsph.harvard.edu/magazine/magazine_article/america-is-failing-its-black-mothers/

Royal College of Obstetricians and Gynaecologists. (2020, March 6). *RCOG position statement: Racial disparities in women's healthcare*. https://www.heart.org/en/news/2019/02/20/why-are-black-women-at-such-high-risk-of-dying-from-pregnancy-complications

Sharma, S., Teijlingen, E. V., Hundley, V., et al. (2016). Dirty and 40 days in the wilderness: Eliciting childbirth and postnatal cultural practices and beliefs in Nepal. *BMC Pregnancy and Childbirth*, *16*, 147.

Smith, P. H. (2018). Social justice at the core of breastfeeding protection, promotion, and support: A conceptualization. *Journal of Human Lactation*, *34*, 220–225.

Smylie, J., Kirst, M., McShane, K., et al. (2016). Understanding the role of Indigenous community participation in Indigenous prenatal and infant-toddler health promotion programs in Canada: A realist review. *Social Science & Medicine*, *150*, 128–143.

Smylie, J., O'Brien, K., Beaudoin, E., et al. (2021). Long-distance travel for birthing among Indigenous and non-Indigenous pregnant people in Canada. *CMAJ*, *193*(25), E948–E955.

Society of Obstetricians and Gynecologists of Canada (SOGC). (2010). SOGC policy statement no. 251, December 2010. Returning birth to Indigenous, rural, and remote communities. *Journal of Obstetrics and Gynaecology Canada*, *32*(12), 1186–1188.

Spencer, B. S., & Grassley, J. S. (2013). African American women and breastfeeding: An integrative literature review. *Health Care for Women International*, *34*(7), 607–625.

Srinivasan, S. (2018). Transnationally relocated? Sex selection among Punjabis in Canada. *Canadian Journal of Development Studies/Revue Canadienne Deludes du Développement*, *39*(3), 408–425.

Statistics Canada. (2016). *Immigrant women*. https://www150.statcan.gc.ca/n1/pub/89-503-x/2015001/article/14217-eng.htm#a14

Statistics Canada. (2017). *Ethnic and cultural origins of Canadians: Portrait of a rich heritage*. Statistics Canada Catalogue no. 98-200-X2016016.

Statistics Canada. (2019). *Maternal mental health in Canada, 2018/2019*. Component of Statistics Canada catalogue no. 11-001-X. https://www150.statcan.gc.ca/n1/daily-quotidien/190624/dq190624b-eng.htm

Subedi, R., Greenberg, L., & Turcotte, M. (2020). *COVID-19 mortality rates in Canada's ethno-cultural neighbourhoods*. Statistics Canada Catalogue no. 45280001.

Tabobondung, R. (2014). A story of Indigenous birth justice. *MICE [Moving Image Culture Etc.]*, Issue 02. https://micemagazine.ca/issue-two/story-indigenous-birth-justice

Teo, C., Chia, A. R., Colega, M. T., et al. (2018). Prospective associations of maternal dietary patterns and postpartum mental health in a multi-ethnic Asian cohort: The growing up in Singapore towards healthy outcomes (GUSTO) study. *Nutrients, 10*(3), 299.

The Center: The Lesbian Gay Bisexual Transgender Community Center. (2021). *What is LGBTQ?* https://gaycenter.org/about/lgbtq/

Truth and Reconciliation Commission of Canada (TRC). (2015). *Truth and Reconciliation Commission of Canada: Calls to action.* http://trc.ca/assets/pdf/Calls_to_Action_English2.pdf

Turpel-Lafond. M. E. (2020). *In plain sight: Addressing Indigenous-specific racism and discrimination in B.C. Health Care.* Government of British Columbia. https://engage.gov.bc.ca/app/uploads/sites/613/2020/11/In-Plain-Sight-Full-Report.pdf

UNICEF. (2018). *From the first hour of life: Making the case for improved infant and young child feeding everywhere.* https://www.unicef.org/media/49801/file/From-the-first-hour-of-life-ENG.pdf

United Nations Children's Fund, & Gupta, G. R. (2013). *Female genital mutilation/cutting: A statistical overview and exploration of the dynamics of change.* https://www.unicef.org/reports/female-genital-mutilation-cutting

United Nations Population Fund. (2018). *Brief on the medicalization of female genital mutilation.* https://www.unfpa.org/resources/brief-medicalization-female-genital-mutilation

Vanier Institute of the Family. (2017). *In context: Understanding maternity care in Canada.* In Context series. https://vanierinstitute.ca/in-context-understanding-maternity-care-in-canada/

Vedam, S., Stoll, K., Taiwo, T. K., et al.(2019). The Giving Voice to Mothers study: Inequity and mistreatment during pregnancy and childbirth in the United States. *Reproductive Health, 16*(1), 1–18.

Watson, H., Harrop, D., Walton, E., et al. (2019). A systematic review of ethnic minority women's experiences of perinatal mental health conditions and services in Europe. *PLoS ONE, 14*(1), 1–19.

Winquist, B., Muhajarine, N., Ogle, K., et al. (2016). Prenatal screening, diagnosis, and termination of pregnancy in First Nations and rural women. *Prenatal Diagnosis, 36*(9), 838–846.

World Health Organization (WHO). (2015). *WHO statement on caesarean section rates. Sexual and reproductive health.* WHO Human Reproduction Program. https://www.who.int/reproductivehealth/publications/maternal_perinatal_health/cs-statement/en/

World Health Organization (WHO). (2018). *Guideline: Counselling of women to improve breastfeeding practices.* https://www.who.int/publications/i/item/9789241550468

World Health Organization (WHO) & UNICEF. (2020). *Protecting, promoting, and supporting breast-feeding in facilities providing maternity and newborn services: The revised Baby-friendly Hospital initiative. 2018 Implementation guidance: Frequently asked questions.* https://www.who.int/publications/i/item/9789240001459

CHAPTER 13

Cultural Considerations at the End of Life

Laurie Clune and Robert Edralin

As we write this chapter, death and death rituals worldwide are changing because of the global COVID-19 pandemic. Factors contributing to these changes include travel advisories, social distancing requirements, masking, hospital rules that restrict visiting people with life-limiting conditions in their homes and hospital, and funeral size restrictions. Mandated restrictions prevent families and friends from gathering for funeral and ceremonial rituals acknowledging a person's passing. Video streaming of such ceremonies allows people from around the world the opportunity to participate virtually in events. Unfortunately, global society will be dealing with this phase of the COVID-19 pandemic for many months to come. The long-term impact of absent or altered traditions is yet to be understood; however, the pandemic has highlighted the importance of rituals during this phase of life, along with the need and ability to adapt.

Like other aspects of life, how the end of life and death is experienced is culturally constructed. In this chapter, we will discuss how health care providers can work with people and their families as they approach the end of life. We begin with a discussion on the impact of death and end-of-life care on the care provider. This is important, as self-awareness is a foundational aspect of culturally appropriate quality care. The discussion on cultural considerations in death highlights aspects of end-of-life care that are particularly sensitive to cultural nuances. These include the understanding of a "good death," the meaning of suffering, and how critical life and death decisions are made. We offer examples of specific cultural patterns as illustrations and examples only. Being an expert in different cultures is neither possible nor desired. Providers need to understand cultural variations and patterns in order to be attuned to patient needs and preferences, particularly those different from needs of the provider or the system. However, labels of culture should not be used to make assumptions or stereotypes. There are always variations within and across cultures, groups, and populations. Intentional conversations are an important part of all end-of-life care, particularly in palliative care. Medical Assistance in Dying (MAiD), an end-of-life option for eligible persons making a voluntary request, will be described within the Canadian context. The chapter ends with a brief exploration of bereavement and the importance of rituals to support grief.

Recognizing Care Providers' Need for Support in Dying

Caring for a person, their family, and loved ones at the end of life has an impact on health care providers (McGilton et al., 2013; Muskat et al., 2019; Niehaus et al., 2020; Rapoport et al., 2017; Shi et al., 2019). Often, providers feel they are ill prepared to deal with the care of people experiencing dying and death (Brown et al., 2020). New graduates, in particular, may experience negative feelings such as nervousness, powerlessness, stress, guilt, and frustration (Zheng et al., 2016). Education has a significant influence on health care providers' attitudes and comfort levels with life-limiting illnesses and death (Chan et al., 2020; Gonella et al., 2020; Niehaus et al., 2020; Shi et al., 2019). While many educational programs devote some curricular attention to palliative approaches to care, most providers report feeling that they have insufficient preparation for working with individuals and families experiencing a life-limiting illness (McMorrow & Wiltse, 2019; Miller et al., 2008). Health education programs typically focus on *doing* something for the patient to sustain life, with minimal consideration to end-of-life care. Hence, providing care for people in the palliative and end-of-life specialty requires shifting away from *doing* to a *comfort-focused* approach or simply *being with* or supporting people in ways that are most meaningful to them.

Health care providers need to know their personal views and beliefs concerning dying and death to effectively provide care to individuals and their families (McMorrow & Wiltse, 2019; Rasheed, 2015). **Self-awareness** is an important therapeutic tool for a solid relationship between the patient and health care providers. "Self-awareness is the continuous process of understanding and knowledge of one's own identity, beliefs, thoughts, traits, motivations, feelings and behaviour and to recognize how they affect others in different ways" (Rasheed, 2015, p. 212). Self-awareness is achieved through self-reflection. Knowing one's values, beliefs, unique strengths and limitations makes health care providers better equipped to form a therapeutic relationship with a patient. Table 13.1 lists some reflective questions to enhance self-awareness.

TABLE 13.1 ■ Understanding Your Own Views on Death

Below are some questions that can be used for self-reflection:

- When did you first experience a death in your family, a group of friends, or your community?
- In your family, how do people behave when there is a death?
- What are your beliefs about death? Are they similar to or different from beliefs evident in your family or among your colleagues?
- What are your beliefs about life after death?
- Are there specific traditions or activities that have helped you cope with death?
- Have you participated in or observed traditions or activities that are different from your own that have been important to others?

The physical demands of providing care combined with the emotional load of supporting a patient's and family's journey as they progress through a trajectory toward end-of-life can significantly impact health care providers (Alderson et al., 2015; Cheung et al., 2015). Hence, health care providers must engage in self-care to promote personal health and well-being (Linzitto & Grance, 2017; Mills et al., 2018; Shariff et al., 2017). Table 13.2 shows some self-care activities that can be undertaken to manage stress and potential burnout.

Cultural Considerations in Care

Recognizing a Need for Support

Elizabeth is a critical care unit (CCU) nurse. For the last 3 weeks, she has been caring for a patient who is rapidly declining and treatments are ineffective. Elizabeth leaves work feeling upset and often crying because her efforts to keep the patient comfortable are not working. The situation is further complicated by the patient's family calling often and asking if the team is doing all they can. She is not sleeping well and feels emotionally exhausted.

During a lunch break Elizabeth tells you how she has been affected by providing care for her patient.
- How would you respond to Elizabeth?
- What can Elizabeth do to support herself?
- What can Elizabeth do to support the family?
- What factors may be contributing to the family's questions and concerns?

It is important to recognize that health care providers caring for patients at the end of life are at risk for compassion fatigue overall and need to contend with their views on death and dying. In a review of the literature on death anxiety among health professionals, Sharif et al. (2017) note that death anxiety is a normative experience across health care providers and impacts the care provided. In addition to personal coping and self-care strategies, the authors recommend education programs on death that increase health care providers' ability to have conversations about death with patients and family members. Nolte et al. (2017) examined compassion fatigue in nurses and noted that the work environment plays an important role. Strategies such as the ability to talk to and debrief with the team, education on compassion fatigue, and role modelling from leaders and senior staff can be effective in overcoming and preventing compassionate fatigue (Nolte et al., 2017).

TABLE 13.2 ■ Self-Care Activities

Physical activities	Any movement activity including running, brisk walking, hiking, Pilates, Zumba, skating, skiing, curling, swimming, dancing, martial arts, cycling, team sports, walking the dog, horseback riding
Hobbies	Cooking, baking, painting, reading, writing, gardening, music, drumming, travelling, sewing, knitting, crochet, weaving, macramé, video games
Cultural and spiritual activities	Guided imagery, yoga, mindfulness meditation, prayer, pausing and breathing, journaling, gratitude practice activities, nature walks, spiritual retreat, speaking to a faith leader, attending a religious event
Social activities	Meeting friends and family; joining a group activity such as a knitting circle, prayer group, Bible group, or team sport; taking a class; taking part in local community activities and festivals; book club; quilting circle; watching, attending, or participating in sports

Cultural Considerations and Death

Canada is a cultural mosaic with people from many cultures and homelands blending and integrating into existing communities. This trend requires health care providers to reflect on their own learned and established views and then be prepared to embrace death and dying practices specific to the individual's unique values, beliefs, and desires. Contextual factors such as culture, social and political influences, and even geography all impact how an individual responds to the end of life and dying (Cohen-Mansfield et al., 2018; Glaser & Strauss, 1968). As Srivastava and Srivastava (2019) suggest, culture encompasses commonly understood learned traditions and unconscious rules of engagement. One's thoughts and approaches to death are shaped by factors such as ethnicity, religion, birthplace, gender, familial traditions, and personal experiences. However, it is vital for health care providers to recognize that how people think about dying, death, and the afterlife is unique, and thus to not make stereotypical assumptions based on such factors.

VIEWS ON DEATH AND DYING

It is important to recognize that views on death and dying in Western cultures are strongly influenced by Christianity (Laungani & Laungani, 2015), where death is generally regarded as an end of a person's life. Upon death, the focus may be on the celebration of the person's life or the mourner's grief or both. In many cultures, however, death is viewed as a transition to another identity or phase, and thus attention is also directed toward ensuring a smooth transition for the deceased.

For some, death is understood as a private event, affecting largely the immediate family, whereas in other communities, death may be seen to affect the broader community. A public view of death may be accompanied by a more public expression of bereavement and grief. Culture and religion are interconnected, and such connections may become stronger toward the end of life and impending death. Individuals and families may prefer to have support from religious or spiritual leaders; however, this cannot be assumed. It is important to inquire about what supports are desired or welcomed, as many people are more secular or express their faith privately and directly with their God (Alladin, 2015).

RITUALS FOR CARE OF THE DECEASED AND FAMILY

Various practices and rituals surround the end of life and death. Culture and religion shape one's understanding of the end of life, death, the afterlife, ceremony, and burial practices (Gire, 2014). When someone dies, a signal is made to the local community for various social roles and responses to be assumed, and expectations specific to burial are enacted. Death is culturally structured and triggers rituals and traditions around the care of the deceased body and supporting the loved ones left behind. Rituals are a way of caring for the family and, for some, undertaking the tasks of transition for the deceased soul. Cultural norms may dictate how the body of the deceased person is treated. It may be important to maintain quiet around the body (Buddhists) or there may be chanting of religious songs or words. Traditions may determine how the body is washed and by whom. Touching or patting of the head carries particular significance and should be done only after checking with the family (Gaun, 2015; Laungani & Laungani, 2015). There may be a desire to have the deceased body placed on the floor or mat (Parkes, 2015). Members of the Jewish faith may wish to have a friend or family member stay with deceased person and not leave the body alone (Levine, 2015). For each patient and family, the preferences and needs will be determined by their unique circumstances. Health care providers can play an important and supportive role by inquiring about and being open and responsive to such needs.

Cultural norms also dictate the period of mourning, the colour of clothing to be worn or avoided, and the activities and ways in which families and community members conduct themselves (Rosenblatt, 2015). For example, in Hinduism there may be a *havan* ceremony that serves the purpose of praying for the smooth passage for the departed soul as well as peace and comfort for the family left behind. People of Jewish faith may practise *Shiva*, which is traditionally a 7-day period of grieving when the family may not leave the house and community members visit to offer condolences and food (Sinai Chapels, 2021). For Hindus the designated mourning ritual is 13 days, when family members are isolated at home and often do not cook, rather the community provides support and condolences by visiting and bringing food. The colour of mourning in Western traditions is black, whereas for Hindu and Buddhist communities this may be traditionally white, although black may be accepted given the context of Canadian society. Grief and mourning are intensely personal, thus such knowledge must not lead to assumptions or stereotypes. It is important for providers to understand what family members may be anticipating and engage in culturally sensitive conversations in such matters as they arise. Often an inability to perform rituals according to what an individual believes are the prescribed methods can lead to feelings of guilt and add to the burden of grieving; again, support from providers can be helpful.

LANGUAGE AND DEATH

Different cultures, locations, countries, religions, languages, dialects, and social situations cause people to speak and communicate about death in different ways (Table 13.3). Expressions often reflect the underlying values or emotions attached to a phenomenon. Providers should take their cue from patients and families, with respect to how death (or impending death) is being experienced. Expressions such as "was called home" or "went to heaven" may be very comforting and relevant to some and quite confusing to others. The complexities may be compounded if patients and families have limited English proficiency or are unfamiliar with cultural terms used. Often people will be comfortable with words such as "lost the battle" when referring to death following an illness such as cancer, but may be uncomfortable with the same terminology in reference to death by suicide or overdose.

> **Cultural Considerations In Care**
>
> *Reflections on Language*
>
> Reflect on some common expressions or language that you use to say someone has died. Discuss with a partner.
> - What did you learn?
> - Why might people use the particular phrases that they use?

TABLE 13.3 ■ Common Expressions for Death

At peace	Gone to the promised land	Slipped away
At rest	Kicked the bucket	Struck down
Croaked	Lost the battle	Succumbed
Demise	Lost their life	Is with the Creator
Deceased	Met the maker	Is in a better place
Departed	No longer with us	Has been promoted to glory
Didn't make it	Passed	Has gone to the grave
Died	Passed on	Joined the choir eternal
Eternal rest	Passed away	Took their last breath
Expired	Pushing up daisies	Was called home
Gave up the ghost	Resting in peace	Went to be with the Lord
Gone to a better place	Sent into eternity	Went to heaven

A GOOD DEATH

What constitutes a good death? The answer may well depend on who you ask. Literature indicates that there are differences in views of patients, families, caregivers, and health care providers as to what constitutes a good death (Krikorian et al., 2020; Rainsford et al., 2016). From a professional perspective, the concept of **"a good death"** is associated with hospice and palliative care and is synonymous with dying peacefully, dying well (Krikorian et al., 2020). It is a crucial goal of palliative and end-of-life care (Rice, 2019).

Krikorian et al. (2020) undertook a systematic review of patient perspectives on notions of a good death and identified six core elements that captured most of the descriptions. These are (1) control of pain and symptoms; (2) clear decision making; (3) a feeling of closure; (4) being seen and perceived as a person; (5) preparation for death; and (6) being able to give something to others. The authors also note that the specific themes within these core elements are influenced by factors such as culture, religion, life circumstances, age, financial situation, and illness or disease. While there was general agreement with regard to pain and symptom control, there were cultural variations in the degree of autonomy and control for decision making, the desire for being awake and alert or dying in sleep, the desire for spiritual support and the ability to carry out traditions associated with food, and care of the body after death. Rainsford et al. (2016) undertook a scoping review of a good death from the perspective of residents in rural areas and identified similar themes of a good death being peaceful and pain free, controlled (control over symptoms, place of death, decision making, manner of death, and remaining independent), timely (after a well-lived life and with opportunity to say goodbye), and dignified and social (with friends and family present). Both reviews note that the desired experience is very individual and influenced by emotional, spiritual, and cultural factors. Familiarity of place also emerged as a factor for consideration through desire to die at home or at least within the home community. A good death may also be influenced by factors that ease the transition to the afterlife—whether that be dying with sounds of prayers in one's consciousness, facing an auspicious direction, or during a particular time in the seasonal cycle.

MEANING OF SUFFERING

Culture mediates both meaning of and response to suffering. Religious beliefs influence whether suffering is seen as an inherent reality of life that should be accepted or an intrusion on life that should be avoided, prevented, or eliminated (Cain & Denny, 2018; Gielen, 2016). Suffering may be seen as a result of karma (for Hindu and Buddhist people) and thus attributed to one's actions, or as a punishment from God for transgressions as per some Christian views (Gielen et al., 2016; Hall & Hill, 2019). Thus, some patients may look to suffer in silence, and endure pain and suffering as a test of faith or atonement for karma in this life rather than carrying it over to the next life. Patients may also rely more heavily on religious coping than on managing it through medications. In addition to culture and religion, individual life circumstances may also influence the approach to pain management. For a family with a history of addiction and substance use, there may be a reluctance to accept opioids as a form of comfort (Cain et al., 2018). It is imperative that health care providers understand the variability that can exist across cultures and life circumstances and engage with patients and families to understand their perspective. This is essential to provide support in ways that are respectful but also promote informed decision making (see Chapter 4 for further discussion of strategies of validation, accommodation/negotiation, or reframing).

DECISION MAKING AND DISCLOSURE

Western culture privileges the value of individual autonomy with respect to care management and decision making. However, this is inconsistent with many worldviews and thus can place patients and families in a conflictual relationship with health care providers and the system. For some cultures, family involvement in decision making is normal and essential, sometimes to the point where "the patient may be left out of decision making" (Gielen et al., 2016, p. 577), whereas for others decision making is expected from the "expert" providers. Some patients want to know everything about their illness trajectory and prognosis, while others may not want direct communication on poor prognosis and impending death (e.g., many Asian and Indigenous cultures) (Ohr et al., 2017).

While talking about impending death is accepted in some cultures, it is rejected in others. For example, in traditional Chinese culture, specific discussions about death and using the word *death* are not appropriate. There is superstition and a belief that bad luck is associated with using the word *death*. Instead, phrases such as "they are no longer with us" are used. Similarly, in Somali culture people with cancer often hide their diagnosis from others (Canadian Virtual Hospice, 2021). Such taboos and reluctance must be understood from the perspective of the values, beliefs, and worldviews as well as from the perspectives of power, social location, and historical legacy of injustice and racism. Cain et al. (2018) note that "preferences are complex and stem from both cultural and structural factors. Availability, accessibility, acceptability, and knowledge about options also fundamentally influence preferences … [and] cultural meanings emanate within multiple social locations, based on social, historical, and political circumstances" (p. 1409). Thus a reluctance or "preference" to avoid some discussions may be influenced by mistrust of the system, and the real issue may not be that the topic is taboo, but rather the hesitation is based on with whom and how to have the conversation.

Differences may also exist with respect to sources of information. While some patients rely on their care team, others will access information on the Internet and other published resources, and still others may seek out information from family. In emphasizing the importance of communication in hospice and palliative care, Herbstsomer and Stahl (2021) note that minority and non-Western patients rely on multiple sources of information, including family, friends, and spiritual and religious leaders. Seeking such information, rather than relying on the health care team, may be reflective of an inherent mistrust of the system. Providers need to be sensitive to such dynamics and work with spiritual, cultural, and community leaders and navigators to facilitate the needed conversations to support a good death.

The varying approaches to disclosure and decision making can become particularly challenging in navigating issues such as "do not resuscitate" or advance directives. Some patients and families may be willing to engage in the dialogue but not put such wishes in writing—either because they are steeped in oral traditions or because they lack trust in the health care provider or system (Cain et al., 2018; Semlali et al., 2020). The mistrust may be due to poor communication and relationship with the current provider(s) or based on "historic patterns of slavery, racism, and research abuses" (Cain et al., 2018, p. 1411) and fear that such a directive could lead to poor care or neglect. Religious beliefs may be another factor impacting discussions of poor prognosis, as ultimately decisions regarding life and death are seen to be in hands of God, and thus health care providers' estimations of time to impending death may be viewed as insulting and met with anger.

CRUCIAL CONVERSATIONS IN DEATH

Canadian pediatric palliative care expert Dr. Christine Newman identifies critical discussion points that individuals (as young as 8 years old) and their health care teams should have to plan for a good death (CBC, 2010). These crucial conversation points assist in the advance care planning process. Newman cautions that individual wishes for a good death can change throughout the continuum of life. Understanding a patient's notion of a good death happens through an ongoing series of conversations (Muskat et al., 2019, 2020; Newman et al., 2014). As noted in the earlier discussion on disclosure and decision making, such conversations must be viewed through a cultural lens and may need to be mediated by family or other individuals who understand the patient's culture as well as the professional culture of care (cultural brokers).

Newman identifies key topics for crucial conversation that health care providers must have with people (including children as young as 8 years old) as they enter palliative care (CBC, 2010).

1. *Am I dying?*

   The individual must know that they are dying to reflect on their life and contribute to the planning of their good death (Anderson et al., 2019; Rice, 2019). Families may not want to tell the patient that they are dying for fear the loved one will give up hope or stop fighting. Researchers have found individuals usually know they are dying because of the apparent decrease in their overall strength, energy level, and functional abilities (Cohen-Mansfield et al., 2018; Reese et al., 2020; Weaver & Wiener, 2020).

   To prepare for the end of life, some patients will create an **advance directive**—a document that expresses a person's wishes about critical care or life-sustaining medical treatments in the event of incapacitation. The Western values of autonomy and choice shape these documents and the directives. By creating advance directives, the individual ensures that their wishes and values guide decision making during end-of-life discussions. Selecting a substitute decision maker is needed. This person will carry out the dying person's wishes when they become incapacitated. It is important to remember that developing this type of document may not be appropriate in some cultures.

2. *What will my death look like?*

   The patient must know what death will look like as the patient progresses on the illness trajectory. While a precise estimation of the course may not be possible, generalities about what to expect must be presented. This description should provide details of expected symptoms such as pain, respiratory difficulties, or the inability to eat. As well, a discussion about symptom management is necessary.

Cultural Considerations In Care

Traditional Medicine

We must recognize that some patients may want to use traditional medicines for symptom management at the end of life. In Indigenous culture, tobacco, sweet grass, sage, and cedar are some of the medicines that may be used when someone is sick. Individuals and their families find comfort from ceremonies such as visits from Elders, prayers, smudging, sweats, dancing, drumming, healing circles, and a traditional diet of game, fish, nuts, and berries (Canadian Virtual Hospice, 2021). (See https://livingmyculture.ca/culture/first-nations/traditional-medicines-at-end-of-life/.)

3. *Where will I die?*

   In palliative care people may have choices of where they would like to die—hospital, hospice, or home (Gonella et al., 2020). However, these choices may be limited by geographic region, as not all communities have palliative care hospital units or hospice spaces available. When people choose care in the home setting, medical services such as nursing, a respiratory therapy visit, and medical equipment, such as a hospital bed, oxygen, intravenous pumps, and fluid supplements, are brought to the home. The home may be a contentious site depending on the family composition and deterioration of the patient. When small children are in a home, there is evidence to suggest that the death of a parent may harm the child's mental health unless proper supports are in place (Bergman et al., 2017). Hence, the topic of where one's death will occur must be reconsidered often.

4. *Who can be with me?*

The identification of key individuals in the dying patient's life is essential. It is assumed that a spouse, parent, or relation by bloodline takes this role. Health care providers need to remember that the patient must identify the individuals who are their support team and who they wish to be present at the time of death.

In some communities, such as the Haisla Nation (an Indigenous community in British Columbia, Canada), a chief or Elder may be the spokesperson (Terrace/Kitimat and Indigenous Health Improvement Committee, 2016). Family members are supported by the community, which provides a network of comfort and care. Community members provide families with food, support, prayer, and cultural duties associated with death. When death occurs, the whole community comes to the hospital. This gathering is a sign of respect and a way for the community to say goodbye to the person.

5. *How do I say goodbye?*

When two people say goodbye it can be an intensely emotional encounter. Research indicates that acknowledging relationships and saying goodbye to parents, siblings, extended family members, friends, and colleagues can assist in the end of life and grieving process (Grant et al., 2020; Neimeyer et al., 2014). Often people do not know how to say goodbye. The following are some suggestions that could be provided to the patient or family.

■ Reminisce about the relationship
■ Talk about fond memories
■ Watch a favourite movie or listen to music together
■ Visit a special place
■ If the individuals are religious, pray or take part in a ceremony together

6. *How will I be honoured?*

People who are dying may want to actively participate in how they will be remembered through ceremony or the future actions of loved ones. Funerals, for example, are influenced by cultural and religious traditions, family preferences, and costs. Some patients may wish to preorganize a religious service by selecting music, scriptures, coffins or urns, and burial site. Others will leave these matters to the family and community, and for some, knowing that traditions will be upheld by family can be very comforting.

Cultural Competence in Action

More Crucial Conversation Approaches and Questions

Each health care provider needs to formulate their way of speaking with a patient about the end of life. The answers that the patient provides will shape how the health care team provides care.

Beginning the Conversation

"I want to make sure we are always doing the things that help you. We never want to do anything you do not want. I need to know what things are most important to you, given your illness."

"(Patient name), I am part of the care team that will be looking after you as your disease progresses. I want to ask you some questions so we can provide you with the care you want."

Beliefs

- How can I honour your spiritual and cultural beliefs as death approaches?
- Are there any specific ways you want the physical environment to be as death approaches?
- Where do you want to die?
- What is the role of religion or culture when making decisions about illness and treatment?
- Are there any cultural beliefs or traditions that you adhere to that I need to respect as I care for you?

Continued

- Have you made any decisions about advance directives and treatment options at the end of life?
- Are there any specific people you want present as death approaches?
- How do you want to say goodbye to important people in your life?

Support System

- Do you have specific family members or important people in your life that you would like to be involved in your care?
- What is the role of your family or important people in your care?
- Are there any people who you do not want to visit or see you?
- Are there specific people who will direct your care or make decisions if you are no longer able to do so?
- Are there any religious or other leaders who will be involved with your care at the end of life?
- If your condition changes may people still visit?

Pain

- How do you manage comfort and pain?
- How would you like me to help you in managing your pain?

Death

- Are there specific people who you want or do not want present for the death?
- What do they believe about the body after death?
- When death happens, how is your body to be treated?
- Who will make the final plans?

The questions above were created based on the following resources: Rapoport, A., Shaheed, J., Newman, C., et al. (2017). Physician-patient end-of-life care discussions: Correlates and associations with end-of-life care preferences of cancer patients – A cross-sectional survey study. *Palliative Medicine, 30*(3), 253–259; Saccomano, S. J., & Abbatiello, G. A. (2014). Cultural considerations at the end of life. *Nurse Practitioner*, 39(2), 24–31. https://doi.org/10.1097/01.NPR.0000441908.16901.2e.

Palliative Care

The terms *end-of-life care* and *palliative care* are often used interchangeably by health care providers. However, there are distinct differences in these care approaches (Krau, 2016). **Palliative care** focuses on improving the quality of life of patients with serious illnesses, by treating symptoms and providing emotional support (Canadian Nurses Association [CNA], 2017; World Health Organization, 2020). The primary goals of palliative care are (1) treating a person with an illness when a cure or recovery is impossible, and (2) prolonging what the person believes is a life of quality and active living as the disease progresses. Creating an environment for optimal quality of life for the individual and significant people involved in their life may include controlling persistent, distressing, and progressing symptoms. Across the continuum of the individual's illness, attention to all life dimensions, including physical, social, spiritual, and psychological needs, is paramount.

End-of-life care is a phase of palliative care when active dying replaces active living. In this phase, the goal of care is for health care team members to provide supportive care to the individual and their support system as the end of their life nears. A significant component of end-of-life care is the focus on enabling patients to die with dignity (Krau, 2016). Pinpointing when this phase will begin is difficult. Most consider this phase to happen in the last year of life (Lewis, 2018). **Hospice care** refers to care provided to a person with a life-limiting illness that emphasizes pain control and emotional support in the last few months of life (CNA, 2017; Matzo & Sherman, 2014). Hospice care may be provided at home or at an institution, often designed for such care and services.

It is essential for health care providers to begin discussing their wishes for a good death throughout the trajectory of palliation and end of life. The palliative and end-of-life trajectory begins when a patient is diagnosed with a life-limiting illness and continues along the entire continuum of care, to home, hospice, and end-of-life care, and finally to family bereavement after death.

Foundational to a palliative care approach is (1) open, transparent, and honest communication between the health care team and patient and family and (2) enhancing quality of life. The cultural considerations related to end-of-life care and death extend across all end-of-life care and death circumstances, whether death is sudden or expected, with or without palliative and hospice support.

It is important to remember that culture is both patterns and power (see Chapter 1), thus the health inequities that exist in other aspects of health care extend to palliative and hospice care. In a scoping review on barriers to providing culturally competent cancer-related palliative care to LGBT patients, Haviland et al. (2021) note that "LGBT patients and their caregivers experience homophobia, exclusion, social isolation, criminalisation, persecution and fear of discrimination. Additionally, lack of provider knowledge has led to negative patient perceptions by [providers] when providing palliative care" (p. 316). The authors highlight the importance of affirming cultural identity, particularly for patients who may experience a change in their social networks or experience conflict between the chosen family and biological family.

Patients who identify as a racial/ethnic minority tend to underutilize palliative care services and thus bear a greater burden of pain and poor symptom management, which impacts the quality of life (Alderson et al., 2015; Gazaway et al., 2019). Factors impeding the use of services include mistrust of the system, lack of knowledge of disease progression and available care modalities, cultural and language barriers leading to ineffective conversations, and health care providers' lack of understanding of religious and cultural beliefs and preferences.

Gazaway et al. (2019) call for a model of care that integrates palliative care into the chronic illness continuum. The proposed four-phase model includes early palliative care, which consists of education on disease progression, symptom management, and psychological support; episodic palliative care provided during a medical crisis by an interprofessional team; late palliative care where the focus may be on advance care planning; and finally, hospice care for a good death with dignity. Throughout these phases, a trusting relationship between a client and the health care team develops. Critical to the success of this relationship is time for discussion, regular contact, and compassion.

It is also important to recognize the role that culturally specific agencies can play at this critical phase of life. For example, Casey House, Canada's first and only stand-alone hospital/hospice for people with HIV/AIDS with a multidisciplinary approach to health and well-being, opened in 1988. Until this time, people with HIV/AIDS received care from providers dressed in hazmat suits. The philosophy of Casey House was different. The multidisciplinary team at Casey House provided holistic care in a nonjudgemental and stigma-free way. In this home-like setting patients and their loved ones were cared for and treated with respect and dignity. Today, Casey House provides care and services through inpatient and day programs, community care and outreach, social community programming, research, and education (see www.caseyhouse.com).

Another example is All Nations' Healing Hospital, owned and operated by the File Hills Qu'Appelle Tribal Council and Touchwood Agency Tribal Council in Saskatchewan, which has one bed devoted to palliative care services and a home care program. The organization's philosophy of care focuses on delivering safe holistic health care services that embrace First Nation culture and traditions. In addition, traditional medicines, healing rooms, and smudging are available for patients and their families. (See https://allnationshealinghospital.ca/.)

Medical Assistance in Dying: A New End-of-Life Option in Canada

Medical Assistance in Dying (MAiD) is an end-of-life care option available to Canadians who meet a set of legal requirements, which are assessed by authorized health care providers such as

---

TABLE 13.4 ■ **Milestones in Legalization of Medical Assistance in Dying**

- In February 2015, the Supreme Court of Canada ruled in favour of exempting health care providers who participated in the delivery of medications to end a person's life from any clinical liability (Versluis, 2020). Following this, a new timeline set by the Supreme Court gave the federal government until June 6, 2016, to establish new legislation.
- On June 17, 2016, the federal government passed eligibility criteria and safeguards through Bill C-14. This historic motion meant that it was no longer illegal for physicians and nurse practitioners to assist individuals in ending their life, given that all legislative requirements are met. The term *MAiD*, Medical Assistance in Dying, was coined, capturing the role and scope of both physicians and nurse practitioners who are permitted to determine eligibility and administer the medications (Beuthin et al., 2018). Pharmacists were also included in the new laws, allowing for a transparent safeguard of the intended prescriptions prepared for the purposes of MAiD.
- On October 5, 2020, the Minister of Justice and Attorney General of Canada introduced Bill C-7: An act to amend the *Criminal Code (Medical Assistance In Dying)* in Parliament, which proposed changes to Canada's law on medical assistance in dying (Government of Canada, 2021).
- On March 17, 2021, the Canadian Parliament passed the proposed changes to legislation, and Bill C-7 received royal assent. Two new pathways for individuals requesting MAiD had emerged, which all individuals follow to access the process of assessment.

---

medical or nurse practitioners.[1] Eligible persons may choose from one of two routes to receive prescribed medications intended to end their life, including clinician-administered (e.g., intravenous) or self-administered (e.g., oral).

The development of MAiD can be attributed to community pressure. In the early 1990s Sue Rodriguez, a Canadian living with amyotrophic lateral sclerosis (ALS, or Lou Gehrig's disease), petitioned Canadian courts for the legal right to have a physician's help in ending her life at a time of her choosing. At this time, assisting with a suicide was illegal and would result in a prison sentence. This case, while controversial, sparked conversations across Canada about dying with dignity and having the choice to end one's life due to medical circumstances.

In the *Carter vs. Canada* decision, the Court ruled that the Criminal Code provisions infringed on the Charter of Rights and Freedoms. Specifically, this contended with the option of a physician-assisted death for a competent adult person who can clearly consent to the termination of life and who has a grievous and irremediable medical condition (including an illness, disease, or disability) that causes enduring suffering that is intolerable to the individual in the circumstances of their condition. Milestones in the legalization of MAiD are shown in Table 13.4. Table 13.5 shows MAiD eligibility criteria as of March 17, 2021.

TWO-TRACK APPROACH

The revised law in Bill C-7 has introduced a two-track approach to procedural safeguards for clinicians to follow. Each track is identified by the MAiD assessor, who will determine whether a person's natural death is reasonably foreseeable.

---

[1]Under Canadian federal law, all requests for MAiD must be assessed by two independent health care providers, either physicians or nurse practitioners. "To be considered independent means that neither of them:
- Holds a position of authority over the other
- Could knowingly benefit from your death
- Is connected to the other or to you in a way that could affect their objectivity"
  https://www.canada.ca/en/health-canada/services/medical-assistance-dying.html

TABLE 13.5 ■ **Eligibility Criteria and Safeguards as per Bill C-7**

MAiD Eligibility Criteria as of March 17, 2021

Persons who wish to receive MAiD must satisfy the following eligibility criteria:
- Be 18 years of age or older and have decision-making capacity
- Be eligible for publicly funded health care services
- Make a voluntary request that is not the result of external pressure
- Give informed consent to receive MAiD, meaning that the person has consented to receiving MAiD after they have received all information needed to make this decision
- Have a serious and incurable illness, disease, or disability
- Be in an advanced state of irreversible decline in capability
- Have enduring and intolerable physical or psychological suffering that cannot be alleviated under conditions the person considers acceptable

MAiD, Medical Assistance in Dying.
From Nicol, J., & Tiedemann, M. (2021). *Legislative summary of Bill C-7: An act to amend the Criminal Code (Medical Assistance in Dying)*. Library of Parliament Research Publications. https://lop.parl.ca/sites/PublicWebsite/default/en_CA/ResearchPublications/LegislativeSummaries/432C7E; The College of Nurses of Ontario. (2021). *Guidance on nurses' roles in medical assistance in dying*. https://laws-lois.justice.gc.ca/eng/acts/C-46/page-53.html#docCont.

For persons whose natural death is reasonably foreseeable, procedural safeguards have been eased, no longer including a 10-day reflection period as indicated in previous MAiD law.

For persons whose natural death is not reasonably foreseeable, new and strengthened safeguards are in place to promote adequate timing and expert consultation during the MAiD assessment process (Table 13.6).

MENTAL ILLNESS AND MAiD

Persons requesting MAiD who have a sole diagnosis of mental illness are currently not eligible. As per Bill C-7, this exclusion will last until March 17, 2023, which provides the federal government time for further examination and planning of the appropriate safeguards. This also includes additional reviews from experts within related fields, where in turn, new recommendations will be developed for consideration toward the potential changes to MAiD legislation.

CULTURAL IDENTITIES IN MAiD

Federal reporting requirements about persons requesting MAiD have been limited to demographic metrics such as age, diagnosis, gender, and location. Nationwide consultation of proposed changes in MAiD have provoked concerns around marginalized populations, where there was the possibility of inequitable access to MAiD, specifically for vulnerable persons. Bill C-7 has introduced new federal reporting. Changes in the new law related to data collection include race, Indigenous identity, and disability, as well as seeking to determine the presence of individual or systemic inequality or disadvantage in the context or delivery of MAiD (Government of Canada, 2021).

Given the data limitations, it is not surprising that literature on cultural considerations in MAiD is limited, largely theoretical, and anecdotal. Hart (2020) talks about the impact on clergy, Isgandarova (2018) discusses MAiD challenges for Muslim health care providers, and Larm (2019) discusses perspectives on MAiD and dying well at Thrangu Monastery Canada. The key points that

TABLE 13.6 ■ Procedural Safeguards in Medical Assistance in Dying as of March 17, 2021

Safeguards for Persons Whose Natural Death Is Reasonably Foreseeable

The following procedural safeguards now apply to persons whose natural death **is** reasonably foreseeable:

- Request for Medical Assistance in Dying (MAiD) must be made in writing after the person is informed that they have a grievous and irremediable medical condition.
- A written request must be signed by one independent witness (this can be a paid professional person, or a health care worker can be an independent witness).
- Two independent doctors or nurse practitioners must complete an assessment that confirms all of the eligibility requirements are met.
- The person must be informed that they can withdraw their request at any time, in any manner.
- The person must be given an opportunity to withdraw consent and must expressly confirm their consent immediately before receiving MAiD (in certain circumstances, there may be an opportunity to waive the "final consent" requirement, which can be arranged in writing between the MAiD provider and person).

Safeguards for Persons Whose Natural Death Is Not Reasonably Foreseeable

The following procedural safeguards now apply to persons whose natural death **is not** reasonably foreseeable (*indicates safeguards specific to those requests):

- Request for MAiD must be made in writing after the person is informed that they have a grievous and irremediable medical condition.
- A written request must be signed by one independent witness (this can be a paid professional person, or a health care worker can be an independent witness).
- Two independent doctors or nurse practitioners must complete an assessment that confirms all of the eligibility requirements are met.
  - If neither of the two practitioners who assesses eligibility has expertise in the medical condition that is causing the person's suffering, they must consult with a practitioner who has such expertise.
- The person must be informed that they can withdraw their request at any time, in any manner.
- The person must be informed of available and appropriate means to relieve their suffering, including counselling services, mental health and disability support services, community services, and palliative care, and must be offered consultations with professionals who provide those services.
- The person and the practitioners must have discussed reasonable and available means to relieve the person's suffering, and agree that the person has seriously considered those means.
- The eligibility assessments must take at least 90 days, but this period can be shortened if the person is about to lose the capacity to make health care decisions, as long as both assessments have been completed.
- Immediately before MAiD is provided, the practitioner must give the person an opportunity to withdraw their request and ensure that they give express consent.

From Government of Canada. (2021). *Bill C-7: An act to amend the Criminal Code (Medical Assistances in Dying)*. https://parl.ca/DocumentViewer/en/43-2/bill/C-7/royal-assent.

emerge in these discussion are as follows: (1) the literature to date looks at MAiD from a theological perspective; more information and understanding from a practice perspective are needed; (2) religious perspectives are interpreted by people in various ways, and the values of compassion, mitigating suffering, and dignity are among the reasons MAiD may be acceptable to people of different faiths; and (3) there is a need for more open dialogue around MAiD to promote awareness (self-awareness and information about MAiD), decrease feelings of isolation and secrecy, and increase opportunities for support for those encountering MAiD as patients, family members, or providers.

A SNAPSHOT OF MAiD

A person may initiate a request for MAiD through their primary care provider, health care specialists, or provincial MAiD coordination service. The preliminary stages of the process will include the completion of two independent assessments to determine eligibility, as well as a written request form for MAiD signed in front of one independent witness. With all subsequent requirements satisfied, a person may choose to plan details surrounding their death with the MAiD provider and their loved ones, which may include religious, spiritual, personal, or cultural practices throughout the process. Because MAiD is planned in advance, there is an opportunity to openly discuss a person's end-of-life preferences and to help support their vision of what a good death means to them. The date and time of MAiD is generally decided by the person, with consideration of the MAiD provider's availability, who can assist with ordering the required medications.

Cultural Considerations in Care

Medical Assistance in Dying Provides Opportunity for Affirmation

The following scenarios have been adapted from practice experiences, to share insights and preserve confidentiality.

1. **A gay man in his 60s**. During enactment of Medical Assistance in Dying (MAiD), the patient's partner and the patient's parents were present together. This was significant as initially the parents struggled with their son's homosexuality and were not accepting. Over time, their relationships improved and togetherness at the final moments was seen as an affirmation of identity and an opportunity for togetherness that would continue between the parents and partner. The patient also compared this new end-of-life option to the impact of the legalization of same-sex marriage.
2. **A woman chose MAiD after breast cancer diagnosis and metastasis**. The Christian faith community had always been very important to her, and she initially struggled with how her decision would be perceived by her faith community and how to seek blessing from her faith leader at this important time in her life. Through dialogue with the team, she was comforted by the reassurance of confidentiality and privacy. The death certificate did not show MAiD, thus her choices regarding MAiD were not at risk for disclosure through records. She also found the courage to reach out to her faith leader, who was very supportive and was present during the MAiD procedure. She did not want to have this done at home, so as not to have home associated with her death or the burden of aftercare to fall to her family. She died peacefully, with her family and clergy present in hospital.
3. **Hispanic patient for whom English was not their first language**. This patient became aware of MAiD through the media. Although this was what he wanted, the family was against this. Over time, with the support of the care team, the family came to accept the patient's wishes and felt prepared to visit the patient in hospital. The patient was very concerned for his family as he understood their difficulties and prioritized their needs and comfort over his wishes. He shared the date with his family but decided not to disclose the time of the MAiD procedure. Interestingly, the family called the patient that day and upon learning of the timing, they chose to come in and be with the patient during the provision of MAiD. The patient's family expressed gratitude to the care team for respecting his wishes and appreciated that this was what he wanted.

MAiD AND HEALTH CARE PROVIDERS

While physicians and nurse practitioners are legally permitted to determine eligibility and provide MAiD, other health care providers may not always have a clear scope as it relates to the MAiD process. Despite the lack of role clarity, professional colleges and associations encourage their members to continue providing routine and optimal care and to remain practising within their scope of practice. Assistance from various health professions such as nurses, social workers, personal support workers, ethicists, and spiritual care practitioners, may create opportunities to collaborate in providing support to persons and their families throughout the MAiD process. While legislation allows for this, attention has not been afforded to health care providers who must participate in MAiD (Versluis, 2020). More attention must be paid to assisting all health providers in addressing moral dilemmas that can arise from MAiD procedures (Canadian Medical Association, 2017). Health professional schools and health care organizations must work with students and providers to reflect on this new end-of-life care intervention and how to cope with emotional and social distress that may arise. Bruce and Beuthin (2020) explored how nurses' overall experience of suffering is shaped by participating in MAiD and note that MAiD provided opportunities for "transformation" of the struggles and frustrations that often accompany the "suffering" and "failure to do more" associated with end-of-life care into narratives of beautiful death characterized by peaceful dying and gratitude. The participants also noted "potential harms if assisted dying is not implemented with the utmost care" and wondered if the "sacredness of dying [would be] diminished over time" and expressed concern about potentially becoming desensitized (Bruce & Beuthin, 2020, p. 273).

The MAiD process can occur in a variety of locations: a home, a hospital, a hospice, a medical office, or care facility (British Columbia Coroners Service, 2017); however, accessibility to MAiD in the these settings may slightly differ or pose significant barriers, which in turn, introduces potential process delays. For instance, patients may be required to undergo an additional assessment from a MAiD provider who works in a different setting, as part of that MAiD provider's own legal safeguard to ensure eligibility is confirmed. When possible, physicians and nurse practitioners involved with an individual's assessments and provision of MAiD are generally aligned with the identified location of MAiD, which promotes continuity of care and streamlines safeguards and documentation.

Bereavement

When a patient dies, the attention of health care providers turns to the family and loved ones who begin the stage of bereavement. In this stage, people experience a variety of reactions to the loss of a loved person by death. *Bereavement* and *grief* are sometimes used interchangeably. Grief is not limited to death; it is an emotional and psychological reaction to loss (Grant et al., 2020; Silverman et al., 2020).

Like other aspects of life and death, bereavement and grief are also shaped by cultural patterns and individual characteristics. As discussed earlier, cultures and communities often have traditions that are designed to create time and space for grieving (the period of mourning) and support from others (memorial service, visitation, bringing food). The traditions vary across all cultures and not all individuals desire or experience the traditions the same way. Each person responds to bereavement and grief in different ways.

Health care providers often do not know what to say to family members following a death. Table 13.7 provides some suggestions to consider. This is not an exhaustive list, and we invite readers to reflect on their experiences of how to support family and community at times of bereavement and grief.

THE POWER OF RITUALS

Doka (2015) notes the importance of rituals throughout illness, death, and the mourning period. Rituals can be public or private, cultural or individual. When individuals don't have traditional rituals that are meaningful to them, they can be invited to create rituals for themselves.

TABLE 13.7 ■ What to Say When You Don't Know What to Say

Below are some statements that can be used by health care providers to begin the conversation at times of bereavement.

1. **I am so sorry for your loss**.
   It is important that health care providers not pretend to understand how another person is feeling. Do not pretend to understand the pain or the significance of the loss.

2. **Refer to the person by name**.
   Language is particularly important when discussing the death of a loved one with family. Do not use words such as "the deceased," "your dead husband" and so on. For example, if a family member asks a nurse, "Where will you be taking him now?", respond using the patient's name: "I will be taking Mr. Y to the morgue once you have said your goodbyes. The funeral home will pick him up from there."

3. **Ask: "What do you need? May I ..."**
   The extreme emotion and shock that engulf a family member at the time of a loved one's death may be overwhelming, whether the death is anticipated or unanticipated. It is important for health care providers to ask how they can help. Often people are unaware of the help that they may need. Some suggestions:
   - Calling other family members
   - Providing a medical letter for their employer or school
   - Giving the contact information for the local funeral home

4. **Offer "memory-making" options, if culturally appropriate.**
   Often family members wish to have a part of the person as a keepsake or engage in a ritual (e.g., touching the feet of a relative as a sign of respect). Things such as a lock of hair or a thumb-hand- or footprint, or a picture of the person can be meaningful for some family members. For others, time, privacy, and support may be most meaningful.

5. **Make connections to support services, if culturally appropriate.**
   Immediately following the death of a loved one, people are in shock and may not recognize a need for assistance as they work through their grief. Most communities have resources to assist people with their grief following the loss of a loved one. These may be found through the following:
   - Faith leaders
   - Community grief recovery support groups
   - Social workers and counsellors
   - Employee assistance benefits
   - Employer or school
   - The local funeral home

Rituals, when used beyond the immediate death traditions, such as funeral and mourning period, can serve as a vehicle for continuity with deceased relatives. For some this may be in the form of a celebration or toast to mark an anniversary, and for others it may be more elaborate, such as annual worship or ceremonies that pay respect to ancestors. Such ceremonies exist across cultures. Such "*rituals of continuity* reaffirm a continuing bond with the deceased—recognition that the relationship is retained even in death" (Doka, 2015, p. 240). This continuity and connectedness can extend to a continuing relationship with God (Gielen et al., 2016). Doka also identifies *rituals of transition* that facilitate movement in the grief process and *rituals of reconciliation* that facilitate finding ways of addressing unfinished business. Expressing remorse or forgiveness can be an example of a reconciliation ritual. *Rituals of affirmation* are like those of reconciliation but focus on affirming the value or support the deceased person(s) has provided through opportunity or the impact of their legacy (Doka, 2015).

> **Cultural Considerations in Care**
>
> *Wiping the Tears*
>
> Elder Elva Jameson experienced grief following her daughter's death. She attended counselling but it did not help. This caused her to return to her people. The *wiping the tears ceremony* was done in her home. Elder Elva believes the ceremony was effective because it was at the spirit level—not a mental, emotional, or cognitive level. For her community, the connection between people is at the spirit level. She feels that the songs of the ceremony are powerful and have an impact on the entire body. Since her experience she has utilized the ceremony to help others through their grief. See https://livingmyculture. ca/culture/first-nations/wiping-the-tears-ceremony/.

Summary

Health care providers must understand that each person has different needs surrounding death and dying. Culture can shape how people experience and respond to the end of a life. Caring for a person and their family experiencing the end of life must be done with kindness, compassion, respect, and sensitivity.

The act of assisted dying in Canada is relatively new compared to other end-of-life care approaches, which highlights this timely need to better understand the impact of culture in an individual's decision to pursue MAiD and how the role of culture influences the planning of one's death. While the topic of MAiD may still be considered unconventional or unfamiliar, this evolving topic continues to incite and provoke meaningful discussions across Canada, especially as MAiD legislation is evaluated with the potential of revised changes. Ultimately, improving access to optimal end-of-life care and resources will support individuals with informed decision making that will foster a person-centred approach in their care journey with their families, loved ones, and health care team.

The physical and psychosocial demands of caring for people at the end of life can impact health care providers and potentially compromise care. Health care providers need to engage in personal health and wellness activities in order to care for people and their families at the end of life.

 evolve.elsevier.com/Srivastava/culturalcompetence/.

Questions for Review and Discussion

1. What self-care activities do you engage in on a regular basis? Are there additional activities you would like to get support for?
2. A patient expresses their concerns to you about suffering near their end of life and shares that they do not want to be in pain when they die. Reflecting on the themes in this chapter, how would you continue supporting this patient?
3. Reflect on a recent experience you have had with death of a family member, friend, or patient. What factors influenced the decisions and activities that happened upon death?
4. Visit the website https://livingmyculture.ca/topic/after-death-and-ceremonies. Choose a culture you are unfamiliar with and watch a video clip. How are the views presented similar to or different from yours? What can health care providers do to support a family with that perspective?

Group Experiential/Reflection Activity

CRUCIAL CONVERSATIONS ROLE PLAY ACTIVITY (30 MINUTES)

As a nurse you need to participate in crucial conversations with patients about their end-of-life expectations. The aim of this activity is to give you practice in having a crucial conversation.

1. Person 1 assumes the role of the patient.

2. Person 2 assumes the role of the nurse.

3. Others can be observers and/or may switch roles partway through the role play.

Preparation (5 minutes):

1. Create a script of questions and responses that you anticipate are needed when having a conversation about the end of life with a patient.

2. Think about how you might respond in the upcoming activity.

Role play activity (10 minutes):

The conversation begins with (1) the nurse initiating the discussion and (2) the patient responding.

Debrief and discussion (15 minutes):

- How did each of you feel about this conversation?
- What went well?
- Re-examine the conversation. Where is improvement needed?
- If you were to have a conversation with a real patient, how would you approach the crucial conversation?

References

Alderson, M., Parent-Rocheleau, X., & Mishara, B. (2015). Critical review on suicide among nurses: What about work-related factors? *Crisis, 36*(2), 91–101. https://doi.org/10.1027/0227-5910/a000305.

Alladin, W. (2015). The Islamic way of death and dying: Homeword bound. In C. M. Parkes, P. Laungani, & W. Young (Eds.), *Death and bereavement across cultures* (2nd ed., pp. 110–132). Routlede. https://doi.org/10.4324/9781315721088.

Anderson, R. J., Bloch, S., Armstrong, M., et al. (2019). Communication between healthcare professionals and relatives of patients approaching the end-of-life: A systematic review of qualitative evidence. *Palliative Medicine, 33*(8), 926–941. https://doi.org/10.1177/0269216319852007.

Beaune, L., & Newman, C. (2003). In search of a good death. *BMJ, 327*(7408), 222–223. https://doi.org/10.1136/bmj.327.7408.222-b.

Bergman, A. S., Axberg, U., & Hanson, E. (2017). When a parent dies – A systematic review of the effects of support programs for parentally bereaved children and their caregivers. *BMC Palliative Care, 16*(1), 39. https://doi.org/10.1186/s12904-017-0223-y.

Beuthin, R., Bruce, A., & Scaia, M. (2018). Medical Assistance in Dying (MAiD): Canadian nurses' experiences. *Nursing Forum, 53*(4), 511–520. https://doi.org/10.1111/nuf.12280.

British Columbia Coroners Service. (2017). *Coroners service death review panel: A review of medically assisted deaths for the period of January 1–December 31, 2016.* https://www2.gov.bc.ca/assets/gov/birth-adoption-death-marriage-and-divorce/deaths/coroners-service/death-review-panel/maid_panel_report_2017_final.pdf

Brown, J., Goodridge, D., & Thorpe, L. (2020). Medical Assistance in Dying in health sciences curricula: A qualitative exploratory study. *Canadian Medical Education Journal, 2020*(6), 79–89. https://doi.org/10.36834/cmej.69325.

Bruce, A., & Beuthin, R. (2020). Medically assisted dying in Canada: "Beautiful death" is transforming nurses' experiences of suffering. *Canadian Journal of Nursing Research, 52*(4), 268–277. https://doi.org/10.1177/0844562119856234.

Cain, C. L., Surbone, A., Elk, R., et al. (2018). Culture and palliative care: Preferences, communication, meaning, and mutual decision making. *Journal of Pain and Symptom Management, 55*(5), 1408–1419. https://doi.org/10.1016/j.jpainsymman.2018.01.007.

Cain, J. M., & Denny, L. (2018). Palliative care in women's cancer care: Global challenges and advances. *International Journal of Gynecology and Obstetrics, 143*, 153–158. https://doi.org/10.1002/ijgo.12624.

Canadian Medical Association. (2017). *CMA policy medical assistance in dying rationale.* https://policybase.cma.ca/documents/policypdf/PD17-03.pdf

Canadian Nurses Association (CNA). (2017). *Palliative and end of life care.* https://www.cna-aiic.ca/en/policy-advocacy/advocacy-priorities/medical-assistance-in-dying

Canadian Virtual Hospice. (2021). *Talking about cancer is taboo.* https://livingmyculture.ca/culture/somali/talking-about-cancer-is-taboo/

CBC. (2010). *Defining a good death: An interview with Dr. Christine Newman*. https://www.cbc.ca/player/play/1898616759

Chan, C. W. H., Chow, M. C. M., Chan, S., et al. (2020). Nurses' perceptions of and barriers to the optimal end-of-life care in hospitals: A cross-sectional study. *Journal of Clinical Nursing, 29*(7–8), 1209–1219. https://doi.org/10.1111/jocn.15160.

Cheung, T., Lee, P. H., & Yip, P. S. F. (2015). Suicidality among Hong Kong nurses: Prevalence and correlates. *Journal of Advanced Nursing, 72*(4), 836–848. https://doi.org/10.1111/jan.12869.

Cohen-Mansfield, J., Skornick-Bouchbinder, M., & Brill, S. (2018). Trajectories of end of life: A systematic review. *The Journals of Gerontology: Series B, 73*(4), 564–572. https://doi.org/10.1093/geronb/gbx093.

College of Nurses of Ontario. (2021). *Guidance on nurses' roles in Medical Assistance in Dying*. https://www.cno.org/globalassets/docs/prac/41056-guidance-on-nurses-roles-in-maid.pdf

Doka, K. J. (2015). Spirituality: QUO VADIS? In J. M. Stillion & T. Attig (Eds.), *Death, dying, and bereavement: Contemporary perspectives, institutions, and practices accounts*. Springer.

Gaun, M. (2015). The Buddhist way of death. In C. M. Parkes, P. Laungani, & W. Young (Eds.), *Death and bereavement across cultures* (2nd ed., pp. 61–72). Routledge.

Gazaway, S., Stewart, M., & Schumacher, A. (2019). Integrating palliative care into the chronic illness continuum: A conceptual model for minority populations. *Journal of Racial and Ethnic Health Disparities, 6*, 1078–1086. https://doi.org/10.1007/s40615-019-00610-y.

Gielen, J. (2016). Education in care ethics: A way to increase palliative care awareness in India. *International Journal of Ethics Education, 1*(1), 15–24. https://doi.org/10.1007/s40889-015-0003-6.

Gielen, J., Bhatnagar, S., & Chaturvedi, S. K. (2016). Spirituality as an ethical challenge in Indian palliative care: A systematic review. *Palliative and Supportive Care, 14*(5), 561–582. https://doi.org/10.1017/S147895151500125X.

Gire, J. (2014). How death imitates life: Cultural influences on conceptions of death and dying. *Online Readings in Psychology and Culture, 6*(2). https://doi.org/10.9707/2307-0919.1120.

Glaser, B. G., & Strauss, A. (1968). *Time for dying*. Routledge.

Gonella, S., Basso, I., De Marinis, M. G., et al. (2020). Communication between healthcare professionals and relatives of patients approaching the end-of-life: A systematic review of qualitative evidence. *Palliative Medicine, 29*(6), 64–74. https://doi.org/10.1177/1755738015581026.

Government of Canada. (2021). *Bill C-7: An act to amend the Criminal Code (Medical Assistances in Dying)*. https://parl.ca/DocumentViewer/en/43-2/bill/C-7/royal-assent

Grant, P. C., Depner, R. M., Levy, K., et al. (2020). Family caregiver perspectives on end-of-life dreams and visions during bereavement: A mixed methods approach. *Journal of Palliative Medicine, 23*(1), 48–53. https://doi.org/10.1089/jpm.2019.0093.

Hall, E. M., & Hill, P. (2019). Meaning-making, suffering, and religion: A worldview conception. *Mental Health, Religion & Culture, 22*(5), 467–479.

Hart, A. E. (2020). *Medical Assistance in Dying and its impact on clergy who have accompanied patients through the procedure. [Unpublished master's thesis]*. Atlantic School of Theology. https://library2.smu.ca/bitstream/handle/01/29494/Hart_April_GRP_2020.pdf?sequence=1&isAllowed=y

Haviland, K., Walters, C., & Newman, S. (2021). Barriers to palliative care in sexual and gender minority patients with cancer: A scoping review of the literature. *Health and Social Care in the Community, 29*, 305–318. https://doi.org/10.1111/hsc.13126.

Herbstsomer, R. A., & Stahl, S. T. (2021). Cross cultural experiences of hospice and palliative care services: A thematic analysis. *OMEGA – Journal of Death and Dying, 84*(2), 551–556. https://doi.org/10.1177/0030222820904205.

Isgandarova, N. (2018). Medical Assistance in Dying: Challenges for Muslim healthcare professionals. *Journal of Pastoral Care & Counseling, 72*(3), 202–211. https://doi.org/10.1177/1542305018796184.

Krau, S. D. (2016). The difference between palliative care and end of life care: More than semantics. *The Nursing Clinics of North America, 51*, ix–x. https://doi.org/10.1016/j.cnur.2016.07.002.

Krikorian, A., Maldonado, C., & Pastrana, T. (2020). Patients' perspectives on the notion of a good death: A systematic review of the literature. *Journal of Pain and Symptom Management, 59*(1), 152–164. https://doi.org/10.1016/j.jpainsymman.2019.07.033.

Larm, J. (2019). Good deaths: Perspectives on dying well and on Medical Assistance in Dying at Thrangu Monastery Canada. *Religions, 10*, 70. https://doi.org/10.3390/rel10020070.

Laungani, P., & Laungani, A. (2015). Death in a Hindu family. In C. M. Parkes, P. Laungani, & W. Young (Eds.), *Death and bereavement across cultures* (2nd ed., pp. 42–60). Routledge.

Levine, E. (2015). Jewish views and customs on death. In C. M. Parkes, P. Laungani, & W. Young (Eds.), *Death and bereavement across cultures* (2nd ed., pp. 76–93). Routledge.

Lewis, R. (2018). End-of-life care in non-malignant conditions. *InnovAiT: Education and Inspiration for General Practice, 11*(1), 41–47. https://doi.org/10.1177/1755738017736910.

Linzitto, J. P., & Grance, G. (2017). Health professionals' quality of life in relation to end of life care. *Current Opinion in Supportive and Palliative Care, 11*(4), 306–309. https://doi.org/10.1097/SPC.0000000000000307.

Matzo, M., & Sherman, D. W. (2014). *Palliative care nursing: Quality care to the end of life* (4th ed.). Springer Publishing Company.

McGilton, K. S., Tourangeau, A., Kavcic, C., et al. (2013). Determinants of regulated nurses' intention to stay in long-term care homes. *Journal of Nursing Management, 21*, 771–781. https://doi.org/10.1111/jonm.12130.

McMorrow, S., & Wiltse, P. (2019). Trauma sensitive training needs for nurses working with families. *International Journal of Caring Sciences, 12*(2), 1213–1217.

Miller, K.-L., Reeves, S., Zwarenstein, M., et al. (2008). Nursing emotion work and interprofessional collaboration in general internal medicine wards: A qualitative study. *Journal of Advanced Nursing, 64*(4), 332–343. https://doi.org/10.1111/j.1365-2648.2008.04768.x.

Mills, J., Wand, T., & Fraser, J. A. (2018). Exploring the meaning and practice of self-care among palliative care nurses and doctors: A qualitative study. *BMC Palliative Care, 17*(1), 63. https://doi.org/10.1186/s12904-018-0318-0.

Muskat, B., Greenblatt, A., Anthony, S., et al. (2020). The experiences of physicians, nurses, and social workers providing end-of-life care in a pediatric acute-care hospital. *Death Studies, 44*(2), 105–116. https://doi.org/10.1080/07481187.2018.1526829.

Neimeyer, R. A., Klass, D., & Dennis, M. R. (2014). A social constructionist account of grief: Loss and the narration of meaning. *Death Studies, 38*(8), 485–498. https://doi.org/10.1080/07481187.2014.913454.

Newman, C., Rapoport, A., & Sangha, G. (2014). Ethical conflicts that may arise when caring for dying children. In R. Zlotnik Shaul (Ed.), *Paediatric patient and family-centred care: Ethical and legal issues. International library of ethics, law, and the new medicine* (pp. 321–335). Springer. https://doi.org/10.1007/978-1-4939-0323-8_18.

Nicol, J., & Tiedemann, M. (2021). *Legislative summary of Bill C-7: An act to amend the Criminal Code (Medical Assistance in Dying)*. Library of Parliament Research Publications. https://lop.parl.ca/sites/PublicWebsite/default/en_CA/ResearchPublications/LegislativeSummaries/432C7E

Niehaus, J. Z., Palmer, M., LaPradd, M., et al. (2020). Pediatric resident perception and participation in end-of-life care. *American Journal of Hospice and Palliative Medicine, 37*(11), 936–942. https://doi.org/10.1177/1049909120913041.

Nolte, A. G. W., Downing, C., Temane, A., et al. (2017). Compassion fatigue in nurses: A metasynthesis. *Journal of Clinical Nursing, 26*, 4364–4378. https://doi.org/10.1111/jocn.13766.

Ohr, S., Jeong, S., & Saul, P. (2017). Cultural and religious beliefs and values, and their impact on preferences for end-of-life care among four ethnic groups of community-dwelling older persons. *Journal of Clinical Nursing, 26*(11–12), 1681–1689. https://doi.org/10.1111/jocn.13572.

Parkes, C. M. (2015). Help for the dying and bereaved. In C. M. Parkes, P. Laungani, & W. Young (Eds.), *Death and bereavement across cultures* (2nd ed., pp. 166–177). Routledge.

Rainsford, S., Macleod, R. D., & Glasgow, N. J. (2016). Place of death in rural palliative care: A systematic review. *Palliative Medicine, 30*(8), 745–763. https://doi.org/10.1177/0269216316628779.

Rapoport, A., Shaheed, J., Newman, C., et al. (2017). Physician-patient end-of-life care discussions: Correlates and associations with end-of-life care preferences of cancer patients—A cross-sectional survey study. *Palliative Medicine, 30*(3), 253–259. https://doi.org/10.1177/1527154416642664.

Rasheed, S. (2015). Self-awareness as a therapeutic tool for nurse/client relationship. *International Journal of Caring Science, 8*(1), 211–216.

Reese, D. J., Buila, S., Cox, S., et al. (2020). Truth telling as an element of culturally competent care at end of life. *American Journal of Hospice and Palliative Medicine, 34*(6), 181–188. https://doi.org/10.1177/1043659615606203.

Rice, M. (2019). *A good death*. Murdoch Books Pty Limited.

Rosenblatt, P. C. (2015). Grief in small scale societies. In C. M. Parkes, P. Laungani, & W. Young (Eds.), *Death and bereavement across cultures* (2nd ed., pp. 23–41). Routledge.

Saccomano, S. J., & Abbatiello, G. A. (2014). Cultural considerations at the end of life. *Nurse Practitioner*, *39*(2), 24–31. https://doi.org/10.1097/01.NPR.0000441908.16901.2e.

Semlali, I., Tamches, E., Singy, P., et al. (2020). Introducing cross-cultural education in palliative care: Focus groups with experts on practical strategies. *BMC Palliative Care*, *19*, 171. https://doi.org/10.1186/s12904-020-00678-y.

Shariff, A., Olson, J., Salas, A. S., et al. (2017). Nurses' experiences of providing care to bereaved families who experience unexpected death in intensive care units: A narrative overview. *The Canadian Journal of Critical Care Nursing*, *28*(1), 21–29.

Shi, H., Shan, B., Zheng, J., et al. (2019). Knowledge and attitudes toward end-of-life care among community health care providers and its influencing factors in China: A cross-sectional study. *Medicine*, *98*(45). e17683–e17683. https://doi.org/10.1097/MD.0000000000017683.

Silverman, G. S., Baroiller, A., & Hemer, S. R. (2020). Culture and grief: Ethnographic perspectives on ritual, relationships and remembering. *Death Studies*, *45*(1), 1–8. https://doi.org/10.1080/07481187.2020.1851885.

Sinai Chapels. (2021). *Shiva customs: A guide to Jewish funerals & customs*. https://jewishfunerals.com/shiva-customs/

Srivastava, R., & Srivastava, R. (2019). Impact of cultural identity on mental health in post-secondary students. *International Journal of Mental Health and Addiction*, *17*. https://doi.org/10.1007/s11469-018-0025-3.

Terrace/Kitimat and Indigenous Health Improvement Committee. (2016). *Cultural practices around death* [Video]. Haisla Nation. Indigenous Health, Northern Health. YouTube. https://www.youtube.com/watch?v=gdjnSp3Wxd8&feature=youtu.be

Versluis, D. (2020). Spotlight on unique advanced practice roles in Canada: MAiD. In E. Staples, R. Pilon, & R. A. Hannon (Eds.), *Canadian perspectives in advanced practice nursing* (2nd ed., pp. 538–539). Canadian Scholars.

Weaver, M. S., & Wiener, L. (2020). Applying palliative care principles to communicate with children about COVID-19. *Journal of Pain and Symptom Management*, *60*(1), e8–e11. https://doi.org/10.1016/j.jpainsymman.2020.03.020.

World Health Organization (WHO). (2020). *Palliative care* [Fact sheet]. https://www.who.int/news-room/fact-sheets/detail/palliative-care

Zheng, R., Lee, S. F., & Bloomer, M. J. (2016). How new graduate nurses experience patient death: A systematic review and qualitative meta-synthesis. *International Journal of Nursing Studies*, *53*, 320–330. https://doi.org/10.1016/j.ijnurstu.2015.09.013.

CHAPTER 14

Cultural Considerations in Mental Health Practice

Ann Pottinger and Stephen G. Lincoln[1]

At the end of this chapter, the learner will be able to:

- Explain how culture influences views on mental health and mental illness
- Recognize the value of integrating the expertise of patients and families to enhance care
- Discuss the following core areas of cultural influence and their implications for mental health providers:
  - Views of mental health and illness
  - Emotional expression and concepts of distress
  - Communication and its context
  - Influence of collectivism
  - Experiences of racism, oppression, and trauma
  - Working with families and communities
  - Program development and working with families
- Assess some clinical tools, including cultural (clinical) formulation, for culturally competent mental health practice

6Ps care planning grid	Cultural idiom of distress	LEARN
Collectivism	Cultural mindedness (CM)	Self-reflexivity
Critical reflection	Cultural safety	Social stressors
Cultural explanations	Culturally adapted	Somatization
Cultural formulation interview (CFI)	cognitive behaviour therapy (CA-CBT)	
Cultural identity	Explanatory model	

---

[1] The authors acknowledge Hung-Tat (Ted) Lo, the former co-author of this chapter, some of whose ideas continue to be reflected in this updated chapter.

Culture shapes our health beliefs and practices, including what experiences are considered illnesses and how or whether they should be treated. Consistent with these notions, culture influences our views of mental health, mental illnesses, and addiction, and these views, in turn, shape how particular health conditions are both conceptualized and experienced. Beliefs about mental illnesses are intricately connected with religion, spirituality, and tradition, which are components of culture. For example, if psychosis is viewed as a manifestation of evil possession, then the action might be to exorcise.[2] If depression is perceived as "laziness," then the response might be some form of exclusion or efforts aimed at improving work ethic. Whereas when a mental illness is viewed as an imbalance of some kind, such as a chemical imbalance, then efforts focus on achieving balance by some means, including the use of psychotropic medication. Culture, including the religious aspect of culture and other social norms, may determine if an addiction is considered an illness. The view may be that the individual has control over the use of a substance and therefore substance abuse is not an illness.

Another way in which culture influences our views is related to how mental health is understood in itself; whether it even exists, and, if it exists, whether it is understood separate from physical, spiritual, or overall health. Across cultures, mental illnesses are accompanied by stigma. However, how stigma is enacted or experienced is also shaped by culture. For instance, while a family with a mostly individualist worldview may be negatively impacted by stigma due to an individual's illness, in a highly collectivist family where the smallest unit of identity is the family, the illness is experienced by the family unit who, in turn, may experience significant exclusion from key aspects of a community, depending on the culture (also see Chapter 7).

Mental health treatment, and the settings in which treatment takes place, varies from culture to culture. Culture not only influences our views about mental health, mental illnesses, and addictions, but it also has a notable impact on health-seeking behaviours and treatment options. Mental health care and psychiatry have their own cultures that have included confinement, institutionalization, and the violation of rights of groups of people. Addiction treatment has its own culture that includes an emphasis on self-help. It is important to recognize the culture of the organization or services providing care and support. Culture influences the attitudes of patients, families, and care providers, and the settings and systems within which care is provided (Gopalkrishnan, 2018). The effectiveness of that care is shaped by the impact it has on the patient throughout the entire care process, based on complex cultural nuances of both patient and setting. Some of these cultural subtleties exist in the areas of emotional expression, shame, power dynamics, and spiritual beliefs (Hechanova & Waelde, 2017), as well as in communication styles. The day-to-day experiences of interacting with the world are all subject to being filtered and interpreted through culture. At the same time, mental health assessments significantly depend on observation and assessment techniques, which are products of the subjective experience of the assessor who must work with few objective tools such as radiographs or blood work. In other words, the clinician is also the diagnostic and therapeutic instrument, and the culture of the clinician can significantly shape the interaction. The development of clinical competency to work effectively with patients from diverse cultures is thus an essential part of professional development for any mental health care provider in the increasingly diverse environments in which we work. In this chapter, we discuss seven core areas of diverse cultural influences that have implications for mental health practice. The vital concepts of power dynamics, safety, and trust are examined throughout the chapter, along with the need for critical reflection and self-reflexivity. These core areas and vital concepts are put forth and proposed to ultimately guide mental health practice that is culturally congruent.

---

[2] *Exorcism* generally refers to the forcing out or attempts to force out evil spirits from a person or place using rituals that may involve prayer or magic.

Core Areas for Cultural Competence in Mental Health Practice

Culturally competent mental health practice requires awareness, knowledge, and, ultimately, the use of skills in some key areas at various stages throughout therapeutic encounters. Some core areas require consideration when providing mental health care across cultures, when working within specific ethnocultural communities (Filmer & Herbig, 2018), or when addressing mental health issues across clinical populations. Table 14.1 shows the seven core areas that require careful consideration in mental health. The concepts of power dynamics, trust, and safety are paramount among and throughout these areas.

Views of Mental Health and Illnesses

It is critical to understand diverse cultural views on mental health and illnesses as they influence both the paths of help that are sought and the types of treatment considered acceptable (Chander et al., 2019). As discussed in the introduction, such views influence what is considered a mental illness and the causes of mental illnesses. For example, in Syria, notions of psychological well-being and mental health are typically associated with negative implications, and suffering is viewed as a normal part of life that generally does not require intervention, except when severe and debilitating (Hassan et al., 2015). Some behaviours that are suggestive of mental illness to health care providers may be viewed by some groups and communities as a "curse," "weakness," or "dangerousness." On the other hand, some behaviours may be viewed as an individual being highly religious, spiritual, or gifted. As health care providers, we need to appreciate and acknowledge that not all members of a group endorse the views or adhere to the norms of their group, or they may do so to varying degrees. For instance, it would not be unusual for views and practices to vary across generations of a group or because of processes such as acculturation. The immigrant and refugee experience–including events leading up to, involved in, and following the actual physical move–shapes people's worldviews. For example, a refugee patient may harbour distrust toward government institutions, which should not be misinterpreted as paranoia (Kronick, 2018). As such, some historical and sociopolitical knowledge of specific immigrant communities will help in the assessment, and some knowledge of local community resources will be crucial in formulating a plan of care. Therefore, specific cultural knowledge, like that of the refugee hearing process, is important when working with these populations (Kronick, 2018) (see Chapter 11).

While knowledge about various views on mental health is important, health care providers must not use this knowledge to make assumptions or stereotype. Like culture, views about mental health are not static and do not remain fixed throughout a group's or individual's lifetime. As well, some groups share similar views of mental health, and some groups express distress in similar ways.

TABLE 14.1 ■ **Seven Core Areas for Cultural Consideration in Mental Health Care**

In mental health care, core areas for cultural consideration include the following:

1. Views of mental health and illnesses
2. Emotional expression and concepts of distress
3. Influence of collectivism
4. Communication and its context
5. Experiences of racism, oppression, and trauma
6. Working with families and communities
7. Program development and working with communities

Emotional Expression and Concepts of Distress

The various ways in which emotions and distress are expressed across cultures is a core area for consideration in mental health practice. Presentation needs to be understood as part of the assessment and to determine further assessment. A lack of health care providers' understanding of mental health conceptualizations by non-Western cultures potentially compromises the effectiveness of mental health treatment and programs. To promote understanding and address such concerns, the *Diagnostic and Statistical Manual of Mental Disorders*, fifth edition (DSM-5), presents cultural impacts on mental disorders in a multifaceted manner that includes the notion of cultural concept of distress (CD), composed of three types of cultural features of mental health experiences: cultural syndromes, cultural idioms of distress, and cultural explanations or perceived causes (American Psychiatric Association [APA], 2013). **A cultural idiom of distress** is an expression of psychological distress and problems which are, in part, culturally specific. Cultural idioms of distress thus may or may not relate to a label or diagnosis of mental illness from the patient's perspective or as determined by Western diagnosis of mental illness (APA, 2013).

Somatization is a cultural idiom of distress and refers to the phenomenon in which emotional or mental distress is expressed as a physical complaint and is an expression shared by several groups. For example, in keeping with cultural norms of emotional expression, a Chinese woman suffering from depression may present with complaints of pressure on the chest. Similarly, in Syria, where the concepts of psychological state and mental health are not commonly understood and are associated with mostly only negative connotations, people typically first present with physical complaints to medical settings before attending to psychological and mental health issues (Hassan et al., 2015). Thus when assessing the cause of the physical symptom, a more holistic assessment is needed. Conversely, assessment of mental illness could begin with an assessment of physical illness for a more comprehensive assessment, as well as beginning with areas that are more easily described and discussed. Again, while specific cultural knowledge is important, it is equally important to avoid assumptions that the knowledge held applies to all individuals in a particular group.

Communication and Its Context

Effective communication is vital to an accurate mental health assessment. Styles and rules of interaction vary across cultures (Liu, 2016). A core aspect of culturally competent mental health care is understanding the context of communication and the role of such context in shaping meaning. A group may share certain cultural elements with other groups, and yet it may have elements distinct from those of other groups. These common elements and dimensions of variability are sometimes classified as *high-* and *low-context features* (Hall & Whyte, 1960) (also see Chapter 5). High-context communication involves indirect use of verbal communication and relies on the context to convey meaning (Yang et al., 2021). In other words, what is spoken is less important than the context. The meaning of communication depends on the physical and social environment and the listener or receiver must attend to context to determine meaning. Whereas in low-context cultures, what is said is most important and usually has the same meaning in all contexts. In low-context communication the speaker has the responsibility of selecting particular words and attends to the order of words to ensure that what and how they speak conveys the intended meaning. Japanese people, as an example of a high-context culture, generally use words with meanings specific to the social situation. By contrast, North Americans, as an example of low-context culture, will use words with the same meaning regardless of the social situation. Therefore, in a high-context culture, depending on the situation, an individual may say "yes" or express agreement out of politeness or a desire not to openly disagree; and thus yes may mean, "Yes, I hear you" rather than, "Yes, I agree." Whereas in a low-context culture, yes is more likely to mean agreement under all situations. This contrast of high- and low-context culture is relevant here, in that clinicians must be sensitive to these kinds of differences in meaning and how these differences may manifest themselves in the presentation, assessment, and treatment of mental illness. Low-context cultures are more likely to provide specific details of their situation, whereas high-context individuals may expect the provider to have the inferred understanding and may require more probing and validation to determine the complete picture. Refer to Chapter 5 for further discussion of high- and low-context communication.

Cultural Considerations In Care

Reflection on Mental Status Assessment

Consider the assessment of mental status and how certain observations such as eye contact and communication style are interpreted. It is crucial to examine any assumptions on which these and other aspects of an assessment are interpreted.

What are the different ways to interpret the avoidance of eye contact?

- A show of respect
- A demonstration of shame
- A manifestation of shyness and withdrawal
- A manifestation of disinterest in one's surroundings
- A manifestation of dishonesty
- A manifestation of …

What are the different ways to interpret detailed storytelling in response to a question for which there seems to be a simple and direct response?

- A demonstration of an altered thought process—circumstantiality
- A demonstration of a particular communication style—high context
- A manifestation of a need for language interpretation
- A manifestation of an area of significant importance

Ask yourself, what was my first thought or interpretation? What might the impact be if that first interpretation is inaccurate? Reflect on these questions following each of your assessments.

The assessment of mood (affective) and thought disorders is particularly challenging in varying cultural contexts. Health care providers are encouraged to conduct all interactions from a position of curiosity with a willingness to ask questions about the patient's background and beliefs (Yager & Kay, 2020) and to listen carefully to the responses to these questions. Yager and Kay (2020) encourage providers to go beyond simple curiosity about patients and encourage "self-reflective curiosity [that] addresses questions concerning how trainees' own past positive and adverse experiences have impacted memory and learning, shaped present feelings about themselves and their worlds, and in turn influence how they respond to people, including patients and events" (p. 92).

Language support is another important aspect of care in all areas of health care and especially in mental health care given the quantity of verbal communication and reliance on the clinical interview in assessment and care. Even when the patient speaks some English (or the dominant language), often it is desirable to work with a cultural interpreter to promote full expression. It is essential that both health care providers and interpreters have training in the health care field (Krystallidou et al., 2018) and, in particular, in the specialty areas of mental health and addictions, especially given the stigma and double-stigma that accompany these areas. It needs also to be recognized that interpreters are cultural beings with their own feelings about the patient and the health care provider, as well as their own views of mental illness.

Health care providers should consider engaging interpreters for the purpose of deciphering behaviours outside of formal assessments. For example, if a hospitalized patient is talking aloud to themselves in another language, the health care provider might call on an interpreter to understand the content of the expression, rather than automatically labelling the behaviour as psychotic or mere "babbling."

In addition to an interpreter, it is often helpful to have the assistance of cultural consultants. These are professionals who are familiar with the patient's cultural background and can help the health care provider contextualize behaviours and ideas within the patient's ethnocultural background. They might be involved in the assessment or provide consultation to the health care provider afterward. Without this understanding, it may be impossible to conduct accurate mental health assessments. Health care providers are encouraged to work with resources such as cultural consultants to negotiate treatment and care in complex situations, to address the interplay of cultural, historical, and systemic factors in a manner that preserves the patient's values and fosters resiliency.

Influence of Collectivism

Collectivism refers to the practice of prioritizing the overall needs or interests of a group above those of one or more individuals within that group. There are both benefits and disadvantages to collectivist cultures or approaches. Collectivism often enables a group to grow and does so through sacrifices made by individuals within a group. Whereas globally many cultures espouse the value and principle of collectivism, Western health care is underpinned by the principles of individualism and individual autonomy, which also have advantages and disadvantages. As previously mentioned, with respect to families, the smallest unit of identity in a collectivist culture is the family.

Whereas individualism is associated with low power distance, collectivism is associated with high power distance. *Power distance* refers to the extent to which power is expected to be distributed equally (or not) within the family and society (see Chapters 3 and 5).

In collectivism, where there is the tendency for high power distance, there is generally less expectation of consultation and greater expectation that those in authority can tell others what to do. In high power distance cultures, society's level of inequality is endorsed by the followers as much as by the leaders (Hofstede, 2011). This has potential implications for how patients might engage with providers with respect to questions and engagement in care decisions. Patients with a collectivist orientation may be hesitant in expressing disagreement with a proposed plan of care and treatment and have greater expectations for the provider to determine treatment goals and interventions.

Thoughtful reflection and planning are especially needed when working with collectivist families. On one hand, there needs to be recognition and preservation of the key values of the collective; on the other hand, there needs to be consideration of the needs of an individual member, including matters of safety and risk. The needs of the family are as important to the individual as are their own needs, with the priority placed on the family's need. But individuals may be making tremendous sacrifices that are ultimately negatively impacting their mental health. Ultimately, the health of the family is also likely negatively affected, but this link is not always seen or acknowledged by an individual member or family. While the collectivist family often fosters coping and resilience and serves as a protective factor, collectivism can be a risk factor (Gopalkrishnan, 2018). The individual patient as well as the family may require assessments and, at the same time, cultural norms and expectations may make certain topics inappropriate. Cultural competence means bridging gaps and working across differences for care to be effective and help people. Such competence does not mean nonadherence or lessening of other professional competencies or standards. Yet, it is necessary to also recognize that standards are underpinned by values and a particular worldview.

Cultural Consideration In Care

Respect for Collectivist Families and Assessments

A South Asian adolescent is receiving care at a mental health outpatient clinic. They describe their family as loving, and their mother as their advocate and part of their circle of care. Their experience includeds psychosis and occasional thoughts of suicide. They have attendance problems at school and declining grades.

Wanting to be family centred and respectful of the collectivist cultural norm associated with South Asian families, the primary clinician readily includes the mother in all conversations and, at some points, relies heavily on the mother's reports of how her adolescent child is doing rather than direct assessment of the patient. The patient's mother reports that the patient is going to school and things are fine. The patient leaves the home each morning with the intention to go to school, which serves as a sign to the mother that "things are getting better." In fact, things are not fine. The patient is not going to school regularly and their use of illicit substances is also increasing.

Considering this scenario, what could the clinician do to be respectful of the collectivist cultural norms as well as ensure accurate assessments?

As you reflect on this scenario, keep the following in mind:

- It is important to recognize that the mother's portrayal of things getting better is likely influenced by her dreams for her child, the value of education, views on mental illness, and her hope for the future. In light of such dynamics and hope, it is not uncommon to present the family in the best possible way.
- It is essential to recognize that regular family involvement does not mean complete reliance on the family.
- Suicide could be the potential consequence of inaccurate assessments. What is the role of increasing substance use as a risk factor for suicide?
- The standard of care requires a direct assessment of the patient.

Experiences of Racism, Oppression, and Trauma

In the provision of mental health care, cultural knowledge also encompasses the understanding and acknowledgement of the significant impact of historical trauma, discrimination, colonization, and racism on the mental health of specific populations (Abramovich & Pang, 2020). For example, Indigenous people share the experiences of colonization and residential schools. Jewish people share the experiences of antisemitism and the Holocaust. Black people share the experiences of colonization and the history of slavery. Members of the lesbian, gay, bisexual, transgender, queer, two-spirit+ (LGBTQ2S+) communities share experiences of discrimination within societies dominated by heteronormative culture. These collective experiences, as well the traumatic experiences of other groups, impact mental health and well-being. Interestingly, such experiences may be more common in many cultures, but may not emerge, simply because they are not disclosed. A meta-analysis of 293 studies indicated that racism is significantly related to poorer health, with the relationship being twice as large for poorer mental health than the correlation with poorer physical health (Paradies et al., 2015).

It is critical for providers to have awareness of some specific disparities and knowledge of their sources and the structures or systems that play a major role in maintaining them. In Canada, one example of an area for awareness is the understanding that the suicide rates for young people in specific Indigenous communities are higher than for non-Indigenous communities along with the contributory factors. It is estimated that suicide rates are five to seven times higher for Indigenous youth compared to non-Indigenous youth in Canada (Government of Canada, 2018). Death by suicide for Indigenous people also occurs at higher rates in other countries, for example, in Australia, where statistics indicate that the suicide rate for Indigenous children and young people is almost five times the rate of non-Indigenous people of the same age (Ralph & Ryan, 2017), and where the overall suicide rate for Indigenous people are double that of non-Indigenous people (Australian Bureau of Statistics, 2019; Australian Institute of Health and Welfare, 2019). There is a need to appreciate and address the ongoing social and structural dynamics that influence these high rates of suicide (Ansloos, 2018).

This specific cultural knowledge, and in particular the historical trauma and other current contributing factors to suicide, is essential to the health care provider's ability to demonstrate humility and to foster cultural safety. "**Cultural safety** comes from recognizing colonial histories and systems of racialized identity and discrimination, domination, marginalization and exclusion, and working to redistribute power to achieve equity" (Kirmayer & Jarvis, 2019, cited in Kirmayer, 2019, p. 1132). The impact of historical trauma endured by Indigenous people, which includes deliberate practices such as residential schooling to remove their language and culture, is still felt today (Hiller et al., 2020, 2021) and necessitates reflection, sensitivity, and the profound need for culturally safe care. In culturally safe health care encounters and settings, people feel safe and respected for who they are in the present, how they are shaped and situated by their past, and for their expectations for their futures. The authors (we) believe, based on our experiences, that a main objective of cultural competence is for patients and families to experience care processes as culturally safe. Likewise, awareness of lower suicide rates among Indigenous communities with greater self-governance (First Nations Health Authority [FNHA], 2011) allows for a focus on resiliency. Communities with greater levels of knowledge of traditional languages, and in which Indigenous languages are widely spoken, are among those that reported over 50% fewer suicides than those that had effectively lost their languages. Other factors that foster resilience for both individuals and communities include "cultural continuity" and the control and administration of health services (Chandler & Lalonde, 2008).

Similarly, there is strong evidence that Indigenous youth are more likely to engage in early-onset substance use than their non-Indigenous counterparts. "In Canada, culturally appropriate prevention programs are needed for Indigenous youth in [as early as] elementary school" (Maina et al., 2020). Further, "[m]aking Indigenous values, beliefs, languages, images and worldviews central to the prevention curriculum enhanced the effectiveness, appropriateness, and sustainability of prevention programs. Indigenous communities are the best positioned to facilitate cultural tailoring without compromising the fidelity of evidence-based prevention programs" (Maina et al., 2020).

The impact of discrimination embedded throughout heteronormative society and its potential impact on the mental health of LGBTQ2S+ persons further reflects the importance of awareness and specific knowledge. The findings of an ethnographic study (Abramovich & Pang, 2020) of LGBTQ2S+ homeless youth in York Region (Ontario, Canada) indicate that at least 3 in 4 youth had overdosed in the last year and almost 4 in 10 had attempted suicide. Youth in the study indicated that they experienced significant family rejection when coming out, which resulted in low self-esteem, fear, anxiety, and stress. While it takes courage to discuss an addiction, in the same study one respondent stated, "I'm more comfortable telling people about my heroin addiction than I am telling people I'm gay" (Abramovich & Pang, 2020, p. 27). This statement highlights the need for cultural safety as it relates to sexuality and sexual identity.

The impact of historical trauma, systemic racism, and everyday microaggressions on the mental health and well-being of Black people is an especially profound example of the importance of culturally specific knowledge. The negative experiences, for example, of many young Black males with law enforcement and the criminal justice system demand a culturally specific and radically different understanding of fear, suspicion, and distrust. "There are several barriers to psychopolitical safety that Black men must cope with and/or resist. The term *psychopolitical* emphasizes the inseparable nature of psychological and political aspects of wellness" (Mosley et al., 2017, p. 165). The sociohistorical context of racism influences the responses of Black men and may reflect healthy or protective adaptations that present as paranoid-like behaviours (Mosley et al., 2017).

According to a 2020 national survey, approximately 3 in 10 (28%) of 1 000 surveyed Canadian adults indicated that they had been the victim of racism (Ipsos Reid Survey, 2020). "While racial discrimination is associated with negative mental health consequences for both genders, male and female Black youth differ (for example) in the effect of an increase in discrimination on deterioration of psychological symptoms. Among those transitioning to young adulthood in economically disadvantaged areas, male Black youth seem to be more susceptible than females to the psychological effects of increased racial discrimination over time" (Assari et al., 2017). Awareness of such issues and experiences is important if a health care provider is to provide competent care. Research for Black females and psychological health is limited. In a study using epidemiological survey data for Blacks residing in the United States, Lacey et al. (2015) identified severe physical intimate partner violence, discrimination, and neighbourhood problems (to a lesser extent) as important predictors of Black women's health (Lacey et al., 2015). More research and contextual understanding is needed for this population.

Cultural Considerations In Care

Assumptions, Harm, and Therapeutic Alliance

In the scenario that follows, consider what the clinician can do when assessing the patient who is a member of a group who has experienced historical and ongoing oppression.

A young Black male is referred to a mental health clinic for assessment due to possible anxiety, depression, substance abuse, intermittent suicidal ideation, and potential legal issues. For the initial assessment, the patient reported feeling dismissed because of one of the initial questions asked by the clinician, "How long did you spend in prison?" (the question was likely asked because of an assumption made on the basis of a particular prior assessment in the patient's health record). The patient did not answer the question initially and thus the question was repeated multiple times. The patient indicated that they left the appointment feeling worse to the point of feeling suicidal. They reported that they did not get a sense that the clinician cared about them or their mental health. Rather, the focus was on a narrative often attributed to Black men and was prejudicial.

Consider the above situation from several perspectives:

1. What is the impact on the patient with respect to future health seeking?
2. How could this situation have been approached differently for a more positive outcome?
3. Does the standard of care, at a minimum, require efforts to establish therapeutic rapport that involves the demonstration of some empathy and the gaining of trust?

As outlined earlier, health care providers also need to understand the influence of social processes on patients. Racism has been identified as a factor contributing to misdiagnosis and inferior treatment of members of Black communities in many countries (Alang, 2019). Similarly, to be ignorant of, disregard, or minimize the impact of colonialism on the mental and physical health of Indigenous people will lead to inadequate care and further marginalization. Indigenous populations have a high prevalence of mental health and substance use concerns that are linked to cultural oppression and marginalization (Turner & Luna Sánchez, 2020), and yet these factors as the sole narrative of Indigenous people contribute to further marginalization.

There is a link between varied experiences of oppression and poor mental health or mental illness. Gay, lesbian, and transgendered individuals, for example, have shared values and concerns, including stress related to issues such as identity, the coming-out process, and substance use (Charbonnier et al., 2018). These may lead to depression and low self-esteem in response to stigma and internalization of society's view of their sexual identities. Beyond the need for knowledge of the experience of groups with various forms of oppression, mental health care providers need to put this knowledge "into action" by making thoughtful inquiries into these areas in their assessments to determine their impact on the behaviours and mental health of patients.

Interestingly, the need for specific cultural competencies also raises the issue of ethnic and cultural matching (discussed in Chapter 2) of health care provider and patient, and how such matches have the potential to enhance patient outcomes. While such matching along with racial matching may be considered one aspect of culturally competent care, the evidence of this practice in terms of actual clinical outcomes is at best inconclusive. Yet, anecdotal patient accounts suggest that cultural matching may contribute to initial engagement in and the likelihood of remaining in therapy. We, the authors, understand that, in clinical reality and especially in the diverse environment that is Canada, it is impossible to provide ethnic matching for all patients. Furthermore, an ethnic match does not guarantee a cultural match for reasons that may include variation in ethnocultural identification and degree of acculturation (Chenot et al., 2019). In fact, possessing a sound knowledge of all cultures one could encounter in one's practice is a formidable task in and of itself. It is thus imperative that all health care providers acquire some degree of generic competence such that they can provide quality and effective clinical care for any patient in a multicultural environment and recognize the need for further support when needed. Further, for some patients, a cultural match may not provide either the safety or confidentiality they require, particularly when they may wish to discuss what they consider the negative aspects of their culture. Yet for other patients, such a match and the need for ethno-specific or culturally specific services is highly important given their experiences around trust, distrust, and those historical events and circumstances that may have resulted in a more profound need for cultural safety when accessing care and across the continuum of care.

Working With Families and Communities

The meaning of family and the role of individuals within families also vary across cultures. Culture shapes all aspects of family life, including communication and decision-making processes. In many cultures, it is the norm for an individual to sacrifice autonomy for the benefit of the family. The health care provider needs to understand patients' and families' worldviews and how their views and values relate to stigma, safety and risk, treatment options, decision making, and informed consent. Engagement of the family is of utmost importance in working with most ethnocultural communities, and family therapy models also must accommodate cultural differences in order to be culturally responsive.

Working with ethnic families and communities is a skill that was seldom taught in professional schools and in recent years is being given more attention in educational programs. Health care providers require this kind of skill when they need the assistance of interpreters or cultural consultants or want to refer to community agencies. It also is an important asset when developing programs for such communities. As in any hospital–community collaboration, the importance of respect and thoughtfulness cannot be overstated.

Consider here that that although the nuclear family structure is often perceived as a typical family type in Western society, this structure may not resonate with other cultures, including Indigenous populations (Tam et al., 2017). More specifically, perceptions of the Indigenous family may be framed through a personal or institutional perspective. "At the personal level, the perception of [the] indigenous family [is] influenced by culture, specifically social ties, language, childrearing practices, and residential location. At the institutional level, the perception of [the] indigenous family [is] defined through demographic [and] legal terms, and influenced by temporal change, though generally through a non-Indigenous lens" (Tam et al., 2017, p. 243). As such, standard Western definitions of the family may not accurately represent Indigenous families. And while institutional definitions of family may serve specific purposes, cultural influences need to be considered.

Respecting and working with Indigenous families therefore requires an understanding of cultural differences in identity, kinship, language, and mobility. Standard terms may be limited here because of "factors influencing family boundary ambiguity such as multiple caregivers, ambiguities in legal status, complex households, and different perceptions of defining family" (Tam et al., 2017, p. 247). The notions of privacy and individual autonomy that are aspects of the individualist culture of mental health care often negatively impact families, especially collectivist families. Families are challenged when trying to understand how their family member, when faced with mental illness that affects thinking and relationships, has the right to not include their families in care. In such situations, health care providers are encouraged to consider how they can honour individual patients' rights and at the same time respond empathically to families' distress. Some options include asking the family what it is like for them to be in this situation where the information they are requesting cannot be provided, and what supports may be helpful to them. While providers cannot share information about the patient with the family members, they can convey messages of love, support, concern, and so on, from the family to the individual patient. Another option is to connect the family with other resources such as a hospital's family engagement service or a community mental service that provides education and support about mental illness and addictions to families. Simply referring to the "privacy legislation" in a detached manner can be quite harmful.

Program Development and Working With Communities

Mental health programs must include systems and processes that provide information about the needs and worldviews of diverse groups. Developing programs for cultural groups requires the thoughtful incorporation of the cultural values of those groups, and ideally with direct input from community members. Health care providers need to consider the assumptions on which services are based, and the impact of such assumptions on the accessibility and care provided to diverse patients. For example, conventional mental health services that are based on mainstream Western values and assumptions are seldom effective for First Nations, Inuit, Métis, Black, and some immigrant and refugee communities. There is clear evidence that control of mental health programs by the communities they serve contributes to better health outcomes (Nelson & Wilson, 2017), making collaborative program development vital. More specifically, research indicates that the inclusion of traditional healing methods is integral to improved health outcomes. And, importantly, an understanding of the intergenerational historical trauma and the effects of trauma are critical considerations in any understanding of "stressed human capacity" in Indigenous communities (O'Neill et al., 2018). When developing programs for any community, it is essential that the community participates in and informs development. Table 14.2 lists some key questions to consider when developing programs for any community.

Cultural Considerations In Care

Example of a Program Co-Designed With Communities

Just over two decades ago, a team of Indigenous social workers and an Elder formed the first team at the Centre for Addiction and Mental Health (CAMH) to support the unique needs of First Nations, Inuit, and Métis patients. In the fall of 2020, CAMH officially launched Shkaabe Makwa—a unique and integrated co-designed centre that aims to transform health outcomes through the advancement of research, training, and innovative healing models that combine traditional knowledge and medical expertise. Leadership at the centre explained that "we believe that culture is central to healing and wellness–and we are committed to bringing about change in ways that respect and honour traditional knowledge and community expertise" (Linklater, 2020). Also see https://www.camh.ca/en/driving-change/shkaabe-makwa for further information.

TABLE 14.2 ■ Important Questions for Program Planners to Consider

Important questions for program planners to ask on an ongoing basis are the following:

1. What is the mental health culture and how do the values of this culture compare to values of diverse groups? How are power differentials addressed?
2. How do health care providers communicate?
   - Are educational materials provided in various languages?
   - How frequently do health care providers work with interpreters?
3. Does the patient group reflect the diversity of the general population? Are our program services accessible?
4. Are members from diverse groups involved in, or do they have input into, planning the program?
5. Is the program meeting the needs for the group or groups for which it was designed to serve? For programs for diverse groups, are there barriers for some groups? For group-specific programs, are there barriers for subgroups withing the group for which the program was designed to serve?

Unlike the example of a co-designed program in the preceding Cultural Considerations in Care box, when there has been little input into planning and services, the cultural mix among patients in the program may lead to certain conflicts. Members of the treatment team often are equally diverse, and the cultural dynamics among them is another important area for planners and leaders to consider. Any such discord may readily lead to disruption in patient care.

Finally, it is worth noting that in Canada, despite an abundance of health research documenting inequalities in morbidity and mortality rates for Indigenous people, notably less research has focused on mental health. The research that does relate to the mental health of Indigenous communities reflects some important tendencies, including an overwhelming concern with issues related to colonialism in mental health services, but with several significant gaps; an overemphasis on suicide and problematic substance use that can have negative implications; and an under-representation of certain population groups, including Métis people and urban or other Indigenous people who do not live on a reserve (Nelson & Wilson, 2017).

Culture and Mental Illness Treatments and Therapies

Cultural competence and cultural safety are essential to effective mental health care. Cultural considerations may require modification in treatment methods such as psychopharmacology and psychotherapy. Treatment plans may need to be devised specifically with the help of cultural resources—for instance, by working with healers and traditional medicines.

It may be necessary to make use of cultural resources to customize treatment and care. Such consultations may include the use of herbal remedies or the involvement of shamans and healers. Health care providers need to become knowledgeable in various cultural practices to negotiate comfortably and respectfully across differences when working with patients. In addition to having knowledge of cultural resources and complementary therapies, health care providers need to consider relevant aspects, such as professional standards, competence, organizational policies, and scope of practice in determining the extent to which they will be involved in such therapies or practices. They are also encouraged to critically reflect on the extent to which the cultural norms of the profession are codified within the profession, its documents, and processes.

PSYCHOPHARMACOLOGY

It is important to appreciate that while the area of psychopharmacology has advanced, it has done so with little recognition of cultural variance. It is only in recent years that drug trials are beginning to include considerations of cultural groupings in sampling. However, there is an increasing body of knowledge of and a recognition that drug metabolism may be influenced by ethnic, genetic, and psychosocial characteristics. While ethnicity represents a factor in influencing response to psychotropic medication, information remains limited on the specific possible impacts of ethnicity on psychopharmacology (Marazziti et al., 2020). Such impacts may manifest as unexpected adverse effects for a low dose of antipsychotic medication in a younger Asian man or, inversely, as a lack of progress despite a high dose in a slender Mexican woman. Some groups tend to be more sensitive to the effects of some drugs, while others are less sensitive. Based on a comparative study of a small sample of Senegalese and Italian men, the researchers suggest thoughtful consideration when administering psychotropics compounds in non-European individuals (Marazziti et al., 2020). Such caution should not be interpreted as avoidance of administering psychotropics but rather careful attention to aspects such as the time taken to metabolize these medications and their potential adverse effects. As well, the way in which medication is viewed varies among cultures, and the potential role of the interaction of diet and medications needs to be considered.

PSYCHOTHERAPY AND COUNSELLING

Cultural aspects of psychotherapy and counselling and how dominant Western perspectives underpin and are embedded within these approaches require examination. Psychotherapy is a cultural product of nineteenth-century Europe and still may be regarded with suspicion by many cultures. More recently, greater attention has been given to complementary approaches to care in North America (refer to Chapter 8). Complex cultural issues must be considered in order to competently provide various types of counselling, including psychotherapies and group and family therapies. There have been efforts to culturally adapt some therapies.

Cognitive behaviour therapy (CBT) was developed within Western culture as a treatment for people with specific mental illnesses such as depression and social anxiety. As early as the mid-1990s, the need to attend to cultural influences with respect to CBT strategies was identified (Hays, 1995). While some concepts of CBT may not directly translate from one language to another, "CBT concepts of 'schemas', 'automatic thoughts', and 'distortions' may readily translate across some cultural groups" (Dobson, 2018, p. 121). Modification may be required to make such concepts understandable and acceptable within non-Western cultures. **Culturally adapted cognitive behaviour therapy (CA-CBT)** refers "to a systematic modification of CBT protocol to consider language and cultural context to promote compatibility with patients' values" (Naeem, 2012, as cited in Naeem et al., 2019, pp. 388–389). The CA-CBT for Indigenous people within North America typically has embedded Indigenous concepts, beliefs, or values within the protocol or approach (Kowatch et al., 2019). Some common concepts included in the adapted versions of these CBT programs include community connections, connections to tradition, and engagement in ceremony throughout treatment. The Medicine Wheel is frequently included in adaptations. The Medicine Wheel, as noted in Chapter 8, emphasizes the notion that physical, emotional, mental, and spiritual domains are foundational for health and wellness.

CBT has been adapted for various groups, including traumatized refugees and ethnic minority groups (Hinton et al., 2012), Latino women with treatment-resistant post-traumatic stress disorder (PTSD) (Hinton et al., 2011), Southeast Asian groups (Hinton & Jalal, 2019), and English-speaking people of Caribbean origin in Canada (Centre for Addiction and Mental Health [CAMH], 2011). All CA-CBT has common adaptations that consider the context and values of the groups for which they were adapted. The CBT for English-speaking people of Caribbean origin emphasizes cultural safety with attention to power dynamics related to ethnic and racial status within the dominance of a Eurocentric context (CAMH, 2011). It considers how historical and current practices have contributed to members of this group's perceptions of mental health services and poorer clinical encounters. Overall, culturally adapted psychotherapies improve outcomes; however, the impact is greater for some groups than for others. It also improves outcomes for substance misuse treatment. As well, culturally adapted treatments for ethnocultural and racialized youth are promising practices (Mental Health Commission of Canada, 2016).

Clinical Tools

One of the difficulties in developing cultural competence is the lack of concrete tools to bridge the gap between having cultural awareness and incorporating it into everyday practice. The other challenge is the ease with which tools facilitate the integration of cultural considerations into the overall assessments. In the sections that follows, the authors describe tools that may be helpful in mental health practice.

CULTURAL FORMULATION INTERVIEW

Cultural formulation is a tool included in the previous version of the *Diagnostic and Statistical Manual of Mental Disorders* (DSM) IV (APA, 1994) as Appendix I, just before the list of contributors; therefore, even those who use the DSM daily could easily overlook it. However, it represented a hard-won victory for a small group of advocates within the American psychiatric community. The historical development of the DSM itself demonstrates how much of a cultural artifact the document is in and of itself, with each version reflecting the cultural norms of the period during which they were developed. For example, homosexuality as a disorder was removed from the DSM in 1973, in part as a response to the changing sociopolitical climate. At the same time, there is benefit to be found in the fluidity of the DSM and the processes involved in its revisions. The latest version, DSM-5 (APA, 2013), has updated criteria to reflect variations in clinical presentations across cultures. It provides detailed information of cultural concepts of distress and acknowledges cultural variations in how symptoms are exhibited and explained. The DSM-5 includes a **cultural formulation interview (CFI)** tool meant to facilitate comprehensive assessments that are person focused. The CFI tool indicates several areas for inquiry and consists of 16 questions that fall under four domains:
1. Cultural definitions of the problem
2. Cultural perceptions of cause, concept, and support
3. Cultural factors affecting self-coping and past help-seeking behaviour
4. Cultural factors affecting current help-seeking

Questions in these domains involve inquiries in areas such as cultural understandings of problems and perceptions of their causes (explanatory models), cultural identities, psychosocial stressors, coping and areas of vulnerability and resilience, help-seeking behaviours, and cultural aspects of the clinician–patient relationship. The domains are briefly discussed in the following sections, and specific tools and strategies are presented that may be helpful in exploring these areas.

Cultural Definitions of the Problem

The focus within this domain is the person's description and understanding of the "problem." It is essential to keep in mind that the person may not view their situation as a "problem" and may name their situation differently. Understanding the person, their situation, and what matters most to them is of utmost importance. Approach and willingness to learn directly from the patient will be of tremendous value. As a health care provider, **self-reflexivity**, awareness of one's biases and prejudices (Shepherd et al., 2019), will be essential prior to, throughout, and following the interview. During the interview, it is suggested that clinicians focus on deep listening with consideration for any "blind spots" or assumptions they themselves have about the "problem." One aspect to ponder is that the interview is focused on individuals in accordance with the Western values of autonomy and self-determination that underpin practice. For some groups with collectivist worldviews, it would be the group at this stage that answers the questions within this domain.

Cultural Perceptions of Cause, Concept, and Support

This domain includes questions in the subcategories of causes, stressors, and supports, and the role of cultural identity. The **explanatory model** (Kleinman, 1988) is used to elicit the person's views regarding the cause(s) of their problem, situation, or illness. **Cultural explanations** are meanings, beliefs, and attitudes that a culture ascribes to a particular phenomenon. Kleinman (1988) formulated the idea that in different cultures, there may be different languages of distress, like somatization, and different explanatory models of illnesses. He proposed a series of questions to clarify the explanatory model with the aim of eliciting the person's view of the nature, cause, consequences, and treatment of the problem or situation. To respond to differences between the models of the patient and the health care provider, Srivastava, in Chapter 4, proposes an adaptation of Leininger's (1995) three paths of action:

1. *Validation/Preservation:* respecting and preserving the values where possible
2. *Accommodation/Negotiation:* accommodating and negotiating across preferences and worldviews where needed
3. *Reframing/Repatterning:* creating new options and approaches for the patient, health care provider, or system

The CFI questions in the areas of stressors and supports are used to obtain information on the person's life context, including areas of stress, resources, supports, and strengths. **Social stressors** are events or experiences that are connected to and impact individuals' social conditions, including their positions, roles, and relationships. Immigration status, discrimination, and stigma could be identified as stressors, while religion, spirituality, and family could be seen as strengths, stressors, or both.

There are significant connections between mental health and **cultural identity**, which is the sense of belonging to a group or culture based on shared characteristics with other members of the cultural group. The health care provider needs to ask the individual to reflect on the most salient elements of their cultural identities. Since identities cannot be based solely on appearance, it is important to ascertain identity from the patient as part of the assessment. Mental health care providers need to be mindful that identities are not static. Groen et al. (2018) suggest that clinicians, in order to grasp and address the complexity of cultural identity, consider the divisions of personal, ethnic, and social identity. Most important, these researchers suggest that clinicians, when working with refugees who have experienced trauma, aim to assess any changes to identity that result from stress and other issues related to acculturation. Please refer to the discussion on identity in Chapter 3, which includes three key features of identity that are also relevant in mental health practice: perceived identity, ascribed identity, and intersectional identities.

It is helpful to ascertain the patterns of acculturation, intersections of identities, and the aspects of identity that matter most to a patient in a particular situation and their implications for mental health. For example, a biracial patient with a Black father and a White mother may need to actively explore one or the other side of their heritage to arrive at a cohesive sense of self, which is essential to one's mental health. In addition, a person's gender identity is not always evident from their appearance. It is equally important to remember that the same identity issues, along with their implications for interactions, apply to health care providers and to everyone they encounter in practice, including families, interpreters, and colleagues. Identity is an important aspect of mental health well-being not only for individuals but also for communities.

Cultural Factors Affecting Self-Coping and Past Help-Seeking

In this domain, as the title suggests, the focus is on learning from the person what they do to cope, and where, when, and with whom they seek help. Various sources of help include medical care, support groups, mental health treatment, work-based counselling, and religious or spiritual counselling. Many patients rely on and seek out traditional healers and various forms of healing, some of which may be considered alternative by other health care providers within "mainstream" health care. The help that people and their families seek or use is often related to their beliefs about the causes of the problem. For example, the family who believes that "possession" is the main cause of psychosis may consider an exorcism for their loved one. The point is that regardless of what or who has been sought out for help, health care providers need to listen to their patients and acknowledge these alternatives that may differ from their own views and care recommendations. Another aspect to consider is that once a person presents to the "mainstream" mental health care system, traditional treatments may not be working or no longer work to the extent desired by the patient. Health care providers need to explore social barriers to past help-seeking, access to care, and engagement in treatment (CFI; APA, 2013), as well as potential barriers to current help-seeking.

Cultural Factors Affecting Current Help-Seeking

How people perceive needs and their expectations along with those of their social network can affect their help-seeking behaviours during encounters with health care providers. Notably, cultural elements of the patient and health care relationship affect help-seeking. Aside from language and cultural differences having an obvious impact on assessment and treatment, they also influence and serve as part of the context for therapeutic relationships. Since both patients and health care providers have a culture, practitioners are encouraged to reflect on the role of culture and power differences within the therapeutic relationship, and how they relate to the notions of trust, transference, and countertransference. The therapeutic pairings (which scholars call *dyads*) are shown in Fig. 14.1. Majority (M) and minority (m) refer to power dynamics and do not necessarily indicate numbers, so that a White health care provider working in a Black neighbourhood would still be considered a member of the majority culture.

With a majority therapist and minority patient (Mm), the patient may be more trusting of the health care provider, feeling that a majority health care provider is more educated than a minority one, leading to a positive transference; or the patient may feel discriminated against by the majority health care provider because of past experience, leading to negative transference. On the other hand, the health care provider may feel good to be helping a minority patient, contributing to positive countertransference; or the health care provider may harbour preconceived ideas that the patient may be lazy and uneducated—negative countertransference. Different types of dynamics could emerge with different pairings, and it is even more complicated with "mm" because of the many possible variations—the patient and health care provider may be from the same

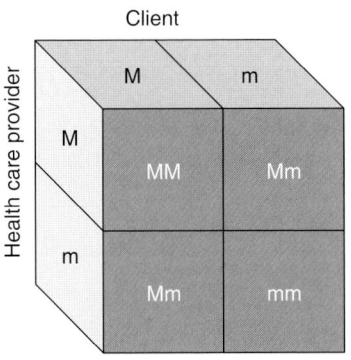

M = Majority culture; m = Minority culture

Fig. 14.1 Psychodynamics of the Health Care Provider–Patient Relationship.

ethnic group or two different minority groups. Attention must be given to the power gaps that exist between patient and health care provider; these power gaps must be assessed and explicitly discussed. The initial goal is to develop trust and promote safety, and these are facilitated through honest and transparent dialogue that addresses power, safety, and fear as perceived and experienced by patients.

6Ps CARE PLANNING GRID

The **6Ps care planning grid** is a tool that allows the health care provider to incorporate all the clinical data into an overall assessment of the patient. The authors present an expanded version (see Table 14.3) of the holistic bio-psycho-social grid approach (Engel, 1977)—where "bio" refers to the biological and physiological; "psycho," the thinking and feeling aspects; and "social," to social networking, which includes cultural aspects and cultural identities, and a spiritual dimension added to include the spiritual issues often prominent in and important to various ethnocultural groups.

> ### Cultural Considerations In Care
>
> *Care Planning Grid: An Overview of All Relevant Information*
>
> The 6Ps in each dimension (biological, psychological, social/cultural and spiritual) are:
> - A *presenting* column, to summarize the clinical features as presented
> - A *predisposing* column, to summarize past contributing factors and experiences, for example, genetic, trauma, oppression, racism
> - A *precipitating* column, summarize current triggering stressors and factors
> - A *perpetuating* column, to summarize ongoing stressors and factors
> - A *protective* column, to consider strengths and foster resiliency, for example, spirituality, religion
> - A *plan* column, to indicate types of actions and interventions
>
> Reflect: What is the plan I (we; the health care team) am recommending versus the plan to which the patient agrees? Am I/we assuming agreement?

The 6Ps care planning grid provides a way of capturing, in clinical assessments, all relevant information—cultural included—that will guide intervention or care planning.

The use of the grid is illustrated in Table 14.3 by planning care for the hypothetical scenario of Kyoko, a single Japanese woman 39 years of age, who immigrated to Toronto 1 year ago. She managed to find work and has done well. However, she is quite shy, and without her family for the first time, she felt lonely and became depressed. Then her family doctor told her that she had a breast lump, possibly cancer. Her mother died of breast cancer 6 years earlier, and Kyoko often felt she did not do enough for her. She had to wait for the specialist to give her the diagnosis and prognosis. She could not tell anyone about the possibility of breast cancer and became obsessed with its potential consequence and the associated fear and stigma. She used to pray at a temple but had not been to one in Toronto. She was referred to a White male therapist. She had difficulty expressing herself in English and was also reticent in discussing her negative emotions. Refer to Table 14.3 for an example of how the 6Ps care planning grid is used to capture relevant information, including cultural information, in this hypothetical scenario of Kyoko.

THE LEARN APPROACH TO NEGOTIATING ACROSS DIFFERENCES

It is essential for health care providers to engage in cross-cultural communication to negotiate care across differences between their and their patients' views. As discussed in Chapter 4, the tool **LEARN** (Ladha et al., 2018, adapted from Berlin & Fowkes, 1983) may be used to help with such

TABLE 14.3 ■ The 6Ps Care Planning Grid for Kyoko

	Presenting	Predisposing	Precipitating	Perpetuating	Protective	Plan
Biological	Insomnia	Family history of cancer	Breast lump	Cancer diagnosis unclear	Healthy otherwise	Antidepressant
Psychological	Depressed	Shyness, guilt about mother	Manner in which she was given the diagnosis/prognosis	Difficulty expressing emotion	Lack of trust in therapist	Encouraged to seek therapy and support
Social	Withdrawal Japanese	Alone in Canada		Further isolation	Working well	Advocacy with specialist
Spiritual	Confused			Not using religious resource	Prays at home	Seek out temple

Note: Some items can be put in different categories, and some categories can be left blank if information is not available. Cultural identity may be included under the Presenting column in the Social Section.

negotiation. *LEARN* refers to **L**isten to understand, **E**xplain your perspective, **A**cknowledge differences, **R**ecommend options, and **N**egotiate care. When using the LEARN tool it is important remember the following:

1. The order in which things are done is important. The health care provider must first listen before explaining or "educating."
2. Acknowledging the perspective of the patient does not mean that the health care provider agrees with that perspective. What is essential are validation and clarification of what was understood through listening.
3. The recommendation of options does not mean that a patient will agree to any of the options. Health care providers are encouraged to engage patients in the discussion and the possible modification of those options.
4. The demonstration of listening, acknowledgement, and respect by the health care provider can provide options for patients to access the system in the future, even when they may not agree to any option. Lack of respect or any dismissive behaviour could potentially serve as a barrier to accessing the system in the future, as health care practitioners, consciously or unconsciously, represent the health systems in which they work.

Cultural Considerations In Care

LEARN: Negotiation Across Differences

A patient of West Indian descent who had been living in Canada for 35 years started to experience "no energy, difficulty sleeping at night, and trouble with waking up in the morning." The patient described feeling "sluggish" and "lazy" and reported taking a tonic (with "minerals and lots of iron") to help with the lack of energy and sluggishness. However, the patient indicated that "tonic seemed to work for a few weeks but no longer works as good as it first did." The primary health care practitioner (PHCP) indicated to the patient that the symptoms they were experiencing suggested depression. The patient's view was that no one from their country of origin had this condition, and in fact expressed their belief that such a condition is a "North American notion." When asked about the name that would be given to what they were experiencing, the patient responded, "laziness" and maybe "too much stress." However,

Continued

the patient was uncertain as to whether they were lazy. The PHCP acknowledged that there was a difference between the patient's view and their view of the situation, and indicated that the diagnosis based on assessment was clinical depression. The PHCP explained their view of clinical depression and how it is caused by an imbalance of chemicals in the brain.

The patient firmly believes that they are not suffering from depression and thinks the only things out of balance are their energy, sleep, and tiredness, likely caused by stress. The patient is concerned because their ability to work is affected. The PHCP explains that it appears that similarities between their views are that they are both concerned and want a resolution to the "lack of energy, poor sleep, and tiredness" and suggests that a medication classified as an antidepressant that impacts serotonin levels in the brain could potentially improve energy and sleep. The PHCP also suggests a certain type of counselling. The patient responds that God is their counsellor and initially declines such therapy. However, with continued dialogue, the patient decides to try the medication and is provided with information on the medication, including potential adverse effects. The patient continues to take the medication and regularly explains that while the medication is an antidepressant, they are not taking it for depression but taking it for their stress and to improve their sleep and energy so they can go to work. The patient reports that the medication works for them.

1. What might have been the result if the PHCP had insisted on the patient's acceptance of the diagnosis or the label of depression?
2. Despite the nonacceptance of the label of depression, was the patient provided with health teaching and did they provide informed consent?
3. What might be a culturally appropriate way to describe cognitive behaviour therapy ("certain type of counselling") to this patient? How might the discussion continue? Perhaps the PHCP could acknowledge that the counselling is not intended to replace or oppose God as the patient's counsellor?

CRITICAL REFLECTION AND SELF-REFLEXIVITY TOOLS

Given factors such as the nature of ethnocentrism, power associated with the role of mental health providers, and the notion of "blind spots," the authors (we) recommend a focused and disciplined approach to self-reflexivity and critical reflection. "**Critical reflection** is a process of constantly analyzing, questioning, and critiquing established assumptions of oneself" (Liu, 2015, p. 144) along with the assumptions, social, and political implications of contexts and systems in which one delivers care. The goal of such reflection is to understand vulnerabilities and behaviour change toward the achievement of more equitable care delivery and services. It is crucial to take opportunities to learn and improve and recognize that the good intentions of health care providers are insufficient and could have devastating outcomes. There are various tools available, and we recommend two approaches that can be used individually or within a group as well as during clinical supervision: Kluckhohn triangle and cultural mindedness.

Kluckhohn Triangle

The concepts of universality, similarity, and individuality are introduced in Chapter 3. Another way of understanding the importance of these concepts is to consider the following quote and its application in practice. "Every [person] is in certain respects like all other [persons], like some other [persons], and like no other [person]" (Kluckhohn & Murray, 1953, p. 388).

This quotation may be helpful in conceptualizing the nature of culture. "Like all other [persons]" represents the universal, "like some other [person]" represents the cultural, and "like no other [person]" represents the individual. Envisaged as a triangle with three layers, it is a graphic reminder for us as health care providers to consider the influence that culture has at all levels of our interactions with patients.

For the uninitiated, there are only two layers, the individual and the universal; one would consider the presentation of any clinical data from the individual patient by comparing it with ourselves—our own universal view, for example, our own views of mental health, mental illness, and addictions, is assumed to be applicable to all. Subsequently, we are likely to intervene in ways

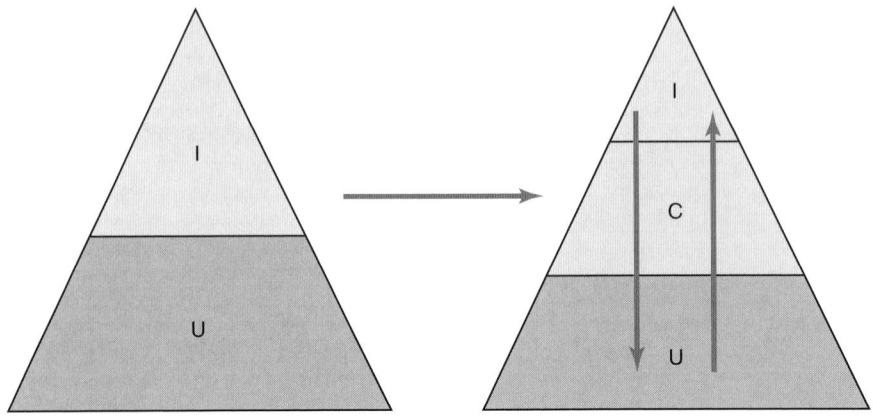

I = Individual   U = Universal   C = Cultural

Fig. 14.2 The Kluckhohn Triangle. (Based on Kluckhohn, C., & Murray, H. A. [Eds.]. [1953]. *Personality in nature, society and culture* [p. 53]. Knopf.)

that are thought to be universally valid. By introducing the cultural layer, we would have three layers; the information from the patient would then be filtered through the cultural layer, and we would interpret it with our cultural knowledge, always remembering to check our interpretations with the patient so as not to engage in stereotyping. For example, we would not assume that the avoidance of eye contact indicates a depressed mood or a demonstration of the person having something to hide. Instead, we would elicit and be open to the patient's explanation that their avoidance of eye contact symbolizes respect. Only after checking out observations with patients would we be able to arrive at a position to truly understand and use our professional knowledge to intervene. However, the intervention again needs to pass through the cultural layer so that it is culturally appropriate and capable of accomplishing the desired goal (Fig. 14.2).

Cultural Considerations In Care

Using the Culture Layer—Checking With the Patient

Scenario: Mr. Chan, a 65-year-old Chinese man, became depressed with various somatic preoccupations after his retirement and immigration to Canada. He has discontinued his antidepressant medication.

What might be a common response by a health care provider?

The health care provider might consider Mr. Chan as being nonadherent when he did not continue taking his antidepressants.

What might be the health care provider's understanding when the culture level is applied?

Using the cultural layer, one might appreciate that depression has not been a known illness in Chinese culture. One might also find out that Mr. Chan was scared by the dizziness he was experiencing, which he interpreted as sign of a serious illness. Besides, he could not see how his problem could be helped by medication.

What might be the health care provider's newly informed understanding of the universal level?

The health care provider could subsequently understand that a patient would not take anything that is scary without being convinced of its usefulness (the result of having new eyes and new ears—see Chapter 3).

What action might the health care provider take following cultural filtration?

The health care provider could proceed to explain Mr. Chan's condition to him, using the concept of neurasthenia, which is well established in Mr. Chan's culture, and present the medication as a "tonic" and reassure him that the dizziness was not serious and would not last long.

Cultural Mindedness

The authors (and previous co-author) of this chapter believe that people vary in their aptitude for dealing with cross-cultural encounters and refer to this aptitude as **cultural mindedness (CM)**.[3] Cultural mindedness is what health care providers bring to their encounters with patients. Part of that aptitude is derived from nature, but part of it also can be purposefully nourished. We consider this aptitude to be the basis of clinical cultural competence and enhancing our CM will further develop it. A conceptualization of CM, with some of its domains, is as follows in Table 14.4.

To enhance one's CM, the health care provider should ask the following questions on an ongoing basis:

- Before any encounter, ask: "Do I want to connect with this person in a respectful manner?"
- At the encounter, ask: "Am I aware that we have different worldviews? How might the patient experience the power differential between us?"

TABLE 14.4 ■ Cultural Mindedness: Domains and Self-Reflexive Questions

Cultural Mindedness (CM) Domain	Self-Reflexive Questions
Attitude Certain attitudes contribute to CM:	
a. **Curiosity**—propels us to inquire into the culture of another person	*Ask: What motivates me to inquire into the culture of another person?*
b. **Respect**—guides our interaction so that the other person does not feel encroached upon or intimidated	*Ask: How do I know what the other considers to be respectful? How are my presence and approach experienced? Have I asked for this feedback?*
c. **Desire** to connect—assess that you have the desire to connect	*Ask: How am I genuinely trying to connect with the other person?*
Awareness Certain areas of awareness contribute to CM: Awareness of worldviews of other Awareness of worldviews of self Awareness of dynamics of difference (described in Chapter 3)	*Ask: Am I aware of the fact that the other person has their own worldview, including views on mental health and causes of mental illnesses?* *Am I aware that as a person and health care provider I also have a distinctive worldview? What assumption might I make because of these views? How might I use knowledge grounded in my own worldview to offer opportunities and options to others?* *Have I given close attention to power dynamics, power gaps, and their impact on the relationship between myself and the patient? Have I used my power to impose views, to offer options, or to help patients negotiate new contexts and sources of knowledge?*
Autobiography or Personal Experience The health care provider's unique life experience powerfully contributes to CM: a. Past (e.g., the health care provider may have a bicultural heritage or experience of being a member of a minority group) b. Present (e.g., current social network, exposure to other cultures through the media) c. Future (e.g., aspirations and direction in life)	*How do my experiences and my aspirations factor into the way I assess and plan care with the patient?*

[3] The notion of cultural mindedness described here is similar to the concept of cultural sensitivity discussed in Chapter 3.

- In what ways can I promote cultural and psychological safety?
- What historical and contextual trauma and factors must I consider?

■ At all times, ask oneself: "Am I living a 'culturally conscious' life? Do I have the patient's trust?" We often ask—do we have time? And do we have tools? Most important and foundational, we need to ask about trust, which is fundamental to cultural safety.

These questions can be a useful tool in developing cultural competence and can be used during reflective practice and clinical supervision of health care providers involved in mental health care.

Summary

Cultural safety is both a process and an outcome and serves as the foundation for culturally competent mental health practice. Cultural competence enables health care providers to understand individuals as unique cultural beings. Health care providers need to focus on patients' perspectives and use their wishes and views to guide care and treatment. Even with different patients from a similar cultural background, there is no single approach or intervention that will always work. Culturally competent mental health care is also holistic care: all the bio-psycho-social and spiritual spheres are considered. Cultural safety serves as the foundation for developing culturally competent and effective mental health programs. Such safety can only be cultivated when attention is given to historical trauma that results from oppression, current oppression, and systems that are built on oppressive histories, which all impact mental health. Cultural competence as well as culturally competent programs are needed to provide care across diverse cultures. As well, specific knowledge is needed to work competently with particular groups, especially those groups who have experienced trauma and mistrust a system, and who may see health care providers representing a system in which their trauma is embedded and codified.

In this chapter we identified key issues within mental health care that are influenced by culture and presented specific and generic competencies that are necessary for health care providers. Cultural identity and cultural explanations are two important areas that require assessment before appropriate interventions can be determined. Power dynamics between health care providers and patients are highlighted through a discussion on the psychodynamics of this relationship and its potential impact on the therapeutic relationship. The chapter presents a care formulation exercise that illustrates how this tool can be used to incorporate the relevant clinical data into an overall assessment and plan of care.

Although the discussion in this chapter focused on the individual health care provider involved in mental health care, culturally competent individuals can exert little influence if the system in which they work is not culturally competent. Conversely, to develop a culturally competent mental health system, individual health care providers also must be trained and supported in their development of cultural competence. This inter-relationship cannot be overstated in view of the uneven development in the field.

Although the development of cultural competence may be an ethical responsibility and a practical necessity, it also serves as a source of tremendous personal rewards. Cultural competence fosters a unique perspective on the full richness of the human experience. Developing cultural competence is an ongoing journey with no specific end point, a journey that the reader is encouraged to embark on. Critical reflection and self-reflexivity are essential to cultural competence, and we recommend a focused and structured approach when engaging in these activities. As part of this journey, we emphasize the value of learning directly from the expertise of patients, families, and communities as part of this journey.

 evolve.elsevier.com/Srivastava/culturalcompetence.

Questions for Review and Discussion

1. What are some various views on mental health or mental illness that you have encountered? Consider how you will respond or have responded to a patient who has a particular view that is different from yours.
2. What are some ways that you can integrate the expertise of diverse patients and families to enhance cultural safety throughout care?
3. Consider the role that context has in your professional communication. Is your communication reflective of high context or low context?
4. What are ways that you examine systemic biases and blind spots in the provision of mental health care?
5. How would you describe to a peer the impacts of racism, oppression, trauma, and stigma on the mental health of individuals and groups?

Group Experiential/Reflection Activity

Working in pairs or as a group, complete the 6Ps on the *care planning grid* for a patient who was referred to a community mental health clinic with a diagnosis of depressive disorder and who is said to be experiencing suspiciousness and paranoia. The patient belongs to a historically oppressed group. They do not trust mental health providers and do not believe in taking "a lot of medications" or in going to counselling. The patient states their belief that God is their counsellor and will help them with their current situation, which they view as "no longer having enough energy to work or endure workplace politics." They do not think that they can be helped at this clinic because it is work they have a problem with, not their mental health. The patient decides to attend the first appointment because they want to appease their doctor of several years who made the referral and with whom they have a good relationship.

References

Abramovich, A., & Pang, N. (2020). *Understanding LGBTQ2S youth homelessness in York region.* https://www.homelesshub.ca/resource/understanding-lgbtq2s-youth-homelessness-york-region

Alang, S. (2019). Mental health care among blacks in America: Confronting racism and constructing solutions. *Health Services Research, 54*(2), 346–355. https://doi.org/10.1111/1475-6773.13115.

American Psychiatric Association. (1994). *Diagnostic and statistical manual of mental disorders* (4th ed.). American Psychiatric Association.

American Psychiatric Association. (2013). *Diagnostic and statistical manual of mental disorders* (5th ed.). American Psychiatric Association.

Ansloos, J. (2018). Rethinking indigenous suicide. *International Journal of Indigenous Health, 13*(2), 8–28. https://doi.org/10.32799/ijih.v13i2.32061.

Assari, S., Moazen-Zadeh, E., Caldwell, C., et al. (2017). Racial discrimination during adolescence predicts mental health deterioration in adulthood: Gender differences among Blacks. *Frontiers in Public Health, 5*(Article 104), 1–10. https://doi.org/10.3389/fpubh.2017.00104.

Australian Bureau of Statistics. (2019). *Intentional self-harm (suicides), key characteristics.* https://www.abs.gov.au/statistics/health/causes-death/causes-death-australia/latest-release#intentional-self-harm-suicides-key-characteristics

Australian Institute of Health and Welfare. (2019). *Deaths by suicide amongst Indigenous Australians.* https://www.aihw.gov.au/suicide-self-harm-monitoring/data/populations-age-groups/suicide-indigenous-australians

Berlin, E., & Fowkes, W. (1983). A teaching framework for cross-cultural health care. Application in family practice. *Western Journal of Medicine, 139*(6), 934–938.

Centre for Addiction and Mental Health (CAMH). (2011). *Cognitive-behavioural therapy for English-speaking people of Caribbean origin: A manual for enhancing the effectiveness of CBT for English-speaking people of Caribbean origin in Canada.* https://www.porticonetwork.ca/documents/43843/277768/CBT-Anglophone_English.pdf/ba2f1c1c-5a55-40a9-95f5-000e48abff09

Chander, K., Manjunatha, N., Binukumar, B., et al. (2019). The prevalence and its correlates of somatization disorder at a quaternary mental health centre. *Asian Journal of Psychiatry*, *42*, 24–27. https://doi.org/10.1016/j.ajp.2019.03.015.

Chandler, M., & Lalonde, C. (2008). Cultural continuity as a protective factor against suicide in First Nations youth. *Horizons—A Special Issue on Indigenous Youth, Hope or Heartbreak: Indigenous Youth and Canada's Future*, *10*(1), 68–72.

Charbonnier, E., Dumas, F., Chesterman, A., et al. (2018). Characteristics of stress and suicidal ideation in the disclosure of sexual orientation among young French LGB adults. *International Journal of Environmental Research and Public Health*, *15*(2), 290. https://doi.org/10.3390/ijerph15020290.

Chenot, D., Benton, A., Iglesias, M., et al. (2019). Ethnic matching: A two-state comparison of child welfare workers' attitudes. *Children and Youth Services Review*, *98*, 24–31. https://doi.org/10.1016/j.childyouth.2018.12.008.

Dobson, K. S. (2018). Dissemination: Science and sensibilities. *Canadian Psychology/Psychologie Canadienne*, *59*(2), 120–125. https://doi.org/10.1037/cap0000143.

Engel, G. L. (1977). The need for a new medical model: A challenge for biomedicine. *Science*, *196*, 129–136.

Filmer, T., & Herbig, B. (2018). Effectiveness of interventions teaching cross-cultural competencies to health-related professionals with work experience: A systematic review. *The Journal of Continuing Education in the Health Professions*, *38*(3), 213–221. https://doi.org/10.1097/CEH.0000000000000212.

First Nations Health Authority (FNHA). (2011). *Our history, our health.* http://www.fnha.ca/wellness/our-history-our-health

Gopalkrishnan, N. (2018). Cultural diversity and mental health: Considerations for policy and practice. *Frontiers in Public Health*, *6*. 179–179. https://doi.org/10.3389/fpubh.2018.00179.

Government of Canada. (2018). *Suicide prevention.* Government of Canada–Health Canada. https://www.sac-isc.gc.ca/eng/1576089685593/1576089741803#wb-cont

Groen, S., Richters, A., Laban, C., et al. (2018). Cultural identity among Afghan and Iraqi traumatized refugees: Towards a conceptual framework for mental health care professionals. *Culture, Medicine and Psychiatry*, *42*(1), 69–91. https://doi.org/10.1007/s11013-016-9514-7.

Hall, E., & Whyte, W. (1960). Intercultural communication: A guide to men of action. *Human Organization*, *19*, 5–12.

Hassan, G., Kirmayer, L. J., MekkiBerrada, A., et al. (2015). *Culture, context and the mental health and psychosocial wellbeing of Syrians: A review for mental health and psychosocial support staff working with Syrians affected by armed conflict.* United Nations High Commissioner for Refugees. http://www.unhcr.org/55f6b90f9.pdf

Hays, P. (1995). Multicultural applications of cognitive-behavior therapy. *Professional Psychology: Research and Practice*, *26*(3), 309–315. https://doi.org/10.1037/0735-7028.26.3.309.

Hechanova, R., & Waelde, L. (2017). The influence of culture on disaster mental health and psychosocial support interventions in Southeast Asia. *Mental Health, Religion & Culture*, *20*(1), 31–44. https://doi.org/10.1080/13674676.2017.1322048.

Hillier, S., Winkler, E., & Lavallée, L. F. (2020). Decolonising the HIV care cascade: Policy and funding recommendations from Indigenous people living with HIV and AIDS. *International Journal of Indigenous Health*, *15*(1), 47–59. https://doi.org/10.32799/ijih.v15i1.33909.

Hiller, S., Winkler, E., & Lavallee, L. (2021). Colonisation, suicide, and resilience: Storying with First Nations people living with HIV and AIDS. *Journal of Indigenous Wellbeing Te Mauri-Pitmatisiwin*, *6*(2), 2H–13H.

Hinton, D., Hofmann, S., Rivera, E., et al. (2011). Culturally adapted CBT (CA-CBT) for Latino women with treatment-resistant PTSD: A pilot study comparing CA-CBT to applied muscle relaxation. *Behaviour Research and Therapy*, *49*(4), 275–280. https://doi.org/10.1016/j.brat.2011.01.005.

Hinton, D., & Jalal, B. (2019). Dimensions of culturally sensitive CBT: Application to Southeast Asian populations. *American Journal of Orthopsychiatry*, *89*(4), 493–507. https://doi.org/10.1037/ort0000392.

Hinton, D. E., Rivera, E. I., Hofmann, S. G., et al. (2012). Adapting CBT for traumatized refugees and ethnic minority patients: Examples from culturally adapted CBT (CA-CBT). *Transcultural Psychiatry*, *49*(2), 340–365. https://doi.org/10.1177/1363461512441595.

Hofstede, G. (2011). Dimensionalizing cultures: The Hofstede model in context. *Online Readings in Psychology and Culture*, *2*(1). http://scholarworks.gvsu.edu/orpc/vol2/iss1/.

Ipsos Reid Survey. (2020). *Majority (60%) see racism as a serious problem in Canada today, up 13 points since last year.* https://www.ipsos.com/en-ca/majority-60-see-racism-serious-problem-canada-today-13-points-last-year

Kirmayer, L. (2019). The politics of diversity: Pluralism, multiculturalism and mental health. *Transcultural Psychiatry, 56*(6), 1119–1138. https://doi.org/10.1177/1363461519888608.

Kirmayer, L., & Jarvis, G. (2019). Culturally responsive services as a path to equity in mental healthcare. *HealthcarePapers (Toronto), 18*(2), 11–23. https://doi.org/10.12927/hcpap.2019.25925.

Kleinman, A. (1988). *The illness narratives: Suffering, healing and the human condition.* Basic Books.

Kluckhohn, C., & Murray, H. A. (Eds.). (1953). *Personality in nature, society and culture.* Knopf.

Kowatch, K., Schmidt, F., & Mushquash, C. (2019). Review of culturally-adapted cognitive behavioral therapy interventions for North American Indigenous children and youth. *Journal of Concurrent Disorders, 1*(3), 5–22.

Kronick. R. (2018). Mental health of refugees and asylum seekers: Assessment and intervention. *The Canadian Journal of Psychiatry, 63*(5), 290–296. https://doi.org/10.1177/0706743717746665.

Krystallidou, D., Van De Walle, C., Deveugele, M., et al. (2018). Training "doctor-minded" interpreters and "interpreter-minded" doctors: The benefits of collaborative practice in interpreter training. *Interpreting: International Journal of Research and Practice in Interpreting, 20*(1), 126–144. https://doi.org/10.1075/intp.00005.kry.

Lacey, K. K., Parnell, R., Mouzon, D. M., et al. (2015). The mental health of US Black women: The roles of social context and severe intimate partner violence. *BMJ Open, 5,* e008415. https://doi.org/10.1136/bmjopen-2015-008415.

Ladha, T., Zubairi, M., Hunter, A., et al. (2018). Cross-cultural communication: Tools for working with families and children. *Paediatrics & Child Health, 23*(1), 66–69. https://doi.org/10.1093/pch/pxx126.

Leininger, M. (1995). *Transcultural nursing: Concepts, theories, research & practices.* McGraw-Hill, Inc.

Linklater, R. (2020). *Shkaabe Makwa: Connecting communities and service providers.* Centre for Addiction and Mental Health (CAMH).

Liu, K. (2015). Critical reflection as a framework for transformative learning in teacher education. *Educational Review (Birmingham), 67*(2), 135–157. https://doi.org/10.1080/00131911.2013.839546.

Liu, M. (2016). Verbal communication styles and culture. *Oxford Research Encyclopedias: Communication.* https://doi.org/10.1093/acrefore/9780190228613.013.162.

Maina, G., Mclean, M., Mcharo, S., et al. (2020). A scoping review of school-based indigenous substance use prevention in preteens. *Substance Abuse Treatment, Prevention and Policy, 15*(1), 1–74. https://doi.org/10.1186/s13011-020-00314-1.

Marazziti, D., Stahl, S., Simoncini, M., et al. (2020). Psychopharmacology and ethnicity: A comparative study on Senegalese and Italian men. *The World Journal of Biological Psychiatry, 21*(4), 300–307. https://doi.org/10.1080/15622975.2019.1583373.

Mental Health Commission of Canada. (2016). The case for diversity: Building the case to improve mental health services for immigrant, refugee, ethno-cultural and racialized populations. https://www.mentalhealthcommission.ca/wp-content/uploads/drupal/2016-10/case_for_diversity_oct_2016_eng.pdf

Mosley, D., Owen, K., Rostosky, S., et al. (2017). Contextualizing behaviors associated with paranoia: Perspectives of Black men. *Psychology of Men & Masculinity, 18*(2), 165–175. https://doi.org/10.1037/men0000052.

Naeem, F. (2012). *Adaptation of cognitive behaviour therapy for depression in Pakistan.* Lambert Academic Publishing.

Naeem, F., Phiri, P., Rathod, S., et al. (2019). Cultural adaptation of cognitive-behavioural therapy. *British Journal of Psychological Advances, 25*(6), 387–395. https://doi.org/10.1192/bja.2019.15.

Nelson, S., & Wilson, K. (2017). The mental health of Indigenous people in Canada: A critical review of research. *Social Science & Medicine (1982), 176,* 93–112. https://doi.org/10.1016/j.socscimed.2017.01.021.

O'Neill, L., Fraser, T., Kitchenham, A., et al. (2018). Hidden burdens: A review of intergenerational, historical and complex trauma, implications for Indigenous families. *Journal of Child & Adolescent Trauma, 11*(2), 173–186. https://doi.org/10.1007/s40653-016-0117-9.

Paradies, Y., Ben, J., Denson, N., et al. (2015). Racism as a determinant of health: A systematic review and meta-analysis. *PloS One, 10*(9). e0138511–e0138511. https://doi.org/10.1371/journal.pone.0138511.

Ralph, S., & Ryan, K. (2017). Addressing the mental health gap in working with indigenous youth: Some considerations for non-Indigenous psychologists working with Indigenous youth. *Australian Psychologist, 52*(4), 288–298.

Shepherd, S. M., Willis-Esqueda, C., Newton, D., et al. (2019). The challenge of cultural competence in the workplace: Perspectives of healthcare providers. *BMC Health Services Research, 19*, 135. https://doi.org/10.1186/s12913-019-3959-7.

Tam, B., Findlay, L., & Kohen, D. (2017). Indigenous families: Who do you call family? *Journal of Family Studies, 23*(3), 243–259. https://doi.org/10.1080/13229400.2015.1093536.

Turner, B., & Luna Sánchez, S. (2020). The legacy of colonialism in Guatemala and its impact on the psychological and mental health of Indigenous Mayan communities. *International Review of Psychiatry (Abingdon, England), 32*(4), 313–319. https://doi.org/10.1080/09540261.2020.1751090.

Yager, J., & Kay, J. (2020). Clinical curiosity in psychiatric residency training: Implications for education and practice. *Academic Psychiatry, 44*(1), 90–94. https://doi.org/10.1007/s40596-019-01131-w.

Yang, X., Hou, J., & Arth, Z. W. (2021). Communicating in a proper way: How people from high-/low-context culture choose their media for communication. *The International Communication Gazette, 83*(3), 238–259. https://doi.org/10.1177/1748048520902617.

CHAPTER 15

Cultural Considerations in Pain Management

Monakshi Sawhney

At the end of this chapter, the learner will be able to:

- Discuss the definition of pain
- Understand how history impacts the current environment of pain and addiction
- Explain the concept of pain threshold and how this is experienced among different cultural groups
- Discuss variations in the affective responses to pain among various cultural groups
- Understand how to provide culturally sensitive pain care

KEY TERMS

Acute pain	Pain assessment tools	Pain tolerance level
Chronic pain	Pain catastrophizing	Stoic
Pain	Pain threshold	

 evolve.elsevier.com/Srivastava/culturalcompetence/.

Pain is an unpleasant sensation experienced by all people from all cultures, regardless of age, sex, and socioeconomic status. It is a "universal experience of human existence" (Khan et al., 2015). Pain is a subjective experience, and there are variations in the way that people perceive, interpret, and respond to pain. Culture can influence many pain-related factors, such as how people communicate about the pain they are experiencing, pain intensity and tolerance, beliefs about coping with pain, and pain catastrophizing (Sharma et al., 2018).

The International Association for the Study of Pain (IASP) defines **pain** as "an unpleasant sensory and emotional experience associated with, or resembling that associated with, actual or potential tissue damage" (Raja et al., 2020). This definition of pain is supported by six additional key concepts that expand on the definition for a more complete understanding. The six additional concepts are as follows (Raja et al., 2020):

1. Pain is a personal experience and is influenced by biological, psychological, and social factors.
2. Pain is more than a neurological response (i.e., it is more than the activity of sensory neurons).
3. An individual's understanding of pain changes over the lifespan and through life experience.
4. Clinicians need to respect the individual's experience of pain.
5. Pain can be a catalyst for adaptation but it can also have negative effects on function, social, and psychological well-being.
6. There are many ways to express pain (verbal and behavioural).

This definition allows pain to be described as a phenomenon that affects a patient's physical and psychosocial well-being. Pain is a subjective experience that cannot be determined by tissue damage alone. The emotional experience associated with a patient's pain needs to be considered just as carefully as the physical experience.

A definition of pain that highlights its subjective and personal nature comes from McCaffery and Pasero (1999). They state that "pain is whatever the experiencing person says it is, existing whenever [they say] it does" (McCaffery & Pasero, 1999, p. 17). This definition helps us to remember that each patient is an expert when it comes to their own pain (McCaffery & Pasero, 1999).

Acute pain is defined as "the physiologic response to and experience of noxious stimuli that can become pathologic, is normally sudden in onset, time limited, and motivates behaviours to avoid potential or actual potential tissue injury" (Kent et al., 2017, pp. 950; Health Quality Ontario, 2018a).

Chronic non-cancer pain is defined as pain that lasts beyond the typical healing time following an injury, or pain that lasts 3 months or longer. Chronic non-cancer pain has a negative effect on quality of life, and it interferes with activities of daily living (Fillingim et al., 2014; Health Quality Ontario, 2018b). In Canada, 19% of the population reports living with chronic pain (Cragg et al., 2018).

Pain is also a safety mechanism in that it can provide an early warning of illness, and it can provide information on how to adapt or protect ourselves (Woolf, 2010). Unfortunately, there is a small group of people who are diagnosed with congenital insensitivity to pain (CIP), an extremely rare genetic phenotype in which no pain of any type is experienced during an affected individual's lifetime (Drissi et al., 2020). The inability to feel pain is dangerous and leads to repeated injuries and prevents normal healing.

Cultural Considerations In Care

Assessing for Safe Patient-Centred Care

Uthman, a 65-year-old man from Egypt, moved to Canada 20 years ago and underwent a total knee arthroplasty yesterday. His health history reveals he has severe osteoarthritis of the knee and mild lower back pain; he is otherwise healthy and does not take any prescription medications. After surgery this man will be taking an anticoagulant for 14 days to prevent a deep vein thrombosis (DVT), and analgesics to help manage postoperative pain (Bircher & Chowdhury, 2020; Chou et al., 2016).

He asks the health care team members when he can resume having cupping treatments for his back pain and general health. Further assessment reveals Uthman uses massage and dry cupping treatments to help promote well-being, increase circulation, and improve his immune system.

What steps need to be taken to ensure that the care provided is safe and patient centred?

As countries continue to grow in cultural diversity, greater attention is being placed on understanding how culture influences the experience of pain. Psychosocial factors that are influenced by culture are an important part of the assessment and management of pain. Mark Zoborowski (1952) was one of the earliest researchers to examine cultural differences in the response to pain, and he recognized that pain acquires specific social and cultural significances and that reactions to pain should be examined in this light. Understanding group attitudes toward pain may be helpful in the understanding of individual reactions (Zoborowski, 1952) and can help health care providers in providing culturally focused pain management. However, the way culture and beliefs influence an individual's behaviour regarding pain and pain management varies from "place to place and person to person" and what may be culturally acceptable to one person may be unacceptable to another person, even if they share the same cultural background (Ovienloba, 2017, p. 31).

The purpose of this chapter is to provide guidance on culturally sensitive pain management practice. This chapter begins with a review of historical concepts of pain management among cultural groups, as well as the differences in how various cultural groups experience and express pain. Concepts of pain threshold, tolerance, catastrophizing, and stoicism along with differences in affective response to pain are highlighted along with a discussion of factors that have an impact on access to pain care.

History, Philosophy, Religion, and Politics: Impact on Pain

The history of the meaning of pain can and does shape our current understanding of the term. There are philosophical, religious, and political meanings of pain that existed before health care providers began to study this phenomenon. Pain has been depicted in religion and philosophy for centuries. An understanding of, or belief about, pain and its management in the general population is still influenced by these early views. Philosophers and historians have depicted pain as both a physical sensation and an emotion. Socrates and Kant both described the need for an individual to experience pain in order to fully understand and experience pleasure (Khan et al., 2015). They described the need to experience the contrast between pain and pleasure to truly appreciate both.

An understanding of, or belief about, pain and its management in the general population continues to be influenced by religious views. Religious beliefs can play an important role in an individual's response to the experience of pain In the religious context, pain is a common image in Judeo-Christian teaching and includes stories of the test of religious faith (Khan et al., 2015; Meldrum, 2003). Many people hold the view that pain has been inflicted on them to atone for previous wrongdoings. In the Hindu religion pain is thought to be experienced as a result of Karma, or for past actions either in the current life or a past life (Barbato, 2017). Prayer and religious beliefs have been used to help manage pain for centuries and are still being used today. Research studies have demonstrated that focusing or meditating on religious images, regardless of the religion, can reduce the intensity of pain in followers of the respective religion (Barbato, 2017). A study that examined the impact of religious prayer as compared to secular prayer on pain during the application of painful electrical stimulation reported that pain intensity was reduced by 11% and pain unpleasantness by 26% with religious prayer, when compared to secular prayer (Elmholdt et al., 2017). It is important for health care providers to explore the impact of religious beliefs and effectiveness of religious coping strategies, including prayer, on the patient's pain experience.

In addition to religious teachings, the political climate throughout the world has an influence on current beliefs about pain. The use of opioids in pain management is one example of a treatment option that has been affected by historical and political events. The events of the First and Second World Wars, Prohibition, and the ongoing fight against street drugs continue to shape our current attitudes about pain and its management. Today, throughout the world, health care providers individuals, and governments have a heightened concern about opioid misuse and addiction. However, until the late 1800s, opioids were unregulated and readily available at the local pharmacy. Opioids were the standard treatment for the management of acute pain, chronic pain, and cancer or palliative pain. This changed in the 1870s when physicians became concerned about the misuse of opioids (Jones et al., 2018). Today, many people (and health care providers) fear that addiction to opioids or opioid-related death will occur with the use of opioids for managing pain. One of the reasons why pain continues to be undertreated in Canada and in other countries is this fear of creating addiction (Government of Canada, 2019; Webster et al., 2019). The opioid crisis is becoming a global concern, expanding from North America to other parts of the world, including Australia. For further information, see Belzak and Halverson (2018), Vadivelu et al. (2018), and Tomazin (2020).

The history of systemic racism in the use of pain medicine has resulted in the unnecessary suffering of many patients, simply because of their cultural or ethnic background. Anti-Black racism, anti-Indigenous racism, and racism against people of colour have highlighted how the social construct of race has impacted the ability of people from different cultures to obtain effective pain management (Hoffman et al., 2016; Patrick, 2020). Such treatment is based on the concept of a false belief, an internal cognitive representation that is not supported by evidence (Schweikart, 2018). False beliefs, such as that the bodies of Black people (people of African descent) are biologically different from the bodies of White people, and that Black people have a thicker skull and thicker skin and are therefore less sensitive to pain, have been supported by scientists and physicians to justify the inhumane treatment of Black people in medical research. These false beliefs continue to influence the treatment of pain in people who are Black, in Indigenous people, and in other persons of colour (Hoffman et al., 2016; Mack et al., 2018).

Indigenous people in Canada, Australia, and throughout the world experience difficulties accessing health care services, including appropriate pain assessment and effective pain management. The barriers to accessing health services include difficulty in obtaining quality care, long wait times to be assessed by health care providers, and experiences of racism and discrimination. Indigenous people have reported that health care providers may not believe reports of pain and may deny analgesics to treat pain because of concerns regarding substance misuse in Indigenous communities (Latimer et al., 2018; Nelson & Wilson, 2018; Strong et al., 2015; Turpel-Lafond, 2020). Stereotypes and implicit bias practised by health care providers continue to impact the delivery of effective pain management for persons of colour (Health Canada, 2021).

Cultural Considerations in Care

Personal Views on Pain

Think about the past 6 months and any experiences of pain that you or a family member experienced.

- How was the pain experienced and managed? How was this influenced by understanding the cause of the pain (e.g., injury, chronic illness, or uncertain etiology)?
- Was the pain managed by medications or non-pharmaceutical strategies? What factors influenced these choices?
- Did others understand and acknowledge your (or your family member's) pain experience? What supports were (or could have been) helpful?

Pain Threshold, Tolerance, Catastrophizing, and Stoicism

Why do different people or different groups of people experience and express pain in different ways? Are there differences in the pain thresholds of various cultural groups? The following definitions review experiences and expression of pain that health care providers may witness. These experiences or expressions of pain may be part of a cultural norm. While it is important to understand these definitions, it is equally important to remember that pain is a subjective and individual experience. In pain research, the **pain threshold** is defined as the "minimum intensity of a stimulus that is perceived as painful" (IASP, 2017), and **pain tolerance level** is the greatest level of pain that an individual is "willing to accept in a given situation" (IASP, 2017). It is important to note that both pain threshold and pain tolerance level are the subjective experiences of the individual (IASP, 2017). **Pain catastrophizing** is defined as "an exaggerated negative mental set brought to bear during actual or anticipated painful experience" (Sullivan et al., 2001). Being **stoic** is defined as a "firmly restraining response to pain or distress" (Merriam-Webster Online Dictionary, 2005). Stoic behaviour on the part of a patient does not necessarily mean that within the patient's culture there is a high tolerance for pain, rather it may be a reflection of cultural norms that determine how pain should be expressed. Conversely, an emotional response to pain does not mean the patient is seeking analgesics. Health care providers should avoid cultural stereotyping associated with pain threshold, pain tolerance, catastrophizing, and stoicism when assessing and managing pain. It is important to individually assess each patient who is experiencing pain (Raja et al., 2020).

There are very few Canadian published studies that examine pain within different cultural groups or pain in persons who are socially marginalized. Therefore, this chapter draws largely from data from the United States. Kim and colleagues (2017) conducted a meta-analysis examining racial and ethnic differences in pain sensitivity in the United States and including people who identified as Black (African American), Asian, White (European), or Hispanic. The authors reported that people who self-identified as Black, Asian, or Hispanic had a lower pain tolerance than that of White people when a cold pain stimulus was applied. When heat was used as a painful stimulus, people of Asian descent had a lower heat pain threshold and reported higher pain scores compared with White and Hispanic people. Black people reported higher heat pain sensitivity compared to White people (Kim et al., 2017). When heat pain (thermal sensory testing) was compared in healthy volunteers in three distinct East Asian populations—Chinese, Malaysian, and Indian—Yosipovitch et al. (2004) found no significant differences in pain thresholds between the three populations.

Studies that examined experimental pressure pain reported no difference in pain threshold between African American, Hispanic, and White people. When experimental pressure pain was examined in people from different Asian countries (China, Japan, and India) as compared to people from European countries (Denmark, Sweden), White Europeans had a higher pain threshold than that of Asians (Kim et al., 2017). Studies examining the tolerance level of people within various cultural groups have found that African American subjects rated cutaneous heat (heat applied to the skin, increasing temperature) and tourniquet pain as more unpleasant and more intense than did White individuals, indicating that African Americans had a lower pain tolerance (Kim et al., 2017). Similarly, the Orofacial Pain: Prospective Evaluation and Risk Assessment (OPPERA) study reported that women were significantly more pain-sensitive than men and White people were less pain-sensitive than Blacks, people of Hispanic descent, and Asian individuals (Ostrom et al., 2017).

These studies indicate that different people experience variations in pain tolerance, but they do not show a difference in pain threshold based on culture or ethnicity. It is important to note that all of these studies had a small sample size, thereby limiting a broad application of the findings to the general public. The identification that a specific stimulus is painful (e.g., a thermal probe at 30°C), also known as pain threshold, does not indicate how long that painful stimulus will be tolerated, or the severity of the pain an individual will experience. There is no strong evidence that pain threshold varies among cultural groups, yet stereotypes continue to influence the practice of health care providers (Hoffman et al., 2016). Each individual has personal beliefs and preconceptions about pain that are based on cultural, sociological, and ethnic factors. Social and cultural norms within an ethnic group often dictate how and to what degree pain behaviour is expressed (Yosipovitch et al., 2004). We can learn more about these norms in response to pain from clinically based, observational studies that focus on affective responses to pain.

Differences in Affective Responses to Pain

As stated earlier, Mark Zoborowski (1952), one of the first researchers to examine the influence of cultural norms on pain, concluded that differences exist among varying cultural groups. However, similar reactions to pain by members of different cultural groups do not necessarily reflect similar attitudes toward pain, and similar reactions toward pain may have different functions or meanings in various cultures (Zoborowski, 1952).

Zoborowski's early study has been the basis of other studies that explore cultural influence on pain. A pilot qualitative study conducted in the United States, which examined cultural differences in pain experience, found that African American and Hispanic participants were more likely than Asian and White participants to say they openly expressed pain symptoms. The participant's response to pain was similar to their family members' response to pain (Liao et al., 2016). See Table 15.1 for some examples that may help health care providers understand how people from different cultural backgrounds respond to pain and manage pain.

TABLE 15.1 ■ **Examples of Responses to Pain**

Group	Response to Pain
Hispanic descent	Traditional Hispanic cultures view pain and illness as punishment from God. Many will use religion or prayer to cope with pain (Gagnon et al., 2014; Hollingshead et al., 2016). Pain may be viewed as a positive experience as it helps with spiritual growth (Liao et al., 2016).
	People of Cuban, Mexican, Puerto Rican, South or Central American, or other Spanish culture descent living in the United States may report fewer pain conditions and less pain-related interference with activities of daily living as they focus on maintaining their level of functioning so they can maintain their social roles. In addition, they may wait until pain is severe before asking for help to manage their pain, because of fears of addiction or adverse effects of medications (Hollingshead et al., 2016).
	Regarding chronic pain, some may use pain catastrophizing as a way of describing pain and coping with pain (Gagnon et al., 2014; Meints et al., 2019).
African descent (African American, Black Canadian)	African Americans may express a greater severity of pain than Americans of White European descent (Kim et al., 2017).
	Prayer, hoping, and emotion-focused coping may be used as a coping strategy (Miller-Matero et al., 2017; Orhan et al., 2018). When asked what pain means to them, it is described as a sensory experience or "hurt."
	African Americans may wait until the pain is severe before asking a doctor or nurse for assistance (Liao et al., 2016).
Women from Arabic cultures during childbirth	Women of Arab descent are verbally expressive during labour, often crying and screaming. They will accept analgesics to manage pain during childbirth (Kridli, 2002). However, these women gain comfort and support from their religious faith and other female members of their family (Callister et al., 2003).
Hindu South Asian	Hindu South Asians in Canada may prefer to define pain in relation to how much it interferes with daily functioning or work (Bostick et al., 2020; Holt & Waterfield, 2018). They may change their diet and eat foods that are known to decrease inflammation, or use traditional remedies to help manage pain (Bostick et al., 2020).
	In a study of South Asian women in the United Kingdom living with chronic pain, the women described having to continue their work despite having pain, to care for their families and community (Mustafa et al., 2020).
Chinese descent	Patients of Chinese descent may be reluctant to express pain, as revealing and admitting to pain is a sign of weakness. They may endure pain and not report it until it becomes unbearable.
	They may be reluctant to discuss pain out of the belief that talking about the problem to someone outside of the family will bring shame to them. This can make it difficult to assess the patient's pain accurately. In addition, health care providers are perceived as people of high social status, therefore it may be culturally inappropriate to bother them (Tung & Li, 2015). Some may believe good patients do not complain and may present themselves as the "perfect patients" by suppressing their emotions even if they experience severe pain (Tung & Li, 2015). Patients may also have negative beliefs about opioids and their related adverse effects.
Indigenous people in Canada	In some Indigenous communities in Canada and the United States, the Medicine Wheel is an important concept in health and well-being. It consists of four dimensions of well-being: physical, mental, emotional, and spiritual (Latimer et al., 2018).
	Indigenous youth and adults may hide their pain from health care providers and members of their family in an effort to remain reserved and be respected (Duwe, 2019). They may be reluctant to report pain and only use vague descriptions when they are reporting pain.
	A qualitative study that examined the pain experience of Indigenous youth described situations in which participants tried to manage their pain on their own by lying down, ignoring the pain, and rubbing the painful location (Latimer et al., 2018).

In summary, people with different cultural backgrounds express pain in various ways and attach different meanings to the pain they experience. Health care providers should recognize that some people adapt or assimilate to the culture into which they migrate. Health care providers should not assume that every person affiliated with a specific cultural group will display the pain behaviours of that cultural group. An understanding of these affective responses to pain should help health care providers to recognize the variations in the way pain is expressed and be amenable to these variations.

Complementary and Alternative Pain Management Treatments

Some people include traditional Chinese medicine (TCM), Ayurvedic medicine, and complementary and alternative medicine (CAM) into their pain-management regimens (these forms of healing are also discussed in Chapter 8).

TCM has existed for more than 5 000 years and involves an understanding of the human body based on the circulation of the universe (a person and heaven are one entity) (Yuan et al., 2015). It involves balancing the energy within and around the individual. It includes treatments such as acupuncture, acupressure, moxibustion (in which the mugwort herb moxa is burned near the skin), massage, and diet (Harvie et al., 2019). There is evidence that acupuncture, acupressure, and cupping are effective in relieving neck pain and low back pain and pain from migraines (Harvie et al., 2019; Yuan et al., 2015).

Cupping therapy has been used for centuries in the Middle East and Asia to treat a number of health care problems including pain. Cupping involves applying cups to selected skin points and creating a subatmospheric pressure, either by heat or by suction, to increase blood flow and decrease inflammation, thereby promoting blood flow and improving the immune system (Aboushanab & AlSanad, 2018; Al-Bedah et al., 2018). Cupping therapy has been reported to show benefits in the treatment of lower back pain, neck and shoulder pain, headache and migraine, and knee pain. Based on the available evidence, patients who have cancer, patients with organ failure, patients who have pacemakers, patients with hemophilia or sickle cell disease, patients with acute infection, and patients who are using anticoagulants, have heart disease, or are pregnant should not receive cupping treatments (Aboushanab & AlSanad, 2018; Al-Bedah et al., 2018).

TCM bears similarities to Hindu Ayurvedic medicine, which has also provided a traditional perspective on the management of pain. Ayurvedic medicine is a comprehensive medical system that has been part of the traditional system of health care in India for more than 5 000 years. It is similar to TCM in that it focuses on establishing and maintaining balance of the life energies within an individual, rather than focusing on individual symptoms. Ayurvedic treatments include meditation, yoga, massage, herbs, and diet. Herbal treatment can include the application of ointments, including "pain ointments." The number of studies evaluating the effect of Ayurvedic treatments has been increasing; many studies report positive effects of Ayurvedic treatments, with minimal adverse effects (Kessler et al., 2015). Topical Ayurvedic treatments, such as Rumalya, have been shown to be effective to manage pain from osteoarthritis (Kessler et al., 2015). Yoga, which is also considered a form of exercise, can be effective for improving pain, function, and stiffness (Cramer et al., 2017).

The use of curcumin or turmeric as either an oral supplement or added to food has increased in popularity for the management of pain caused by inflammation. A randomized controlled trial examined the effectiveness of curcumin (turmeric) and the combination of curcumin and boswellic acid as compared to placebo on pain in patients with osteoarthritis. This trial reported that the use of curcumin alone and the combination of curcumin and boswellic acid reduced pain in patients with osteoarthritis (Haroyan et al., 2018). The effectiveness of curcumin in reducing osteoarthritis-related pain has been compared to the non-steroidal anti-inflammatory drug

(NSAID) diclofenac in an open-label study (Shep et al., 2019). This study reported that patients taking curcumin had similar reduction in pain as compared to the patients taking diclofenac, indicating that curcumin could be an alternative analgesic for people who cannot take NSAIDs; however, more research is needed (Shep et al., 2019).

Acknowledging that patients may be using traditional medicine or CAM as part of their pain management plan is important. Approximately 10% of Canadians, 30% of Americans, and over 50% of Australians use CAM (Canizares et al., 2017; Nahin et al., 2016; Steel et al., 2018). For pain management, this includes, but is not limited to, treatments such as acupuncture, massage, chiropractic care, and homeopathy or naturopathy. The body of evidence for CAM in pain management is increasing, and as its use increases, health care providers can review the evidence associated with these treatments, as they may be expected to answer patients' questions about the potential value of CAM in the management of pain. Health care providers should routinely assess patients' use of CAM to help manage their pain and be open to evaluating the usefulness of these therapies as well as partnering with culturally based healers. This requires health care providers to be aware of their own biases and views on pain management, along with an approach that reflects the view that the patient is the expert in their pain management.

Access to Pain Care in North America

Chronic pain is pain that has persisted for at least 3 to 6 months more than the time of expected tissue healing. Chronic pain, in Canada, is more common among older persons, females, Indigenous people, veterans, and populations affected by social inequities and discrimination (Government of Canada, 2019). In Canada, chronic pain is reported most frequently by persons of low income, with a mean health care cost (hospitalizations, drugs, and physician care) of $5 177 per person each year and costs increasing each year (Hogan et al., 2016).

In the United States it is estimated that 50 million adults experience chronic pain that interferes with daily life or work activities. The cost of pain is estimated at between $560 billion and $635 billion annually (U.S. Department of Health and Human Services, 2019). These cost estimates are based on direct care costs and do not include less quantifiable costs, such as quality of life. Australian data indicate that, in 2016, one in five Australians (1.6 million people) had chronic pain, at an estimated 2018 cost of $139 billion due to loss of productivity and reduced quality of life (Australian Institute of Health and Welfare, 2020). Mills et al. (2019) note that globally, chronic pain is among the leading causes of disease and disability and that the burden of chronic pain is increasing worldwide.

Although the burden of chronic pain is significant across societies, access to care is inconsistent. Many factors contribute to the inadequate availability of pain care in communities across Canada and the United States. Socioeconomic and cultural barriers may impede access to effective interprofessional pain care (Health Canada, 2020; U.S. Department of Health and Human Services, 2019). Evidence exists of racial and ethnic disparities in pain treatment and treatment outcomes; however, few interventions have been designed to address these disparities. Lower quality pain care may be related to many factors, including barriers to accessing health care, lack of insurance, discrimination, lower likelihood to be screened or receive treatment, and environmental barriers that impede self-management (Health Canada, 2020; U.S. Department of Health and Human Services, 2019). Individualized patient-centred care that includes physical, psychological, and pharmacological therapies to manage acute and chronic pain is vital.

Table 15.2 highlights the barriers that people from different cultures may face when accessing care related to their pain. Although the literature cited in the table is limited to Canada and the United States, the issues are global, and readers are encouraged to seek out information for the populations they serve.

TABLE 15.2 ▪ Common Barriers to Accessing Pain Care

Barrier	
Inconsistent pain assessment and treatment	Studies of culturally diverse populations have found that there is a high prevalence of unrelieved pain among minority groups. In a study of nursing home residents, non-Hispanic Black residents were less likely to have either their self-reported pain or pain behaviours documented than were non-Hispanic White residents. Black residents also received less analgesics than White residents (Mack et al., 2018). In other studies, Hispanic Americans reported that health care providers did not believe their reports of pain, and sometimes these patients did not receive analgesics when hospitalized (Hollingshead et al., 2016).
Language barrier	Language barriers, lack of interpreter services, and cultural differences in communication styles are commonly reported by both health care providers and patients in management of acute pain and chronic pain (Bostick et al., 2020; Lor et al., 2020; Meints et al., 2019; Sharma et al., 2016). A study examining the documentation of pain intensity for hospitalized Spanish-speaking patients compared to English-speaking patients reported that Spanish speakers' pain was assessed and documented significantly less frequently than English speakers' pain. This suggests an insufficient use of interpreter services (McDonald et al., 2015).
Fear of addiction	Health care providers fear the possibility of opioid misuse and addiction and need to balance the risk of opioid misuse with effective pain management (Health Canada, 2020; Webster et al., 2019). Fear of addiction also creates a reluctance on the part of the patient to take opioids to manage pain, when taking them would be appropriate.
Lack of knowledge	The assessment and management of pain are affected by the health care providers' knowledge and attitudes regarding pain and pain management. Surveys of health care providers have documented knowledge deficits and attitudinal barriers related to the control of pain (Bouya et al., 2019; Health Canada, 2020; Hroch et al., 2019; Smeland et al., 2018; Ung et al., 2016).

Providing Culturally Sensitive Pain Care

To enhance cultural sensitivity, health care providers should assess and discuss patients' understanding of and beliefs about pain. This assessment can occur with patients and their families so that mutual goals are identified and are taken into account (Bostick et al., 2020; Lor et al., 2020). The following approaches can be used to help provide culturally sensitive pain care.

BE AWARE OF PERSONAL VALUES THAT MAY AFFECT THE ASSESSMENT AND TREATMENT OF PAIN

It is important for health care providers to explore their implicit biases or personal values regarding pain management so they can differentiate their own values from the values of those for whom they provide care. The patient's ethnic background may unconsciously influence health care providers' decisions regarding pain management. Studies of health care providers' accuracy in assessing patients' pain have found that medical and nursing personnel underestimate patients' pain and may limit use of analgesics (Ruben et al., 2015).

When the health care provider and the patient who is experiencing pain share a common language and values regarding the expression and meaning of pain, there may be less misunderstanding regarding pain experiences and management (Lor et al., 2020). However, when the values regarding the expression and meaning of pain are different, conflict can arise when it comes to determining the most effective pain-management plan.

Western society values a stoic response to pain. When patients are expressive of their pain, they may be seen as unable to cope and may be identified as "bad" or "uncooperative" patients. Health care providers must be aware of biases and stereotypes when assessing and managing pain

(Hoffman et al., 2016). One way to assist in the elimination of negative patient labels is to avoid using the phrase "complaints of pain." A more objective way to communicate a patient's pain, either verbally or in writing, would be to cite "the client's report of pain" and use objective measures to assess pain (Scher et al., 2018).

Cultural Competence In Action

Patient's Topical Ointment Preference

Patients may have treatment preferences that health care providers need to understand, as is the case with Savita, a 62-year-old woman of East Indian descent who has been admitted to the hospital for the treatment of community-acquired pneumonia.

Savita also has painful chronic rheumatoid arthritis in her right knee. At home, she managed the pain in her knee with a topical "pain ointment" that her younger brother sent from India. She has experienced decreased mobility since being admitted into the hospital, which she attributes to the pain in her knee. However, Savita refuses to take the oral analgesic that was prescribed as she feels it would be unnecessary if she were able to use her own pain ointment.

Although, based on your personal beliefs, you think Savita should use oral analgesics as the first-line treatment for her pain, you understand that the topical treatment is her preference. After researching the literature regarding this topical treatment for the management of arthritis pain, you find limited but positive evidence to support this practice. You then advocate on behalf of the patient that she be allowed to continue her topical treatment for her painful rheumatoid arthritis while in the hospital. Savita's family is happy to bring the pain ointment to the hospital for her to use as necessary.

This example highlights how personal beliefs regarding the treatment of pain may differ, but how discussion and research can help health care providers to incorporate personal and cultural preference into the plan of care for their patients.

BE CONSCIOUS OF VARIATIONS IN AFFECTIVE RESPONSES AND THE MEANING OF PAIN AMONG CULTURES

How pain is experienced and expressed varies across cultural groups. This may be due to cultural values of stoicism or fear of being misjudged and disrespected on the basis of health care provider biases. It is therefore important to be mindful of one's own assumptions, to intentionally assess pain using validated tools, and to assess for efficacy of pain management strategies in a patient-centred manner.

Use Established Pain Assessment Tools To Assist In Measuring Pain

Patients from many different cultures may be assessed using similar validated pain assessment tools, and the findings will have similar meanings across cultures. Behavioural expression of pain may differ among cultural groups; however, pain ratings and tools to assess pain can be applied across cultures with success. Many validated pain assessment tools have been translated into different languages and have been tested in different countries around the world. Self-report of the intensity of pain should be measured using valid and reliable tools. Examples of **pain assessment tools** include, but are not limited to, the numeric rating scale (NRS), faces scales, and verbal descriptors of pain, as well as behavioural and observational tools to assess pain in infants and non-verbal adults (Herr et al., 2004; Hicks et al., 2001; Karcioglu et al., 2018; Scher et al., 2018).

Pain Intensity Scales

An NRS of pain intensity consists of a range of numbers from 0 to 10 (see Fig. 15.1A). Individuals are informed that 0 represents "no pain" and 10 represents "worst pain imaginable." The NRS may be used either verbally or visually. A patient with pain would state or record the number that best represents their level of pain intensity. Another way to assess the intensity of pain is by using the word descriptor scale. This consists of asking the patient if the pain is none, mild, moderate, or severe (Karcioglu, et al., 2018).

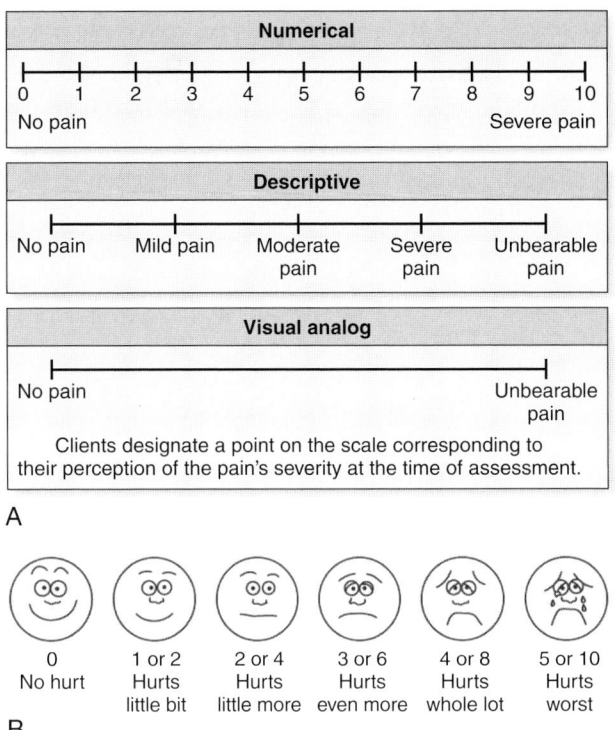

Fig. 15.1 Pain Assessment Scales. (A) Numerical, descriptive, and visual analogue scales. (B) Wong-Baker FACES Pain Rating Scale. ([B] Wong-Baker FACES Foundation. [1983]. www.WongBakerFACES.org. Used with permission. Originally published in Hockenberry, M. J., & Wilson, D. (2018). *Whaley & Wong's nursing care of infants and children*. Elsevier Inc.)

The Faces Pain Scale—Revised

Faces pain scales present the patient with drawings of facial expressions, representing increasing levels of pain intensity (Hicks et al., 2001; Karcioglu et al., 2018). The patient is asked to select the face that best represents their pain intensity (or level), and the resulting score is the corresponding number (rank order) of the expression chosen. Patients do not see the numbers; these are shown in Fig. 15.1B only for reference purposes. The Faces Pain Scale—Revised (FPS-R) is available in 22 languages (https://www.iasp-pain.org/resources/faces-pain-scale-revised/). It was developed to assess pain intensity in children but can also be used with adults, even when a language barrier exists.

Additional Pain Assessment Tools

A multidimensional tool can be used when a more comprehensive pain assessment is necessary. The McGill Pain Questionnaire and the Brief Pain Inventory are two examples of comprehensive pain assessment tools. Both of these validated assessment tools are available online and have been used with patients from a variety of cultural backgrounds (Cleeland et al., 1996; Greenwald, 1991; Lasch, 2000; Melzak, 1975; Saxena et al., 1999).

Remember that a patient's self-report of pain is the most reliable indicator of the presence and intensity of pain and its impact on function and quality of life. In addition to the established pain assessment tools, Table 15.1 presents questions that may assist the health care provider in obtaining a culturally sensitive pain assessment.

TABLE 15.1 ■ Questions You Can Ask to Assess an Individual's Beliefs About Pain

- What do you call your pain? What name do you give it?
- Why do you think you have this pain?
- What does your pain mean for your body?
- How severe is it? Will it last a long or short time?
- Do you have any fears about your pain? If so, what do you fear most about your pain?
- What are the chief problems that your pain causes for you?
- What kind of treatment do you think you should receive? What are the most important results you hope to receive from the treatment?
- What cultural remedies have you tried to help you with your pain?
- Have you seen a traditional healer for your pain? Do you want to?
- Who, if anyone, in your family do you talk to about your pain? What do they know? What do you want them to know?
- Do you have family and friends that help you because of your pain? If so, who helps you?

From Lasch, K. E. (2000). Culture, pain, and culturally sensitive pain care. *Pain Management Nursing,* *1*(3 Suppl. I), p. 19.

BIOLOGICAL DIFFERENCES IN THE METABOLISM OF MEDICATIONS

Patients' genetic makeup, as influenced by their ethnic background, can have an impact on how medication is metabolized. For example, codeine (a prodrug), a weak opioid analgesic, is metabolized in the liver and converted to its active analgesic form, which is morphine. It is converted from codeine into morphine using a cytochrome P-450 enzyme, CYP 2D6. This is also true for tramadol, which is a prodrug that is metabolized by cytochrome P-450 (CYP), enzymes CYP2D6, and CYP3A4 to its more potent opioid analgesic metabolites, particularly O-desmethyltramadol (Crews et al., 2012; Miotto et al., 2017). However, some people produce only a small amount of the enzyme CYP 2D6 and are not able to break down (metabolize) codeine into morphine, or tramadol into O-desmethyltramadol. If a patient cannot metabolize these analgesics they will be ineffective (Miotto et al., 2017).

About 5–10% of individuals are poor metabolizers. In these individuals, codeine and tramadol will provide little or no pain relief. Poor metabolizers are more commonly found among White Europeans and their descendants (Dean, 2021). There are also people who are ultra-rapid (very fast) metabolizers, and they experience an increase in the production of active ingredients (metabolites) of codeine (which is morphine) and tramadol (which is O-desmethyltramadol). It is estimated that 1–2% of individuals are ultra-rapid metabolizers, but this can vary widely in different ethnic groups. It is estimated that up to 28% of North Africans, Ethiopians, and Arabs; up to 10% of White people; 3% of African Americans; and up to 1% of Hispanics, Chinese, and Japanese are ultra-metabolizers

---

Cultural Competence In Action

Assessment, Bias, and Assumptions

Christopher, a 26-year-old Black Canadian man, undergoes emergency surgery for appendicitis. He has been admitted to the inpatient surgical unit, and he returned from surgery 8 hours ago. Following his appendectomy surgery, he is receiving codeine, acetaminophen, and celecoxib to manage his pain. Using the numeric rating scale, he rates his pain at rest as 6/10, and 8/10 when he moves. He informs you that the codeine he is receiving is not effective in managing his pain and is asking if his pain medicine can be changed to something stronger. When you leave his room, you can hear him talking on the phone and laughing.

1. What would you document for Christopher's pain intensity?
2. What are the possible reasons for Christopher's request for a stronger or different opioid?
3. What next steps would you take regarding Christopher's pain management?

(Dean, 2021). In children who are ultra-rapid metabolizers, the use of codeine or tramadol can lead to oversedation, respiratory depression, and death (Fortenberry et al., 2019). Switching to an opioid that is not activated by CYP2D6 may provide more effective pain relief. Examples of such opioids include morphine, hydromorphone, oxycodone, and fentanyl (Owusu Obeng et al., 2017; Smith et al., 2019).

INCLUDE CULTURALLY SPECIFIC AND PATIENT-CENTRED PRACTICES INTO THE PAIN MANAGEMENT PLAN

The health care team must communicate, with both the patient and the family, how culturally specific practices can be included into the plan of care. This type of discussion can help to clarify which methods of treatment the patient would find helpful, or not helpful, to manage their pain. Understanding the common beliefs about pain in various cultures is helpful for providing culturally sensitive pain management. When health care providers educate themselves regarding cultural diversity, cultural awareness, and cultural sensitivity, they are better able to provide holistic, inclusive, culturally safe patient-centred care.

Summary

Pain is a subjective experience that has different meanings for different people. As cultural diversity increases, health care providers will be required to care for individuals from many backgrounds that are different from their own, with pain management being an important aspect of the care provided. It is important to recognize that different cultural groups express pain in a variety of ways: some groups allow for free expression of pain, while others value stoicism. Different cultural groups also ascribe different meanings to their pain. Individuals who have immigrated may adopt their new homeland's common expression and meaning of pain, leaving behind their traditional cultural values. There are also many barriers to accessing effective care of acute and chronic pain. It is important for health care providers to take a culturally sensitive, client patient-centred approach to the assessment and management of pain that recognizes the cultural differences in pain experiences and also the sociocultural barriers to effective pain care.

When assessing pain in clients from different cultural backgrounds, knowledge of cultural patterns may be useful for making generalizations about populations; however, these generalizations should not be used to predict individual behaviour (Crawley et al., 2002). One way to help avoid making these generalizations in pain assessment and management is to remember the definition of pain: pain is an individual, subjective experience, with both emotional and sensory components. Only the individual who is experiencing the pain can describe it and indicate when it occurs. Nonverbal cues to determine the presence and intensity of pain may not always be present. Using valid and reliable pain assessment tools and asking questions that can assist in obtaining a culturally sensitive pain assessment will aid health care providers in determining the presence and intensity of the pain, and the best treatment plan.

Questions for Review and Discussion

1. What are some of the pain-related factors that culture can influence?
2. How can health care providers avoid personal bias when assessing pain?
3. How can health care provides utilize knowledge about cultural groups' views toward pain?
4. Identify three strategies to improve pain management when caring for patients from diverse cultural groups.

Group Experiential/Reflection Activity

1. Working in small groups, review the Cultural Considerations in Care box "Assessing for Safe Patient-Centred Care" near the beginning of the chapter. Discuss and identity actions

to support Uthman's request to use cupping as a method to manage pain. List all actions suggested by group members. Place these actiovns in order of priority. Eliminate actions or steps that do not support culturally safe care and patient-centred care.

Did your answers include:

- Understanding what cupping is
- Seeking evidence regarding how cupping is helpful to manage pain and improve health
- Determining if there are any absolute or relative contraindications for cupping

In your follow-up, you have learned that a *relative contraindication* for cupping is anticoagulant use, and you are aware that the protocol calls for anticoagulant use for 14 days after surgery. Discuss ways to approach this potential conflict. (Hint: consider modes of decision making discussed in Chapter 4).

2. Review the report "In Plain Sight" (Turpel-Lafond, 2020) for examples of discriminatory experiences in pain care. Discuss in small groups how health care providers can address this to improve pain care. Have you witnessed examples similar to those cited? If you did, what actions can you take? (Hint: see Chapter 4 section on allyship and advocacy). Reflect on stereotypes or bias that health care providers may have that can impact the pain assessment or pain management of a client.

References

Aboushanab, T. S., & AlSanad, S. (2018). Cupping therapy: An overview from a modern medicine perspective. *Journal of Acupuncture and Meridian Studies, 11*(3), 83–87. https://doi.org/10.1016/j.jams.2018.02.001.

Al-Bedah, A., Elsubai, I. S., Qureshi, N. A., et al. (2018). The medical perspective of cupping therapy: Effects and mechanisms of action. *Journal of Traditional and Complementary Medicine, 9*(2), 90–97.

Australian Institute of Health and Welfare (2020) *Chronic pain in Australia.* https://www.aihw.gov.au/getmedia/10434b6f-2147-46ab-b654-a90f05592d35/aihw-phe-267.pdf.aspx?inline=true

Barbato, M. (2017). Interreligious resources for pain management. *The Journal of Interreligious Studies, 20,* 80–89.

Belzak, L., & Halverson, J. (2018). The opioid crisis in Canada: A national perspective. *Health Promotion and Chronic Disease Prevention in Canada : Research, Policy and Practice, 38*(6), 224–233. https://doi.org/10.24095/hpcdp.38.6.02.

Bircher, A., & Chowdhury, A. (2020). Current DVT prophylaxis: A review. *Orthopaedics and Trauma, 34*(3), 161–167. https://doi.org/10.1016/j.mporth.2020.03.010.

Bostick, G. P., Norman, K. E., Sharma, A., et al. (2020). Improving cultural knowledge to facilitate cultural adaptation of pain management in a culturally and linguistically diverse community. *Physiotherapy Canada, 73*(1), 19–25. https://doi.org/10.3138/ptc-2019-0027.

Bouya, S., Balouchi, A., Maleknejad, A., et al. (2019). Cancer pain management among oncology nurses: Knowledge, attitude, related factors, and clinical recommendations: A systematic review. *Journal of Cancer Education, 34*(5), 839–846. https://doi.org/10.1007/s13187-018-1433-6.

Callister, L. C., Khalaf, I., Semenic, S., et al. (2003). The pain of childbirth: Perceptions of culturally diverse women. *Pain Management Nursing, 4*(4), 145–154.

Canizares, M., Hogg-Johnson, S., Gignac, M., et al. (2017). Changes in the use practitioner-based complementary and alternative medicine over time in Canada: Cohort and period effects. *PloS One, 12*(5), e0177307.

Chou, R., Gordon, D. B., de Leon-Casasola, O. A., et al. (2016). Management of postoperative pain: A clinical practice guideline from the American Pain Society, the American Society of Regional Anesthesia and Pain Medicine, and the American Society of Anesthesiologists' Committee on Regional Anesthesia, Executive Committee, and Administrative Council. *The Journal of Pain, 17*(2), 131–157. https://doi.org/10.1016/j.jpain.2015.12.008.

Cleeland, C. S., Nakamura, Y., & Mendoza, T. R. (1996). Dimensions of the impact of cancer in a four-country sample: New information from multidimensional scaling. *Pain, 67,* 267–273.

Cragg, J. J., Warner, F. M., Shupler, M. S., et al. (2018). Prevalence of chronic pain among individuals with neurological conditions. *Statistics Canada: Health Reports, 29*(3), 11–16.

Cramer, H., Klose, P., Brinkhaus, B., et al. (2017). Effects of yoga on chronic neck pain: A systematic review and meta-analysis. *Clinical Rehabilitation, 31*(11), 1457–1465. https://doi.org/10.1177/0269215517698735.

Crawley, L. M., Marshall, P. A., Lo, B., et al. (2002). Strategies for culturally effective end-of-life care. *Annals of Internal Medicine, 1*(9), 673–679.

Crews, K. R., Gaedigk, A., Dunnenberger, H. M., et al. (2012). Clinical Pharmacogenetics Implementation Consortium (CPIC) guidelines for codeine therapy in the context of cytochrome P450 2D6 (CYP2D6) genotype. *Clinical Pharmacology and Therapeutics, 91*(2), 321–326. https://doi.org/10.1038/clpt.2011.287.

Dean, L. (2021). Codeine therapy and *CYP2D6* genotype. In V. M. Pratt, S. A. Scott, M. Pirmohamed, et al. (Eds.), *Medical genetics summaries*. National Center for Biotechnology Information (US).

Drissi, I., Woods, W., & Woods, C. G. (2020). Understanding the genetic basis of congenital insensitivity to pain. *British Medical Bulletin, 133*, 65–78. https://doi.org/10.1093/bmb/ldaa003.

Duwe, E. A. G. (2019). Suffering like a broken toy: Social, psychological, and cultural impacts for urban American Indians with chronic pain. *International Journal of Indigenous Health, 14*(2), 150–168. https://doi.org/10.32799/ijih.v14i2.32958.

Elmholdt, E. M., Skewes, J., Dietz, M., et al. (2017). Reduced pain sensation and reduced BOLD signal in parietofrontal networks during religious prayer. *Frontiers in Human Neuroscience, 11*, 337. https://doi.org/10.3389/fnhum.2017.00337.

Fillingim, R. B., Bruehl, S., Dworkin, R. H., et al. (2014). The ACTTION-American Pain Society Pain Taxonomy (AAPT): An evidence-based and multidimensional approach to classifying chronic pain conditions. *The Journal of Pain, 15*(3), 241–249. https://doi.org/10.1016/j.jpain.2014.01.004.

Fortenberry, M., Crowder, J., & So, T. Y. (2019). The use of codeine and tramadol in the pediatric population—What is the verdict now? *Journal of Pediatric Health Care, 33*(1), 117–123. https://doi.org/10.1016/j.pedhc.2018.04.016.

Gagnon, C. M., Matsuura, J. T., Smith, C. C., et al. (2014). Ethnicity and interdisciplinary pain treatment. *Pain Practice, 14*(6), 532–540. https://doi.org/10.1111/papr.12102.

Government of Canada. (2019). *Canadian Pain Task Force report: Chronic pain in Canada: Laying a foundation for action.* https://www.canada.ca/en/health-canada/corporate/about-health-canada/public-engagement/external-advisory-bodies/canadian-pain-task-force/report-2019.html

Greenwald. H. P. (1991). Interethnic differences in pain perception. *Pain, 44*(2), 157–163. https://doi.org/10.1016/0304-3959(91)90130-P.

Haroyan, A., Mukuchyan, V., Mkrtchyan, N., et al. (2018). Efficacy and safety of curcumin and its combination with boswellic acid in osteoarthritis: A comparative, randomized, double-blind, placebo-controlled study. *BMC Complementary and Alternative Medicine, 18*(1), 7. https://doi.org/10.1186/s12906-017-2062-z.

Harvie, A., Steel, A., & Wardle, J. (2019). Traditional Chinese medicine self-care and lifestyle medicine outside of Asia: A systematic literature review. *Journal of Alternative and Complementary Medicine (New York, N.Y.), 25*(8), 789–808. https://doi.org/10.1089/acm.2018.0520.

Health Canada. (2020). *Working together to better understand, prevent, and manage chronic pain: What we heard. A report by the Canadian Pain Task Force.* https://www.canada.ca/content/dam/hc-sc/documents/corporate/about-health-canada/public-engagement/external-advisory-bodies/canadian-pain-task-force/report-2020-rapport/report-2020.pdf

Health Canada. (2021). *An action plan for pain in Canada.* https://www.canada.ca/en/health-canada/corporate/about-health-canada/public-engagement/external-advisory-bodies/canadian-pain-task-force/report-2021.html#_Toc67582196

Health Quality Ontario. (2018a). *Opioid prescribing for acute pain.* http://www.hqontario.ca/Evidence-to-Improve-Care/Quality-Standards/View-all-Quality-Standards/Opioid-Prescribing-for-Acute-Pain

Health Quality Ontario. (2018b). *Opioid prescribing for chronic pain.* http://www.hqontario.ca/Evidence-to-Improve-Care/Quality-Standards/View-all-Quality-Standards/Opioid-Prescribing-for-chronic-Pain

Herr, K. A., Spratt, K., Mobily, P. R., et al. (2004). Pain intensity assessment in older adults: Use of experimental pain to compare psychometric properties and usability of selected pain scales with younger adults. *Clinical Journal of Pain, 20*(4), 207–219. https://doi.org/10.1097/00002508-200407000-00002.

Hicks, C. L., von Baeyer, C. L., Spafford, P. A., et al. (2001). The Faces Pain Scale-Revised: Toward a common metric in pediatric pain measurement. *Pain, 93*(2), 173–183. https://doi.org/10.1016/S0304-3959(01)00314-1.

Hoffman, K. M., Trawalter, S., Axt, J. R., et al. (2016). Racial bias in pain assessment and treatment recommendations, and false beliefs about biological differences between blacks and whites. *Proceedings of the National Academy of Science of the United States of America, 113*(16), 4296–4301. https://doi.org/10.1073/pnas.1516047113.

Hogan, M. E., Taddio, A., Katz, J., et al. (2016). Incremental health care costs for chronic pain in Ontario, Canada: A population-based matched cohort study of adolescents and adults using administrative data. *Pain, 157*(8), 1626–1633.

Hollingshead, N. A., Ashburn-Nardo, L., Stewart, J. C., et al. (2016). The pain experience of Hispanic Americans: A critical literature review and conceptual model. *The Journal of Pain, 17*(5), 513–528. https://doi.org/10.1016/j.jpain.2015.10.022.

Holt, S., & Waterfield, J. (2018). Cultural aspects of pain: A study of Indian Asian women in the UK. *Musculoskeletal Care, 16*(2), 260–268. https://doi.org/10.1002/msc.1229.

Hroch, J., VanDenKerkhof, E. G., Sawhney, M., et al. (2019). Knowledge and attitudes about pain management among Canadian nursing students. *Pain Management Nursing, 20*(4), 382–389. https://doi.org/10.1016/j.pmn.2018.12.005.

International Association for the Study of Pain (IASP). (2017). *Pain terminology.* https://www.iasp-pain.org/Education/Content.aspx?ItemNumber=1698

Jones, M. R., Viswanth, O., Peck, J., et al. (2018). A brief history of the opioid epidemic and strategies for pain medicine. *Pain Therapies, 7*, 13–21.

Karcioglu, O., Topacoglu, H., Dikme, O., et al. (2018). A systematic review of the pain scales in adults: Which to use? *The American Journal of Emergency Medicine, 36*(4), 707–714. https://doi.org/10.1016/j.ajem.2018.01.008.

Kent, M. L., Tighe, P. J., Belfer, I., et al. (2017). The ACTTION-APS-AAPM Pain Taxonomy (AAAPT) multidimensional approach to classifying acute pain conditions. *Pain Medicine, 18*(5), 947–958. https://doi.org/10.1093/pm/pnx019.

Kessler, C. S., Pinders, L., Michalsen, A., et al. (2015). Ayurvedic interventions for osteoarthritis: A systematic review and meta-analysis. *Rheumatology International, 35*(2), 211–232. https://doi.org/10.1007/s00296-014-3095-y.

Khan, M. A., Raza, F., & Khan, I. A. (2015). Pain: History, culture and philosophy. *Acta Medico-Historica Adriatica: AMHA, 13*(1), 113–130.

Kim, H. J., Yang, G. S., Greenspan, J. D., et al. (2017). Racial and ethnic differences in experimental pain sensitivity: Systematic review and meta-analysis. *Pain, 158*(2), 194–211. https://doi.org/10.1097/j.pain.0000000000000731.

Kridli, S. A. (2002). Health beliefs and practices among Arab women. *MCN: The American Journal of Maternal Child Nursing, 27*(3), 178–182. https://doi.org/10.1097/00005721-200205000-00010.

Krupić, F., Čustović, S., Jašarević, M., et al. (2019). Ethnic differences in the perception of pain: A systematic review of qualitative and quantitative research. *Medicinski Glasnik, 16*(1), 108–114. https://doi.org/10.17392/966-19.

Lasch, K. E., Wilkes, G., Montuori, L. M., et al. (2000). Using focus group methods to develop multicultural cancer pain education materials. *Pain Management Nursing, 1*(4), 129–139.

Lauche, R., Hunter, D. J., Adams, J., et al. (2019). Yoga for osteoarthritis: A systematic review and meta-analysis. *Current Rheumatology Reports, 21*(9), 47. https://doi.org/10.1007/s11926-019-0846-5.

Latimer, M., Sylliboy, J. R., MacLeod, E., et al. (2018). Creating a safe space for First Nations youth to share their pain. *Pain Reports, 3*(Suppl 1), e682. https://doi.org/10.1097/PR9.0000000000000682.

Liao, Y. H., Henceroth, M., Lu, Q., et al. (2016). Cultural differences in pain experience among four ethnic groups: A qualitative pilot study. *Journal of Behavioral Health, 5*(2), 75–81. https://doi.org/10.5455/jbh.20160204094059.

Lor, M., Rabago, D., & Backonja, M. (2020). "There are so many nuances …": Health care providers' perspectives of pain communication with Hmong patients in primary care settings. *Journal of Transcultural Nursing, 32*(5), 575–582. https://doi.org/10.1177/1043659620959437.

Mack, D. S., Hunnicut, J. N., Jesdale, B. M., et al. (2018). Non-Hispanic Black-White disparities in pain and pain management among newly admitted nursing home residents with cancer. *Journal of Pain Research, 11*, 753–761.

McCaffery, M., & Pasero, C. (1999). *Pain clinical manual* (2nd ed.). Mosby.

McDonald, D. D., Ambrose, M., & Morey, B. (2015). Hispanic inpatient pain intensity. *Western Journal of Nursing Research, 37*(11), 1479–1488. https://doi.org/10.1177/0193945914540056.

Meints, S. M., Cortes, A., Morais, C. A., et al. (2019). Racial and ethnic differences in the experience and treatment of noncancer pain. *Pain Management*, *9*(3), 317–334. https://doi.org/10.2217/pmt-2018-0030.

Meldrum. M. (2003). A capsule history of pain management. *Journal of the American Medical Association*, *290*(18), 2470–2475.

Melzak. R. (1975). The McGill pain questionnaire: Major properties and scoring methods. *Pain*, *1*, 277–299.

Merriam-Webster Online Dictionary. (2005). *Stoic*. http://www.m-w.com/dictionary/stoic

Miller-Matero, L. R., Chipungu, K., Martinez, S., et al. (2017). How do I cope with pain? Let me count the ways: Awareness of pain coping behaviors and relationships with depression and anxiety. *Psychology, Health & Medicine*, *22*(1), 19–27. https://doi.org/10.1080/13548506.2016.1191659.

Mills, S., Nicolson, K. P., & Smith, B. H. (2019). Chronic pain: A review of its epidemiology and associated factors in population-based studies. *British Journal of Anaesthesia*, *123*(2), e273–e283. https://doi.org/10.1016/j.bja.2019.03.023.

Miotto, K., Cho, A. K., Khalil, M. A., et al. (2017). Trends in tramadol: Pharmacology, metabolism, and misuse. *Anesthesia and Analgesia*, *124*(1), 44–51. https://doi.org/10.1213/ANE.0000000000001683.

Mustafa, N., Einstein, G., MacNeill, M., et al. (2020). The lived experiences of chronic pain among immigrant Indian-Canadian women: A phenomenological analysis. *Canadian Journal of Pain*, *4*(3), 40–50. https://doi.org/10.1080/24740527.2020.1768835.

Nahin, R. L., Boineau, R., Khalsa, P. S., et al. (2016). Evidence-based evaluation of complementary health approaches for pain management in the United States. *Mayo Clinic Proceedings*, *91*(9), 1292–1306. https://doi.org/10.1016/j.mayocp.2016.06.007.

Nelson, S. E., & Wilson, K. (2018). Understanding barriers to health care access through cultural safety and ethical space: Indigenous people's experiences in Prince George, Canada. *Social Science & Medicine*, *218*, 21–27.

Orhan, C., Van Looveren, E., Cagnie, B., et al. (2018). Are pain beliefs, cognitions, and behaviors influenced by race, ethnicity, and culture in patients with chronic musculoskeletal pain? A systematic review. *Pain Physician*, *21*(6), 541–558.

Ostrom, C., Bair, E., Maixner, W., et al. (2017). Demographic predictors of pain sensitivity? Results from the OPPERA Study. *The Journal of Pain*, *18*(3), 295–307.

Ovienloba, A. A. (2017). Anthropological synthesis of spirituality and pain management: How spirituality affects pain outcomes and copings. *Journal of Health and Human Experience*, *3*(1), 103–114.

Owusu Obeng, A., Hamadeh, I., & Smith, M. (2017). Review of opioid pharmacogenetics and considerations for pain management. *Pharmacotherapy*, *37*(9), 1105–1121. https://doi.org/10.1002/phar.1986.

Patrick, J. O. (2020). A concern for the human race. *Journal of Health and Human Experience*, *4*(3), 135–141.

Raja, S. N., Carr, D. B., Cohen, M., et al. (2020). The revised International Association for the Study of Pain definition of pain: concepts, challenges, and compromises. *Pain*, *161*(9), 1976–1982. https://doi.org/10.1097/j.pain.0000000000001939.

Ruben, M. A., van Osch, M., & Blanch-Hartigan, D. (2015). Healthcare providers' accuracy in assessing patients' pain: A systematic review. *Patient Education and Counseling*, *98*(10), 1197–1206. https://doi.org/10.1016/j.pec.2015.07.009.

Saxena, A., Mendoza, T., & Cleeland, C. (1999). The assessment of cancer pain in North India: Validation of the Hindi Brief Pain Inventory–BPI-H. *Journal of Pain and Symptom Management*, *17*(1), 27–41.

Scher, C., Meador, L., Van Cleave, J. H., et al. (2018). Moving beyond pain as the fifth vital sign and patient satisfaction scores to improve pain care in the 21st century. *Pain Management Nursing*, *19*(2), 125–129. https://doi.org/10.1016/j.pmn.2017.10.010.

Schweikart, S. J. (2018). Constitutional regulation of speech (and false beliefs) in health care. *AMA Journal of Ethics*, *20*(11), E1041–E1048. https://doi.org/10.1001/amajethics.2018.1041.

Sharma, S., Abbott, J. H., & Jensen, M. P. (2018). Why clinicians should consider the role of culture in chronic pain. *Brazilian Journal of Physical Therapy*, *22*(5), 345–346. https://doi.org/10.1016/j.bjpt.2018.07.002.

Sharma, S., Pathak, A., & Jensen, M. P. (2016). Words that describe chronic musculoskeletal pain: Implications for assessing pain quality across cultures. *Journal of Pain Research*, *9*, 1057–1066. https://doi.org/10.2147/JPR.S119212.

Shep, D., Khanwelkar, C., Gade, P., et al. (2019). Safety and efficacy of curcumin versus diclofenac in knee osteoarthritis: A randomized open-label parallel-arm study. *Trials*, *20*(1), 214. https://doi.org/10.1186/s13063-019-3327-2.

Simpson, C. A. (2006). Complementary medicine in chronic pain treatment. *Physical Medicine and Rehabilitation Clinics of North America, 17*(2). 451–472, viii. https://doi.org/10.1016/j.pmr.2005.11.006.

Smeland, A. H., Twycross, A., Lundeberg, S., et al. (2018). Nurses' knowledge, attitudes and clinical practice in pediatric postoperative pain management. *Pain Management Nursing, 19*(6), 585–598. https://doi.org/10.1016/j.pmn.2018.04.006.

Smith, D. M., Weitzel, K. W., Elsey, A. R., et al. (2019). CYP2D6-guided opioid therapy improves pain control in CYP2D6 intermediate and poor metabolizers: A pragmatic clinical trial. *Genetics in Medicine, 21*(8), 1842–1850. https://doi.org/10.1038/s41436-018-0431-8.

Steel, A., McIntyre, E., Harnett, J., et al. (2018). Complementary medicine use in the Australian population: Results of a nationally representative cross-sectional survey. *Scientific Reports, 8*(1), 17325. https://doi.org/10.1038/s41598-018-35508-y.

Strong, S., Nielsen, T. M., Williams, M., et al. (2015). Quiet about pain: Experiences of Indigenous people in two rural communities. *Australian Journal of Rural Health, 23*(3), 181–184. https://doi.org/10.1111/ajr.12185.

Sullivan, M. J. L., Thorn, B., Keefe, F. J., et al. (2001). Theoretical perspectives on the relation between catastrophizing and pain. *Clinical Journal of Pain 2001, 17*, 52–64.

Tomazin, F. (2020). Australia's opioid crisis: Deaths rise as companies encourage doctors topresceibe. *The Age*, February 4. https://www.theage.com.au/national/australia-s-opioid-crisis-deaths-rise-as-companies-encourage-doctors-to-prescribe-20200203-p53x72.html

Tung, W. C., & Li, Z. (2015). Pain beliefs and behaviours among Chinese. *Home Health Care Management, 27*(2), 95–97.

Turpel-Lafond M. E. (2020). *In plain sight: Addressing Indigenous-specific racism anddiscrimination in BC health care. Full report, November 2020*. https://engage.gov.bc.ca/app/uploads/sites/613/2020/11/In-Plain-Sight-Summary-Report.pdf

Ung, A., Salamonson, Y., Hu, W., et al. (2016). Assessing knowledge, perceptions and attitudes to pain management among medical and nursing students: A review of the literature. *British Journal of Pain, 10*(1), 8–21. https://doi.org/10.1177/2049463715583142.

U.S. Department of Health and Human Services. (2019, May). *Pain Management Best Practices Inter-Agency Task Force Report: Updates, gaps, inconsistencies, and recommendations.* https://www.hhs.gov/sites/default/files/pain-mgmt-best-practices-draft-final-report-05062019.pdf

Vadivelu, N., Kai, A. M., Kodumudi, V., et al. (2018). The Opioid Crisis: A Comprehensive Overview. *Current Pain and Headache Reports, 22*(16). https://doi.org/10.1007/s11916-018-0670-z.

Webster, F., Rice, K., Katz, J., et al. (2019). An ethnography of chronic pain management in primary care: The social organization of physicians' work in the midst of the opioid crisis. *PLoS One, 14*(5), e0215148. https://doi.org/10.1371/journal.pone.0215148.

Woolf, C. (2010). What is this thing called pain? *The Journal of Clinical Investigation, 120*(11), 3742–3744. https://doi.org/10.1172/JCI45178.

Yosipovitch, G., Meredith, G., Chan, Y. H., et al. (2004). Do ethnicity and gender have an impact on pain thresholds in minor dermatologic procedures? A study on thermal pain perception thresholds in Asian ethnic groups. *Skin Research and Technology, 10*, 38–42.

Yuan, Q. L., Guo, T. M., Liu, L., et al. (2015). Traditional Chinese medicine for neck pain and low back pain: A systematic review and meta-analysis. *PLoS One, 10*(2), e0117146. https://doi.org/10.1371/journal.pone.0117146.

Zoborowski, M. (1952). Cultural components in responses to pain. *Journal of Social Issues, 8*, 15–30.

CHAPTER 16

The Impact of Social and Structural Determinants on Community Health: A Focus on the African Nova Scotian Experience

Barbara-Ann Hamilton-Hinch and Nancy MacVicar

As an eighth-generation Indigenous African Nova Scotian[1] I am reminded of the pervasiveness of racism and discrimination in all systems and structures. In this chapter I wanted to share some of the experiences of people of African descent, particularly that of Indigenous African Nova Scotians, so you, the reader, can share in the journey of change. You will note the use of Black, Indigenous African Nova Scotian, and African Canadian within this chapter; it is important that we respect how groups and individuals choose to be identified.

Barb Hamilton-Hinch

As a White settler woman, I was challenged as I wrote elements of this chapter. I recognize that I have not experienced racism or struggled against the determinants of health or power imbalances. I want to encourage you, like me, to keep on listening about how power imbalances have shaped the health of many Canadians. Let us engage and work together to improve health by addressing the social and structural determinants of health.

Nancy MacVicar

LEARNING OBJECTIVES

At the end of this chapter, the learner will be able to:

- Reflect an understanding of the experiences of Indigenous African Nova Scotians and other people of African descent living in Canada
- Identify and describe the social and structural determinants of health and health inequities affecting people of African descent living in Nova Scotia
- Describe how to examine both personal and societal bias when engaging a community to develop strategies to improve population health
- Describe how unintended consequences can be created by population health strategies intended to improve health
- Explore strategies to promote health equity and improve individual and population health
- Describe how COVID-19 has affected specific populations in Canada and how it has exacerbated health inequities

---

[1] *Indigenous African Nova Scotian* is a term that describes identity for Black Nova Scotians who have a history and experiences distinct from the immigrant Black experiences of people from the United States, the Caribbean, and Africa. The term is not meant to be disrespectful of the Indigenous Mi'kmaq people and is further discussed in the chapter.

KEY TERMS

African Nova Scotians	Health promotion	Social justice
Community engagement	Health protection	Structural determinants of
Environmental racism	Public health	health
Health	Social determinants of	Structural racism
Health inequity	health	

As stated throughout this book, health care providers must develop cultural competence when working within health systems and community settings. The focus of this chapter is to illustrate the impact of social and structural determinants of health as experienced by people of African descent living in Nova Scotia. The insights are applicable to other diverse populations. This chapter was written during a worldwide pandemic, so it would be incomplete if the impact of COVID-19, particularly on diverse populations, was not discussed. A significant portion is devoted to evidence-informed resources about African Nova Scotians, public health, and cultural competence. **African Nova Scotians**/Indigenous Blacks can be defined as "a Distinct People who descend from free and enslaved Black Loyalists, Black refugees, Maroons, the Planters, and other Black people who inhabited the original 52 land-based Black communities in Mi'kma'ki" (Williams et al., 2018, p. 1). This definition is based on "unique cultural, social, economic, political, spiritual and social traditions, practices, institutions and ways of relating" (p. 1) and "has been developed based on literature reviews, community consultations, how we self-identify and how our institutions have defined us as a People over time" (p. 1).

The chapter begins with an exploration of the history and development of public health. It describes how public health evolved from a focus on individual health to population health with an emphasis on social and structural determinants of health using a social justice framework. **Social justice** is a societal concept, based on concepts of human rights and equity, that promotes treating individuals and groups fairly and fosters an equitable share of the benefits of society (Public Health Agency of Canada [PHAC], 2021c). The chapter provides examples of health promotion efforts to address health inequities at an individual, community, and societal level. The impact of the social and structural determinants of health is illustrated by describing some of the colonized history of African Nova Scotians. Learnings from the experiences of African Nova Scotians can be applied when considering other populations that may be subject to the social and structural determinants of health. The chapter argues the need to improve racialized data collection and health indicators so that Canadians can understand and address issues that negatively affect the health status of African Nova Scotians and Black Canadians, as it is impossible to focus on issues that are not measured.

It would be remiss to begin this chapter without acknowledgement of the pervasive nature of privilege, particularly White privilege, within Canadian society. This privileged status means Eurocentric ideologies, beliefs, and traditions have become normalized in structures, institutional practices, and principles. These norms result in routine mistreatment of racialized individuals (Hamilton-Hinch, 2016; James et al., 2010; Veenstra & Patterson, 2016; Waldron, 2016, 2018a, b, c, 2020; Waldron et al., 2015). Health care providers need to be cognizant that health inequities can increase when health promotion interventions overtly target the majority population rather than focusing on populations struggling with the social and structural determinants of health (Trinh-Shevrin et al., 2015). Consequently, health care providers and health care teams need to become culturally competent to provide safe, culturally appropriate care. Cultural competence is a journey—not an end point.

Public Health

Public health is an approach "to maintaining and improving the health of populations that is based on principles of social justice, attention to human rights and equity, evidence-informed policy and practice and addressing the underlying determinants of health" (Canadian Public Health Association, 2017, p. 4). Public health interdisciplinary teams include physicians, epidemiologists, environmental health officers, enhanced home visitors, health promoters and educators, nurses, nutritionists, policy analysts, dental hygienists, social workers, therapeutic recreation specialists, and others who focus on health protection, health promotion, population health surveillance, healthy development, and the prevention of death, disease, injury, and disability. Improving population health requires engaging the public and community sectors in defining the issue, developing interventions, and evaluating the results. It is also important to recognize that public health continues to evolve (Canadian Public Health Association, 2017).

Health protection safeguards individuals, groups, and populations from infectious diseases like COVID-19 or tuberculosis, and non-infectious environmental hazards such as second-hand smoke or lead (PHAC, 2021c). Older pipes and paint are sources of lead poisoning. Environmental health standards have been implemented to remove lead from gasoline, pipes, and paint (Health Canada, 2021). **Health promotion** improves the health of populations through initiatives such as smoking bylaws, improving food security, increasing access to affordable housing, and increasing the minimum wage (PHAC, 2021c).

Health status was once attributed to environmental, biological, genetic, cultural, or lifestyle choice (Lalonde, 1974). However, the Canadian Institute for Advanced Research estimates that only 25% of health of the population is attributable to the health care system, while 15% is due to biology and genetic factors, 10% results from the physical environment, and 50% is attributable to social and economic environments (Canadian Medical Association, 2022; Raphael, 2016). Health inequalities among populations result from systematic differences in health status because of unequal exposure to the social determinants of health along a gradient (Farrer et al., 2015; Lucyk & McLaren, 2017; Trinh-Shevrin et al., 2015; Veenstra & Patterson, 2016; Waldron et al., 2015; Walker et al., 2016).

A government white paper, *A New Perspective on the Health of Canadians* (Lalonde Report), issued in 1974, proposed that modifying lifestyle behaviours or social and physical environments would improve the health status of Canadians. This report resulted in several highly successful programs that increased public awareness of the health risks associated with certain personal lifestyle behaviours (e.g., smoking, alcohol, nutrition, fitness). The Alma Ata Conference reframed health as not only freedom from disease but as a "state of positive wellbeing for all by the end of the 20th century and a combination of promotive, preventive, curative and rehabilitative actions" (World Health Organization, [WHO], 1978). The Alma Ata Declaration deemed that health inequalities between different parts of the world, as well as between and within countries, were unacceptable. While the Lalonde Report was ground breaking, it was criticized for focusing too much on individual responsibilities for health and neglecting the societal issues that resulted in health inequities (Lucyk & McLaren, 2017). **Population health** emerged, with the aim of improving the health of an entire population and reducing health inequities among population groups (PHAC, 2021c). It also became clear that reinforcing change at the individual level could further marginalize those who lacked the financial and social levers to improve their health status (Trinh-Shevrin et al., 2015). A foundational document, the Ottawa Charter for Health Promotion, was developed in 1986. The Charter described **health** as "a complete state of physical, mental and social wellbeing." Health promotion focuses on health equity by combining "diverse but complementary approaches including legislation, fiscal measures, taxation and organizational change" (WHO, 1986). Over recent decades, there has been a recognition that focusing too much on individual responsibilities for health neglects societal issues. Thus addressing social determinants of health is critical to reducing health inequities (Lucyk & McLaren, 2017).

Social and Structural Determinants of Health

While many Canadians enjoy good health, it is not the case across the entire population (PHAC, 2018). Health equity is directly affected by social and structural determinants of health. **Structural**

determinants of health are economic, social, and political systems that produce unequal socio-economic systems that stratify individuals according to income, occupation, gender, race, ethnicity, and other factors leading to the health inequity gradient (PHAC, 2020a). **Health inequity** (sometimes known as health disparity) refers to health differences that are systemic, preventable, and unjust (Arcaya et al., 2015; Trinh-Shevrin et al., 2015). They can be observed across social groups, within the same populations, or as a gradient across a population ranked by social position (McCartney et al., 2019).

SOCIAL DETERMINANTS OF HEALTH

The determinants of health represent an extensive list of personal, environmental, social, and economic factors, which include "income and social status, employment and working conditions, education and literacy, childhood experiences, physical environments, social supports and coping skills, healthy behaviours, access to health services, biology and genetic endowment, gender, culture and race/racism that affect individual and population health" (PHAC, 2020b). The **social determinants of health** refer to a subset of social and economic factors within the broader determinants of health that relate to a person's place in society, including income, education, or employment. Black, Indigenous, and 2-spirit, lesbian, gay, bisexual, transgender, queer, and other sexual identities (2SLGBTQ+) communities also experience racism, discrimination, and historical trauma adding to the social determinants of health (Abdilliha & Shaw, 2020).

Communities can also define their own social determinants of health. Waldron et al. (2015) assisted African Nova Scotian residents of North End Halifax to identify a community-focused list of social determinants of health that included factors found in the Public Health Agency of Canada (PHAC) list, such as race, employment, education, and literacy. Within this list community residents noted that affordable housing was being replaced by affluent middle- and upper-class businesses and homes, displacing people who had lived there for generations. For this reason, participants identified gentrification as a determinant of health. One participant in the study noted: "We can't lose sight of the systemic issues that confront us as people in terms of our health … taking a look at policies, procedures, the systemic things within the system to see how it negatively impacts us" (p. 32).

STRUCTURAL DETERMINANTS OF HEALTH

The determinants of health can be described as operating at three levels: distal, intermediary, and proximal (PHAC, 2018). These levels are differentiated according to proximity to the individual, as seen in Fig. 16.1. This figure identifies some of the structural and social determinants of health that apply to African Nova Scotians.

The structural determinants of health (also known as the distal level) operate furthest away from the individual at the system level, entrenching economic, social, and political power and ensuring that those who already have a privileged position in society maintain it. The economic, social, and political systems are intertwined, producing unequal socioeconomic systems that stratify individuals according to income, occupation, gender, race, ethnicity, and other factors leading to the health inequity gradient. These structural determinants affect the social and physical conditions in which people live, work, and age. The intermediary level of determinants situates a person within the social hierarchy and affects how vulnerable they are to health-compromising situations and protective mechanisms that reduce these issues. The individual level (also known as the proximal level) includes determinants of health such as income, education, and employment (PHAC, 2018). Health care providers can support social justice movements that recognize and strive to change the unfair political and socioeconomic systems so that everyone has access to the same opportunities for health equality (Canadian Public Health Association, 2017).

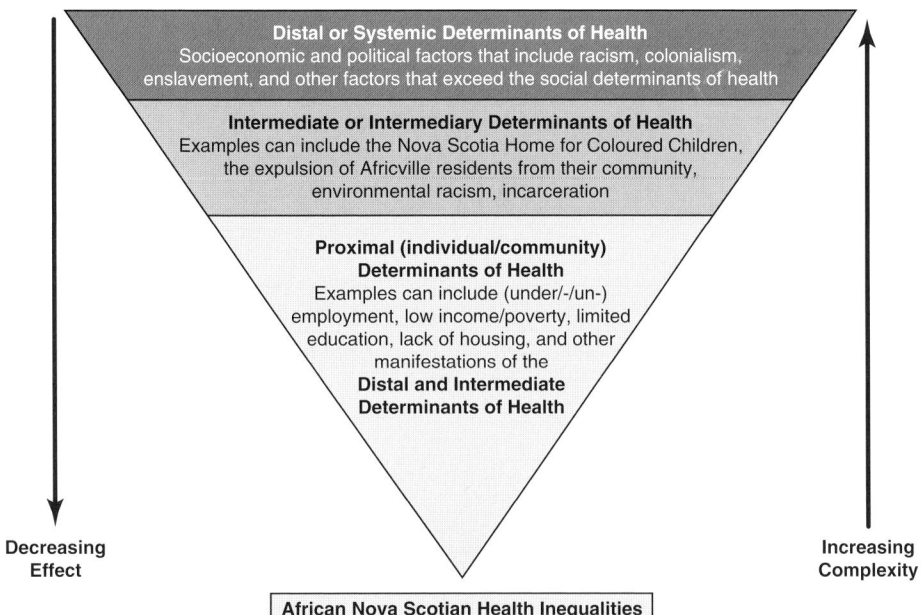

Fig. 16.1   Structural Determinants of Health for African Nova Scotians. (Created by Dr. Barbara-Ann Hamilton-Hinch and Nancy MacVicar. Adapted from World Health Organization [WHO]. [2010]. *A conceptual framework for action on the social determinants of health*. Social Determinants of Health Discussion Paper 2 [Policy and Practice]. https://www.who.int/social_determinants/publications/9789241500852/en/.)

AFRICAN NOVA SCOTIA—ILLUSTRATING THE EFFECTS OF HEALTH INEQUITIES

People of African descent have been residing in Nova Scotia for over 400 years. The majority of African Nova Scotians (77.3%) have been in Canada for three or more generations, representing the largest Indigenous Black/African Nova Scotian community in Canada (Walker, 2015). As they settled in Nova Scotia, African Nova Scotians were given the most inhospitable land and forced to live on the margins of society. In spite of these challenges, people of African descent persevered, and they now live in distinct, historic communities across the entire province (Walker, 2015).

Currently, people of African descent constitute the largest racially visible community, making up nearly 2.4% of the population of Nova Scotia (Office of African Nova Scotian Affairs, 2022). It is important to recognize that a proportion of African Nova Scotians do not feel safe to self-identify as a particular racially visible group in spite of being in the country for generations, because of fear, experiences of discrimination, and targeted racism. Therefore, these reported numbers could be higher (Hamilton-Hinch, 2016). Table 16.1 presents a historical overview of people of African descent in Nova Scotia.

It is important to examine the historical overview of people of African descent in Nova Scotia in order to develop a more comprehensive understanding of the social and structural determinants of health in relation to their health and well-being. These issues can be generalized to other populations that struggle with similar issues, such as new immigrants and Indigenous people.

Social Determinants and Inequities in Health Among African Nova Scotians and Black Canadians

A report by the United Nations Human Rights Council (2017) states that Canada has created human rights legislation but has failed to adopt targeted measures to address barriers Black

TABLE 16.1 ■ **Historical Overview of African Nova Scotia**

Date	Historical Event
1605	Arrival of Mathieu da Costa as part of an expedition that founded Port Royal.
1700s	Small populations of French and English Black people were part of colonial towns, including 300 in Louisburg and early Halifax.
1763	Between 100 and 150 people of African descent were among the new arrivals known as Planters who came from New England after the British gained control over Nova Scotia in 1763.
1782–1795	Approximately 3 500 Black Loyalists fled to what is now Nova Scotia and New Brunswick at the end of the American Revolution in 1776. In return for freedom, they fought for Britain. They lived in Annapolis Royal and other areas such as Cornwallis/Horton, Weymouth, Digby, Windsor, Preston, Sydney, Fort Cumberland, Parrsboro, Halifax, Birchtown, and Port Mouton. Upon arrival in the Maritimes, they were not given the promised land, were forced to work on public projects such as roads and buildings, and were denied equal status with White Loyalists.
1784	Canada's first race riot in Shelburne, Nova Scotia.
1792	One thousand one hundred and ninety men, women, and children left Halifax for Sierra Leone, West Africa. Sixty-five died en route.
1796	Nearly 600 Trelawny Maroons exiled from Jamaica arrived in the Maritimes. They faced miserable conditions and chose to migrate to Sierra Leone in 1800.
1813–1815	About 2 000 American Black people who were refugees from the War of 1812 (under similar conditions to those of the Black Loyalists) moved into the Halifax area and lived in areas including Preston, Hammonds Plains, Beechville, Porters Lake, Lucasville, and Windsor.
1833	Britain officially abolished African chattel slavery in the British Empire, including the Maritimes.
1848	The first records of a Black presence in Africville. The community existed for 150 years with hundreds of individuals and families living there. The community had stores, a school, a post office, and the Seaview Baptist Church.
1854	African United Baptist Association officially established many churches around the province that still exist today.
1916–1918	No. 2 Construction Battalion was formed during WWI — Canada's first and only Black military regiment.
1920s	Hundreds of Caribbean immigrants called "later arrivals" travelled to Cape Breton to work in the coal mines and steel factory.
1954	Legal segregation of schools ended.
1960s	Changes to the Canadian immigration act allowed immigration of Black people directly from Africa and the Caribbean.

From Marshall, T. (2013). *Black Canadians*. The Canadian Encyclopedia, Historica Canada (last edited in 2021). https://www.thecanadianencyclopedia.ca/en/article/black-canadians; Black Cultural Center. (2021). Black migration in Nova Scotia. http://www. https://bccns.com/our-history/.

Canadians experience to achieve parallel social and economic rights to the rest of society. This results in Black Canadians disproportionately suffering from chronic health conditions such as hypertension, diabetes, HIV and AIDS, cancers, mental health issues, and sickle cell disease (United Nations Human Rights Council, 2017). People who struggle with social determinants of health such as racism also experience high levels of physiological and psychological stress. Coping with poor housing, food insecurity, low income, and inadequate working conditions increases health inequities (Mikkonen & Raphael, 2010).

Fair or poor self-perceived health status was reported by 14.2% of Black Canadians compared to 11.3% of White Canadians. Young Black women aged 12–17 reported significantly lower levels

---

TABLE 16.2 ■ Health Disparities Among Black Canadians

- Black respondents were more likely than Whites to report hypertension. This pattern also occurs in the United States, where the prevalence of hypertension in African Americans is the highest in the world. Between 2009 and 2012, the age-adjusted prevalence of hypertension for Black men was 44.9% compared to 32.9% for White men and 46.1% for Black women compared to 30.1% for White women (Spence & Rayner, 2018).
- 2.1 times as many Black Canadian adults as White Canadians are diabetic (Pan-Canadian Health Inequalities Data Tool, 2017).
- 54.2% of White Canadians are moderately active compared to 40.8% of Black Canadians age 18 years and older (Pan-Canadian Health Inequalities Data Tool, 2017).
- As of 2016, Black Canadians had significantly lower rates of heavy alcohol use and smoking compared to White Canadians (Pan-Canadian Health Inequalities Data Tool, 2017).
- African Nova Scotians are less likely to access health services than other groups. Social factors such as unemployment, poverty, racism, and discrimination increase the risk of illness and interfere with obtaining culturally competent medical care (United Nations Human Rights Council, 2017).

---

of "excellent or very good" mental health, at 64.0% compared to 77.2% of young White women (Pan-Canadian Health Inequalities Data Tool, 2017). Canada has not historically collected racialized health data so it lacks a complete understanding of the depth of health inequities among these populations (Dryden & Nnorom, 2021; UN Human Rights Council, 2017). For this reason, Canada has relied on data from the United States and other countries to understand health disparities. For a more detailed description of health disparities among Black Canadians, see Table 16.2.

It is important for health care providers to be aware of these health inequities. Recognizing that these issues are likely the result of social determinants of health can impact care planning and provide additional supports to mitigate issues around food insecurity, housing issues, transportation, and challenges in attending appointments. When taking a patient's history, the health care provider needs to utilize therapeutic communication, avoiding stigma and judgement. It is important to ask open-ended questions, such as "Tell me about …" and "What barriers would make it hard for you to …?" See the following story about Mary to understand cultural considerations in care.

Cultural Considerations In Care

Food Insecurity

Mary had a regular appointment with a nurse practitioner to monitor her diabetes. Her blood glucose was high and she admitted that she was not following her diabetic diet. The nurse practitioner reminded Mary that she needed to follow her diet to remain healthy and brought out the usual handouts on diabetes. She started to review the information and stopped when Mary asked, "Can I buy this stuff at the Dollar Shop?" Suddenly the nurse practitioner realized she needed to sensitively explore the issue of food security with Mary and began to ask where she shopped. Mary had been living with her daughter, who contributed to the rent. After her daughter moved out, Mary had to pay the full rent, leaving only $50 per month for food. Mary was unaware of neighbourhood resources like the Food Pantry and government stipends for which she was eligible because of her diabetes.

This situation illustrates the need for health care providers to understand that patients may not be able to follow health care recommendations because of larger social issues such as food insecurity, lack of affordable housing, and low income. It is critical that health care providers not jump to conclusions but develop communication skills that sensitively explore the systemic issues that contribute to challenges following health care recommendations. There is an opportunity to support communities advocating for affordable housing, proximity to supermarkets, and a livable income.

TABLE 16.3 ■ Social Determinants and Health Inequities Among Black Canadians: A Snapshot

Education	• In 2016, only 1.8% of elementary and high school teachers in Canada were Black (Turcotte, 2020).
	• Black high school students are the most likely to be streamed into lower academic courses, individual program plans, and applied programs and are the least likely to enroll in college and university (Hamilton-Hinch et al., 2017; Turner, 2017).
	• Black youth in Toronto face discrimination and are subject to negative stereotypes and lower expectations (Turner, 2017).
	• In Nova Scotia, the educational inequities are unchanged over 30 years after the end of segregation (United Nations Human Rights Council, 2017).
	• In 2016, Black youth aged 23 to 27 were less likely to have a postsecondary certificate, diploma, or degree than other Canadian youth in that age group (Turcotte, 2020).
Employment and Income	• In 2016, the unemployment rate for the Black population was 9.2%, compared to 5.3% for those in the rest of the population with a postsecondary education (Statistics Canada, 2020).
	• In 2014, 13% of Black Canadians reported experiencing discrimination at work or in the context of a hiring process, compared to 6% of the rest of the Canadian population (Turcotte, 2020). A high level of discrimination at 50% was found in a student survey done in 2011-12 in Quebec by the Community Economic Development and Employability Corporation (CEDEC, 2013). It should be noted that 20% of respondents did not answer the question on discrimination.
	• In 2016, Black men were 1.5 times as likely to be unemployed as White men (Pan-Canadian Health Inequalities Data Tool, 2017).
	• In 2016, the prevalence of low-income households among African Nova Scotian men was 21.9% and for women was 21.7% compared to the rest of Nova Scotia, at 7.9% (Statistics Canada, 2019).
	• In 2016, the unemployment rate for the Black population was 9.2%, compared to 5.3% for those in the rest of the population with a postsecondary education (Statistics Canada, 2019).
Housing	• A common barrier to adequate housing is landlord discrimination against Black tenants (Teixeira, 2008).
	• African Nova Scotians residing in specific areas for 20 years are entitled to be granted ownership of the land. However, the process is onerous and an unfair burden, disenfranchising their right to the land (United Nations Human Rights Council, 2017).
	• As of 2016, 28.6% of Black Canadians were living in unaffordable housing compared to 16.1% of White Canadians (Abdilliha & Shaw, 2020).
Food Insecurity	• Black Canadians reported moderate or severe household food insecurity 2.8 times more often than White Canadians between 2009 and 2012 (Pan-Canadian Health Inequalities Data Tool, 2017).

Table 16.3 describes some specific social determinants of health experienced by Black Canadians and African Nova Scotians.

Experiences with the social determinants of health impact how African Nova Scotians and, to a similar degree, Black/African Canadians interact with the health care system. Health care providers who develop a better understanding of how these experiences have affected African Nova Scotians' ability to trust the health care system will provide improved culturally competent care. The historical trauma of people of African descent has contributed to a history of mistrust. It is well documented that people of African descent have been treated unethically (Beskow, 2016; Brandt, 1978; Qureshi, 2004). For example, African American men were infected with syphilis in medical experiments such as the 1932 Tuskegee Syphilis study (Brandt, 1978), and in

1951 Henrietta Lacks's cells were retrieved and used without her consent (Beskow, 2016). Saartjie Baartman's body parts were put on display in 1815 and finally buried in 2002 (Qureshi, 2004).

Understanding how the Black population was used by society without their consent to further "scientific knowledge" can help health care providers recognize why this population may mistrust the health care system. It is imperative that a space of welcoming and inclusivity is created (a space that reflects the patients), particularly when it comes to health, so that everyone can receive optimal and equitable service regardless of race, ethnicity, sexual orientation, income, or education. Health care providers need knowledge and the tools to provide trauma- and violence-informed care. This includes acquiring an understanding of trauma and violence and their impact on people lives and behaviours, creating an emotionally and physically safe environment, providing choice, collaboration, and connection, and using a strengths-based approach to the provision of patient care (Tebes et al., 2019).

Structural Determinants of Health Among African Nova Scotians

The social determinants of health are created and maintained by the structural determinants of health. For African Nova Scotians, structural determinants of health are related to their experience of significant trauma throughout their 400-year history in Nova Scotia. Some of these experiences include structural racism, colonization, enslavement, the Home for Coloured Children, Africville, environmental racism, and experiences with the criminal justice system (United Nations Human Rights Council, 2017).

STRUCTURAL RACISM

Race has been identified as a social determinant of health (Government of Canada, 2021; Mikkonen & Raphael, 2010; PHAC, 2020b; Waldron et al., 2015). **Structural racism** is "the processes of racism that are embedded in laws (local, state, and federal), policies, and practices of society and its institutions that provide advantages to racial groups deemed as superior, while differentially oppressing, disadvantaging, or otherwise neglecting racial groups viewed as inferior" (Williams et al., 2019). It is promoted by societies, using entrenched political and socioeconomic systems that are historically rooted and culturally normalized over generations. These systems reinforce discriminatory beliefs, values, and distribution of resources, causing adverse health outcomes (Bailey et al., 2017). This affects access to quality education employment, income, and health care and increases exposure to the criminal justice system. While traditional approaches to medicine and health research attributed health disparities in racialized populations to biological, genetic, cultural, or lifestyle choices, it is now recognized that social inequalities and racism are important contributors to health status (Hamilton-Hinch, 2016; James et al., 2010; Public Health Ontario, 2020; Waldron et al., 2015).

There are many reports of anti-Black racism experienced by health care providers within the Canadian health care system (Dryden & Nnorom, 2021; Nourpanah, 2019). This issue is exacerbated by the low proportion of Black physicians in Canada. For example, in Ontario, Black people comprise 2.3% of practising physicians, while 4.5% of Ontarians are Black citizens (Toronto Sinai Health, 2020). Health care providers must develop the skills and language to address these comments within the workplace. They also need to promote systemic changes, including hiring practices, promotion, and inclusion of Black/African Canadians on boards.

COLONIZATION

It is important to recognize and understand that people of African descent living in Canada experienced colonization. Through colonialism, socioeconomic and political power systems have been set up that have embedded within them structural racism (Chambers et al., 2018; Waldron, 2018a, 2018b, 2018c; Waldron et al., 2015). People of African descent arrived or were brought to Nova Scotia through various means—some enslaved, indentured servants, exiled, refugees, and Loyalist (Black Cultural Center, 2021; Cooper, 2006; Pachai, 1990, 1997, 2007; Whitfield, 2006). Through these various passages to Nova Scotia, African Nova Scotians suffered loss of culture, language, family, and community, which resulted in a negative impact on their mental, physical, emotional, and spiritual health and well-being (Beagan & Etowa, 2009, 2011; Beagan et al., 2012; Este & Bernard, 2006; Hamilton-Hinch, 2016; James et al., 2010; McGibbon & Etowa, 2009). African Nova Scotians were not expected to survive as they were given rocky, barren land to farm; substandard living conditions; and limited access to education, employment, and health care (Pachai, 1990, 1997, 2007). In 2020, many African Nova Scotian communities are considered rural and not located near health clinics, hospitals, grocery stores, and educational institutions. Elements of colonization remain and are evident in the historical and generational trauma of having been enslaved and denied knowledge of a rich history.

ENSLAVEMENT

The history of people of African descent does not begin with a history of being enslaved. People of African descent are descendants of kings, queens, orators, mathematicians, scientists, healers, teachers, cultivators, engineers, and architects. However, the historical and generational trauma of having been enslaved is engrained in the psyche of some people of African descent (Hamilton-Hinch, 2016; Leary, 2005). This trauma is passed down from generation to generation, resulting in intergenerational trauma (DeGruy, 2005; Hamilton-Hinch, 2016). Waldron (2018a) describes historical trauma as the relationship between colonialism, structural racism, and poor health outcomes, experienced intergenerationally. Although Canada is often referenced as a place of refuge for the Underground Railroad (a secret network of White abolitionist and free Black people who helped runaways to freedom), slavery did exist in Nova Scotia, Canada (Hamilton, 1994; Whitfield, 2006). Slavery was not abolished until 1833, and even after that date, a semblance of being enslaved continued to exist as some African Nova Scotians became indentured servants to survive, until their deaths. Other African Nova Scotians were not provided with the resources to sustain themselves and their families. In some cases, families had to depend on the government to take care of their children.

HOME FOR COLOURED CHILDREN

> …To the African Nova Scotian community: we are sorry. The struggle of the Home is only one chapter in the history of systemic racism and inequality that has scarred our province for generations. African Nova Scotians are a founding culture in our province – a resourceful people of strength. We must acknowledge that in many ways and for many years we as a province have not adequately met the needs of African Nova Scotian children and their families. We are sorry. As Nova Scotians – as a people, walking together – we must do better. An apology is not closing of the books, but a recognition that we must cast an unflinching eye on the past as we strive toward a better future.
>
> Honourable Stephen Mcneil, Premier of Nova Scotia (Nova Scotia News Release, 2014)

This apology was given by the Premier of Nova Scotia for the mistreatment of many children of African descent while in the care of the Province. While the acknowledgement and apology is a first step, it will not improve health inequities among African Nova Scotians if the status quo continues to exist. The Home for Coloured Children (later named Akoma Family Centre) opened in June of 1921 to provide care for children of African descent who were not accepted or allowed in White care institutions in Nova Scotia. Although seen as a place of safety for some, others at the Home suffered physical, sexual, and emotional abuse. Some former residents of the Home have successfully launched a class action lawsuit against the province of Nova Scotia for their mistreatment. Nonetheless, children of African descent continue to be over-represented in child welfare institutions (Trocme et al., 2004; Turner 2016; Ujima Design Team, 2015; Waldron 2018c). This experience is representative of an intermediary structural determinant of health.

Health care providers need to question why children and families of African descent continue to experience inequities based on their race, community, income, education, and other social and structural determinants of health, including environmental racism. It is critical to also focus on the strengths inherent in the African Nova Scotian population. In spite of these conditions, many African Nova Scotians resisted, survived, and thrived in the many African Nova Scotian communities. Health care providers must consider intergenerational trauma and the provision of trauma- and violence-informed care in any treatment plan (Tebes et al., 2019). It is important to build relationships built on trust and respect to provide effective care. Health care providers need to invite non-traditional health providers into treatment plans, such as Elders, spiritual advisors, and lay counsellors. The health care system has an obligation to work with the community to increase representation of people of African descent at all levels of care and acknowledge the injustices experienced by African Nova Scotians.

AFRICVILLE

The spirit of Africville will never die. Africville was a historical African Nova Scotian community located on the shores of the Bedford Basin. The first records of Black inhabitants are from 1848 (McRae, 2021). It was home to many descendants of enslaved, free, and indentured people of African descent seeking employment, opportunities, and a sense of family. Africville had its own schools, community stores, hardware stores, and, most importantly, the heart of the community, its church, Seaview Baptist Church.

As Irvine Carvery, a resident of Africville, states, "you weren't isolated at any time in Africville. You always felt at home; the doors were always open. This is one of the most important things that has always stayed with me throughout my life" (McRae, 2021). The community of Africville faced countless discriminatory challenges. The city refused to provide many amenities given to other residents of Halifax, including garbage removal, water, and sewage, even though the residents of Africville paid municipal taxes.

The city also built a prison, an infectious disease hospital, and dump near the community. In 1964 the City of Halifax expelled the residents of Africville without meaningful consultation. The city said it wanted to build industry and infrastructure in the area, but this never occurred. Motivated by racism and greed, Africville was destroyed and residents were forced out of their homes—some being moved using garbage trucks—and into government housing (National Film Board, 1991; Remes, 2018; Rutland, 2011).

When living in Africville, residents owned their land and homes and had a strong sense of community. Children had places to play and families had places to gather and worship. The destruction and relocation of the residents of Africville is known locally, nationally, and internationally because of the overt racism, discrimination, environmental racism, and human rights violations (National Film Board, Remember Africaville, 1991; Remes, 2018; Rutland, 2011).

ENVIRONMENTAL RACISM

Environmental racism can be described as the disproportionate placement of environmentally hazardous industry and other activities in Indigenous communities and communities of colour (Waldron, 2018a). Environmental racism is considered a structural determinant of health. Most African Nova Scotian communities are located in rural communities, and many have been exposed to environmental racism through the historical and ongoing location of "garbage dumps" and run-off sewage disposal, which resulted in contaminated and arsenic water (Hudson, 2001; Waldron, 2016, 2018a, b; Waldron et al., 2015). Waldron et al. (2015) have facilitated extensive research examining environmental racism. Waldon's book and subsequent movie, *There's Something in the Water*, have garnered international recognition for Indigenous and African Nova Scotian communities.

As defined by Waldron (2018c p. 36), environmental racism refers to "environmental policies, practices or dierctives that disproportinately disadvantage individuals, groups, or communities (intentionally or unintentionally) based on race or colour." Environmental racism is being linked to various health conditions in people of African and Indigenous descent, such as higher rates of cancers, diabetes, breathing and other respiratory conditions, and allergies, as well as emotional and psychological disorders (Atari et al., 2013; Cryderman et al., 2016; Masuda et al., 2008; Sharp, 2009; Teelucksingh, 2006; Waldron, 2018a). These increased health conditions associated with environmental racism demand more in-depth exploration, attention, and linkage to the social and structural determinants of health. As political discussions are held about where to locate new dumps, or dispose of pollutants, environmental reviews need to examine and address any potential for environmental racism. In addition, another area relevant to people of African descent that demands more exploration is the criminal justice system. This is particularly important given the local, national, and international Black Lives Matter (BLM) Movement elevated in 2020.

THE (BIASED) CRIMINAL JUSTICE SYSTEM

The *Halifax Nova Scotia Street Checks Report* (the Wortley Report) (Nova Scotia Human Rights Commission, 2019) indicated that African Nova Scotians are 5.33 times more likely to be stopped by police and 4.75% more likely to be charged with an offence. The Wortley (Nova Scotia Human Rights Commission, 2021) provided information on progress made addressing the 53 recommendations. An African Nova Scotia Justice Institute designed to create programs and services to addess systemic racism faced by African Nova Scotians in their interactions with the justice system is being developed. People of African descent have a longstanding history of anti-Black racism that is embedded in criminal justice institutions. Similarly, the Sentencing Project (Nellis, 2016) indicated that people of African descent are incarcerated at three times the rate of non-racialized populations (Statistics Canada, 2018). African Nova Scotians constitute 2.6% of the population but represent 11% of admission (or remand) and 12% sentenced custody in adult correctional facilities (NS Adult Admissions to Custody by Ethnicity, 2018). Between March 2003 and March 2013, the White inmate population decreased by 3%, while there was a significant increase in racialized men and women in federal prisons (Pedlar et al., 2018). In addition, the Office of the Correctional Investigator (OCI) indicated that Black inmates are one of the fastest growing populations in federal institutions. This is concerning; given the percentage of Black people in Canada, they should not make up 9.3% of the total federal prison population, as was reported in 2012 (Office of the Correctional Investigator, 2014). The over-involvement of persons of African descent with the criminal justice system is reflective of the structural, social determinants of health and the intergenerational trauma experienced by many people of African descent. In addition, few programs within the criminal justice system and institutions are culturally relevant or recognize the distinct needs of people of African descent. Some programs have been developed to support the Indigenous inmate populations, such as The Indigenous Continuum of Care, Elders, and Spiritual Advisors (Office of the Correctional Investigator, 2015). Health care providers must work to reduce the rate of recidivism and investigate criminal justice–related experiences of people of African descent.

Addressing the Social and Structural Determinants of Health

Improving health disparities requires focusing interventions at the socioeconomic and political levels (Lucyk & McLaren, 2017; Raphael, 2011). A social justice approach is used to close avoidable, unjust, and unfair health equity gaps between populations that are vulnerable and non-vulnerable (Trinh-Shevrin et al., 2015). Advocacy is recognized as a way to promote policies that improve health equity by taking action on the social determinants of health and thus improving the health of groups that have been disadvantaged (Lucyk & McLaren, 2017). A synthesis review by Farrer et al. (2015) examined the literature and grey literature on advocacy for health equity. These authors describe advocacy for health equity as "a deliberate attempt to influence decision-makers and other stakeholders to support or implement policies to improve health equity using evidence" (p. 396). Efforts that support advocacy to address the social and structural determinants of health require timely, succinct qualitative and quantitative evidence from the local level that support arguments for policy development.

The WHO (2010) has recommended three courses of action: (1) improve daily life circumstances; (2) address inequitable distribution of power, money, and resources; and (3) understand the scope of the problem and evaluate interventions utilizing measurement tools. PHAC (2018) notes that it is critical to address systemic approaches that can exacerbate health disparities (e.g., tax benefits that support richer members of society). It has been argued that health promotion has focused on changing individuals, emphasizing lifestyle choices and behaviour change, rather than recognizing and addressing political, social, and economic issues around capitalism that cement the social determinants of health (Baker et al., 2018; Hanson & Metzl, 2016; Raphael, 2011).

Trinh-Shevrin et al. (2015) approach rectifying the structural determinants of health from the perspective of developing partnerships, mobilizing communities, and developing shared goals by both non-health sectors and policymakers. A health equity lens needs to be applied to all policy development by governmental and non-governmental polices for all sectors. Health impact tools are standardized decision support tools that proactively examine the potential impacts of any government plans. A health impact assessment examines the potential effects of a proposed policy or project on population health and makes recommendations to support decision-making. (National Collaborating Centre for Healthy Public Policy, 2015). Policies and interventions in any sector can unintentionally disadvantage specific populations. Therefore, it is critical to examine the effect of a decision on the social determinants of health, looking at the distribution of effects among various populations and listening to the concerns of various groups that are likely affected by the change (National Collaborating Centre for Healthy Public Policy, 2015; St-Pierre, 2015). As Woolf et al. (2016) suggest, aligning stakeholders across sectors will create the incentive to address shared goals. Health care providers can assist communities to speak about potential health effects of various political decisions but must ensure that they do not take over and speak for them. Intuitively, as health care providers, when we know better, we do better.

Frieden (2010) developed the health impact period to illustrate which interventions will have the greatest impact on population health status. Interventions focused on individuals, such as counselling to promote weight loss or increased exercise, require high investment by health care providers but have limited impact on improving societal health. These interventions seldom create long-term change if the underlying social issues are not addressed. Fig. 16.2 demonstrates the impact of various interventions on population health.

Educating a patient about healthy food, without recognizing low income or limited proximity to a grocery store, will not support them in making healthy lifestyle changes. Health care providers can support individuals by providing resources such as information about housing, tenants' rights, or local foodbanks. In addition, health care providers can pressure politicians and others to increase the amount of affordable housing and the minimum wage. While these approaches require forethought and investment, they also have a higher impact on more people.

Universities must support students with supportive strategies that enhance human rights and equity. Dalhousie Univeristy offers the African Nova Scotian Strategy, which provides support for African Nova Scotian students as a distinct people (Dalhousie University, African Nova Scotian Strategy Advisory Council, n.d.; Gagnon, 2021). Other inequities can be tackled through such measures as free tuition for postsecondary institutions. Some provinces, universities, and colleges

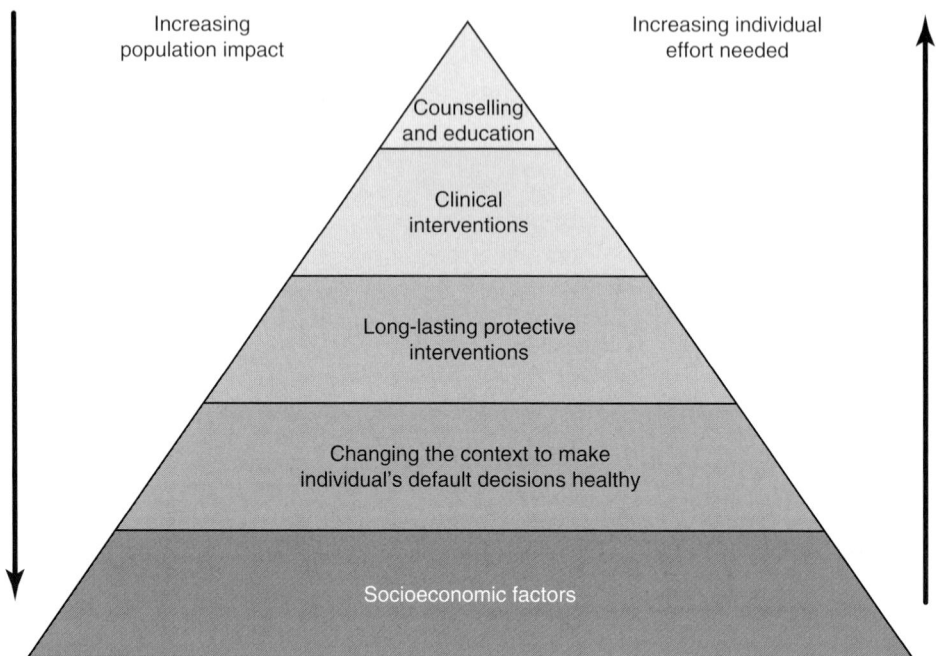

Fig. 16.2 Health Promotion Impact Pyramid. (Frieden, T. [2010]. A framework for public health action: The health impact period. *American Journal of Public Health, 100*[4], 590–595.)

have introduced free tuition for adults who were children within the care system. British Columbia announced that young adults aged 19–27 who had been in care were eligible, and hundreds of students applied to 25 universities in 2018 (BC Government News, 2018). Similarly, Nova Scotia institutions such as Mount St. Vincent University, Dalhousie University, and the Nova Scotia Community College announced similar free tuition progams and supportive programming for 2020-2021 for young adults who had been in foster care (Canadian Broadcasting Corporation, 2020a, 2021b). This provides the opportunity for children who have had difficult childhoods and lack family support systems to obtain postsecondary education and have improved employment prospects. Individuals, including African Nova Scotian children, who have been in care require more assistance than others to have the same opportunities.

Waldron et al. (2015) involved African Nova Scotian community members in participatory research to further their understanding of health and the social and structural determinants of health. While true engagement requires time and effort, the results are meaningful as it helps residents understand and address socioeconomic and political effects on their health. This promotes agency and empowerment, which is critical for populations that have been historically disenfranchised (Woolf et al., 2016).

Health care providers need to understand the community factors affecting patient health (Alicea-Alvarez et al., 2016). Efforts to improve understanding among medical students and other health practitioners have included fieldwork, service learning, programs to increase diversity in health professions, and volunteer opportunities in the curriculum. Health care providers both in the academic setting and as graduates need to be encouraged to look beyond individual issues to the system that builds health inequality and develop advocacy skills to make evidence-informed arguments for changes to socioeconomic structures (Farrer et al., 2015; Hanson & Metzl, 2016). For example, Dalhousie University in Halifax requires that students in medicine, dentistry, and nursing take a course in Indigenous Studies as part of their degree requirements. It also supports two programs with a mandate to increase the number of African Nova Scotian (Dalhousie University, n.d.; Hamilton-Hinch et al., 2017) and Indigenous students in medicine, dentistry, and the health professions (Indigenous Health in Medicine, 2020).

All health care providers need education, exposure to, and acknowledgement of the broad social and structural determinants of health. Some determinants may be unfamiliar, as ignorance or White privilege can blind people to the preservation of racist policies and practices by Eurocentric policies (Teelucksingh, 2018). For that reason, it is important for health care providers to use tools in this book to build an understanding of the social and structural determinants of health and community engagement skills tailored to populations that have been marginalized (Cyril et al., 2015). Effective **community engagement** means that community members directly participate in decision making about developments that affect the community—for example, setting health priorities, making decisions, planning strategies and implementing them (Goverment of Canada, 2021). It is important to not examine health from a "colour-blind" lens, but instead see racial and cultural diversity in order to activate change. It is equally important to apply cultural awareness and sensitivity to empower communities to develop initiatives like the community-based project Hope Blooms.

Cultural Competency In Action

Hope Blooms

Hope Blooms was founded in 2008 by seven young children who began growing tomatoes on a forgotten plot of land in inner Halifax. Now, there are 53 youths aged 5–18 years, older persons, and 35 families participating and are operating an award-winning community garden, greenhouse, and community kitchen. The youth grow approximately 1 814 kg (4 000 lb) of fresh produce yearly, which is turned into herb dressings and specialty teas. They foster a healthy community through their social enterprise, urban organic food gardens, nutrition, and experiential education programs. Funds earned from the sale of the herb dressings and teas are returned to the community. This non-profit creates space for "Halifax youth to become change agents in their community, improving food security, education, social inclusion and disrupting poverty" (Hope Blooms, 2022). In research conducted by the Dalhousie School of Health and Human Performance, Health Promotion Division, 100% of the youth felt that Hope Blooms had increased their ability to provide food for their families, 99% had an increased sense of belonging, and 92% had improved their level of community involvement (O'Reilly, 2017). Funds from Hope Blooms are put toward scholarships. In 2016, a participant was the first person in his family to attend postsecondary school. Four youths graduated from high school in 2018 and are on track for postsecondary education. Another participant who was involved in Hope Blooms since age 10 was shortlisted for the Loran Scholarship of $100, 000. In 2016, four youths received their Masters Organic Gardeners Certification, the youngest people in Canada to receive this university credit. Hope Blooms continues to motivate and support the community even through the COVID-19 pandemic (Hope Blooms, 2018).

The Effects of COVID-19

COVID-19, a novel infectious disease caused by SARS-CoV-2, was identified in humans in China on December 31, 2019. In late January 2020 it reached Canada when a traveller developed symptoms after their arrival and was hospitalized. A month later, there was documented community transmission of COVID-19 in Canada. As of mid-December 2021, COVID-19 had infected over 1.8 million Canadians, leaving more than 30 000 dead (PHAC, 2022a). Knowledge of this virus continues to evolve, but it appears to be more contagious than many other respiratory infectious diseases. During the first year, the only defence against the spread of COVID-19 were public health measures such as physical distancing, handwashing, and masking (PHAC, 2021d). By December 2020 new vaccines had been developed and were beginning to be administered (PHAC, 2022b).

More infectious variants of concern have been identified, including the Omicron variant, which are spreading across the world. Symptoms of COVID-19 can vary from asymptomatic to more serious forms of the disease that require hospitalization and treatment in a critical care unit (CCU). There have also been people documented with sequelae post-infection and potential long-term outcomes.

COVID-19 has not affected the population of Canada equally (PHAC, 2021e; WHO, 2021). Older populations, people with chronic disease, and those who are immunocompromised have experienced higher infection rates of COVID-19 accompanied by more severe outcomes (PHAC, 2022c). Canada has not systematically collected information on ethnicity, race, and associated health disparities (Canadian Institute for Health Information (CIHI), 2020; Thompson et al., 2021). A report by PHAC (2020c) analyzed demographic information as well as neighbourhood characteristics of people who died from COVID-19 across Canada (except for the Yukon). This report utilized information from the 2016 short form Canadian census, 2016 census area profile, and COVID-19 mortality data from Statistics Canada. It discovered that males from the lowest income bracket were more likely to die from COVID-19. An increased number of deaths occurred in populations who lived in apartments in lower income neighbourhoods and individuals who are racially visible, recent immigrants to Canada and speak neither English nor French (PHAC, 2021e). As information describing the disproportionate effects of COVID-19 on Black and Brown populations began to emerge, Ontario, Quebec, and Manitoba collected information from COVID-19 case data information on ethnicity and race (Public Health Ontario, 2020). Data on COVID-19 cases at one Ontario public health unit indicated that Black residents had twice the case numbers and twice the mortality rate. American and British studies also found Black populations were more likely to contract COVID-19 and be hospitalized (Turner-Musa et al., 2020). Warren et al. (2020) stated that Black Americans accounted for 21% of COVID-19 deaths even though they make up only 13% of the US population. In order to better understand the issues and target containment measures including vaccination, PHAC has added a race-based field to the COVID-19 case report form (PHAC, 2021a). Questions on the social determinants of health including housing, pre-existing health conditions, employment, and sexual identity are also included.

Fig. 16.3 illustrates how the structural and social determinants of health interact with COVID-19 transmission and mitigating factors. Critical to this representation is the understanding that there have been longstanding health inequities prior to COVID-19.

A Canadian study that explored social and structural determinants of health associated with COVID-19 suggested that individuals of African descent and individuals who experienced low income were more likely to contract COVID-19 because many used public transport and some had jobs that interfaced with the public (McNeely et al., 2020). Workers paid low wages and lacking paid sick leave find it more difficult to miss work. Living in crowded conditions and intergenerational large households make self-isolation difficult (PHAC, 2022c). Yoshida-Montezuma et al. (2021) found that parents who experienced unemployment, lived in an apartment, and were essential workers had decreased adherence to public health measures. Children in the same families did not demonstrate the same result. In Canada, 74% of patients who contracted COVID-19 had one or more underlying health conditions, primarily cardiovascular disease, hypertension, and diabetes. These underlying illnesses can exacerbate the effects of COVID-19. Many of these underlying conditions are directly connected to long-term exposure to racism and discrimination. Due to historical racism, some Black Canadians have a higher incidence of these comorbidities that are likely to worsen COVID-19 (Abdilliha & Shaw, 2020).

COVID-19 IN LONG-TERM CARE (LTC)

Residents and workers in long term care (LTC) facilities were disproportionately affected by the first wave of COVID-19. The Canadian Institute for Health Information (2021) states that

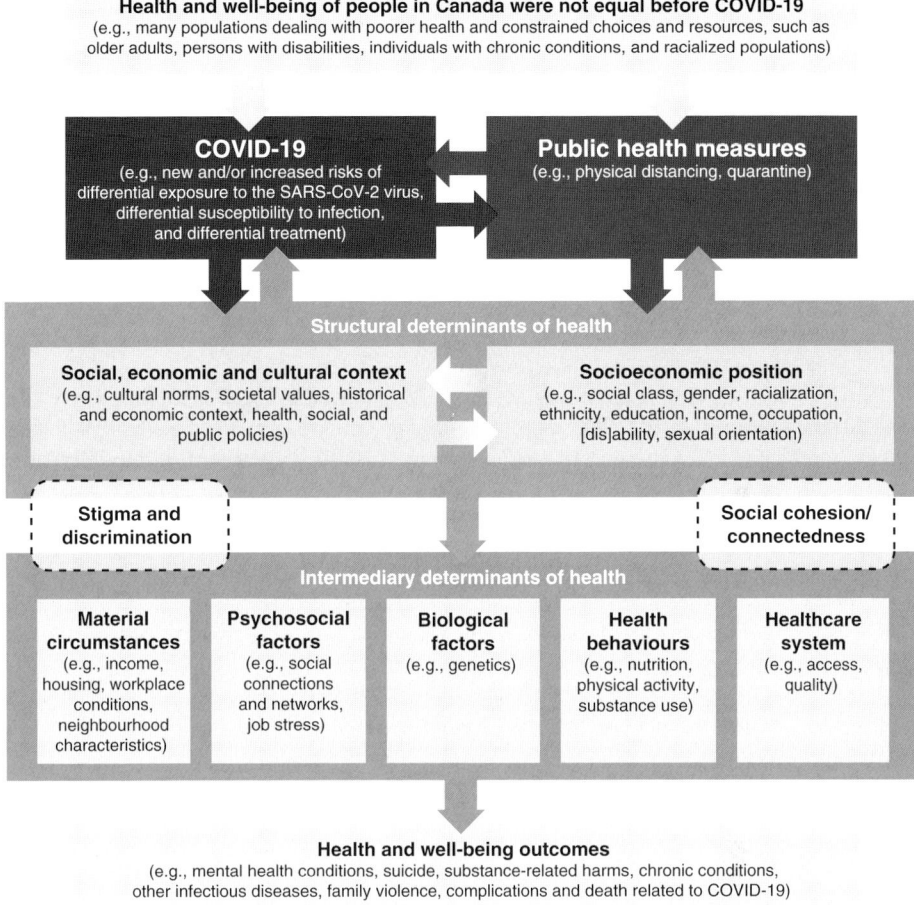

Fig. 16.3 Direct and Indirect Consequences of COVID-19. (© All rights reserved. The Chief Public Health Officer of Canada's Report on the State of Public Health in Canada 2020: From Risk to Resilience: An Equity Approach to Covid-19. Public Health Agency of Canada, 2020. Adapted and reproduced with permission from the Minister of Health, 2021.)

between March 1, 2020 and February 15, 2021, more than 2 500 LTC facilities experienced an outbreak of COVID-19. This resulted in the death of 14 000 residents and close to 30 staff and accounts for over two-thirds of Canada's deaths during that time frame. The proportion of deaths among LTC residents from COVID-19 was 67% and is significantly higher than the international average of 41%. Most staff working in LTC facilities are unregulated care aids or personal support workers who receive low wages, work part-time without benefits, and are contracted through agencies. In addition, workers are 90% women, 60% speak English as a second language, 20–30% work more than one job, and 65% report they are unable to complete care tasks (Estabrooks et al., 2020). Workers are often poor, disproportionately racialized females who are unlikely to speak up because of the threat of job loss. As Dr. Lightman concluded at the Best Brains Exchange held in July 2020, "Care is essential and we socially and economically devalue it"…[We need to] "prioritize employment conditions and compensation for marginalized workers" (PHAC, 2021f,

p. 7). Health care providers can advocate for standards of care, adequate pay, and staffing levels to support both staff and patients in LTC.

STIGMA

As discussed above, COVID-19 has not affected all Canadians equally. Groups most at risk were disproportionately affected by public health measures as access to housing, working from home, and income were not equally distributed (PHAC, 2020c). Social stigma is a negative association between a group of people who share certain characteristics and a specific disease. Race, sexual orientation, ability, sex, gender, religion, or age can reduce social position, which can increase stigma and discrimination. During an outbreak, this can result in labelling, stereotyping, discrimination, and a loss of status negatively affecting those with the disease, their caregivers, friends, families, and communities. Stigma undercuts social cohesion and increases social isolation (WHO et al., 2020). This has the potential to further blame victims.

When the virus arrived in North America, an American politician characterized it as the "China virus" (Turner-Musa et al., 2020). As people became frightened, they targeted persons of Chinese descent, resulting in multiple stories of racism. In June 2020 the Angus Reid Institute, in partnership with the University of Alberta, polled 500 East Asian and Asian people across Canada who described threats, graffiti, and worse since the pandemic was declared (Korzinski, 2020).

This was the very thing that the WHO Director General, Dr. Tedros Ghebreyesus, hoped to avoid when the coronavirus disease was named COVID-19; following best practices, the name did not refer to an animal, individual, or group of people (WHO, 2020).

During outbreaks, community clusters can be identified. This can stigmatize Black or Brown communities who are identifiable by the colour of their skin. Fear and social media have made name calling commonplace. Early in the pandemic, two community clusters of COVID-19 in Nova Scotia were identified in the news—one was an African Nova Scotian community and the other primarily White. The African Nova Scotian community expressed concerns "that the language was problematic since it advanced stereotypes around excessive partying in [Black] communities and that the people there 'just won't listen'" (Canadian Broadcasting Corporation, 2020b). In contrast to the negative stereotype, the community had initiated and developed robust relationships with local public health and had strong community participation at a local testing site to protect their community. After the negative media coverage, African Nova Scotians experienced racism and discrimination when they went into stores or work. As the WHO et al. (2020) document says, words matter. Decisions to reveal the name of communities or specific groups that can be targeted can only be done when it is essential to protect public health. Clear messaging in an article by local medical officers of health asked the public not to stigmatize individuals or communities experiencing outbreaks (Canadian Broadcasting Corporation, 2021a).

Implementation of the COVID-19 Vaccine Program Across Canada

There is a long history of anti-Black and anti-Indigenous systemic racism within the Canadian health care system. This has led to systemic mistrust in these systems contributing to significant COVID-19 vaccine hesitancy among both populations (PHAC, 2022a). This is a critical issue because trust is an important factor in convincing populations to receive the COVID-19 vaccine (Burgess et al., 2020).

Prior to vaccine authorization by Health Canada, the National Advisory Committee for Immunization (2020) developed a list of priority groups for vaccination based on programmatic factors, economics ethics, feasibility, and acceptability. Public health workers across the country have engaged formal and informal leadership within the Black, Indigenous, and other communities and provided them with the opportunity to control the vaccine rollout to specific communities (PHAC, 2022a). By mid-December 2021, 87% of Canadians age 12 years and over were fully vaccinated. It should be noted that booster doses have been rolled out and are not captured in this statistic (PHAC, 2022a).

Across Canada, the initial COVID-19 vaccine rollout was subject to limited supply. Consequently, provinces had to plan carefully to ensure that communities vulnerable to COVID-19 were prioritized. Community-based organizations, leaders, and members worked to build trust in the vaccine, providing culturally appropriate information and addressing misinformation (PHAC, 2020c). Examples where government and health organizations worked collaboratively to address community vaccine priorities include the following:

- Manitoba First Nations traditional healers and knowledge keepers were prioritized for receipt of the vaccine (Government of Manitoba News Release, 2021).
- Cowessess First Nation in Saskatchewan worked with Morning Star Indigenous-led health research lab to provide vaccine information to the community and answer questions (PHAC, 2021b)
- In the Yukon, several First Nations Chiefs led by example by being first in line to receive COVID-19 vaccine (APTN National News, 2021).
- The Black Scientists Task Force on Vaccine Equity hosted a series of town hall meetings in Toronto to counter vaccine distrust and misinformation (Canadian Broadcasting Company, 2021c)
- In Nova Scotia, the Health Association of African Canadians and the Association of Black Social Workers organized COVID-19 response teams and regularly hosted town hall community meetings that included health professionals of African descent to educate and inform communities and create trust around COVID-19 vaccines (PHAC, 2021b).

Health care providers must critically examine data about any chronic or infectious disease to discern the burden of health inequities and underlying social and structural determinants of health. It is important for health care providers to engage with communities to address the socio-economic and political structures that maintain health inequities. When planning disease control measures like vaccination, health care providers must authentically engage community leadership and members to empower them to make decisions and create solutions appropriate to their community. Health care workers need to build relationships with community members to develop an understanding of the community's culture and issues.

The following Cultural Competence in Action case study provides the opportunity to practise and further understand the topics covered in this chapter. Suggested answers are provided to guide learning.

Cultural Competence In Action

Case Study: Community Engagement and Health Promotion

Rose is a relatively new public health nurse who visits new mothers in the Healthy Beginnings Program. The program provides enhanced home visiting to support parents, promote a healthy parent–child relationship, foster healthy childhood development, and link families with community resources, because early childhood development is a determinant of health.

Rose is meeting Andrea and her 2-month-old baby, Max, for the second time. She is there to do an assessment and start the process for intake into the Healthy Beginning Program. Andrea is an 18-year-old African Nova Scotian mother who lives in a small, one-bedroom apartment in the North End of Halifax. Andrea is also a part-time student in her first year of college. Andrea's mother and older brother live 15 km away in Cherry Brook. While Andrea and her mother enjoy a happy relationship, her mother lacks a car, and municipal transit connections between the two places are poor. Max is a healthy baby who is currently breastfed.

Rose knocks on the door of the apartment. There is no answer for a couple of minutes, then the door opens. Andrea looks dishevelled and her eyes are tearstained. Rose asks if she can come in and Andrea nods. Rose looks at Andrea and reassesses the purpose of the visit. Rather than beginning the Healthy Beginnings assessment, she tries to understand what is happening with Andrea and her baby.

Continued

"How are things?" asks Rose, making eye contact with Andrea and sitting down.

"I have to leave this apartment by the end of next month," says Andrea. "Max and I don't have any place to live." She cuddles her baby close to her chest.

Rose says, "Can you tell me more?"

"The landlord says I have to leave because he is going to upgrade the apartment so he can charge more rent. I can't afford to pay any more and pay for my school tuition."

Rose knows that Andrea is on Employment Insurance (EI) since the coffee shop she used to work at part-time closed because of COVID-19. Her EI runs out in 2 months. She is also having trouble getting enough food to eat properly because most of her money is going to rent and there is no nearby grocery store, but she mentions that she plans to visit the local foodbank tomorrow. Rose can see that Andrea is struggling, but recognizes Andrea is beginning to identify some actions. Rose helps her build a plan based on Andrea's priorities and needs that builds on her resilience. Andrea and Rose identify actions and timelines:

1. Andrea and Max will visit the foodbank tomorrow.
2. Rose will obtain contact information for Andrea so she can connect with social services housing at the end of the week.
3. Rose and Andrea will visit the transit office early next week to get a free bus pass (available for everyone on social services).
4. Rose and Andrea will visit the local library in a couple of weeks to look for new job postings online. As the home visit concludes, Andrea looks more relaxed and has begun to make eye contact. She and Rose make a plan to meet next week.

1. Identify which social determinants of health are described and identify what Rose could do to support Andrea in the short term.
2. What should Rose do to improve her own level of cultural competence?
3. What can Public Health do to improve Healthy Beginnings Team cultural competence?
4. What underlying structural determinants of health are described in the case?
5. Describe how the structural determinants of health experienced by Andrea can be changed to reduce inequities.

Summary

This chapter explores the understanding of social and structural determinants of health and health inequities. The chapter focuses on people of African descent living in Nova Scotia for two reasons: (1) to make visible a distinct population in Canada, and (2) to illustrate the impact of historical legacies of racism and discrimination and their ongoing impact on the health of individuals and communities. This understanding can be applied to other communities and populations that have been marginalized. The example of the impact of COVID-19 on these communities further highlights how inequities are compounded during a public health crisis.

We contend that community health interventions are successful when the work is done in partnerships with communities. As the world around us becomes more diverse, our practice must evolve. The provision of equitable care to all requires the exploration of historical and intergenerational trauma, exploration of racism and environmental racism, and a willingness to change "the systems" that currently do not meet the needs of people of African descent and others. Most importantly, it means challenging our personal and professional assumptions and perspectives to look beyond assumptions and Eurocentric perspectives. Applying an anti-Black racism lens, a lens of Afrocentricity, or a lens of Indigeneity will centre the experience of those communities in their care. Achieving health equity through health promotion and community engagement requires understanding of and attention to social and structural determinants of health.

evolve.elsevier.com/Srivastava/culturalcompetence/.

Questions for Review and Discussion

1. Describe a situation that illustrates how societal values underlie the social determinants of health and the structural determinants of health.
2. Describe how you would examine both personal and societal bias when engaging an individual or a community to develop strategies to improve population health. What tools could you use to approach this analysis?
3. Describe how unintended consequences can be created by population health strategies intended to improve health.
4. What strategies can be used to promote health equity and improve individual and population health?

Group Experiential/Reflection Activity

Watch the free National Film Board documentary:
Remember Africville (https://www.nfb.ca/film/remember-africville/).

DISCUSS AS A GROUP

What elements of the social and structural determinants of health are evident in the film? What community strengths are identifiable?

As a health care provider, how would you provide care for patients who experienced historical and generational trauma such as residents who lived in Africville?

Collaboratively develop a culturally relevant interview tool that does not stigmatize, but provides important information relevant to providing health care.

Practise using this tool with a partner so you can develop a comfort level asking these questions.

References

Abdilliha, I., & Shaw, A. (2020). *Social determinants and inequities in health for Black Canadians: A snapshot*. https://www.canada.ca/content/dam/phac-aspc/documents/services/health-promotion/population-health/what-determines-health/social-determinants-inequities-black-canadians-snapshot/health-inequities-black-canadians.pdf

Alicea-Alvarez, N., Reeves, K., Lucas, M. S., et al. (2016). Impacting health disparities in urban communities: Preparing future healthcare providers for "Neighbourhood-Engaged Care" through a community engagement course intervention. *Journal of Urban Health: Bulletin of the New York Academy of Medicine, 93*(4), 732–743.

APTN National News. (2021). *Yukon medical community trying to ease fears around COVID-19 vaccine*. https://www.aptnnews.ca/national-news/yukon-medical-community-covid-19-moderna-vaccine/

Arcaya, M., Arcaya, A., & Subramanian, S. (2015). Inequalities in health: Definitions, concepts and theories. *Global Health Journal, 8*(1), 27106.

Atari, D. O., Luginaah, I., Gorey, K., et al. (2013). Associations between self-reported odour annoyance and volatile organic compounds in 'Chemical Valley' Sarnia, Ontario. *Environmental Monitoring and Assessment, 185*(6), 4537–4549.

Bailey, Z. D., Krieger, N., Agenor, M., et al. (2017). Structural racism and health inequities in the USA. Evidence and interventions. *Lancet, 389*, 1453–1463.

Baker, S. R., Page, L. F., Thomson, W. M., et al. (2018). Structural determinants and children's oral health: A cross-national study. *Journal of Dental Research, 97*(10), 1129–1136.

BC Government News. (2018). *Hundreds of former youth in care take advantage of tuition waiver*. https://news.gov.bc.ca/releases/2019PREM0038-000688

Beagan, B. L., & Etowa, J. B. (2009). The impact of everyday racism on the occupations of African Canadian women. *Canadian Journal Occupational Therapy*, *76*(4), 285–293.

Beagan, B. L., & Etowa, J. B. (2011). The meanings and functions of occupations related to spirituality for African Nova Scotian women. *Journal of Occupational Science*, *18*(3), 277–290.

Beagan, B. L., Etowa, J. B., & Bernard, W. T. (2012). "With God in our lives he gives us the strength to carry on": African Nova Scotia women, spirituality, and racism-related stress. *Mental Health, Religion & Culture*, *15*(2), 103–120.

Beskow, L. M. (2016). Lessons from HeLa cells: The ethics and policy of niospecimens. *Annual Review Genomics Human Genetics*, *17*, 395–417. https://doi.org/10.1146/annurev-genom-083115-022536.

Black Cultural Centre. (2021). *Black migration in Nova Scotia*. http://www. https://bccns.com/our-history/

Brandt, A. M. (1978). Racism and research: The case of the Tuskegee Syphilis Study. *The Hantings Center Report*, *8*(6), 21–29. https://www.jstor.org/stable/3561468

Burgess, R. A., Osborne, R. H., Yongabi, K. A., et al. (2020). The COVID-19 vaccines rush: Participatory community engagement matters more than ever. *The Lancet*, *397*(10268), 8–10. https://doi.org/10.1016/S0140-6736(20)32642-8.

Canadian Broadcasting Corporation. (CBC). (2020a). *Halifax University to cover tuition for former youth in foster care*. https://www.cbc.ca/news/canada/nova-scotia/nscc-waive-tuiton-former-youth-in-care-1.5866755

Canadian Broadcasting Corporation (CBC). (2020b). *Preston group upset premier singled community out for COVID-19 criticism*. https://www.cbc.ca/news/canada/nova-scotia/preston-covid-19-premier-mcneil-nova-scotia-stigma-1.5526032

Canadian Broadcasting Corporation (CBC). (2021a). *Blaming, shaming could lead to more COVID spread, doctors warn*. https://www.cbc.ca/news/canada/nova-scotia/covid-19-public-health-doctors-opinion-letter-stigma-virus-blaming-shaming-1.5892043

Canadian Broadcasting Corporation. (CBC). (2021b). *NSCC covers tuition for former youth in foster care*. https://www.cbc.ca/news/canada/nova-scotia/nscc-waive-tuiton-former-youth-in-care-1.5866755

Canadian Broadcasting Corporation. (CBC). (2021c). *20 townhalls later, here's how Toronto's Black scientists' task force reduced vaccine hesitancy*. https://www.cbc.ca/news/canada/toronto/20-townhalls-later-here-s-how-toronto-s-black-scientists-task-force-reduced-vaccine-hesitancy-1.6064806

Canadian Institute of Health Information (CIHI). (2020). *Proposed standards for race-based and Indigenous identity data*. https://www.cihi.ca/en/proposed-standards-for-race-based-and-indigenous-identity-data

Canadian Institute of Health Information (CIHI). (2021). *The impact of COVID-19 on long-term care in Canada: Focus on the first 6 months*. https://www.cihi.ca/sites/default/files/document/impact-covid-19-long-term-care-canada-first-6-months-report-en.pdf

Canadian Medical Association. (2022). *What makes Canadians sick?* https://www.cma.ca/health-care-canada-what-makes-us-sick

Canadian Public Health Association. (2017). *Public health: A conceptual framework*. https://www.cpha.ca/sites/default/files/uploads/resources/cannabis/cpha_public_health_conceptual_framework_e.pdf

Chambers, L. A., Jackson, R., Worthington, C., et al. (2018). Decolonizing scoping review methodologies for literature with and by Indigenous People and the African Diaspora: Dialoguing with tensions. *Qualitative Health Research*, *28*(2), 175–188. https://doi.org/10.1177/1049732317743237.

Community Economic Development and Employability Corporation (CEDEC). (2013). *African-Canadian Career Excellence undergraduate survey 2011–2012: Summary report*. https://cedec.ca/wp-content/uploads/2021/05/CEDEC_ACCE_Final_Undergraduate_Report_June_26_2013_EN.pdf

Cooper, A. (2006). *The hanging of Angelique: The untold story of slavery in Canada and the burning of Old Montreal*. University of Georgia Press.

Cryderman, D., Letourneau, L., Miller, F., et al. (2016). An ecological and human biomonitoring investigation of mercury contamination at the Aamjiwnaang First Nation. *EcoHealth*, *13*(4), 78e.

Cyril, S., Smith, B. J., Possami-Inesedy, A., et al. (2015). Exploring the role of community engagement in improving the health of disadvantaged populations: A systemic review. *Global Health Action*, *8*, 298642. https://doi.org/10.3402/gha.v8.29842.

Dalhousie University (n.d.) *Support for Black students aspiring to a career in health*. https://medicine.dal.ca/departments/core-units/global-health/plans.html

Dalhousie University: African Nova Scotian Strategy Advisory Council. (n.d.). *African Nova Scotian strategy overview & recommendations*. https://cdn.dal.ca/content/dam/dalhousie/pdf/dalnews/ANS-Strategy%20(1).pdf

Degruy, J. (2005). *Post traumatic slave syndrome: America's legacy of enduring injury and healing.* Uptone Press.

Dryden, O., & Nnorom, O. (2021). Time to dismantle anti-Black Racism in medicine in Canada. *CMAJ*, *11*(193). https://doi.org/10.1503/cmaj.201579.

Estabrooks, C. A., Straus, S., Flood, C. M., et al. (2020). *Restoring trust: COVID-19 and the future of long-term care.* Royal Society of Canada.

Este, D., & Bernard, W. T. (2006). Spirituality among African Nova Scotians: A key to survival in Canadian society. *Critical Social Work*, *7*(1), 1–22.

Farrer, L., Marinetti, C., Cavaco, Y. K., & Costongs, C. (2015). Advocacy for health equity. *The Milbank Quarterly*, *06. 93*(02), 392–437.

Frieden, T. (2010). A framework for public health action: The health impact period. *American Journal of Public Health*, *100*(4), 590–595.

Gagnon, E. (2021). *'A Distinct People': Updated African Nova Scotia strategy get close-up at in-person event.* https://www.dal.ca/news/2021/10/26/-a-distinct-people—updated-african-nova-scotia-strategy-gets-c.html

Government of Canada. (2021). *Social inequalities in COVID-19 deaths in Canada.* https://health-infobase.canada.ca/covid-19/inequalities-deaths/technical-report.html

Government of Manitoba News Release. (2021). *First Nations, Provincial officials release vaccination plans to protect First Nations People from COVID-19.* https://news.gov.mb.ca/news/index.html?item=50543

Hamilton-Hinch, B. (2016). *Surviving the impact of the experience of the racism on health and well-being: An exploration of women of African ancestry living in Nova Scotia.* [Unpublished doctoral dissertation]. Dalhousie University.

Hamilton-Hinch, B., Harkins, M.J., & Seselja, D. (2017). Implementing culturally sensitive pedagogies. *Proceeding of the 2017 Atlantic Universities' Teaching Showcase*, *21*(0): 99–114.

Hamilton, S. (1994). Naming names, naming ourselves: A survey of early Black women in Nova Scotia. In P. Bristow (Ed.), *We're rooted here and they can't pull us up* (pp. 13–40). University of Toronto Press. https://doi.org/10.3138/9781442683273-004.

Hanson, H., & Metzl, J. (2016). Structural competency in the U.S. healthcare crisis: Putting social and policy interventions into clinical practice. *Bioethical Inquiry*, *13*, 179–183. https://doi.org/10.1007/s11673-016-9719-z.

Health Canada. (2021). *Lead information package. Some commonly asked questions about lead and human health.* https://www.canada.ca/en/health-canada/services/environmental-workplace-health/environmental-contaminants/lead/lead-information-package-some-commonly-asked-questions-about-lead-human-health.html

Hope Blooms. (2018). *Dragon's Den pitch.* https://hopeblooms.ca/

Hope Blooms. (2022). *About us.* https://hopeblooms.ca/about/#:~:text=We%20engage%20youth%20in%20the,initiatives%20are%20inclusive%20and%20diverse

Hudson, K. (2001). *The case of environmental racism in the Preston area.* [Unpublished master's thesis]. Dalhousie University.

Indigenous Health in Medicine (IHIM). (2020). *Indigenous Health in Medicine program director looks to build and strengthen connections.* Dalhousie University. https://medicine.dal.ca/news/2020/10/29/indigenous_health_in_medicine_program_manager_looks_to_build_and_strengthen_connections.html

James, C., Este, D., Bernard, W. T., et al. (2010). *Race & well-being: The lives, hopes and activism of African Canadians.* Fernwood Publishing.

Korzinski, D. (2020). *Blame, bullying and disrespect: Chinese Canadians reveal their experiences with racism during COVID-19.* Angus Reid Institute. https://angusreid.org/racism-chinese-canadians-covid19/print

Lalonde. M. (1974). *A new perspective on the health of Canadians.* Minister of Supply and Services Canada. http://www.phac-aspc.gc.ca/ph-sp/pdf/perspect-eng.pdf

Leary, J. D. (2005). *Post traumatic slave syndrome: America's legacy of enduring injury and healing.* Uptone Press.

Lucyk, K., & McLaren, L. (2017). Taking stock of the social determinants of health: A scoping review. *PLoS*, *12*(5), e0177306. https://doi.org/10.1371/journal.pone.0177306.

Masuda, J. R., Zupancic, T., Poland, B., et al. (2008). Environmental health and vulnerable populations in Canada: Mapping an integrated equity-focused research agenda. *The Canadian Geographer*, *52*(4), 427–450.

McCartney, G., Popham, F., McMaster, R., et al. (2019). Defining health and health inequalities. *Public Health*, *172*, 22–30. https://doi.org/10.1016/j.puhe.2019.03.023.

McGibbon, E., & Etowa, J. (2009). *Anti-racist health care practice.* Canadian Scholars Press Inc.

McNeely, C. L., Schintler, L. A., & Stabile, B. (2020). Social determinants and COVID-19 disparities: Differential pandemic effects and dynamics. *World Medical and Health Policy*, *9*(12), 206–217.

McRae, M. (2021). *The story of Africville*. Canadian Museum for Human Rights. https://humanrights.ca/story/the-story-of-africville

Mikkonen, J., & Raphael, D. (2010). *Social determinants of health: Canadian facts*. York University. https://thecanadianfacts.org/the_canadian_facts.pdf

National Advisory Committee for Immunization. (2020). *COVID-19: Preliminary guidance on key populations for early immunization*. https://www.canada.ca/en/public-health/services/immunization/national-advisory-committee-on-immunization-naci/guidance-key-populations-early-covid-19-immunization.html#a10

National Collaborating Centre for Healthy Public Policy. (2015). *Briefing note: When to perform a Health Impact Assessment (HIA)?* https://ccnpps-ncchpp.ca/docs/2015_EIS-HIA_WhenToPerformAHIA_En.pdf

National Film Board. (2021). *Remember Africville*. [Video]. https://www.nfb.ca/film/remember-africville/

Nellis, A. (2016). The colour of justice: Racial and ethnic disparity in state prisons. *The Sentencing Project.org* https://www.jstor.org/stable/resrep27215

Nourpanah, S. (2019). 'Maybe we shouldn't laugh so loud:' The hostility and welcome experienced by foreign nurses on temporary work permits in Nova Scotia Canada. *Labour/Le Travail*, *83*, 105–120.

Nova Scotia Department of Justice. (2018). *NS adult admissions to custody by ethnicity*. https://data.novascotia.ca/Crime-and-Justice/NS-Adult-Admissions-to-Custody-by-Ethnicity/9cqk-8ceu

Nova Scotia Human Rights Commission. (2019). *Halifax, Nova Scotia street checks report*. https://humanrights.novascotia.ca/streetchecks

Nova Scotia Human Rights Commission. (2021). *The Wortley Report*. https://novascotia.ca/just/publications/docs/Wortley-Report-Update.pdf

Nova Scotia News Release. (2014). *Province apologizes to former residents of Nova Scotia Home for Coloured Children*. Government of Nova Scotia. https://novascotia.ca/news/release/?id=20141010002

Office of African Nova Scotian Affairs, Nova Scotia Government. (2022). *African Nova Scotian community*. https://ansa.novascotia.ca/community

Office of the Correctional Investigator (CGI). (2014). *A case study of diversity in corrections: The Black in mate experience in federal penitentiaries*. https://oci-bec.gc.ca/cnt/rpt/oth-aut/oth-aut20131126-eng-aspx?texthighlight=Black+inmates+9/3%

Office of the Correctional Investigator (CGI). (2015). *Annual report of the Office of Correctional Investigator 2014–2015*. https://www.oci-bec.gc.ca/cnt/rpt/pdf/annrpt/annrpt20142015-eng.pdf

O'Reilly, J. (2017). Planting seeds for healthy youth exploring parents percentions of a community-based program in Halifax, Nova Scotia. [Masters thesis]. https://dalspace.library.dal.ca/xmlui/handle/10222/72823

Pachai, B. (1990). *Beneath the clouds of the promised land: The survival of Nova Scotia's Blacks (volume II)*. Lancelot Press Ltd.

Pachai, B. (1997). *Blacks* (2nd ed.). Nimbus.

Pachai, B. (2007). *The Nova Scotia Black experience through the centuries*. Nimbus Publishing Limited.

Pan-Canadian Health Inequalities Data Tool. (2017). A joint initiative of the Public Health Agency of Canada, the Pan-Canadian Public Health Network, Statistics Canada and the Canadian Institute of Health Information. https://health-infobase.canada.ca/health-inequalities/data-tool/index

Pedlar, A., Arai, S., Yuen, F., et al. (2018). *Community re-entry: Uncertain futures for women leaving prison*. Routledge.

Public Health Agency of Canada (PHAC). (2013). *Population health approach: The organizing framework*. https://cbpp-pcpe.phac-aspc.gc.ca/population-health-approach-organizing-framework/#:~:text=Best%20practices%20are%20only%20a%20part%20of%20an,an%20entire%20population,%20or%20a%20sub-population,%20rather%20than%20individuals

Public Health Agency of Canada (PHAC). (2018). *Key health inequalities in Canada: A national portrait*. https://www.canada.ca/content/dam/phac-aspc/documents/services/publications/science-research/key-health-inequalities-canada-national-portrait-executive-summary/key_health_inequalities_full_report-eng.pdf

Public Health Agency of Canada (PHAC). (2020a). *From risk to resilience: An equity approach to COVID-19*. https://www.canada.ca/content/dam/phac-aspc/documents/corporate/publications/chief-public-health-officer-reports-state-public-health-canada/from-risk-resilience-equity-approach-covid-19/cpho-covid-report-eng.pdf

Public Health Agency of Canada (PHAC). (2020b). *Social determinants of health and health inequalities.* https://www.canada.ca/en/public-health/services/health-promotion/population-health/what-determines-health.html

Public Health Agency of Canada (PHAC). (2020c). *Social inequalities in COVID-19 mortality by area- and individual-level characteristics in Canada.* https://health-infobase.canada.ca/src/doc/PDF_COVID-19_Mort_Can_2020_EN.pdf

Public Health Agency of Canada (PHAC). (2021a). *Coronavirus disease (COVID-19) case report form.* https://www.canada.ca/content/dam/phac-aspc/documents/services/diseases/2019-novel-coronavirus-infection/health-professionals/2019-nCoV-case-report-form-en.pdf

Public Health Agency of Canada (PHAC). (2021b). *CPHO Sunday edition: The impact of COVID-19 on racialized communities.* https://www.canada.ca/en/public-health/news/2021/02/cpho-sunday-edition-the-impact-of-covid-19-on-racialized-communities.html

Public Health Agency of Canada (PHAC). (2021c). *Glossary of terms.* https://www.canada.ca/en/public-health/services/public-health-practice/skills-online/glossary-terms.html

Public Health Agency of Canada (PHAC). (2021d). *Individual and community measures to mitigate the spread of COVD-19 in Canada.* https://www.canada.ca/en/public-health/services/diseases/2019-novel-coronavirus-infection/health-professionals/public-health-measures-mitigate-covid-19.html

Public Health Agency of Canada (PHAC). (2021e). *Statement from the Chief Public Health Officer of Canada on July 7, 2021.* https//www.canada.ca/en/public-health/news/2021/07/statemetn-from-the-chief-public-health-officer-of-canada-on-July-7-2021.html

Public Health Agency of Canada (PHAC). (2021f). *Best Brains Exchange proceedings report: Strengthening the structural determinants of health post-COVID-19.* https://www.canada.ca/en/public-health/corporate/publications/chief-public-health-officer-reports-state-public-health-canada/from-risk-resilience-equity-approach-covid-19/best-brains-exchange-proceedings-report.html

Public Health Agency of Canada (PHAC). (2022a). *COVID daily epidemiology update.* https://health-infobase.canada.ca/covid-19/epidemiological-summary-covid-19-cases.html

Public Health Agency of Canada (PHAC). (2022b). *COVID-19 vaccination coverage in Canada.* https://health-infobase.canada.ca/covid-19/vaccination-coverage/

Public Health Agency of Canada (PHAC). (2022c). *People who are at a risk of more severe disease or outcomes from COVID-19.* https://www.canada.ca/en/public-health/services/publications/diseases-conditions/people-high-risk-for-severe-illness-covid-19.html

Public Health Ontario. (2020). *COVID-19 – What we know so far about… social determinants of health.* Queen's Printer for Ontario. https://www.publichealthontario.ca/-/media/documents/ncov/covid-wwksf/2020/05/what-we-know-social-determinants-health.pdf?la=en

Qureshi, S. (2004). Displaying Sara Baartman, the 'Hottentot Venus'. *History of Science, 42*(2), 233–257. https://doi.org/10.1177/007327530404200204.

Raphael, D. (2011). A discourse analysis of the social determinants of health. *Critical Public Health, 21*(2), 221–236.

Raphael, D. (2016). *Social determinants of health: Canadian perspectives* (3rd ed.). Canadian Scholars' Press.

Remes, J. (2018). What we talk about when we talk about Africville. *African American Review, 51*(3), 223–231.

Rutland, T. (2011). Re-remembering Africville. *City, 15*(6), 757–761. https://doi.org/10.1080/13604813.2011.595595.

Sharp, D. (2009). Environmental toxins, a potential risk factor for diabetes among Canadian Indigenouss. *International Journal of Circumpolar Health, 68*(4), 316–326.

Spence, J. D., & Rayner, B. L. (2018). Hypertension in Blacks: Individualized therapy based on renin/aldosterone phenotyping. *Hypertension, 72*, 263–269. https://doi.org/10.1161/HYPERTENSIONAHA.118.11064.

St-Pierre, L. (2015). *When to perform a health impact assessment (HIA)?* National Collaborating Centre for Healthy Public Policy.

Statistics Canada. (2018). *NHS profile, 2011.* https://www12.statcan.gc.ca/nhs-enm/2011/dp-pd/prof/index.cfm?Lang=E

Statistics Canada. (2019). *Census profile, 2016 census. Nova Scotia.* statcan.gc.ca.

Statistics Canada. (2020). *Canada's Black population: Education, labour and resilience.* https://www150.statcan.gc.ca/n1/pub/89-657-x/89-657-x2020002-eng.htm

Tebes, J. K., Champine, R. B., Matlin, S. L., et al. (2019). Population health and trauma-informed practice: Implications for programs, systems and policies. *American Journal of Community Psychology, 64*(3–4). https://doi.org/10.1002/ajcp.12382.

Teelucksingh, C. (2006). *Claiming space: Racialization in Canadian cities.* Wilfrid Laurier University Press.

Teelucksingh, C. (2008). Dismantling White privilege: Barriers and outcomes in the housing searches of new immigrants and refugees: A case study of "Black" Africans in Toronto's rental market. *Journal of Housing and the Built Environment, 23*(4), 253–276.

Teelucksingh, C. (2018). Dismantling white privilege. The Black Lives Matter Movement and environmental justice. *Kalfou, 5*(2).

Teixeira, C. (2008). Barriers and outcomes in the housing searches of new immigrants and refugees: A case study of "Black" Africans in Toronto's rental market. *Journal of Housing and the Built Environment, 23*(4), 253–276.

Thompson, E., Edjoc, R., Atchessi, N., et al. (2021). COVID-19: A case for the collection of race data in Canada and abroad. *Canada Communicable Disease Report, 47*(7/8).

Toronto Sinai Health. (2020). *Black experiences in health care symposium: Bringing together community and health systems for improved health outcomes.* Black Health Alliance, Health Commons Solutions Lab, Sinai Health. https://static1.squarespace.com/static/5a0d40298dd041f9a60bb3a7/t/5ea9a317983eca78fd95ee6d/1588175652047/Full+Report-+Black+Experiences+in+Health+Care+Symposium+2020.pdf

Trinh-Shevrin, C., Islam, N. S., Nadkarni, S., et al. (2015). Defining an integrative approach for health promotion and disease prevention: A population health equity framework. *Journal of Healthcare for the Poor and Underserved, 26*, 46–163.

Trocmé, N., Knoke, D., & Blackstock, C. (2004). Pathways to the overrepresentation of Indigenous children in Canada's child welfare system. *Social Service Review, 78*(4), 577–600.

Turcotte, M. (2020). *Results from the 2016 census: Education and labour market integration of Black youth in Canada. Insights on Canadian Society.* Statistics Canada, Catalogue no. 75-006-X. https://www150.statcan.gc.ca/n1/pub/75-006-x/2020001/article/00002-eng.htm

Turner, T. (2016). *One vision one voice: Changing the Ontario Child Welfare System to better serve African Canadians. Practice framework part 1: Promising practices and implementation toolkit.* Ontario Association of Children's Aid Societies. http://www.oacas.org/wp-content/uploads/2016/09/One-Vision-One-Voice-Part-1_digital_english-May-2019.pdf

Turner, J. C. E. (2017). *Towards race equity in education: The schooling of Black students in the Greater Toronto Area.* York University.

Turner-Musa, J., Ajayi, O., & Kemp, L. (2016). Examining social determinants of health, stigma and COVID-19 disparities. *Healthcare (Basel), 8*(2), 168.

Ujima Design Team. (2015). *The Nova Scotia Home for Colored Children Restorative Inquiry.* Halifax, Nova Scotia.

United Nations Human Rights Council. (2017). *Report of the working group of experts on People of African Descent on its mission to Canada.* A/HRC/36/60/Add.1. https://ansa.novascotia.ca/sites/default/files/files/report-of-the-working-group-of-experts-on-people-of-african-descent-on-its-mission-to-canada.pdf

Veenstra, G., & Patterson, A. C. (2016). Black and White inequalities in Canada. *Journal of Immigrant Minority Health, 18*, 15–57.

Waldron, I. R. G. (2016). *Experiences of environmental health inequities in African Nova Scotian communities.* Dalhousie University.

Waldron, I. R. G. (2018a). Rethinking waste: Mapping racial geographies of violence on the colonial landscape. *Environmental Sociology, 4*(1), 36–53.

Waldron, I. R. G. (2018b). *There's something in the water: Environmental racism in Indigenous and Black communities.* Fernwood Publishing.

Waldron, I. R. G. (2018c). Women on the frontlines: Grassroots movements against environmental violence in Indigenous and Black communities in Canada. *Kalfou, 5*(4).

Waldron, I. R. G. (2020). In your place: And out of your place: Mapping special violence in urban and rural African Nova Scotian communities. *Canadian Review of Sociology, 57*(4), 733–736.

Waldron, I., Price, S., & Grant, J. (2015). *Final study report for north end matters: Using the people assessing their health process (PATH) to explore the social determinants of health in the Black community in the North End.* Dalhousie University.

Walker, J. W. St. G. (2015). *Black Canadians.* The Canadian Encyclopedia, Historica Canada. https://www.thecanadianencyclopedia.ca/en/article/black-canadians

Walker, R. J., Williams, J. S., & Egeda, L. E. (2016). Impact of race/ethnicity and social determinants of health on diabetes outcomes. *American Journal of Medical Sciences*, *351*(4), 366–373.

Warren, R. C., Forrow, L., Hodge, A., et al. (2020). Trustworthiness before trust: COVID-19 vaccine trials and the black community. *New England Journal of Medicine*, *383*, e121. https://doi.org/10.1056/NEJMp2030033.

Whitfield. H. A. (2006). *Blacks on the border: The Black refugees in British North America 1815-1860*. University of Vermont Press.

Williams, D. R., Lawrence, J. A., & Davis, B. A. (2019). Racism and health: Evidence and needed research. *Annual Review of Public Health*, *40*, 105–125.

Williams, M.Y., Adams, Q., Hamilton-Hinch, B., et al. (2018). *Toward an African Nova Scotia strategy for Dalhousie University*. Internal Dalhousie University report [Unpublished].

Woolf, S. H., Zimmerman, E., Haley, A., et al. (2016). Authentic engagement of patients and communities can transform research, practice and policy. *Health Affairs*, *35*(4), 590–594.

World Health Organization (WHO). (1978). *Alma Ata Declaration*. https://www.who.int/publications/almaata_declaration_en.pdf

World Health Organization (WHO). (1986). *The Ottawa Charter for health promotion: First international conference on health promotion*, 21 November 1986. https://www.healthpromotion.org.au/images/ottawa_charter_hp.pdf

World Health Organization (WHO). (2010). *A conceptual framework for action on the social determinants of health*. Social Determinants of Health Discussion Paper 2 (Policy and Practice). https://www.who.int/sdh-conference/resources/ConceptualframeworkforactiononSDH_eng.pdf

World Health Organization (WHO). (2020). *WHO Director-General's remarks at media briefing on 2019-nCoV on 11 February 2020*. https://www.who.int/director-general/speeches/detail/who-director-general-s-remarks-at-the-media-briefing-on-2019-ncov-on-11-february-2020

World Health Organization (WHO). (2021). *Post COVID condition (long COVID)*. https://www.who.int/srilanka/news/detail/16-10-2021-post-covid-19-condition

WHO (2021). Update on the clinical long-term effects of COVID-19. Coronavirus Update 54.

World Health Organization (WHO), UNICEF, & International Federation of Red Cross and Red Crescent Societies (IFRC). (2020). *Social stigma associated with the coronavirus disease (COVID-19)*. https://www.unicef.org/documents/social-stigma-associated-coronavirus-disease-covid-19

Yoshida-Montezuma, Y., Keown-Stoneman, C. D. G., Wantigaratne, S., et al. (2021). The social determinants of health as predictors of adherence to public health preventive measures among parents and young children during the COVID-19 pandemic: A longitudinal cohort study. *Canadian Journal of Public Health*, *112*(4), 552–564. https://doi.org/10.17269/s41997-021-00540-5.

GLOSSARY

2SLGBTQ+ [Ch. 10]: Acronym that stands for **2**-**S**pirit, **L**esbian, **G**ay, **Bi**sexual, **T**ransgender, and **Q**ueer with a + at the end to signify other identities.

6Ps care planning grid [Ch. 14]: A tool that allows the health care provider to incorporate all the clinical data into an overall assessment of the patient. The Ps stand for presenting, predisposing, precipitating, perpetuating, protective factors, and plan.

A good death [Ch. 13]: The concept of "a good death" can vary by culture. It is synonymous with dying peacefully and dying well and is considered a crucial goal of palliative and end-of-life care.

Acculturation [Ch. 7]: The process by which members of a cultural group learn and adopt behaviours of a different culture as a result of close, often continuous, contact.

Active listening [Ch. 5]: Careful and intentional listening to hear the verbal and nonverbal messages in an engaged way.

Activist [Ch. 4]: Someone who works to bring about social or political change.

Acupuncture [Ch. 8]: Therapy that involves insertion of fine needles into specific anatomical points in the body (called *acupoints* or *acupuncture points*) for therapeutic purposes. Acupuncture literally means "needle piercing."

Acute pain [Ch. 15]: Pain that is usually of sudden onset, in response to a particular injury, and time limited.

Ad hoc interpreters [Ch. 6]: People serving as interpreters who have not received any training in interpretation, also known as *informal interpreters*. These individuals can include family, friends, and community volunteers.

Advance directive [Ch. 13]: A document, created in advance, that expresses a person's wishes about critical care or life-sustaining medical treatments in the event of incapacitation.

Advocate [Ch. 4]: Someone who takes on the role of speaking on behalf of others and lobbying for change.

African Nova Scotians [Ch. 16]: Descendants of free and enslaved Black Loyalists, Black refugees, Maroons, the Planters, and other Black people who inhabited the original 52 land-based Black communities in Mi'kma'ki.

Allopathic medicine [Ch. 8]: Also known as *biomedicine*, this is the healing tradition that most people are most familiar with in Canada and the United States as the dominant paradigm.

Ally [Ch. 4]: A person who joins forces with others for a common purpose or cause. The term is often used to indicate commitment toward social justice and addressing racism in all forms.

Allyship [Ch. 4]: Process through which a person in position of power and privilege stands in solidarity with those who are marginalized. The process involves active engagement as well as ongoing learning and unlearning.

Alternative medicine [Ch. 8]: Healing traditions or health practices that are not part of that society's dominant health care system.

Anti-colonial knowledge [Ch. 9]: An approach that recognizes the existence and importance of locally produced knowledge originating from cultural heritage and history, daily human experience, and social interactions.

Anti-oppressive practice [Ch. 9]: A philosphical approach that recognizes the existence of power differences based on history, trauma, and intersecting social identities. Through such practice people work toward equalizing the power imbalance and mitigation of injustices by building on the strengths of individuals and communities.

Anti-racism/anti-oppression [Ch. 2]: An approach or idealogy that recognizes injustice and disadvantage based on race, class, gender, and other marginalized social identities, and challenges power and privilege associated with dominance.

Assimilation [Ch. 2]: A process whereby a minority group gradually adopts the customs and attitudes of the dominant culture while losing its own distinctive features over time.

Ayurveda [Ch. 8]: Ayurveda or Ayurvedic medicine is a comprehensive medical system that originated in India over 5 000 years ago and is viewed as a holistic health care system. The word *Ayurveda* means the knowledge of living or the science of life. Ayurveda provides an integrated approach to preventing and treating illness through lifestyle interventions and natural therapies.

Back translation [Ch. 6]: The process of taking a document that has already been translated into a foreign language and then having an independent translator translate it back to the source or original language to check accuracy of original translation.

Bicultural [Ch. 6]: Belonging to or knowledgeable about two cultures. Bicultural individuals have some legitimacy in both cultures and can serve as brokers between the cultures to bridge the cultural gap and negotiate across cultural misunderstandings.

Bidirectional conversations [Ch. 5]: Conversations in which information flows both ways—from health care provider to patient/family and vice versa, and both parties (health care providers and patients) give as much time to listening as to talking.

Bilingual [Ch. 6]: Proficiency in two languages. In Canada, *bilingualism* refers to the ability to speak the two official languages, English and French.

Biomedicine [Ch. 8]: Also known as allopathic medicine or Western medicine, biomedicine is the dominant healing tradition in Canada and the United States. Biomedicine generally views health as an absence of illness.

Birth evacuation [Ch. 12]: Mandatory birth travel to urban areas for Indigenous pregnant people living in remote communities.

Birth plan [Ch. 12]: A written plan of preferences and desires for the labour and birthing experience.

Black, Indigenous, or People of Colour (BIPOC) [Chs. 1, 12]: The term **BIPOC** gained popularity in 2019–2020 to acknowledge the violence and discrimination experienced by Black and Indigenous people. While the term aspires to be inclusive, the reference to people of colour is controversial as it blends several groups into one and fails to recognize and name people and their experiences.

Chiropractic medicine [Ch. 8]: A system of diagnosis and treatment based on the concept that the nervous system serves as the human body's control mechanism and slight misalignment of the spine could significantly impact a person's health. Considered a complementary medical treatment, this approach now plays a significant role in managing conditions and injuries related to the musculoskeletal system.

Chronic pain [Ch. 15]: Pain that has persisted for at least 6 months more than the time of expected tissue healing.

Cisnormativity [Ch. 10]: A cultural and/or societal assumption of identity in which gender identity matches sex assigned at birth.

Clitoridectomy [Ch. 12]: Type of female genital cutting (FGC) that involves the removal or partial removal of the clitoris.

Collectivism [Chs. 5, 7, 14]: Social pattern in which individuals see themselves as inextricably linked parts of one larger group or community. Individuals are motivated primarily by group norms, duties, and expectations of the group (versus individual preferences and desires). Collectivist cultures focus on the family or group as the smallest unit in society and give importance to social role obligations.

Colonialism [Ch. 9]: The historical and contemporary practice of domination (political, social, economic, and cultural) over people by a foreign power for an extended period of time. In Canada, the term is used in reference to European migrants who became settlers, acquired Indigenous lands, and obliterated Indigenous language and culture, resulting in multigenerational dispossession and dependency on the state by Indigenous people.

Community engagement [Ch. 16]: A deliberate approach to building relationships with individuals and groups in which community members directly participate in decision making about developments that affect the community.

Complementary and alternative medicine (CAM) [Ch. 8]: Healing traditions or health care practices that are not part of that country's traditional or dominant approach to health and health care and can be used together with or instead of the country's dominant healing tradition.

Consecutive interpreting [Ch. 6]: Interpreter session in which the interpreter listens to chunks of information from the health care provider and then interprets in the other language.

Constructivist knowledge [Ch. 9]: Recognition that people construct knowledge through their interactions. Thus knowledge is situated within historical, social, and cultural context and is reflective of individual values and experiences based on their own realities.

Critical reflection [Ch. 14]: A process of constantly analyzing, questioning, and critiquing established assumptions of oneself as well as social and political implications of contexts and systems in which care is delivered.

Cultural awareness [Ch. 3]: In the Culture Care Framework, cultural awareness is seen as a complex set of perceptions and realizations about culture, oneself, and the dynamics associated with issues of difference. Cultural awareness is part of cultural sensitivity and reflects "knowing that"; sensitivity requires a greater degree of proficiency and includes "knowing how."

Cultural bias [Ch. 1]: A preference for a particular culture's values, beliefs, and norms, often with an accompanying belief that it is the superior perspective to guide the situation or decisions.

Cultural blindness [Ch. 1]: Unwillingness or inability to recognize the existence of cultural differences, frequently due to a desire to be unbiased and treat everyone the same way.

Cultural care accommodation/negotiation [Ch. 4]: Refers to actions and decisions that help patients or providers adapt to or negotiate with others for beneficial and meaningful health care outcomes.

Cultural care reframing/repatterning [Ch. 4]: Refers to actions and decisions that help patients reorder, change, or modify their lifeways to discover new possibilities and ways of achieving health goals. Reframing is about seeing something differently; repatterning is about changing our patterns to do things differently.

Cultural care validation/preservation [Ch. 4]: Refers to actions and decisions that acknowledge, and where possible, help patients retain their meaningful care values and preferences for their health and well-being.

Cultural competence [Chs. 1, 9]: Refers to the ability of health care providers to apply knowledge and skills appropriately in interactions with patients in cross-cultural situations to achieve equity in health quality and outcomes. Cultural competence is often described as a process or journey, not as a destination or an outcome. cultural competency is also seen as a "call to action" for health care providers and systems to develop capacity and skills to deliver culturally safe care with Indigenous people.

Cultural competence continuum [Ch. 1]: Description of various stages of cultural competence. The stages present possible ways to respond to cultural difference, including ways that are harmful and destructive. Individuals can be at different stages with different groups.

Cultural destructiveness [Ch. 1]: At the extreme negative end of the cultural competence continuum, this stage refers to attitudes, practices, and organizational policies that focus on the superiority of one culture to the extent that other cultures are dehumanized and destroyed.

Cultural explanations [Ch. 14]: Meanings, beliefs, and perspectives that a culture ascribes to a particular phenomenon.

Cultural formulation interview (CFI) [Ch. 14]: A tool in the DSM-5 with the aim of facilitating comprehensive assessments that consider cultural factors that influence patients and the way in which these factors could affect the working relationship between the patient and health care provider. The CFI tool consists of 16 questions under four domains: (1) cultural definitions of the problem; (2) cultural perceptions of cause, concept, and support; (3) cultural factors affecting self-coping and past help-seeking behaviour; and (4) cultural factors affecting current help seeking.

Cultural humility [Chs. 1, 9]: A concept that focuses on self-awareness, particularly in relation to issues of professional knowledge, power, and privilege. With cultural humility one recognizes the need to learn from others and "unlearn" pre-existing prejudices, biases, and stereotypes.

Cultural identity [Chs. 3, 14]: A sense of belonging to a group or culture, based on characteristics that are shared with other members of the cultural group.

Cultural idiom of distress [Ch. 14]: Expressions of psychological distress and problems that are culturally nuanced, may be culturally specific, and may or may not relate to a label or diagnosis of mental illness as determined by Western diagnosis of mental illness.

Cultural imposition [Ch. 1]: A belief in one's own way of doing things as being superior and thus imposing or forcing it on others.

Cultural incapacity [Ch. 1]: Part of the cultural competence continuum; refers to the inability of health care providers and institutions to help patients from different cultures. Cultural incapacity is characterized by ignorance, stereotypes, and unrealistic fears.

Cultural interpretation [Ch. 6]: Interpretation where an interpreter may offer additional information about potential cultural values and meanings of verbal and nonverbal communication.

Cultural knowledge [Ch. 3]: Recognizes that cultural competence is knowledge-based care and refers to information and understanding needed to understand and accurately interpret cultural expressions and behaviour. Cultural knowledge has two components: generic cultural knowledge or fundamental knowledge that can be applied across cultural and clinical populations, and specific cultural knowledge that is focused on specific cultural populations or the processes of care associated with specific clinical populations.

Cultural literacy [Ch. 2]: Knowledge of a specific cultural group(s), including associated values, beliefs, lifeways, and language (verbal and nonverbal), leading to an ability to understand and interact effectively with that cultural group.

Cultural mindedness (CM) [Ch. 14]: The attitude of and aptitude for cross-cultural interactions and situations; similar to cultural sensitivity and cultural awareness.

Cultural mosaic [Ch. 2]: Term used to describe the wide array of ethnic groups, languages, and cultures that coexist within Canadian society, with each group retaining its distinct heritage.

Cultural pre-competence [Ch. 1]: Part of the cultural competence continuum. At this stage there is an awareness or recognition of needs based on culture; however, the ability to take appropriate action is limited.

Cultural proficiency [Ch. 1]: Final stage of the cultural competence continuum in which providers and organizations value diversity, seek out strengths, and recognize the positive role that culture can play in health and health care. Cultural proficiency creates opportunities for new knowledge, innovative practices, and transformative change.

Cultural racism [Ch. 1]: Asserts the inferiority of non-dominant cultural groups through policies and practices or stereotypical negative representations of values, language, imagery, symbols, and worldviews. Through conscious and unconscious bias, discrimination, prejudice, and exclusionary practices are normalized.

Cultural resources [Ch. 3]: As an element of the Culture Care Framework, cultural resources involve recognition that what happens in a particular clinical interaction depends not only on provider competence but also on the resources available to health care providers in their personal and professional environment.

Cultural safety [Chs. 1, 2, 9, 12, 14]: As an approach, cultural safety is used to call attention to the devastating negative impact of colonization on Indigenous people with respect to all aspects of life and culture—including health. Cultural safety is described as both a process and an outcome, and the degree to which cultural safety exists can only be determined by person(s) receiving care. In culturally safe health care encounters and settings, people feel safe and respected for who they are in the present, how they are shaped and situated by their past, and for their expectations for their futures.

Cultural sensitivity [Ch. 3]: As an element of the Culture Care Framework, cultural sensitivity refers to awareness, understanding, and a respect for culture and its influence on people and processes. Cultural sensitivity focuses on self-awareness and insight and includes the practical "knowing how" used to recognize the dynamics of difference along with cultural ways of being.

Culturally adapted cognitive behaviour therapy (CA-CBT) [Ch. 14]: Refers to a protocol for cognitive behaviour therapy that has been modified to include language and cultural considerations consistent with patients' values.

Culturally congruent care [Ch. 3]: Care that incorporates key values and beliefs of the patient in a given situation.

Culture [Ch. 1]: Culture is a complex, dynamic concept that recognizes shared values and commonly understood, unconscious, learned traditions, and ways of being to navigate one's environment. Culture is about patterns and is reflective of power dynamics associated with privilege and marginalization.

Culture care [Ch. 3]: Reflects the goal of integrating cultural issues into all aspects of health care.

Culture Care Framework [Ch. 3]: The Culture Care Framework is an approach to care that makes culture visible and offers health care providers a way to understand and work with cultural complexities and influences on health and health care. Based on the core concepts in Madeleine Leininger's (1995) Theory of Culture Care Diversity and Universality, the framework is an integrative and practical approach, reflecting the issues of power as well as cultural patterns.

Decolonization [Ch. 9]: A process to undo the impact of colonialism and dominance over Indigenous people.

Discrimination [Chs. 1, 11]: Refers to actions, behaviours, or conditions based on stereotypes and prejudices that reflect unequal, unfair access and unfair treatment of people and that lead to inequitable outcomes. Discrimination may be overt but is often subtle.

Diversity [Ch. 1]: A term used to describe variation between people with respect to a range of characteristics such as ethnicity, national origin, gender, social class, sexual orientation, age, religion, physical abilities, values, and life experiences.

Dosha [Ch. 8]: A concept in Ayurvedic medicine that describes mind and body elements. Doshas interact with other components of the human body to control how the body functions.

Doula [Ch. 12]: A trained health care worker who provides continuous physical and emotional support to a patient before, during, and after birth.

Elder [Ch. 8]: A respected individual within the community who is the holder of wisdom and knowledge in the community. Such knowledge may be acquired through visions, dreams, intuition, or ancestors and is believed to originate in the spirit and ancestral world.

Emic knowledge [Ch. 4]: Local, insider, or Indigenous cultural knowledge.

Environmental racism [Ch. 16]: Disproportionate placement of environmentally hazardous industry and other activities in Indigenous and racialized communities.

Equity [Chs. 2, 3]: Rooted in equal opportunity, equity focuses on equality of outcomes and often requires differential treatment of individuals, based on need, to achieve the same results.

Equity deserving group [Ch. 2]: Refers to groups or communities that have experienced barriers to equal access and opportunities due to discrimination, disadvantage, and historical injustices often used in place of or interchangeably with *equity priority* or *equity seeking groups.*

Ethical space [Ch. 9]: A neutral zone between cultures characterized by mutual respect, humility, honesty, and commitment (which offers an opening for reconciliation).

Ethnic matching [Ch. 2]: An attempt to match patients with health care providers of the same ethnic background.

Ethnicity [Ch. 1]: A group identity based on particular linguistic, historical, geographic, religious, and/or racial homogeneity.

Ethno-specific agencies [Ch. 2]: Agencies serving specific cultural groups.

Ethnocentrism [Ch. 1]: A belief that one's own cultural values, beliefs, and behaviours are the best, preferred, and most superior ways.

Etic knowledge [Ch 4]: Observer's or outsider's (including health care providers') perspective or knowledge on a particular issue or phenomenon.

Everyday racism [Ch. 1]: A concept that highlights the everyday injustices and routine encounters with discriminatory behaviour from the dominant group that permeate people's daily social interactions. Everyday racism can include microaggressions, subtle acts of exclusion, as well as overt, severe racist experiences.

Explanatory model of illness [Chs. 2, 3, 4, 14]: Perceptions and beliefs about the meanings and expectations associated with the illness and the illness experience, including the cause of illness, the severity of illness, the expected treatment, and the prognosis.

Face [Ch. 5]: Refers to the projected image of oneself in a relational situation involving two or more parties. Face is associated with honour and related emotions such as respect, shame, pride, dignity, and guilt.

Familism [Ch. 7]: A social pattern in which family solidarity and tradition have greater value than individual rights and interests.

Family-centred prenatal and newborn care [Ch. 12]: An approach to care that supports the principle of holistic care, recognizing and respecting cultural differences between individuals, families, and communities, and promoting informed decision making based on unique needs and expectations during pregnancy.

Female genital cutting [Ch. 12]: A cultural practice occurring mainly in Africa and parts of the Middle East and Asia that involves procedures on the female genitalia, varying in severity. It is also known as female genital circumcision.

Filial piety [Ch. 7]: Value of conveying respect and deference to elders and authority figures.

Gender binary [Ch. 10]: The classification of gender into two distinct categories of male and female.

Gender dysphoria [Ch. 10]: Distress related to gender assigned at birth, gender expression, or others' perceptions of one's gender.

Gender identity [Ch. 12]: How an individual defines their gender.

Generalizations [Ch. 2]: Common attributes of individuals applied to a group. Generalizations can be a helpful beginning point, indicating trends and patterns that require additional information as to their appropriateness and applicability to specific individuals and situations.

Generic cultural knowledge [Ch. 3]: Fundamental knowledge that can be applied across cultural and clinical populations.

Genocide [Ch. 9]: Deliberate destruction of a large number of people from a particular ethnic or cultural group such as Indigenous people.

Health [Ch. 16]: A state of complete physical, mental, and social well-being, not merely the absence of disease or infirmity.

Health equity [Chs. 1, 16]: The absence of unfair and avoidable or remediable differences in health across different populations. Health equity creates equal opportunities for good health for everyone by (1) decreasing the negative effect of the social determinants of health and (2) improving services to enhance access and reduce exclusion.

Health inequality [Ch. 1]: Differences in health status between different groups. These differences can be attributed to many factors, including biological factors, individual choices, and chance.

Health inequity [Chs. 1, 11, 16]: Differences in health outcomes that can be attributed to unequal distribution of social or economic resources. These factors are therefore considered unfair and unjust.

Health literacy [Chs. 5, 7]: The ability to obtain and act on information to achieve health.

Health promotion [Ch. 16]: Activities undertaken by individuals, consciously or unconsciously, to optimize their health as part of everyday life.

Health protection [Ch. 16]: Refers to public health activities that safeguard individuals, groups, and communities from environmental hazards and infectious diseases.

Healthy immigrant effect [Ch. 11]: A phenomenon in which new immigrants are generally healthier than the Canadian-born population with regard to mental health, chronic conditions, disability, and risk behaviours.

Heteronormativity [Ch. 10]: A cultural and/or societal assumption of exclusively heterosexual expression of sexuality in a gender binary system.

High-context communication [Ch. 5]: Style of communication in which the intent and the meaning of the message are highly dependent on context and less on the words used. The meaning is embedded in how something is said, including what is not said.

Holding knowledge [Ch. 3]: A term coined by Madeline Leininger to describe specific knowledge of cultural patterns that is held by the health care provider and used to reflect on ideas and experiences. Holding knowledge is not to make stereotypical judgements, but it can guide assessment.

Homonormativity [Ch. 10]: A belief that sexual and gender diverse (SGD) people should conform to the societal norms and models of heterosexual relationships, apart from the gender of their sexual partner(s).

Hospice care [Ch. 13]: Refers to care provided to a terminally ill person to provide comfort and emotional support in the last few months of life.

Idioms [Ch. 5]: Phrases or expressions in which meaning is based on cultural understanding rather than the sum of the meanings of each individual word.

Immigrant [Ch. 11]: A person who has been granted the right to live in another country (e.g., Canada) permanently.

Implicit bias [Ch. 1]: Refers to attitudes, beliefs, and perceptions that affect behaviour, interactions, and decision making, but are unintentional and thus often remain unrecognized and unacknowledged. Also known as *unconscious bias.*

Inclusivity [Ch. 2]: Actions aimed at ensuring that everyone has a sense of belonging and the ability to participate.

Indigenous health equity [Ch. 9]: Care for Indigenous people that recognizes the sociocultural factors that lead to culturally safe care, equitable outcomes, and supporting Indigenous people to achieve their full potential.

Indigenous Knowledges [Ch. 9]: Indigenous ways of being, knowing, and doing. The term is pluralized to acknowledge diversity in the knowledge systems of First Nations, Inuit, and Métis peoples in Canada.

Indigenous medicine [Ch. 8]: Traditional healing methods used by Indigenous people for thousands of years that view health as a balance between the physical, mental, emotional, environmental, and spiritual components.

Individualism [Chs. 5, 7]: A social pattern in which individuals are primarily motivated by their own preferences, needs, rights, and desires and view themselves largely as being independent of the larger collective. Individualistic cultures give importance to individual rights with emphasis on self-expression, personal freedom of choice, individual responsibility, and independence.

Infibulation [Ch. 12]: A type of female genital cutting that consists of creating a narrow vaginal orifice by sealing the labia majora to the labia minora.

Inquiring responses [Ch. 5]: Responses that inquire into the patient's perspectives and invite further conversation.

Integrative care [Ch. 8]: An integrated approach to health care that combines knowledge of conventional and traditional treatments in a coordinated manner.

Intercessory prayer [Ch. 8]: Praying on behalf of others.

Intergenerational trauma [Ch. 7]: Trauma that is transmitted across generations in which descendants of a person who has experienced trauma show adverse reactions similar to the person who experienced the trauma. Also known as *historical* or *collective trauma.*

Interpretation [Ch. 6]: Refers to the process of mediating a verbal interaction between people who speak two different languages, without omission, addition, editorializing, or any distortion in meaning.

Intersex/Person with "differences of sexual development" (DSD) [Ch. 10]: A person born with a body that is neither typically male nor female due to ambiguous genitalia or chromosomal anomalies.

Institutional racism [Ch. 1]: Also known as *systemic racism,* institutional racism manifests through organizational policies and practices and leads to negative outcomes for particular populations.

Intersectionality [Chs. 1, 9, 10]: An approach or framework for understanding how multiple social identities such as race, gender, sexual orientation, and disability combine and interact with each other to influence individual experiences of discrimination, marginalization, and privilege.

Joint family [Ch. 7]: In some cultures, the term for the family when parents and adult children and their families live under a single roof. Also known as a *multigenerational family* or *household.*

Language concordance [Ch. 6]: Health care provider speaks the same language as the patient's preferred language.

Layers [Ch. 3]: Like the notion of intersectionality, layers can be described as the various dimensions of a person's identity and life experiences that shape perception. They can include race, ethnicity, gender, age, marital status, education level, socioeconomic status, religion, sexual orientation, profession, political affiliation, and leisure activities. Layers are dynamically intertwined with legacies and contribute to the ideas, beliefs, and perceptions about a variety of situations and issues.

LEARN [Ch. 14]: As a tool to understand and work across cultures, LEARN refers to Listen to understand, Explain your perspective, Acknowledge differences, Recommend options, and Negotiate care.

Legacies [Ch. 3]: Powerful historical events experienced by our ancestors, family, and community of origin that continue to have ripple effects in our lives today.

LGBTQ2 [Ch. 12]: Acronym recognized by the Government of Canada's LGBTQ2 Secretariat and which stands for Lesbian, Gay, Bisexual, Transgender, Queer, and Two-Spirit. It can also stand for Lesbian, Gay, Bisexual, Transgender, Queer/Questioning, and is often used as an umbrella term used to refer to the community as a whole.

Linguistic interpretation [Ch. 6]: Interpretation in which only the spoken word is interpreted.

Lone-parent family [Ch. 7]: Single parent family with at least one child.

Low-context communication [Ch. 5]: Style of communication in which information and meaning are made explicit in the language used. What is said is more important than how it is said.

Marginalization [Ch. 1]: An exclusionary social process that limits a person's ability to be a full participant, thus questioning their right to belong and be full participants, leading to experiences of being left out or silenced.

Masculinity–Femininity [Ch. 5]: The dimension of masculinity and femininity is associated with the degree of competitiveness and defined gender roles. Masculine cultures are associated with assertiveness, competitiveness, independence, and focus on material rewards, whereas feminine cultures focus on consensus, cooperation, modesty, interdependence, and nurturance.

Medical Assistance in Dying (MAiD) [Ch. 13]: An end-of-life care option available to Canadians who meet a set of legal requirements, which are assessed by authorized health care providers.

Medical interpreter [Ch. 6]: Trained professional with skills in interpretation as well as medical terminology.

Meritocracy [Ch. 3]: A belief that individual success is based solely on merit, hard work, ability, and accomplishment without influence from systemic or social factors.

Microaggressions [Ch. 1]: Everyday interactions that communicate a negative bias toward a marginalized group. While on the surface these interactions are usually not a "big deal" (hence the term "micro") and are difficult to challenge, they are nonetheless demeaning and exclusionary and have a significant adverse impact over time.

Minority [Ch. 1]: Existing in proportionally smaller and may not reflect minority in numbers. Within social contexts it is a misleading term to describe non-dominant ethnic identities. Minority group status is usually associated with marginalized status.

Monochronic time (M-time) [Ch. 5]: M-time, or linear time, is associated with low-context cultures and emphasizes schedules, appointments, promptness, and doing things in a structured manner with a "one at a time" focus.

Multiculturalism [Ch. 2]: A condition in which many cultures coexist in society and maintain their cultural differences. Regarded as a fundamental characteristic of Canadian society, multiculturalism also refers to the public policy of managing cultural diversity in a multiethnic society, emphasizing tolerance and respect for cultural diversity.

Multigenerational family [Ch. 7]: At least three generations living in the same household.

Naturopathic medicine [Ch. 8]: A formal system of medicine that is based on the philosophical approach of the healing power of nature, and where disease is due to a departure from natural ways of living.

Non-binary [Ch. 12]: Refers to individuals whose gender identity does not fall under the binary of male or female (also referred to as *gender non-binary*).

Nuclear family [Ch. 7]: A view of the family unit consisting of parents (usually heterosexual but may include reference to same-sex partners) with children.

Oppression [Ch. 9]: Refers to a pressing down, a burdening and an overpowering, because of unjust exercise of power.

Pain [Ch. 15]: An unpleasant sensory and emotional experience associated with actual or potential physical and/or psychosocial injury.

Pain assessment tools [Ch. 15]: These include, but are not limited to, the Numeric Rating Scale (NRS), faces scales, and verbal descriptors of pain, as well as behavioural and observational tools to assess pain in infants and nonverbal adults.

Pain catastrophizing [Ch. 15]: A tendency to exaggerate the threat or impact of pain accompanied by feelings of helplessness in abilities to manage pain.

Pain threshold [Ch. 15]: The level or intensity at which a stimulus is recognized as painful.

Pain tolerance level [Ch. 15]: The greatest level of pain that an individual is able to endure.

Palliative care [Ch. 13]: Care for serious illness that focuses on symptom management, comfort, and emotional support rather than treatment and cure.

Perspectives [Ch. 2]: Perspectives can be thought of as conceptual landscapes or sets of ideas that form the overall picture on a given topic.

Polychronic time (P-time) [Ch. 5]: P-time, or circular time, is associated with high-context culture and Indigenous people, where people are more apt to do several things at once and value involvement with others over schedules and appointments.

Power distance [Chs. 3, 5]: Describes the extent to which power is expected to be distributed equally (or not) within the family and society. Low power distance is associated with individualism, while high power distance is associated with collectivism.

Pregnant person [Ch. 12]: A person who is expecting a baby; also known as a *birthing person.*

Prejudice [Ch. 1]: A belief, feeling, or attitude, usually negative and lacking in legitimacy, about another person or persons.

Pre-session [Ch. 6]: A brief meeting between the health care provider and interpreter before the interpreted session, which can reinforce the role of the interpreter on the team, clarify the purpose of the encounter, and establish necessary ground rules and boundaries for the upcoming session.

Privilege [Ch. 3]: A ubiquitous concept that provides rights, resources, and advantages to members of a particular (generally dominant) sociocultural group. Privilege is a difficult concept to make visible and acknowledge.

Public health [Ch. 16]: An organized approach to improving the health of populations and prevent illness and injury. In Canada, public health is based on principles of social justice, attention to human rights and equity, evidence-informed policy and practice, and addressing the underlying determinants of health.

Qi [Ch. 8]: In traditional Chinese medicine, *qi* (pronounced "chee") is viewed as life energy that flows along different pathways (*jing luo* or meridians) within the body. The presence of a free flow of *qi* directly correlates with health, and blockage leads to illness or disease.

Race [Ch. 1]: Refers to grouping of individuals based on genetically transmitted physical characteristics, such as skin colour, hair type, and body proportions. In contemporary discourse, the concept is recognized as a social construction that is used to categorize people and denote superiority and inferiority between groups.

Racism [Chs. 1, 9]: An attitude as well as specific actions through which one group exercises power over others based on skin colour, heritage, and other social-situated identities (e.g., sexual and gender diversity). The effect is to marginalize and oppress some people while sustaining advantages for others.Refugees [Ch. 11]: Individuals granted permanent resident status on the basis of fear of persecution in their home country, war, armed conflict, natural disaster, or a massive violation of human rights.

Relational practice [Chs. 7, 9]: Practice that is guided by the context of the relationship and recognizes patients with their own unique history and identity. Grounded in principles of partnership, relational practice uses a number of skills such as listening, questioning, empathy, mutuality, reciprocity, self-observation, reflection, and a sensitivity to emotional contexts.

Remote interpreting [Ch. 6]: Refers to situations in which the interpreter is not in the physical presence of the speakers but may be present via virtual video or over the telephone.

Residential school system [Ch. 9]: Schools established by the government in the 1870s with the specific objective of assimilating Indigenous children into the dominant culture by forcibly removing and isolating children from their homes, communities, and culture.

Resiliency [Ch. 10]: The ability to overcome or deal with adversity based on personal attributes and environmental factors.

Restorative justice [Ch. 7]: An approach that seeks to repair harm and promote healing by providing an opportunity for connection between those who have been harmed and those who have contributed to the harm.

Self-awareness [Ch. 13]: The continuous process of understanding, and knowledge of, one's own identity, beliefs, thoughts, traits, motivations, feelings, and behaviour, and recognizing how they affect others in different ways.

Self-determination [Ch. 9]: Refers to the rights of Indigenous people to determine their political, economic, social, and cultural development.

Self-reflexivity [Chs. 3, 14]: Process of critical self-examination one can use to challenge the stance of neutrality and instead examine one's own assumptions, biases, and prejudices.

Settlers [Ch. 2]: People who came from different lands (as migrants) and made Canada their home. In Canadian history, settlers displaced Indigenous communities who were the original inhabitants of the land through colonization.

Sex assigned at birth [Ch. 10]: Determination of a person's sex based on their external genitalia visible at birth.

SGD people [Ch. 10]: Refers to the community of people who do not identify as heterosexual or cisgender but rather as sexually or gender diverse.

Sight translation [Ch. 6]: A process in which a professional interpreter reads written material in one language and then expresses it out loud verbally in another language.

Simultaneous interpreting [Ch. 6]: A nearly instantaneous interpretation of the message from one language to another.

Sixties Scoop [Ch. 9]: Describes cultural genocide in Canada that peaked in the 1960s when thousands of First Nations, Inuit, and Métis children were forcibly removed from birth families and placed with non-Indigenous families or in residential school environments.

Skip-generation family [Ch. 7]: A family in which a grandparent takes on the dual role of parent and grandparent.

Smudging [Ch. 8]: A sacred act that is part of many traditional Indigenous ceremonies and rituals. It involves burning a small amount of traditional medicine, such as sweetgrass, sage, tobacco, or cedar, and the smoke is used to cleanse and purify people and places.

Social determinants of health [Chs. 11, 16]: A subset of social and economic factors within the broader determinants of health that relate to a person's place in society including income, education, or employment.

Social exclusion [Ch. 11]: Lack of access to resources and opportunities to participate fully in society.

Social inclusion [Ch. 11]: Ability to participate in society and contribute to its social, political, cultural, and economic aspects.

Social justice [Ch. 16]: Social justice focuses on fairness and equality in distribution of resources (wealth, opportunity, privilege) across all individuals and groups in society so that avoidable, unjust, and unfair health equity gaps between populations are eliminated.

Social stressors [Ch. 14]: Events or experiences that are connected to and impact individuals' social conditions, including their positions, roles, and relationships.

Somatization [Ch. 14]: A phenomenon in which emotional or mental distress is expressed as a physical complaint.

Specific cultural knowledge [Ch. 3]: In-depth cultural knowledge that is focused on specific cultural populations in their context, or the processes of care associated with specific clinical populations that are sensitive to cultural differences.

Stereotype [Chs. 1, 2]: A preconceived generalization of a group of people that is consciously or unconsciously imposed on members of the group, without regard for individual differences.

Stoic [Ch. 15]: Exercising restraint in expression of emotions and appearing indifferent to pain, grief, joy, or pleasure.

Strengths-based approach [Ch. 9]: Practice that focuses on recognizing positive attributes of individuals and groups to create and sustain health and well-being, while acknowledging systemic health disparities.

Structural competency [Ch. 9]: The ability of health care providers to understand and address the structural determinants of health; includes adaptation of structures and systems that shape clinical interactions.

Structural determinants of health [Ch. 16]: Determinants that function at the system (distal) level (economic, social, and political power) that lead to sustaining privilege for some and to unequal disadvantage for others. The structural determinants affect the social and physical conditions in which people live, work, and age.

Structural racism [Chs. 1, 16]: Refers to broad factors in society (political and socioeconomic systems) that are historically rooted and culturally normalized over generations, leading to inequitable distribution of resources and outcomes, providing advantages to some racial groups, while differentially oppressing and disadvantaging others. Structural racism is insidious and persists even if there is no intent or individual(s) that explicitly expresses these views.

Sweat lodge ceremony [Ch. 8]: A traditional healing ceremony for various Indigenous groups that is led by an Elder and consists of both physical and spiritual purification.

Systemic racism [Chs. 1, 9]: Discrimination enacted through societal systems, structures, and institutions in the form of requirements, conditions, practices, policies, or processes that maintain and reproduce avoidable and unfair inequalities across ethnic and racial groups (also see institutional racism).

Temporary residents [Ch. 11]: People authorized to stay in a country that is other than their home country, for specified periods of time and for a specific purpose (e.g., temporary foreign workers, international students, or visitors).

Terra nullius [Ch. 9]: Principle of "empty lands," asserting that North America was not populated by humans before the arrival of Europeans and thus giving legitimacy to land claims by settlers.

Traditional Chinese medicine [Ch. 8]: A health system with origins in China over 5 000 years ago, which focuses on the idea of balance of opposites (*yin* and *yang*) and adopts a holistic approach to health.

Traditional healing [Ch. 8]: Healing practices, such as fasting, prayer, meditation, ceremony, or traditional medicine, used to achieve health that is inclusive of spiritual connectedness and harmony with nature.

Traditional medicine [Ch. 8]: Medicine that is indigenous to different cultures and uses local (often ancient) knowledge in health maintenance and treatment of illness.

Transgender men [Ch. 12]: Persons who were assigned female gender at birth and who identify as male.

Translation [Ch. 6]: The process of transcribing written documents from one language to another.

Trauma-informed care [Ch. 9]: An approach that promotes a culture of safety, empowerment, and healing by assuming that individuals have past experience of trauma that needs to be recognized to prevent further harm. It shifts perspective from "what is wrong" to "what has happened."

Treaties [Ch. 9]: Formal agreements initiated by the Crown with Indigenous peoples in Canada.

Triadic communication [Ch. 6]: Communication that involves three parties: health care provider, interpreter, and patient.

Trust [Ch. 3]: A valued and critical concept in all relationships, particularly patient–health care provider relationships, based on expectations that the health care provider will be knowledgeable, compassionate, and take responsibility for the care that is needed, leading to good outcomes.

Two-eyed seeing [Chs. 4, 8]: An Indigenous framework that allows health care providers to view and understand medicine through two different lenses: one eye embraces knowledge and strength from the Western system of biomedicine and the other embraces strengths of Indigenous knowledge and ways of being; use of both eyes together leads to an integrative approach. The concept can also be applied to other worldviews.

Uncertainty avoidance [Ch. 5]: Cultural characteristic that refers to tolerance for ambiguity.

Unconscious bias [Chs. 1, 4]: Refers to attitudes, beliefs, and perceptions that affect behaviour, interactions, and decision making, which are subconscious and unintentional and thus are often unrecognized and unacknowledged. See implicit bias.

Unconscious privilege [Ch. 4]: Privilege by its very nature is invisible and generally hidden most from those who have it, thus it often remains unrecognized and unacknowledged.

Unequal risk [Ch. 4]: The inherent power dynamics within a group lead to different experiences of safety and vulnerability based on differences in identity and previous experiences of discrimination. Unequal risk occurs because people who are already vulnerable are often subject to more scrutiny, threat, or disrespect when they raise concerns or challenge a perspective.

Unlearning [Ch. 3]: Refers to making a conscious choice to discard an old belief or mental model and adopt a different one.

Visible minorities [Ch. 1]: A Statistics Canada term that refers to non-Whites, with the exclusion of Indigenous people.

Western culture [Ch. 1]: A broad term that describes values and social norms associated with European culture and Christian religion.

Whispered simultaneous interpreting [Ch. 6]: Interpreter session in which the interpreter is seated next to one or more persons with limited English proficiency and whispers in the target language the content of the speech. Also called *chuchotage*.

White privilege [Ch. 3]: Unearned power that is grounded in values of the dominant White society and allocated to White people without a specific request by individuals. It is associated with economic, social, and environmental advantage and an absence of consequences of systemic racism.

White supremacy [Ch. 9]: A belief that White people are superior and people who are not White are inferior. This ideology is used as justification for maintaining power, wealth, status dominance, and exclusion of people who are not White.

Worldview [Ch. 1]: Beliefs and values about life, people, and the surrounding world that influence how we perceive, interpret, and relate to the world around us.

INDEX

Page numbers followed by *f* indicate figures; *t*, tables; *b*, boxes

A

Aboriginal healers and Elders, 180–181
Accessibility of Ontarians with Disability Act, 134–135
Acculturation, 156–157
Active listening, 125, 126*t*
Acute pain, 364
Ad hoc interpreters, 141–142
Adichie, C. N., 62
Advance directive, end of life, 322
Aelbrecht, K., 133
Africville, 391
Ahmann, E., 171
Albertini, 162
Allopathic medicine, 184–185
Ally, 96–97, 97*b*, 98*t*
Alma Ata Conference, 383
Al Shamsi, H., 133
AM. *See* Ayurvedic medicine (AM)
Anicha, C., 96
Anti Black racism, 87–88, 389, 400–401
Anti-colonial knowledge, 206–207
Anti-oppressive practices, 46–47
   communication, 224–225
   cultural competency, 226
   cultural humility, 225–226, 226*b*
   culturally safe care, 222
   cultural safety, 226–228, 228*t*
   legal requirements, 223
   organizational level, 222–223
   relational practice, 223–228
Anti-racism, 46–47, 67
Ayurveda, 185
Ayurvedic medicine (AM)
   Charak Samhita, 185
   clinical examination, 187
   doshas, 185, 186*f*, 186*t*
   Susrut Samhita, 185
   treatment, 187

B

Back translation, 136
Bansal, A., 23–24
Beagan, B., 37, 243
Benner, P., 58
Bereavement, end of life care, 330–332
Beuthin, R., 329–330
Bicultural interpreters, 140
Bi-directional communication, 110
Bilingual interpreters, 132
Biomedicine, 181, 184
Birth evacuation, 291
Birth plan, 300, 300*t*, 304*b*
Black community, 295
Black, Indigenous, People of Colour (BIPOC), 13, 174, 290, 297

Black Lives Matter (BLM), 6, 11–12, 41, 166, 391–392
Black people, perinatal period, 293–295
Bowen, S., 133
Breastfeeding, 307*f*, 308*b*
   colostrum benefits, 306–307
   dietary changes, 307–308
   racial disparities, 308
Brief Pain Inventory, 373
British North America Act, 208
Brooks, L. A., 123
Browne, A. J., 13
Browne, V., 227
Bruce, A., 329–330

C

CA-CBT. *See* Culturally adapted cognitive behaviour therapy (CA-CBT)
Calgary Family Assessment Model (CFAM), 171–172, 172*f*
CAM. *See* Complementary and alternative medicine (CAM)
CAMH. *See* Centre for Addiction and Mental Health (CAMH)
Canadian Institute for Advanced Research, 383
Canadian Patient Safety Institute (CPSI), 111
Canadian Psychiatric Association (CPA), 240–241
Canadian refugee system, 262–263
Cassidy, C. M., 183
Cazzola, M., 76
CBT. *See* Cognitive behaviour therapy (CBT)
CCF. *See* Culture Care Framework (CCF)
CD. *See* Concepts of distress (CD)
Centre for Addiction and Mental Health (CAMH), 347*b*
CFI. *See* Cultural formulation interview (CFI)
Charak Samhita, 185
Childbirth, 287–288
   complications, 293–294
   medicalization, 288, 302–303
   support during, 302
Chiropractic medicine, 194–196
Chronic non-cancer pain, 364
Chronic pain, 370
Chronic stress, 265
Churchill, M. E., 292–293
CIP. *See* Congenital insensitivity to pain (CIP)
Cisgender, 237
Cisnormativity, 243
Civil Rights Act, 134
Clarke, S., 23–24
Clitoridectomy, 304–305
CM. *See* Cultural mindedness (CM)
Cochran, D., 93
Codeine, 374
Code of ethics, interpreters, 137–138

421